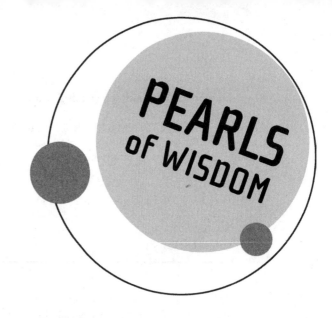

Physician Assistant
EXAM REVIEW

Fifth Edition

Editor-in-Chief
Daniel Thibodeau, MHP, PA-C, DFAAPA

Associate Editor
Scott Plantz, MD

HALF HOLLOW HILLS
COMMUNITY LIBRARY
55 Vanderbilt Parkway
Dix Hills, NY 11746

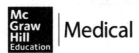

New York   Chicago   San Francisco   Athens   London   Madrid
Mexico City   Milan   New Delhi   Singapore   Sydney   Toronto

Physician Assistant Exam Review, Fifth Edition

Copyright © 2014, 2010, 2006 by McGraw-Hill Education. All rights reserved. Printed in the United States of America. Except as permitted under the United States Copyright Act of 1976, no part of this publication may be reproduced or distributed in any form or by any means, or stored in a data base or retrieval system, without the prior written permission of the publisher.

1 2 3 4 5 6 7 8 9 0 QVS/QVS 19 18 17 16 15 14

ISBN 978-0-07-182136-0
MHID 0-07-182136-8

Notice

Medicine is an ever-changing science. As new research and clinical experience broaden our knowledge, changes in treatment and drug therapy are required. The authors and the publisher of this work have checked with sources believed to be reliable in their efforts to provide information that is complete and generally in accord with the standards accepted at the time of publication. However, in view of the possibility of human error or changes in medical sciences, neither the authors nor the publisher nor any other party who has been involved in the preparation or publication of this work warrants that the information contained herein is in every respect accurate or complete, and they disclaim all responsibility for any errors or omissions or for the results obtained from use of the information contained in this work. Readers are encouraged to confirm the information contained herein with other sources. For example and in particular, readers are advised to check the product information sheet included in the package of each drug they plan to administer to be certain that the information contained in this work is accurate and that changes have not been made in the recommended dose or in the contraindications for administration. This recommendation is of particular importance in connection with new or infrequently used drugs.

This book was set in Adobe Garamond by Aptara, Inc.
The editors were Andrew Moyer and Cindy Yoo.
The production supervisor was Richard Ruzycka.
Project management was provided by Indu Jawwad, Aptara, Inc.
Cover image credit: John Giustina.
Caption: Doctor checking blood pressure.
Quad Graphics Versailles was printer and binder.

This book is printed on acid-free paper.

Cataloging-in-Publication Data

Physician assistant examination review: pearls of wiscom/editor-in-chief, Daniel Thibodeau; associate editor, Scott H. Plantz. – Fifth edition.
    p. ; cm.
    Preceded by Physician assistant: examination review/editor-in-chief, Daniel Thibodeau; associate editor, Scott Plantz. 4th ed. c2010.
    Includes bibliographical references.
    ISBN-13: 978-0-07-182136-0 (pbk. : alk. paper)
    ISBN-10: 0-07-182136-8
    I. Thibodeau, Daniel, editor of compilation. II. Plantz, Scott H., editor of compilation.
    [DNLM: 1. Physician Assistants–Examination Questions. W 18.2]
    R697.P45
    610.76–dc23
                                                            2014003661

McGraw-Hill Education books are available at special quantity discounts to use as premiums and sales promotions or for use in corporate training programs. To contact a representative, please visit the Contact Us pages at www.mhprofessional.com.

DEDICATION

Nothing in this world means anything without the love and support of family and friends.
To all of my family and friends, I am grateful. To my sons—keep the fire of your imagination burning,
and never let any boundary hold you back.

Dan Thibodeau

"If you laugh, you think, and you cry, that's a full day. That's a heck of a day. You do that
seven days a week, you're going to have something special."

Jim Valvano

CONTENTS

Contributors vii

Foreword ix

Preface xi

Acknowledgments xiii

1. Examination Preparation and Test-Taking Strategies. 1

2. Cardiovascular 9

3. Pulmonary 49

4. Endocrine. 97

5. EENT (Eyes, Ears, Nose, Throat). 117

6. Gastrointestinal/Nutritional 141

7. Genitourinary/Nephrology. 163

8. Reproductive 189

9. Musculoskeletal 231

10. Neurology 265

11. Psychiatry/Behavioral Science 289

12.   Dermatology 309

13.   Hematology/Oncology 321

14.   Infectious Disease 327

15.   Pediatrics/Geriatrics 367

16.   Surgery 387

17.   Trauma 415

18.   Pharmacology/Toxicology 437

Index 483

CONTRIBUTORS

Courtney Anderson, MPAS, PA-C
Assistant Professor
Physician Assistant Program
Eastern Virginia Medical School
Norfolk, Virginia
Genitourinary

Anthony E. Brenneman, MPAS, PA-C
Program Director
Clinical Associate Professor
Physician Assistant Program
University of Iowa
Iowa City, Iowa
Hematology

Angela Jean Cerezo, MPAS, PA-C
Assistant Professor
Physician Assistant Program
Eastern Virginia Medical School
Norfolk, Virginia
Endocrine

Angela M. E. Conrad, MPAS, PA-C
Assistant Professor
Physician Assistant Program
Eastern Virginia Medical School
Norfolk, Virginia
Neurology

Kimberly K. Dempsey, MPA, PA-C
Associate Director of Academic Education
Assistant Professor
Physician Assistant Program
Eastern Virginia Medical School
Norfolk, Virginia
Dermatology

Monica Fernandez, MMS, PA-C
Assistant Professor
A. T. Still University PA Program
Mesa, Arizona
Pediatrics/Geriatrics

Travis Kirby, MPAS, PA-C
Assistant Professor
Physician Assistant Program
Eastern Virginia Medical School
Norfolk, Virginia
Gastrointestinal/Nutritional

David J. Klocko, MPAS, PA-C
Associate Professor and Clinical Coordinator
Department of Physician Assistant Studies
UT Southwestern Medical Center
Dallas, Texas
Eyes, Ears, Nose, Throat (EENT)

Alexis Moore, MPH, PA-C
Assistant Professor
Department of Physician Assistant Studies
Elon University
Elon, North Carolina
Infectious Diseases

John Oliphant, MHP, MSEd, PA-C, ATC
Clinical Coordinator
Rochester Institute of Technology
Rochester, New York
Musculoskeletal

Jacqueline Jordan Spiegel, MS, PA-C
Assistant Professor and Clinical Coordinator
Physician Assistant Program
Midwestern University College of Health Sciences
Glendale, Arizona
Reproductive

Daniel Thibodeau, MHP, PA-C, DFAAPA
Assistant Professor
Physician Assistant Program
Eastern Virginia Medical School
Norfolk, Virginia
Examination Preparation and Test-Taking Strategies
    Pulmonary
Pharmacology/Toxicology
Cardiovascular

Tracey Tonsor, MPAS, PA-C
Assistant Professor
Department of Physician Assistant Studies
Elon University
Elon, North Carolina
Psychiatry/Behavioral Science

Jeffrey G. Yates, MPA, PA-C
Associate Professor
Eastern Virginia Medical School
Department of Surgery
Norfolk, Virginia
Surgery Trauma

FOREWORD

"It is not the answer that enlightens, but the question"

—Eugene Ionesco

The Fifth edition of *Pearls of Wisdom*, from my colleague and friend Dan Thibodeau, represents an update of a very novel approach to studying for the PANCE or PANRE examinations. This collection of concise questions and answers allows one to effectively review medical knowledge needed to successfully pass the exams. Each question is based on the content blueprint for the examinations provided by the National Commission on the Certification of Physician Assistants (NCCPA).

Pearls of Wisdom, is a unique text for exam review as it poses relevant questions and provides answers with brief supporting material. This format simulates the experiences of most of us in our PA programs and in our clinical encounters. The process of being confronted with questions and providing acceptable answers is repeated every day in the classroom and the clinic for all PAs. Studying for PANCE and PANRE using *Pearls of Wisdom*, should provide a familiar way of approaching the breadth of medical topics required for success on the examinations.

Additionally, this text is written by Physician Assistants, specifically for our certification and recertification examinations. Several of our colleagues at Eastern Virginia Medical School have contributed to this text, sharing their knowledge and their perspectives as active faculty in a large and successful PA Program. Collectively, they have done a wonderful job bringing together the information that will help you succeed in passing the board exams.

This text will be a great resource for the new physician assistant or the seasoned practitioner. The questions contained here will provide an invaluable source of material for review and to guide further reading and study.

Thomas Parish, DHSc, PA-C
Associate Professor and PA Program Director
Eastern Virginia Medical School
Norfolk, Virginia

PREFACE

Welcome to the fifth edition of the *Pearls of Wisdom Physician Assistant Exam Review*. The authors are delighted that you have chosen this book as a study guide in your quest to pass the national certification examination (PANCE), or for those graduates in passing their recertification (PANRE). This fifth edition will add value to all that prepare for such an important exam. We believe that not only does this book prepare you well for the national examination, but there is also value for the PA student on clinical rotations. Each section is dedicated to a system-based approach that will guide you in a recall of the essential elements that make up the examination. In addition, this format of a bulleted question with a single answer allows you to focus on the necessary information without having to navigate through multiple references to rule out incorrect choices on multiple choice question formats. The rapid-fire method of learning works well for those who need instant feedback into their own study habits.

All practicing physician assistants created this fifth edition. First, we wanted to be sure that we were addressing the necessary content that you will see on the national examination. The structure of this book goes in line with the approach to the blueprint for the national exams. There are a couple of exceptions. In this book, we have taken the time to provide you with a detailed chapter in pharmacology, which should enhance the value of all the other chapters as pharmacology encompasses material into every subject matter. In addition, we have added a short chapter on test preparation as well as test-taking strategies. Many of you are confident with the material that you have faced every day in clinical practice or in school. However, to sit and take a test to assess your knowledge of this material can be difficult for some. The test-taking strategies chapter will try to allow you to see ways of helping choose the best answer on the examination. It will also assist you into helpful tips in preparing for sitting for the examination.

Many of you who are reading this book are coming right out of school and preparing for the PANCE. While you want to feel as prepared as possible for the examination, you will never feel 100% about going in to take a test such as this. Because you have just finished or are about to finish PA school, my advice is to take the examination as soon as you are able. At our institution we encourage our graduates to take the examination no later than three months after graduation. While this has no scientific basis, we have noticed that individuals taking the examination early after graduation perform better than those that wait. The thought is that this may be because of students being fresh off of clinical rotations and test taking as a regular routine in their academic life.

For graduates who need to prepare to take the PANRE, this is a different story. With the recent changes to the administration of the PANRE to be required every ten years instead of six (with new performance improvement requirements added), preparation for a recertification test will be even more important. Because of work restraints and your regular life schedule, it is wise to prepare in a manner that allows you sufficient time to study. Having said that, I would still recommend taking the examination during the first year of eligibility so that by the off chance you do not pass the recertification, you will have enough time to study again and take the test. Vast majorities of PAs (>95%) who take the recertification test pass on the first time.

I want to wish you well in your studies for this examination. The time you spend preparing for the big test will be well worth the time and effort. We certainly hope that the *Pearls of Wisdom* book will be a big reason for you passing the test.

All the best,

Daniel Thibodeau MHP, PAC, DFAAPA

Dan Thibodeau, MHP, PA-C, DFAAPA

ACKNOWLEDGMENTS

I would be remiss if I did not thank the countless number of faces that are responsible for the production of this book. I am grateful for the hard work and dedication to all of my colleagues as contributing authors, and especially to my colleagues here at Eastern Virginia Medical School. I would also like to thank our senior editor Andrew Moyer for all of his guidance on this edition, as well as Cindy Yoo, our senior project development editor. Lastly, I would like to thank Kirsten Funk who was brave enough to give me my first chance at being an author. I thank you for your guidance and support during my first production of this book, and realize that this fifth edition is a result of you having the confidence in me.

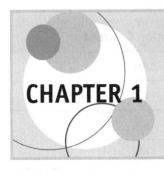

CHAPTER 1

Examination Preparation and Test-Taking Strategies

Daniel Thibodeau, MHP, PA-C, DFAAPA

INTRODUCTION

After you have finished a long and distinguished journey from your physician assistant program, you are now faced with the reality of taking and passing the Physician Assistant National Certification Examination (PANCE). Those who have graduated in the past, that is, practicing PAs, are required to take the Physician Assistant National Recertification Examination (PANRE). Recent changes to the examination time line now have graduates taking the examination every 10 years, with the other certification standards changing to performance improvement CME. The certifying examination is not just another test; it is a comprehensive assessment of the knowledge you have accumulated through courses and clinical experiences. Because we do not take examinations like this on a regular basis, you should have a careful plan of action in preparing to take such an important test. For the graduate who practices in a specialty or focused area of medicine, it is even more important to prepare to take an examination that will have questions you haven't seen since your days as a student. This chapter will help prepare you to sit for this examination—whether it's your first time or you are recertifying for the third time.

ABOUT THE EXAMINATION

The PANCE and PANRE are single-day examinations covering multiple aspects of clinical medicine. The PANCE comprises 360 multiple-choice questions that are broken into six blocks of 60 questions. Each block is 60 minutes long, so you have approximately 1 minute per question. The PANRE comprises 300 questions that are divided into five 60-minute blocks.

The framework of content on the examination is built around a "blueprint." The blueprint focuses on two large areas that the questions will cover—task areas and questions related to organ system. The National Commission on the Certification of Physician Assistants (NCCPA) determines the percentage of the content of questions on the examination. Their most recent blueprint is shown here[1]:

---

[1] *NCCPA Connect.* Retrieved May 1, 2009, from National Commission on Certification of Physician Assistants (www.nccpa.net).

Task Area	Examination Content
History taking and performing physical examinations	16%
Using laboratory and diagnostic studies	14%
Formulating most likely diagnosis	18%
Health maintenance	10%
Clinical intervention	14%
Pharmaceutical therapeutics	18%
Applying basic science concepts	10%
Total	**100%**

Organ System	Examination Content
Cardiovascular	16%
Pulmonary	12%
Endocrine	6%
EENT	9%
Gastrointestinal/nutritional	10%
Genitourinary	6%
Musculoskeletal	10%
Reproductive	8%
Neurological	6%
Psychiatric/behavioral	6%
Dermatologic	5%
Hematologic	3%
Infectious disease	3%
Total	**100%**

The organization of this book is based on the content of the blueprint and covers the majority of topics found in the test. However, the test is random and does not group the type of questions being asked from one section to the next. You must be prepared to answer any question from any category at any time.

You may answer the questions within a given block in any order, and you may review and change responses within a block during the time allotted for that section. As you navigate through the examination, you may encounter a question that is more difficult for you to answer. Try to remember that you must use good time management skills in taking the test. If the question requires more time than normal to think about, skip the question and move on. You can always come back to it later.

As you finish each section, you will be given a summary of that section and if all the questions have been answered. If you have not answered all of the questions for that section, go back and answer every question in the block. A blank answer counts as an error, so it is in your best interest to take an educated guess on every question. Keep in mind that once you exit a block of questions or the time expires for that block, you cannot review or change your answers.

PREPARING FOR YOUR EXAMINATION

We all have different ways of learning. Each of us has different experiences of how we are able to retain knowledge and remember certain items. For new graduates, you have the recent experience of completing a vigorous program in which you have been tested numerous times throughout that the last couple of years. The PANCE, will be an examination similar to your tests at school but much longer and with a lot more at stake. For practicing PAs taking the PANRE, getting back in to the habit of studying may be a bit of a challenge. Because you have been out of school for years, compounded with schedule restrictions such as full-time employment, the thought of preparing for and taking a large test can be intimidating. Here are some suggestions when preparing to study for the examination:

- **Commitment:** You need to pledge to yourself that you will do everything needed to properly prepare for the examination. Your certification/recertification depends upon it. For taking the PANCE just remember that this test is one of a few key hurdles that allow you to practice as a PA. For the graduate the PANRE allows you to continue to practice, so dedicate the time and effort to ensure you'll pass the examination.
- **Confidence:** If you have just graduated from PA school, build confidence from the fact that you were able to successfully handle a lot of complex material. This test is an assessment of the knowledge that you have already obtained while in school. For recertification as a practicing PA, you have gained knowledge in your everyday practice over the past 5 to 6 years (or more) and so apply this experience toward the content of the examination. If you keep a positive attitude about preparing for the examination, you will feel better about going into the examination on a positive note.
- **Time management:** Whether you are a new graduate or a professional recertifying, make the most of your time studying. Consider the amount of material that you will need to prepare for and try to estimate the amount of preparation you will need for those areas. Look at a calendar and plan backward from your examination date to ensure you allow yourself enough time to review. Set up a schedule that you can follow and a routine that you can commit to. If you can keep up with this strategy, you will not feel rushed at the end to cram a lot of material into the last minute.
- **Comfortable environment:** Choose a study area that has the fewest distractions so that you can focus. The content of a test like this is complicated at times. Having a comfortable environment can be helpful to your concentration. Whatever the place, make sure that you can study in this area with your undivided attention.
- **Nutrition and exercise:** Make sure that as you prepare you not only take care of studying but you take care of yourself as well. Proper nutrition and exercise can be very helpful in preparing for a test. Another facet of preparation for the examination is to familiarize you with the testing software. The NCCPA offers a practice self-assessment module for a nominal fee.

EXAMINATION DAY TIPS

The day of the examination will usually start early for you. Here are some important reminders for you to consider:

- When registering for the test, make your time in accordance with your own biological clock. If you are an early riser, think about registering for a morning time slot. If getting up in the morning is tough for you, consider starting at a later time.

- Leave plenty of time getting to the testing facility. Showing up late not only causes unneeded stress on the day, but you could jeopardize being able to take the test if you are late.
- Make sure that you have a good meal before you go into the testing center so you don't tire while taking the examination.
- Take breaks during the examination to refresh you mentally and physically.

You will be taking the test in an independent testing facility called a Pearson Vue Testing Centers. It is important that you be prepared for the examination before you enter the facility. Make sure that you have the following materials with you when entering the testing center:

- Your testing certificate that states you are registered for the examination.
- Two valid forms of photo identification card (driving license, passport).
- Comfortable clothing (dress in layers in case you get warm/cold).

Once you enter the facility and sign in, you will have to verify who you are each time you step into the testing area. Leave any nonessential items in your vehicle because you cannot take anything into the examination room except your identification. You can use a locker to store other personals that you have, but try to bring in as little as possible. You will be asked to empty out your pockets so that you enter the testing area only with the clothes you have on. You will then be asked to give your fingerprint before entering the testing room, and then would be escorted to the computer where you will take the test. From the moment you enter the examination room, you will be videotaped as well as recorded for sound. Once seated, you will be offered some earplugs to drown out noise. I would recommend accepting a pair and holding on to them in case you need them. For some of you who have test-taking anxiety or are easily distracted, remember to prepare yourself for this and try to make sure you get comfortable in the surroundings of the testing center. You will likely be in a room with other individuals taking a test in the same fashion as you. Try to adjust to this environment, zone out any possible distractions you may see or hear, and get your mind set on the task at hand. The testing assistant will help you log on to the computer and you are on your way!

TEST-TAKING STRATEGY

Believe it or not, taking a test like this involves a bit of strategy on your part. You just have to know how to think about answering a question so that you can narrow down your choices. Questions are usually written in a format that follows a consistent formula. For example, you might have a question that focuses on a particular clinical problem. You will be given five choices, all of which will either be a physical examination finding, a diagnosis, a laboratory test to order, or a treatment plan. The hard part for you is to figure out which of these similar answers is correct. This is where test-taking strategy can help. To work on this, let's focus on types of questions, then discuss answer types, and conclude on making the best choice.

Most questions asked on the examination can be placed into certain categories. In general, questions will be based on either a major medical problem or a situation that requires you to think about the next step in a clinical scenario. Before we describe type of questions that will be on the examination, here are some question types that you **will not see** on the examination:

- True/False questions
- Matching
- Questions of negation (i.e., … all of the following EXCEPT …)
- "Type K" questions (i.e., choices that have more than one answer; e.g., A and B)

Almost all of the questions will come in the form of clinical vignettes. These types of questions are used because they can assess an individual's knowledge in many different ways. The questions are generally straightforward and most good questions will test an individual to the general knowledge of a subject. With that in mind, you need to take your time in reading the question carefully to determine what it is asking. The first part of the question that you will read is called the stem. The stem is the precursor to the actual question that will be asked. Take this question for example:

A 22-year-old male patient has a 4-day history of periumbilical pain that has migrated to the right lower quadrant over the last 24 hours. He complains of fever, nausea, and a sharp pain to the right lower quadrant on movement. On examination, he has a temperature of 100.7°F, P: 92, R: 16, BP 133/88; head and neck examination is normal and cardiac examination has a regular rate and rhythm. Abdominal

examination reveals a flat abdomen without scars, normal active bowel sounds are present, and pain on palpation to the right lower quadrant with rebound tenderness at McBurneys point. Laboratory results reveal a WBC count of 12,000/mm^3 with a left shift, urinalysis is negative, and acute abdominal series X-ray has nonspecific bowel gas patterns. Which of the following is the most appropriate diagnosis?

You will notice that the first part of the question is the clinical vignette—this is the stem. By reading the vignette, you should be able to determine that the case is pointing to an acute appendicitis as the most likely diagnosis. The next part of the question, usually the last sentence, is what will determine how you need to answer. On the basis of the last sentence, this same scenario could change and ask you to determine the next step in treatment, or whether or not to give a certain medication, or if evaluation by a surgeon is warranted. Regardless of any question being asked in the last sentence, you should be able to read the vignette (stem), think about the entire clinical situation (symptoms, examination findings, predictable laboratory results, diagnostic tests, and treatment plans), and be able to answer questions that relate to that clinical scenario.

If you notice the question above, you will see that there is a pattern to how the question is written. Most of the questions that are written in clinical vignette format have a basic flow to the stem.

Here are some basics to most clinical scenario questions:

- Patient demographics (age, gender, ethnicity)
- Presenting problem or chief complaint
- Past history including:
  o Medical history
  o Surgical history
  o Medications
  o Family/social history may also be listed
- Details of the physical examination
- Laboratory data and any testing (CT, MRI, X-rays, etc.)

Why is this important to know? If you can learn how questions are written, then you can start to try to understand how to think about what may be asked. A good test taker has the ability to infer all of the necessary information about a clinical scenario from the stem that will be needed to answer any question that comes from the information supplied. In the case of the acute appendicitis question above, while reading the question one should be already thinking about appendicitis and the details associated with the condition: presenting signs and symptoms, typical physical examination findings, differential diagnosis, laboratory and testing findings, and lastly treatment plans and prognosis. By using this technique, you can make a reasonable guess to what possible questions could be asked, and by the time you get to the actual question you have already assessed possible paths that may need to be taken to get to the correct answer. By the time you get to the answer options to the question, you can already have a good idea on the correct choice without having even looked at them yet. This can help minimize making an incorrect choice. As you look to the choices, try to think in terms of the *most* common issue or most commonly treated condition. Try to avoid thinking in terms of what is done sometimes in practice. This may not always be the treatment of choice or standard of care. Some questions will require you to answer about treatment plans. These questions are trying to test you on the gold standard for a condition or treatment of a disease. Remember that these questions are not here to trick you, so be equivocal in your thought process on the best answer. In this type of examination, you should not see questions that would be considered too detailed or too specific in nature. The "zebras" that can be seen in medicine are usually not the type of questions that are asked in an examination such as the PANCE or PANRE. The questions are written to assess your general knowledge of medicine and are written in a way to make sure that you understand the basic concepts of the material that is listed within the blueprint of the examination. They are also written in a way to assess your ability to take a question, think about the question from a standpoint of clinical practicality, and are able to choose the best answer based on the information provided. A majority of the questions that are asked should be formatted in a way where you will be able to have an idea on what the answer is even before looking at the choices given.

Now that we have looked at how questions are presented, let's think about choosing an answer. There will be questions that may have more than one *correct* answer that you can choose. You need to determine not only what you think is correct, but also what is the ***best*** choice available. In many of the questions your objective should be to seek out the answer that is the "most common," "most likely," or "next best step" in regard to the clinical scenario provided. This means that you have to know the general knowledge of a disease or pathology as well as how to prioritize these choices into a list from most correct to least. Let's give some examples of how this works:

The pathogen that is most responsible for community-acquired pneumonia in an outpatient setting is:

A.   *Haemophilus influenza*
B.   *Streptococcus pneumoniae*
C.   *Moraxella catarrhalis*
D.   *Staphylococcus aureus*
E.   *Mycoplasma pneumoniae*

From this question, you can see that there are several correct answers to this question. While it is true that *H. influenza*, *S. aureus*, and *M. pneumoniae* can all cause community-acquired pneumonia, the ***best*** choice for this question is **B** (or *Streptococcus pneumoniae*). To dig a little deeper into the question, you could also consider *M. catarrhalis* as a choice. However, this pathogen is seen more in patients with comorbidity like COPD. You have to consider what the *most likely* pathogen would be. Let's give another example:

What test is the standard test for confirmation of a pulmonary embolus?

A.   **Chest X-ray**
B.   **Ventilation to perfusion scan**
C.   **CT scan**
D.   **Pulmonary angiography**
E.   **MRI**

There are a few correct answers that could be used clinically to find a pulmonary embolus. However, when considering the ***best*** choice and what is considered the gold standard, the answer for this question is **D** (or Pulmonary angiography). This is one of the aspects to this test that you must remember—many of the questions will be looking for the gold standard of care. While you may remember that there are other choices that can be used in everyday medicine to either diagnose or treat a disease, the test question is looking for the *best* choice, not just *any* correct choice. Having clinical experience is very helpful when testing. However, be careful to remember the standards of care as some clinical practices are more advanced than what a question will ask.

For some questions, you may read the entire scenario but still fall short on knowing what the correct answer is. In this situation, try to think about the most common findings that are associated with this clinical question and then look at the choices. In some cases, you may be able to deduce what the best possible guess may be. A goal in the completion of taking the test is to answer every question that is given to you. Not answering a question can mean points against you, thus lowering your overall performance on the examination.

OTHER CONSIDERATIONS

There are aspects to many questions where you will be given an image to evaluate in order to answer the question or test results. Some things you will see on the examination are:

- ECG
- An X-ray, CT scan, or MRI
- Laboratory values (blood, urine, other tests)
- Photographs, usually of a physical examination finding

A question will usually refer to the information provided by these visual aides. It is worth spending a little time discussing what you need to think about when confronted with these types of questions.

Most of the electrocardiograms that will be given to you will have some basic pathology on the ECG. The tracing will either be in a rhythm strip, and in some cases a 12-lead ECG. You should consider a simple approach to determine what the basic problem may be. Think of each ECG in this easy-to-remember rhyme: "Narrow or wide, fast or slow, kill my patient, yes or no." If you can approach the ECG and ask yourself what could be the most life-threatening thing that you may see on the ECG, you should be able to figure out what the question is trying to ask. Try to think about the most common types of ECG rhythms/problems that you will encounter in medicine and have a good general knowledge of their etiology, different presentations, and lastly treatment for the problem. Several questions may be present that will give you one or two views from an X-ray, a CT scan, or an MRI. With regard to X-rays, try to keep a methodical approach in looking at the films. First understand what you are viewing with regard to anatomy and the type of film that was performed. Next, make sure you can identify anatomic reference points on the film that will help you assess the entire film. For example, let's consider a chest X-ray. For starters, think about your **ABCs** as an easy approach.

- **A** (Airway): Look at the airway, alignment, and the lung tissue and note in your mind any abnormalities. Infiltrates, nodules, masses, atelectasis, and loss of lung tissue as in a pneumothorax and any fluid that may be present are some things to consider.
- **B** (Bone): Look at the bony structures for any abnormalities. Look at the contour of the ribs and at spine from the AP view and try to determine if there are any abnormalities that stick out on the film.
- **C** (Cardiac): Look at the cardiac silhouette. Is it large or normal appearance in size? Is there any evidence that there is obstruction of the silhouette by another structure such as a widened mediastinum, mass, or fluid?
- **D** (Diaphragm): Does the diaphragm appear to be normal? Is there an effusion present that obscures your view of the diaphragm, and do the borders anatomically appear to be in the correct position?
- **E** (Everything else): Look at the soft tissue for any abnormalities (free air, foreign body, etc.).

This is one way to try to stay organized while taking the test. That way, as you look at the picture or X-ray on the screen, you can determine what the abnormality is, which can give you a better idea on how to answer the question before you see the choices. In several of the questions you will be given a series of laboratory results, blood, urine, and other tests. Remember, the testing material that you are given will provide you with a list of all laboratory tests and their normal values. These are usually available to you at all times on the test in a separate page on the computer that is easy to pull up at any time. Just remember that if you cannot recall what a normal value is, reference it by utilizing the laboratory value page that is provided. That way, if you get stuck on a question where you may not recall the significance of a laboratory test, you can try to work through the problem by understanding how the laboratory value is abnormal (either elevated, low, positive when a normal value is negative, and so forth). In some cases, you will encounter a photo that will be provided with a question. In most instances the photo will be directly related to the condition that you are being questioned. This will be in the form of a physical examination finding, a blood smear, a gram stain photo, or some other type of photo that will aid in the question. Remember to use a methodical approach in trying to answer in your mind what you are looking at before you make a decision on the choices that will be given.

CONCLUSION

Not everyone is a great test taker. But the good news is, you don't have to be. If you can take a methodical approach to your study time and preparation, along with reminding yourself of some basic test-taking strategies, you can better your chances of improving your test score. Good luck!

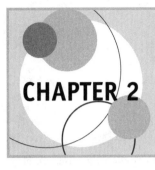

CHAPTER 2 Cardiovascular

Daniel Thibodeau, MHP, PA-C, DFAAPA

CARDIOMYOPATHIES

○ **Which is the most common type of cardiomyopathy?**

Dilated cardiomyopathy (dilation of all the four chambers). This condition is often idiopathic but can be induced by progression of ischemia, myocarditis, alcohol consumption, Adriamycin, diabetes, pheochromocytoma, thiamine deficiency, thyroid disease, and valve replacement. The other type of cardiomyopathies are hypertrophic and restrictive.

○ **What is the abnormality seen in the 2D echocardiogram shown in Figure 2-1?**

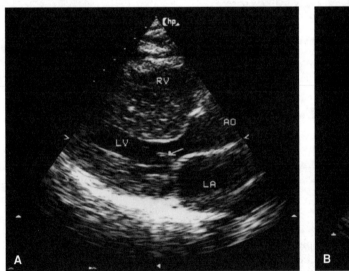 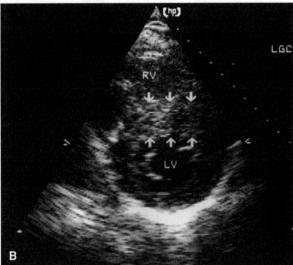

Figure 2-1 (Reproduced, with permission, from Fuster V et al. *Hurst's the Heart.* 12th ed. New York, NY: McGraw-Hill: 2008, Fig. 16-106.)

Hypertrophic cardiomyopathy. Note the very thickened septum.

○ **What drugs have been shown to regress LV hypertrophy and reduce LV mass?**

Beta-blockers, alpha-methyldopa (Aldomet), ACE inhibitors, and thiazide diuretics.

○ **What is the most common mechanism responsible for supraventricular tachycardia (SVT)?**

AV node reentry. The most common form is referred to as typical AV.

○ **What are the common causes of SVT?**

Myocardial ischemia, myocardial infarction, congestive heart failure, pericarditis, rheumatic heart disease, mitral valve prolapse, pre-excitation syndromes, COPD, ethanol intoxication, hypoxia, pneumonia, sepsis, and digoxin toxicity.

○ **What are the physiologic characteristics of dilated cardiomyopathies?**

Reduced ventricular ejection fraction, high end-diastolic filling volumes and pressures, reduced cardiac output, and high pulmonary capillary wedge pressures.

○ **What are the common clinical presentations that can occur with a dilated cardiomyopathy?**

Fatigue, exertional dyspnea, and orthopnea. They commonly have an S_3 and an LV/RV heave. Other presentations that could occur include mitral and/or tricuspid regurgitation, jugular venous distention, rales and edema, low voltage on EKG, and signs of cardiomegaly by CXR.

○ **What are the physiological aspects of restricted cardiomyopathy?**

Normal systolic contractility, reduction in diastolic relaxation and filling capacity, high LV end-diastolic filling pressures, and high pulmonary wedge pressures especially with exercise.

○ **What are the common causes of restrictive cardiomyopathy?**

Most are idiopathic but other causes include infiltrative diseases, for example, sarcoid and amyloid, and storage diseases, for example, hemochromatosis. Other potential causes include radiation exposure and cancer.

○ **What are the common clinical presentations associated with restrictive cardiomyopathy?**

Symptoms are very similar to dilated cardiomyopathy with fatigue, exertional dyspnea, and orthopnea but could present with syncope/near syncope and palpitations. Restrictive cardiomyopathy is more likely to have an S_4 as opposed to S_3. The symptoms often present with a resting tachycardia and typically will not show signs of cardiomegaly on CXR.

○ **What is hypertrophic cardiomyopathy?**

It is a genetic disorder resulting in abnormal hypertrophy of the ventricular walls. It often results in asymmetric hypertrophic changes, which can create outlet obstruction. Typically, there is normal LV systolic contractility but increased diastolic stiffness resulting in reduced LV filling volumes. Patients often present with high pulmonary capillary wedge pressures and pulmonary hypertension.

○ **What are the common clinical presentations of hypertrophic cardiomyopathy?**

In young patients, clinical signs and symptoms may be difficult to ascertain. Commonly, they may present with complaints of palpitations, chest pain, dyspnea, syncope, or dizziness. Sudden death is not an uncommon presentation for this disorder. Resting tachycardia is common.

○ **What are the key management options for patients with hypertrophic cardiomyopathy?**

Patients may be advised to avoid vigorous physical activity. Avoid preload and afterload reducing agents and positive inotropes such as digoxin. Beta-blockers and calcium channel blockers may be used to slow the heart rate. Myomectomy and septal ablation by catheter or chemical means may be needed to decrease outflow tract obstruction. ICDs are often considered because of the increased risk for ventricular dysrhythmias in these patients. Also, the immediate family should be screened for undiagnosed individuals at risk.

CONDUCTION DISORDERS

○ **What are the common causes of multifocal atrial tachycardia?**

COPD, CHF, sepsis, valvular heart disease, and methylxanthine toxicity. Treat the arrhythmia with magnesium, verapamil, or beta-blocking agents. Overall management is to treat the underlying cause of the MAT.

○ **How is atrial flutter treated?**

Initiate AV nodal blockade with beta-blockers, calcium channel blockers, or digoxin. If necessary, treat a stable patient with chemical cardioversion by using a class IA agent, such as procainamide or quinidine, after digitalization. If this treatment fails or if the patient is unstable, electrocardiovert at 25 to 50 J.

○ **What are some causes of atrial fibrillation?**

Hypertension, rheumatic heart disease, pneumonia, thyrotoxicosis, ischemic heart, pericarditis, ethanol intoxication, PE, CHF, valvular heart disease, and COPD.

○ **How is atrial fibrillation treated?**

Control rate with beta-blocker or calcium channel blocker (such as verapamil or diltiazem), and then convert with procainamide, quinidine, or verapamil. Digoxin may be considered for rates that are not controlled with the typical first-line drugs, although its effect will be delayed. Synchronized cardioversion at 100 to 200 J should be performed on an unstable patient. In a stable patient with a-fib of unclear duration, anticoagulation should be considered for 3 weeks prior to chemical or electrical cardioversion. *A transesophageal echocardiogram is commonly used to determine the timing of cardioversions.* Watch for hypotension with the administration of negative inotropes.

○ **What is the treatment of SVT caused by digitalis toxicity?**

Stop the digitalis, treat hypokalemia, and administer magnesium or phenytoin. Provide digoxin-specific antibodies to the unstable patient. Avoid cardioversion.

○ **What is the treatment for stable SVT not caused by digitalis toxicity or WPW syndrome?**

Vagal maneuvers, adenosine, verapamil, or beta-blockers.

○ **Describe the key feature of Mobitz I (Wenckebach) second-degree AV block:**

A progressive prolongation of the PR interval until the atrial impulse is no longer conducted. If symptomatic, atropine and transcutaneous/transvenous pacing may be required.

○ **Describe the key feature of Mobitz II second-degree AV block:**

A constant PR interval in which one or more beats fail to conduct.

○ **What is the treatment for Mobitz II second-degree AV block?**

Atropine and transcutaneous/transvenous pacing, if symptomatic.

○ **Carotid massage or Valsalva maneuver is useful for slowing supraventricular rhythms. When is carotid massage contraindicated?**

With ventricular dysrhythmias, digitalis toxicity, stroke, syncope, seizures, known carotid artery disease, or in those with a carotid bruit.

○ **What are some common vagal maneuvers?**

Breath holding, Valsalva (bearing down as if having a bowel movement), stimulating of the gag reflex, squatting, pressure on the eyeballs, and immersing the face in cold water.

○ **What is more common: premature atrial beats or ventricular beats?**

Premature atrial beats. Palpitations that occur because of premature atrial beats are generally benign and asymptomatic. Reassurance is the only treatment. Less frequent but more serious causes of atrial premature beats include pheochromocytoma and thyrotoxicosis. Random unifocal PVCs are also benign but common in the general population. Runs of PVCs and/or associated symptoms of dyspnea, angina, or syncope require investigation and are most likely related to an underlying heart disease.

○ **How do the fixed-rate demand modes of pacemakers differ?**

Fixed-rate mode produces an impulse at a continuous specific rate, regardless of the patient's own cardiac activity. Demand mode detects the patient's electrical activity and triggers only if the heart is not depolarizing.

○ **What is the treatment for ventricular fibrillation in a patient with a pacemaker?**

Defibrillation, but be sure to keep the paddles away from the pacemaker.

○ **What is the average lifespan of a pacemaker battery?**

7 to 15 years.

○ **What are the most common causes of multifocal atrial tachycardia (MAT)?**

COPD with exacerbation is the most common cause, followed by CHF, sepsis, and methylxanthine toxicity. Treatment consists of treating the underlying disorder as well as the use of verapamil, magnesium, or digoxin for slowing the arrhythmia.

○ **What are the most common causes of atrial fibrillation?**

Coronary artery disease with myocardial ischemia and hypertensive heart disease are the most common causes. Other common causes are mitral or aortic valvular heart disease, cor pulmonale, dilated cardiomyopathy, hypertrophic cardiomyopathy (particularly the obstructive type), alcohol intoxication or "holiday heart syndrome," hypo- or hyperthyroidism, pulmonary embolism, sepsis, hypoxia, pre-excitation syndrome, and pericarditis.

○ **How is atrial fibrillation treated?**

The treatment of atrial fibrillation consists of three major considerations:

1. Control of ventricular rate
2. Conversion, if possible or feasible, to sinus rhythm
3. Prevention of thromboembolic events, particularly CVA

Rate control is best managed with beta-adrenergic blocker or calcium channel blockers (diltiazem or verapamil), or less desirable, digoxin. Digoxin should be used in patients with poor LV systolic function and those with a contraindication to beta-blockers and calcium channel blockers. Digoxin provides good rate control at rest, but often suboptimal rate control during exertion. For conversion to sinus rhythm, in the stable patient with a duration of symptoms <48 hours, it is best managed, initially, with antiarrhythmic agents (amiodarone, ibutilide, propafenone, or procainamide). In the unstable patient or the patient with acute ischemia, hypotension or pulmonary edema, immediate synchronized electrical cardioversion, starting at 200 J should be performed without interruption of antiarrhythmic therapy. Patients with atrial fibrillation of 1 year duration or longer, or those with left atrial size of >5 cm on echocardiography cardioversion, are not recommended this therapy because of its low success rate. Patients with recent atrial fibrillation >2 days duration should be started on warfarin and anticoagulated to an INR between 2 and 3 for at least 3 weeks, before any attempt to cardiovert to sinus rhythm because of the significant risk for embolic CVA. Earlier cardioversion attempts could be considered if the patient is at adequate anticoagulation levels and no evidence of intrachamber thrombus by transesophageal echocardiography. Those patients with chronic atrial fibrillation should be on lifelong warfarin unless an absolute contraindication to warfarin exists or the patient cannot reliably take warfarin.

○ **What percentage of patients with atrial fibrillation converted to sinus rhythm will revert into atrial fibrillation?**

50% will revert to atrial fibrillation within 1 year of cardioversion, regardless of medical therapy.

○ **What is the risk of CVA in patients with atrial fibrillation, with or without anticoagulation?**

Patients with atrial fibrillation, not anticoagulated with warfarin, have a 25% incidence of CVA within 5 years (5% per year). Those patients anticoagulated to therapeutic levels have a 4% incidence of CVA within 5 years (0.8%). Aspirin is a clearly inferior substitute to warfarin, but is much more preferable to no anticoagulant or antithrombotic therapy.

○ **What risk calculation score can be used to evaluate stroke in those patients with atrial fibrillation?**

The CHADS$_2$ score. This stands for Congestive Heart Failure, Hypertension, Age (>75), Diabetes, and history of Stroke. All give one point score with 2 points for stroke totaling 6 possible total points. A score of 6 would give a patient a 19% chance of stroke in the first year with atrial fibrillation.

○ **What is the recommendation for patients with sustained atrial fibrillation and a CHADS$_2$ score of 3?**

The recommended treatment would be dual antiplatelet therapy with aspirin and clopidogrel or a Factor X inhibitor like dabigatran, rivaroxiban, or edoxiban.

○ **What is the key feature of Mobitz I second-degree AV block (Wenckebach)?**

A progressive prolongation of the PR interval until the atrial impulse is no longer conducted through to the ventricle, resulting in a dropped QRS. Almost always transient, atropine and transcutaneous/transvenous pacing is required for the rare instances of symptoms or cardiac stability.

○ **What is the feature of Mobitz II second-degree AV block?**

A constant PR interval until one sinus beat fails to conduct through the ventricle, resulting in a dropped QRS. Because this rhythm is indicative of His bundle damage, and 85% of patients with this rhythm eventually develop complete heart block, temporary pacing followed by permanent pacing is usually required.

○ **A 57-year-old male is scheduled for a total colectomy for ulcerative colitis. He has a history of stable angina for several years, as well as hypertension. His preoperative EKG reveals normal sinus rhythm (NSR), left ventricular hypertrophy (LVH), and a first-degree AV block. What is the likelihood of a high-degree AV block occurring during the perioperative period?**

Patients with first-degree AV block have an extremely low incidence of developing high-degree AV block in the perioperative period. Thus, no temporary pacing in the perioperative period is required.

○ **A 26-year-old man presents to your clinic for an insurance physical. An EKG reveals Wolff–Parkinson–White syndrome. He is asymptomatic and has no history of palpitations or arrhythmia. What is the most appropriate management of this patient?**

No therapy or work-up is required at this time since there is no evidence that the risk of sudden death can be safely mitigated or that individuals with asymptomatic WPW can be reliably risk stratified with regard to sudden death. The appropriate management is observation in this situation.

○ **What is the most commonly occurring form of ventricular tachycardia?**

Ventricular tachycardia (VT) occurring in patients with healed myocardial infarction. Other causes include bundle branch reentry VT, VT of right ventricular outflow tract origin, idiopathic left ventricular tachycardia, drug-induced VT (proarrhythmia), and VT caused by right ventricular dysplasia. Rare causes include long QT syndrome and lymphocytic myocarditis.

○ **A 48-year-old male patient with no history of angina, MI, or other cardiac symptoms is referred to you for evaluation of palpitations. A 24-hour Holter monitor reveals 4 three-beat runs of ventricular tachycardia without any symptoms. The patient has no risk factors for coronary artery disease, is not a smoker, and has a normal resting EKG. His echocardiogram is normal. What is the best management strategy for this patient?**

No therapy or further work-up is required. The patient should be reassured that the risk of sudden death is very low and that medical therapy will either worsen his arrhythmia or be of no significant benefit.

○ **A 28-year-old male patient with two previous episodes of palpitations and shortness of breath in the last year is brought in the emergency department by EMS presenting with severe palpitations, hypotension, and shortness of breath. His BP is 90/55 and HR is 195 bpm. A rhythm strip reveals narrow QRS complex tachycardia. A 12-lead EKG reveals what appears to be atrial fibrillation. Synchronized cardioversion is successful in terminating the arrhythmia, and the postcardioversion EKG reveals Wolff Parkinson White syndrome. What is the most appropriate management strategy in this patient?**

Electrophysiology testing with intracardiac mapping, followed by catheter ablation of the accessory conduction pathway.

○ **A 67-year-old woman with severe three-vessel coronary artery disease with very small distal vessels, deemed inoperable, is brought into the emergency department following a syncopal episode. The paramedics caught the final beats of what looked like a wide QRS complex tachycardia on a rhythm strip and you confirm this on inspection of the tracing. She is now awake, alert, and breathing comfortably. An echocardiogram performed 1 month ago revealed a dilated left ventricle with poor systolic function (estimated ejection fraction is 20%–25%). What is the most appropriate management strategy for this patient?**

Empiric therapy with amiodarone.

○　**What medications, used to maintain sinus rhythm in a patient recently cardioverted from atrial fibrillation, should be avoided in patients with stress test proven myocardial ischemia?**

Class IC antiarrhythmics, such as flecainide and propafenone, and class IA agents, such as quinidine and procainamide. They can lead to lethal proarrhythmia in patients with active myocardial ischemia. Amiodarone, an agent that has anti-ischemic properties, is the preferred agent.

○　**What drugs can increase serum digoxin levels?**

Quinidine, procainamide, verapamil, and amiodarone.

○　**What are the end points in procainamide loading infusion for patient with unstable VT?**

Hypotension, QRS widened more than 50% of pretreatment width, arrhythmia suppression, or a total of 17 mg/kg.

○　**If a defibrillator is available, what is the immediate treatment of a patient with ventricular fibrillation?**

Unsynchronized countershock at 200 J (biphasic) or 360 J (monophasic).

○　**What is the differential diagnosis for pulseless electrical activity (PEA)?**

- Hypoxia/hypovolemia/hyper- or hypokalemia/hyperthermia
- Acute MI/acidosis
- Tension pneumothorax/tamponade/thrombosis (pulmonary)/tablets (drug overdose)

○　**What is the differential diagnosis of asystole?**

Drug overdose, acidosis, hyperkalemia, hypothermia, hypokalemia, and hypoxia.

○　**What is the treatment for unstable supraventricular tachycardia?**

Synchronized cardioversion.

○　**A patient in the emergency department suddenly demonstrates ventricular fibrillation on the monitor. The patient is alert and has a pulse. What should you do first?**

Check the monitor leads and first determine if the monitor tracing is accurate.

○　**Inferior wall MIs commonly lead to what two types of heart block?**

First-degree AV block and Mobitz I second-degree AV block (Wenckebach). Sinus bradycardia can also occur. Progression to complete AV block is not common. The mechanism for this is damage to autonomic fibers in the atrial septum giving increased vagal tone impairing AV node conduction.

○　**Anterior wall MIs may directly damage intracardiac conduction. This may lead to which type of arrhythmias?**

A Mobitz II second-degree AV block that can suddenly progress to complete AV block.

○　**Which type of drug is contraindicated for the treatment of Torsades de pointes?**

Any drug that prolongs repolarization (QT interval). For example, class IA antiarrhythmics, such as quinidine and procainamide, are contraindicated for treating torsades de pointes. Other drugs that share this effect include TCAs, disopyramide, and phenothiazine.

○ **What is this cardiac arrhythmia shown in Figure 2-2?**

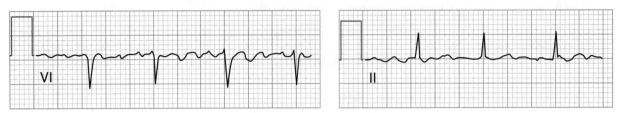

Figure 2-2 (Reproduced, with permission, from Fauci AS, Braunwald E, Kasper DL, et al., eds. *Harrison's Principles of Internal Medicine.* 17th ed. New York, NY: McGraw-Hill; 2008, Fig. 226-4A.)

Atrial fibrillation.

○ **What is the cardiac arrhythmia seen in Figure 2-3?**

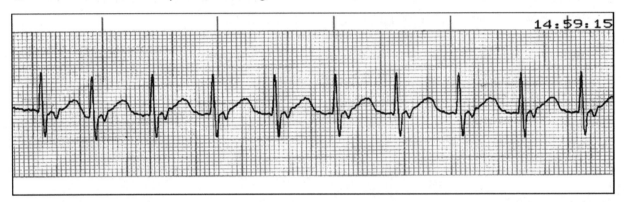

Figure 2-3

Accelerated junctional rhythm with retrograde P waves.

○ **What is the cardiac arrhythmia seen in Figure 2-4?**

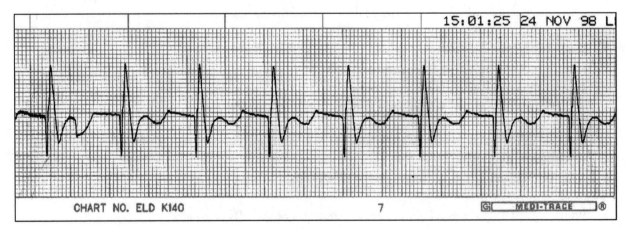

Figure 2-4

Ventricular pacemaker rhythm.

○ **What is the cardiac arrhythmia seen in Figure 2-5?**

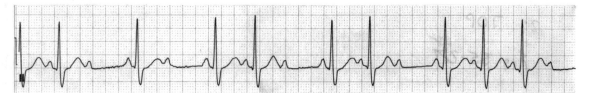

Figure 2-5 (Reproduced, with permission, from Stone CK, Humphries RL. *Current Diagnosis & Treatment Emergency Medicine*. 6th ed. New York, NY: McGraw-Hill, 2008, Fig. 33-28.)

Mobitz type II second-degree AV block.

○ **What is the EKG rhythm abnormality seen in Figure 2-6?**

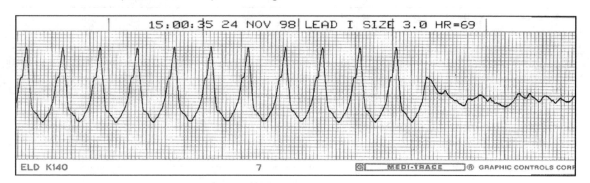

Figure 2-6

Ventricular tachycardia degrading into ventricular fibrillation.

○ **What is the cardiac arrhythmia seen in Figure 2-7?**

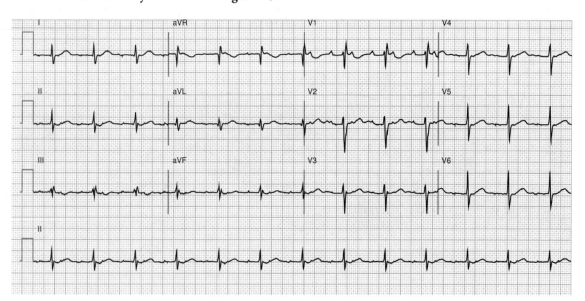

Figure 2-7 (Reproduced, with permission, from Fauci AS, Braunwald E, Kasper DL, et al., eds. *Harrison's Principles of Internal Medicine*. 17th ed. New York, NY: McGraw-Hill; 2008, Fig. e21-11.)

2:1 AB block.

○ **What is the abnormality seen in the EKG in Figure 2-8?**

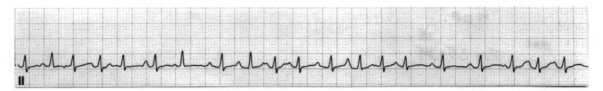

Figure 2-8 (Reproduced, with permission, from Stone CK, Humphries RL. *Current Diagnosis & Treatment Emergency Medicine.* 6th ed. New York, NY: McGraw-Hill; 2008, Fig. 33-15.)

Multifocal atrial tachycardia. Notice the change of the p-wave morphology.

○ **What is the abnormality seen in the EKG in Figure 2-9?**

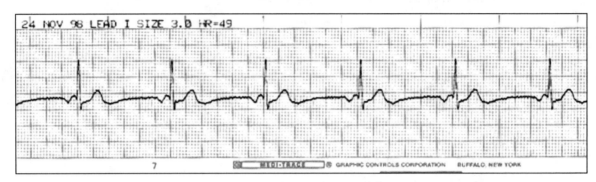

Figure 2-9

Junctional rhythm.

○ **What is the abnormality seen in the rhythm strip in Figure 2-10?**

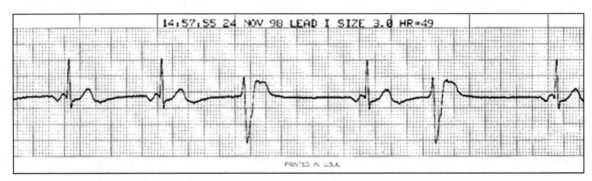

Figure 2-10

Junctional rhythm with escape ventricular beat.

○ **What is the abnormality seen in the rhythm strip in Figure 2-11?**

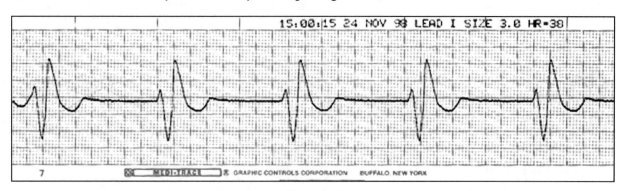

Figure 2-11

Idioventricular rhythm.

○ **What is the abnormality seen in the rhythm strip in Figure 2-12?**

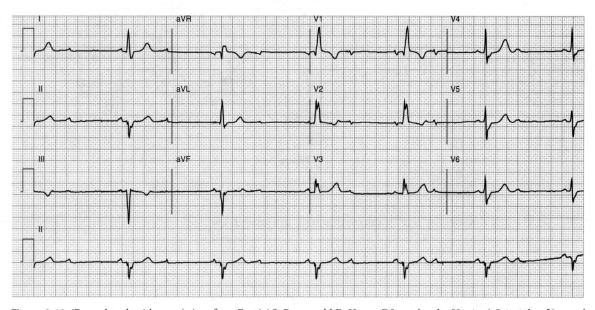

Figure 2-12 (Reproduced, with permission, from Fauci AS, Braunwald E, Kasper DL, et al., eds. *Harrison's Principles of Internal Medicine*, 17th ed. New York, NY: McGraw-Hill; 2008, Fig. e21-4.)

2:1 AV block.

○   **What is the abnormality seen in the rhythm strip in Figure 2-13?**

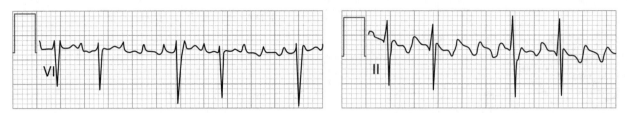

Figure 2-13 (Reproduced, with permission, from Fauci AS, Braunwald E, Kasper DL, et al., eds. *Harrison's Principles of Internal Medicine,* 17th ed. New York, NY: McGraw-Hill; 2008, Fig. 226-4B.)

Atrial flutter.

○   **What is the abnormality seen in the rhythm strip in Figure 2-14?**

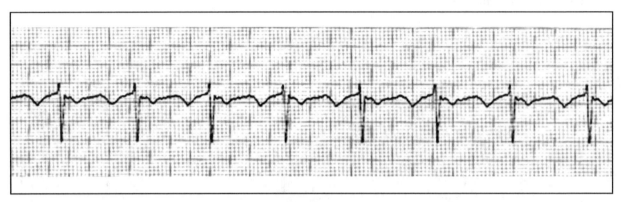

Figure 2-14

Rhythm strip erroneously mounted upside down. When viewed with right side up, it shows normal sinus rhythm.

○   **What is the abnormality seen in the rhythm strip in Figure 2-15?**

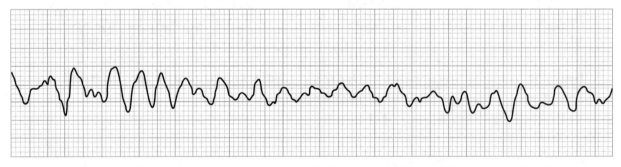

Figure 2-15 (Reproduced, with permission, from Gomella LG, Haist. *Clinician's Pocket Reference,* 11th ed. New York, NY: McGraw-Hill, 2007, Fig. 19.18.)

Ventricular fibrillation.

○ **What is the interpretation of the EKG shown in Figure 2-16?**

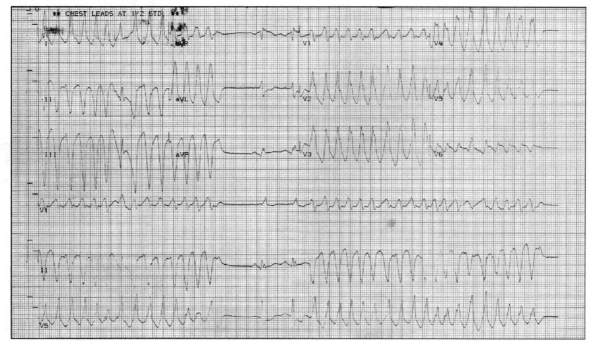

Figure 2-16

Ventricular tachycardia.

○ **What is the interpretation of the EKG shown in Figure 2-17?**

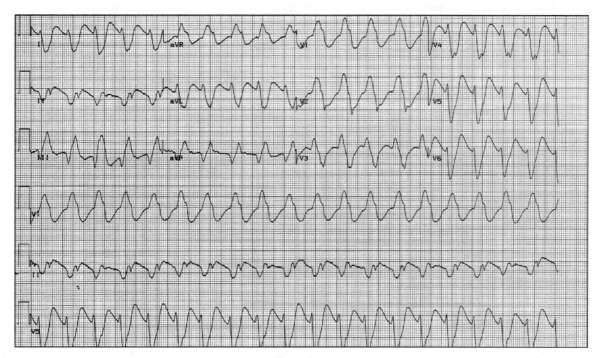

Figure 2-17

Ventricular tachycardia with hyperkalemia. Note the very wide QRS complex with the early stages of a "sine wave."

○ **What is the interpretation of the EKG shown in Figure 2-18?**

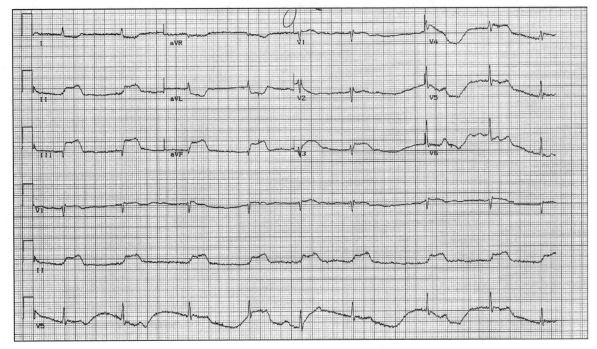

Figure 2-18

Acute inferior myocardial infarction with posterior wall involvement, and atrial fibrillation with slow ventricular rate.

○ **What is the interpretation of the EKG shown in Figure 2-19?**

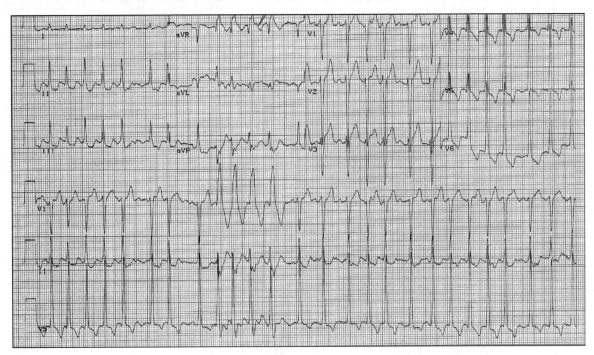

Figure 2-19

Atrial fibrillation with rapid ventricular rate of 155 bpm, LVH, and ischemic-type ST depression in the inferior and lateral leads.

○ **What is the interpretation of the EKG shown in Figure 2-20?**

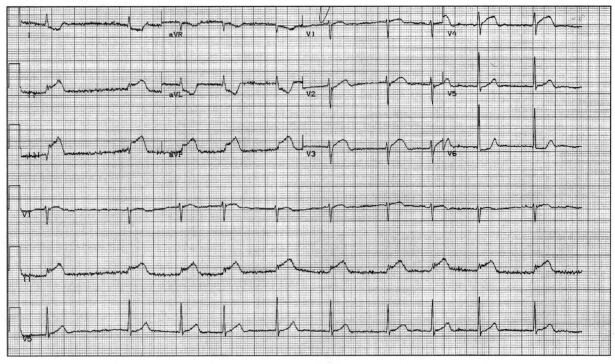

Figure 2-20

Acute inferior myocardial infarction and atrial fibrillation with slow ventricular rate.

○ **In the EKG shown in Figure 2-20, does the patient absolutely have myocardial ischemia?**

Not necessarily. Patients with supraventricular tachycardia of any type with ST depression can have "ischemic" appearing ST depression without having myocardial ischemia. The ST depression can be as a result of abnormal repolarization that occurs in any tachydysrhythmia. Nonetheless, it would be incorrect to automatically assume that this patient's ST depression is not caused by myocardial ischemia.

○ **What is the interpretation of the EKG shown in Figure 2-21?**

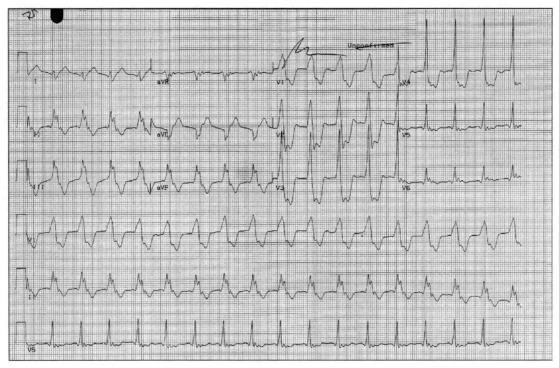

Figure 2-21

Ventricular tachycardia with a ventricular rate of 103 bpm. Note the VA conduction evidenced by the retrograde P waves, which occur in the early part of the ST segment.

○ **What is the interpretation of the EKG shown in Figure 2-22?**

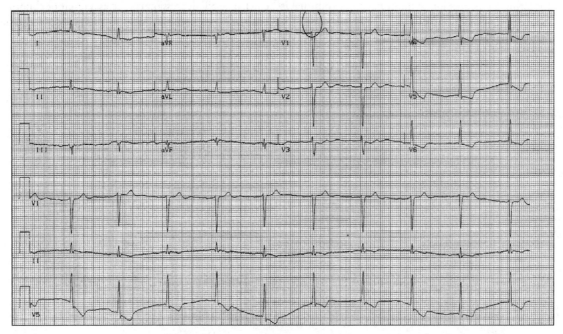

Figure 2-22

Ectopic atrial rhythm with an old inferior infarction and nonspecific ST-T abnormality.

○ **What is the interpretation of the EKG shown in Figure 2-23?**

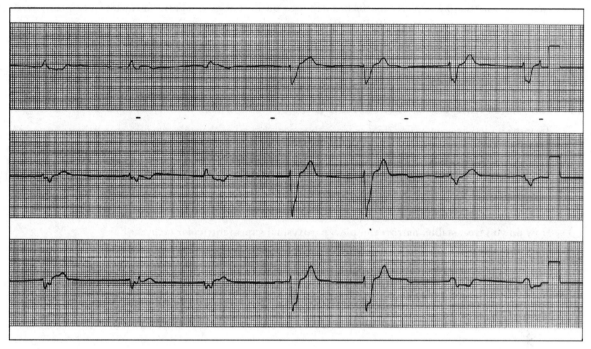

Figure 2-23

Idioventricular rhythm (rate of 40 bpm).

○ **What is the interpretation of the EKG shown in Figure 2-24?**

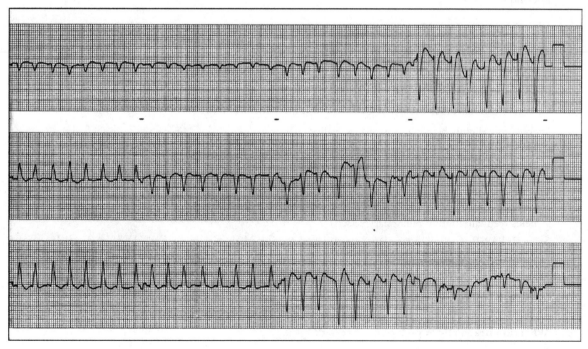

Figure 2-24

Supraventricular tachycardia.

○ **How do you treat ventricular fibrillation and pulseless ventricular tachycardia?**

Defibrillate at 360 J monophasic for the first and subsequent shocks. Continue CPR with an emphasis on chest compressions to respirations at a 30:2 ratio for 2 minutes between shocks. Epinephrine should be given at 1 mg IV/IO every 3 to 5 minutes or vasopressin 40 IU IV/IO × once and in place of the first two doses of epinephrine. Consider antidysrhythmic medications such as amiodarone 300 mg IV/IO or lidocaine (if amiodarone is not available) at 1 to 1.5 mg/kg.

○ **How do you treat pulseless electrical activity?**

Treat the underlying causes first (hypovolemia, hypoxia, hyper/hypokalemia, hypothermia, acidosis, acute MI, tamponade (cardiac), tension pneumothorax, thrombus (pulmonary), and drug overdose). If unknown cause or unsuccessful attempts to treat underlying cause, then give 1 mg of epinephrine IV/IO every 3 to 5 minutes or vasopressin 40 U IV/IO once and in place of the first two epinephrine doses. Atropine can be attempted for slow rates at 1 mg IV/IO every 3 to 5 minutes up to 3 mg maximum.

○ **How do you treat stable, narrow complex, paroxysmal supraventricular tachycardia?**

First attempt vagal maneuvers; but if there is no success, then use adenosine 6 mg rapid IV push (this can be repeated two more times up to 12 mg if needed). If adenosine fails and the ventricular function is preserved (EF >40), then use diltiazem. Other drugs could include beta-blockers, digoxin, DC cardioversion, procainamide, amiodarone, and sotalol. If the ventricular function is compromised (EF <40), then do not attempt cardioversion but attempt chemical conversion with diltiazem, amiodarone, or digoxin.

CONGESTIVE HEART FAILURE

○ **Which is the most common type of cardiac failure: high or low output?**

Low output failure. Reduced stroke volume, lowered pulse pressure, and peripheral vasoconstriction are all signs of low output failure.

○ **What is the most common cause of low output heart failure in the United States?**

Coronary artery disease. Other causes include congenital heart disease, cor pulmonale, dilated cardiomyopathy, hypertension, hypertrophic cardiomyopathy, infection, toxins, and valvular heart disease.

○ **Compare the mortality rate from CHF between men and women:**

Women fare slightly better. The 5-year mortality rate for women with CHF is 45% as compared to 60% for men. The majority of deaths from CHF result from ventricular dysrhythmias.

○ **Describe the three stages of chest radiographic findings in CHF:**

Stage I: Pulmonary arterial wedge pressure (PAWP) of 12 to 18 mm Hg. Blood flow increases in the upper lung fields (cephalization of pulmonary vessels).

Stage II: PAWP of 18 to 25 mm Hg. Interstitial edema is evident with blurred edges of blood vessels and Kerley B lines.

Stage III: PAWP >25 mm Hg. Fluid exudes into alveoli with the generation of the classic butterfly pattern of perihilar infiltrates.

○ **What do nitrates affect: preload or afterload?**

Predominantly preload.

○ **What does hydralazine affect: preload or afterload?**

Afterload.

○ **Do captopril, nifedipine, and prazosin affect afterload?**

Yes.

○ **When is dobutamine used in congestive heart failure?**

When heart failure is not accompanied with severe hypotension. Dobutamine is a potent inotrope with some vasodilation activity.

○ **When is dopamine selected in congestive heart failure?**

When a patient is in shock. Dopamine is a vasoconstrictor and a positive inotrope.

○ **What is the most common cause of right heart failure?**

Left ventricular heart failure.

○ **Match the sign or symptom with the most likely associated type of heart failure—left (L) or right (R):**

1. Hypotension
2. Hepatomegaly
3. Orthopnea
4. Cough
5. Dyspnea on exertion
6. Abdominal distention
7. Paroxysmal nocturnal dyspnea
8. Hemoptysis
9. S_3 gallop
10. Early satiety
11. Jugular venous distention
12. Ascites
13. Rales

(1) L, (2) R, (3) L, (4) L, (5) L, (6) R, (7) L, (8) L, (9) L, (10) R, (11) R, (12) R, (13) L.

HYPERTENSION

○ **What hypertensive medications should be used with caution in diabetic patients?**

Diuretics and beta-blockers should be used with caution because they may increase insulin resistance. If considered for the management of hypertension, they should not be a choice for first-line agent and be chosen only if there is a compelling indication such as heart failure or synergistic blood pressure management. ACE inhibitors and ARBs are the preferred first-line drugs of choice in diabetic patients.

○ **What antihypertensive class is most likely to present with a cough as a side effect?**

ACE inhibitors may cause a dry, persistent cough in up to 15% of patients who use them.

○ **What percentage of hypertension is secondary?**

Approximately 5%. Secondary hypertension should be suspected in patients younger than 35 years, those with sudden-onset hypertension, and those without a family history for hypertension.

○ **What is the most common cause of secondary hypertension?**

Renal parenchymal disease. In women, the most common cause is oral contraceptives. In patients older than 50 years, secondary hypertension can usually be contributed to renal artery stenosis. Other causes include pheochromocytoma, coarctation of the aorta, drugs (such as cocaine), hyperthyroidism, aldosteronism, and Cushing disease.

○ **What percentage of patients with aortic dissection are hypertensive?**

70% to 90%.

○ **What percentage of hypertensive patients are afflicted with left ventricular hypertrophy?**

50%. This is the primary reason that hypertension is a major risk factor for MI, CHF, and sudden death.

○ **What are the side effects of thiazide diuretics?**

Hyperglycemia, hyperlipidemia, hyperuricemia, hypokalemia, hypomagnesemia, and hyponatremia.

○ **Which drugs should be administered to lower the BP in a patient with thoracic aortic dissection?**

Sodium nitroprusside. A beta-blocker should also be used to reduce the dp/dt (propagation speed).

○ **A patient has a history of episodic blood pressure elevations. She complains of headache, diarrhea, and skin pallor. What is the most probable diagnosis?**

Pheochromocytoma.

○ **What is the most common complication of nitroprusside?**

Hypotension. Thiocyanate toxicity accompanied by blurred vision, tinnitus, change in mental status, muscle weakness, and seizures is more prevalent in patients with renal failure or prolonged infusions. Cyanide toxicity is uncommon. However, this type of toxicity may occur with hepatic dysfunction, after prolonged infusions, and in rates greater than 10 mg/kg/min.

○ **Define a hypertensive emergency:**

In general, a blood pressure of ≥180/115 with evidence of end-organ dysfunction or damage.

○ **How quickly should a patient's blood pressure be lowered in a hypertensive emergency?**

Gradually over 2 to 3 hours to 140–160 systolic and 90–110 diastolic. To prevent cerebral hypoperfusion, the blood pressure should not be decreased by more than 25% of the mean arterial pressure.

○ **What drug is preferred for the treatment of a hypertensive emergency?**

Sodium nitroprusside. It assists in relaxing smooth muscle tissue through the production of cGMP. As a result, there is decreased preload and afterload, decreased oxygen demand, and a slightly increased heart rate with no change in myocardial blood flow, cardiac output, or renal blood flow. The duration of action is 1 to 2 minutes. Sometimes, beta-blocker is required to treat rebound tachycardia.

○ **Define a hypertensive urgency:**

In general, a blood pressure of ≥180/115 without evidence of end-organ dysfunction or damage. Blood pressure reduction in these individuals should be done gradually over 24 to 48 hours.

○ **What laboratory findings can assist in confirming end-organ compromise in a hypertensive emergency?**

- Urinalysis: RBCs, red cell casts, and proteinuria
- BUN and CR: Elevated
- X-ray: Cardiomegaly, aortic dissection, pulmonary edema, or coarctation of aorta
- EKG: LVH and cardiac ischemia

○ **What are the signs of symptoms of hypertensive encephalopathy?**

Nausea, vomiting, headache, lethargy, coma, blindness, nerve palsies, hemiparesis, aphasia, retinal hemorrhage, cotton wool spots, exudates, sausage linking, and papilledema. Treat with labetalol or sodium nitroprusside and lower the mean arterial pressure to approximately 120 mm Hg.

○ **What is the first-line pharmacologic therapy for a 40-year-old obese White woman with uncomplicated mild hypertension?**

ACE inhibitors or a thiazide diuretic. Beta-blockers, ARBs, or calcium channel blockers could be considered if contraindications to ACEI or diuretics.

○ **What is the preferred choice of antihypertensive therapy for a 58-year-old White man with severe COPD and mild hypertension?**

Long-acting calcium channel blockers such as amlodipine, diltiazem, or nifedipine. These agents are particularly useful in patients with a likelihood of pulmonary hypertension. If pulmonary hypertension is suspected, verapamil should be avoided because of its significant negative inotropic effects.

○ **What is the agent of choice in diabetic patients with hypertension?**

ACE inhibitors or ARBs.

○ **Which agent is more likely to cause bradycardia: verapamil or diltiazem?**

Diltiazem. Diltiazem blocks conduction through both the SA and AV node, whereas verapamil blocks only the AV node.

○ **What antihypertensive agents are preferred agents to use in a 63-year-old obese, African American man?**

Calcium channel blockers. Diuretics and/or ACE inhibitors can be considered too.

○ **What is the most common side effect of esmolol, labetalol, and bretylium?**

Hypotension.

○ **What side effect can occur with a rapid infusion of procainamide?**

Hypotension. Other side effects include QRS/QT prolongation, ventricular fibrillation, and torsades de pointes.

○ **What is one of the most common side effect of antihypertensive medications that patients should be warned about?**

Orthostatic hypotension.

○ **How long can ST and T *wave changes* persist after an episode of pain in unstable angina?**

Several hours.

○   **What are the diagnostic criteria for a Q wave?**

More than 0.04 seconds and at least one-quarter the size of the R wave in the same lead. Beware, EKGs can be normal in up to 10% of all acute MIs.

○   **What is the cause of Prinzmetal angina?**

Coronary artery vasospasm with or without fixed stenotic lesions. Prinzmetal angina is more often associated with ST segment elevation than with depression. Calcium channel blockers are the drugs of choice to treat this condition. Beta-blockers are contraindicated in patients with vasospasm without fixed stenotic lesions.

○   **Eighty to ninety percent of patients who experience sudden nontraumatic cardiac death are in what rhythm?**

Ventricular fibrillation. Early defibrillation is the key. In an acute MI, the infarction zone becomes electrically unstable. Ventricular fibrillation is most common during original coronary occlusion or when the coronaries begin to reperfuse.

○   **What is the rate of restenosis after percutaneous transluminal coronary angioplasty (PTCA)?**

20% to 30% within the first 6 months, but bare metal and drug-eluding stents have greatly reduced restenosis rates. PTCA is now rarely used by itself but commonly used prior to stent placement. In most situations it is imperative that patients are treated at a minimum of three months of aspirin and clopidogrel.

○   **What two drugs are commonly used to reduce thrombosis formation in a patient who has received an intracoronary stent?**

Aspirin and clopidogrel.

○   **What is the restenosis rate of coronary vessels following a coronary artery bypass graft (CABG)?**

When using venous grafts, there is a 50% restenosis rate within 5 to 10 years. When an artery is used, such as the internal mammary artery, the restenosis rate drops to 5% at 10 years. Occlusion of the grafts is caused by anastomy, trauma to the vessel, postoperative adhesions, or atherosclerosis.

○   **How are acute MI, angina pectoralis, and Prinzmetal angina differentiated?**

The pain is similar but typically differs in radiation, duration, provocation, and palliation. Obtaining an accurate history is the most important tool for diagnosing chest pain.

- Angina pectoralis is aggravated by exercise, cold, and excitement but is relieved with rest and nitroglycerin.
- Prinzmetal angina occurs at rest during normal activity, and generally at night or in the early morning. It lasts longer than angina pectoralis.
- Acute MIs produce pain with a greater radius of radiation that may last for hours.

○   **Which type of myocardial infarction is more often associated with thrombosis: transmural or subendocardial?**

Transmural. Thrombolytic therapy increases left ventricular ejection fraction post-MI, reduces the development of postinfarction CHF, and can reduce early MI mortality by 25%.

○   **How much aspirin should a post-MI patient take daily to reduce the incidence of reinfarction?**

75 to 150 mg daily.

○ **What is the most common cause of death during the first few hours of a MI?**

Cardiac dysrhythmias, generally ventricular fibrillation.

○ **When treating early MIs, beta-blockers decrease the risk of reinfarction. Which patients should not receive beta-blockers?**

Patients presenting with hypotension, congestive heart failure, severe left ventricular dysfunction, AV block, bradycardia, asthma, or other bronchospastic disease.

○ **How common are PVCs in post-MI patients?**

90% will have PVCs within the first few weeks. Concern arises if the PVCs are complex, which is the case in 20% to 40% of MI patients. Risk of sudden death in post-MI patients with complex PVCs increases two to five times.

○ **What percentage of the LV myocardium must be damaged to induce cardiogenic shock?**

40%. Twenty-five percent or greater damage to the heart typically results in heart failure.

○ **What percentage of MIs are clinically unrecognized?**

5% to 10%.

○ **A non–Q-wave infarction is usually associated with what?**

Subsequent angina or recurrent infarction. Non–Q-wave infarctions also have lower in-hospital mortality rate compared to Q-wave MIs.

○ **Why do T waves invert in an acute myocardial infarction?**

Infarction or ischemia causes a reversal of the sequence of repolarization, for example, endocardial-to-epicardial as opposed to normally epicardial-to-endocardial.

○ **What EKG changes arise in a true posterior infarction?**

Large R wave and ST depression in V_1 and V_2.

○ **What conduction defects commonly occur in an anterior wall MI?**

The dangerous kind. Damage to the conducting system results in a Mobitz type II second- or third-degree AV block.

○ **How should PSVT be treated during an acute myocardial infarction?**

Adenosine, cardioversion, or vagal maneuvers could be attempted. Stable patients may be able to tolerate negative inotropes such as calcium channel blockers (verapamil) or even beta-blockers.

○ **A patient presents 1 day after discharge for an acute myocardial infarction with a new harsh systolic ejection murmur along the left sternal border and pulmonary edema. What is the diagnosis?**

Ventricular septal rupture. Diagnosis is made by either a Swan–Ganz catheterization or echocardiogram. These patients often present with cardiogenic shock.

○ **When does cardiac rupture usually occur in patients who have suffered acute MIs?**

50% arise within the first 5 days and 90% occur within the first 14 days post-MI.

○ **Which type of infarct commonly leads to papillary muscle dysfunction?**

Inferior wall MI. Signs and symptoms include a mild transient systolic murmur and pulmonary edema.

○ **A patient presents 2 weeks post–acute MI with chest pain, fever, and pleuropericarditis. A pleural effusion is detected on chest radiography. What is the diagnosis?**

Dressler (post–myocardial infarction) syndrome. This syndrome is caused by an immunologic reaction to myocardial antigens.

○ **What percentage of patients older than 80 years' experience chest pain with an acute myocardial infarction?**

Only 50%. Twenty percent experience diaphoresis, stroke, syncope, and/or acute confusion.

○ **What three secondary processes resulting in myocardial deterioration occur following acute myocardial infarction?**

Ventricular remodeling, typically following Q-wave infarctions; infarct expansion, occurring most frequently from anteroapical infarctions and results in thinning of the left ventricular wall; and ventricular dilatation, an early and progressive response to acute myocardial infarction that is an important predictor of increased mortality following myocardial infarction.

○ **What is the most common cause of death related to acute myocardial infarction?**

Ventricular fibrillation, usually occurring within the first hour following symptoms.

○ **What percentage of patients with acute myocardial infarction develop cardiogenic shock?**

10%.

○ **What percentage of arteries successfully opened with thrombolytic therapy for acute myocardial infarction, reocclude?**

15% of arteries successfully opened reocclude during the first few days following thrombolytic therapy.

○ **What is the mortality benefit from aspirin alone in acute myocardial infarction with thrombolytic therapy and in subsequent reinfarction?**

Aspirin reduced mortality from acute myocardial infarction by 23% and reduced nonfatal reinfarction by 49%. When used with thrombolytic therapy, there was a 40% to 50% reduction in mortality from acute myocardial infarction.

○ **A 63-year-old man presents to the emergency department with moderate substernal chest pressure and lightheadedness for 90 minutes. His BP on admission is 80/40 and his HR is 110 bpm and regular. Physical examination reveals JVD to the angle of the jaw, a right parasternal S_3 gallop, an apical S_4 gallop, and clear lungs on auscultation. EKG reveals 2-mm ST elevation in leads II, III, and aVF with reciprocal ST depression in V_1 through V_3. What is the most likely diagnosis and what is the most appropriate initial therapy?**

Inferior wall myocardial infarction with right ventricular infarction. Initial therapy includes 325 mg of aspirin administration, thrombolytic therapy, and a large bolus of intravenous saline followed by a moderately high infusion rate of saline. If the patient remains hypotensive despite adequate infusion of saline (typically measured by development of lung congestion on auscultation), then intravenous dobutamine is indicated.

○ **A 70-year-old man is admitted to the hospital with chest pain of 3 hours duration. EKG demonstrates anterior ST elevation for which he is given aspirin, r-TPA, heparin, and intravenous nitroglycerin. His symptoms resolve. Serum chemistries reveal a peak CPK of 1,800 and CK-MB fraction of 15%. The patient is eventually transferred out of the CCU and his hospitalization is uneventful until day 5, when he develops sudden, severe shortness of breath. BP is 110/75 and his pulse is 125 bpm and regular. Examination reveals a new systolic murmur. What would the most appropriate therapeutic intervention be?**

Intravenous sodium nitroprusside. This patient is most likely suffering from rupture of the left ventricular septum and subsequent defect—a not uncommon complication of MI. Afterload reduction is key to stabilization until surgical repair of the VSD can be performed, usually in about 8 to 12 weeks, after the infarct has healed. If nitroprusside fails to stabilize the patient, intra-aortic balloon counterpulsation and intravenous nitroglycerin should be employed.

○ **A 60-year-old patient suffers an acute inferior myocardial infarction. Three hours after he arrives in the hospital, he develops ventricular fibrillation and is successfully defibrillated back to normal sinus rhythm within 30 seconds. He makes a full recovery and has no further post-MI complications. What does his ventricular fibrillation episode indicate with regard to subsequent risk for sudden death?**

This episode has no bearing on his subsequent risk of sudden death. Ventricular fibrillation in the immediate setting of an acute myocardial infarction has no prognostic significance.

○ **A 65-year-old female patient presents to the hospital with sudden crushing chest discomfort and moderate shortness of breath. Her initial EKG reveals 2-mm ST depression in leads V_1 through V_4 and inverted T waves. She has bibasilar rales in the lower half of both lungs on auscultation. CXR reveals moderate pulmonary edema. Serial EKGs, CPKs, and troponins confirm a non–Q-wave myocardial infarction. With diuretics, her pulmonary edema resolves within 24 hours. What is the most appropriate management strategy at this point?**

Cardiac catheterization with coronary angiography. A non–Q-wave MI that results in pulmonary edema signifies a larger amount of myocardium at risk for reinfarction within the next year.

○ **What arrhythmias that occur in patients with acute myocardial infarction require temporary pacing?**

Complete heart block; new left bundle branch block; new bifascicular block; marked sinus bradycardia with ischemic pain, hypotension, CHF, frequent PVCs or syncope despite atropine; and Mobitz II second-degree AV block.

○ **A 54-year-old man, admitted 2 days ago with an acute anterolateral myocardial infarction, suddenly develops atrial fibrillation with a ventricular rate of 135 bpm. He subsequently complains of substernal chest discomfort. His BP is 135/70. What is the most appropriate immediate action to be taken?**

Synchronized DC cardioversion.

○ **What percentage of patients with acute myocardial infarction develop paroxysmal atrial fibrillation?**

10% to 15%.

○ **A 58-year-old man is admitted with an acute anteroseptal myocardial infarction. He is in pulmonary edema clinically, confirmed by chest radiography. His blood pressure is 122/76, his HR is 122. Despite two doses of 80 mg of intravenous furosemide, he remains in pulmonary edema. A Swan–Ganz pulmonary artery catheter is inserted and his initial hemodynamics reveal a cardiac output of 3.1 L/min and a pulmonary capillary wedge pressure of 27 mm Hg. What is the most appropriate pharmacologic agent in this setting?**

Intravenous dobutamine, at a dose of 5 to 20 g/kg/min.

○ **What are the major complications of left ventricular aneurysms?**

LV thrombus formation (with subsequent risk of thromboembolic events), CHF, and ventricular arrhythmias.

○ **What is the current recommended therapy for patients with large anterior myocardial infarctions?**

Reperfusion therapy with thrombolytics, beta-blockers, intravenous nitroglycerin, and ACE inhibitors to limit and retard ventricular remodeling. Intravenous heparin in a sufficient dose to prolong the APTT to 1.5 to 2 times control should be started on admission and continued to discharge. In patients with large akinetic apical segments or mural thrombi, oral anticoagulation with warfarin is indicated for at least 6 months.

○ **What is the significance of pericarditis following acute myocardial infarction?**

Pericarditis occurs in about 20% of patients with acute myocardial infarction, more likely in Q-wave infarcts than non–Q-wave infarcts. Patients with pericarditis usually have significantly larger infarcts, lower ejection fractions, and a higher incidence of congestive heart failure. The presence of pericarditis and/or pericardial effusion following acute myocardial infarction is associated with higher mortality.

○ **A previously healthy 65-year-old man is admitted with an acute inferior myocardial infarction. Within several hours, he is hypotensive (BP 90/60) and oliguric. Insertion of a pulmonary artery catheter reveals the following pressure: pulmonary artery wedge pressure, 3 mm Hg; pulmonary artery, 21/3 mm Hg; and mean right atrial pressure, 11 mm Hg. What is the best treatment for this man?**

Fluids until his wedge pressure is between 16 and 20 mm Hg.

○ **A 60-year-old man with a recent syncopal episode is hospitalized with congestive heart failure and chest pain. His BP is 165/85 mm Hg, his pulse is 85 bpm, and there is a grade III/VI harsh systolic murmur at the apex and aortic area. An echocardiogram reveals a disproportionately thickened septum and anterior systolic motion of the mitral valve. What is this patient's diagnosis and what physical findings would most likely be present?**

Idiopathic obstructive hypertrophic cardiomyopathy (IHSS). The murmur typically decreases with handgrip and squatting and increases with Valsalva, vasodilators, standing, nitroglycerin, diuretics, and digoxin. Mitral regurgitation is frequent as a result of anterior systolic motion of the mitral valve. Congestive heart failure is present because of diastolic dysfunction, thus an S_4 gallop is common.

○ **In patients with coronary artery disease, which patients have been shown to benefit from revascularization with bypass grafting?**

Patients with left main coronary artery disease (>50% stenosis) and those with three vessel coronary artery disease (>70% stenosis) with depressed LV function (<40% EF).

○ **What are the classic EKG results associated with posterior MI?**

A large R wave in leads V_1 and V_2, ST depression in leads V_1 and V_2, Q waves in the inferior leads and, occasionally, ST elevation in the inferior leads.

○ **What is the most common complication of extracorporeal circulation?**

Stroke occurs in 1% to 2% of patients after open heart operations. Other postoperative complications are arrhythmias, bleeding, renal failure, and respiratory complications.

○   **What drug is used to reverse heparin after open heart surgery?**

Protamine sulfate.

○   **In 90% of the population, the right coronary artery terminates as the:**

Posterior descending artery.

○   **The left main coronary artery gives rise to which two coronary arteries?**

The left anterior descending artery and the left circumflex coronary artery.

○   **What is the vessel of preference in coronary bypass grafting?**

The internal mammary artery. Other artery grafts such as the radial artery are preferred too. Arterial grafts tend to have higher rates of patency at 10 years compared to venous grafts. Venous grafts are also more susceptible to atherosclerotic disease.

VASCULAR DISEASE

○   **Are aortic aneurysms more common in men or women?**

Men (10:1 male-to-female ratio). Other risk factors include hypertension, atherosclerosis, diabetes, hyperlipidemia, smoking, syphilis, Marfan disease, and Ehlers–Danlos disease.

○   **A patient presents with sudden-onset chest and back pain. Further work-up reveals an ischemic right leg. What is your diagnosis?**

Suspect an acute aortic dissection when chest or back pain is associated with ischemic and/or neurologic deficits.

○   **What physical findings suggest an acute aortic dissection?**

Blood pressure and pulse differences between arms and/or legs, cardiac tamponade, and aortic insufficiency murmur.

○   **What CXR findings occur with a thoracic aortic aneurysm?**

Change in aortic appearance, mediastinal widening, hump in the aortic arch, pleural effusion (most commonly on the left), and extension of the aortic shadow.

○   **A 74-year-old male patient presents with acute-onset testicular pain. Ecchymosis is present in the groin and scrotal sac. What is the diagnosis?**

A ruptured aortic or iliac artery aneurysm.

○   **What X-ray study should be ordered for a patient with an abdominal mass and a suspected ruptured abdominal aortic aneurysm?**

None! The patient should go to the operating room immediately. About 60% of AAAs occur with calcification and appear on a lateral abdominal X-ray.

○   **What may an X-ray of a patient with an aortic dissection reveal?**

Widening of the superior mediastinum, a hazy or enlarged aortic knob, an irregular aortic contour, separation of the intimal calcification from the outer aortic contour that is greater than 5 mm, a displaced trachea to the right, and cardiomegaly.

○ **What is the most common symptom of aortic dissection?**

Interscapular back pain. Many patients will complain of a "ripping" sensation in their backs as the dissection is taking place.

○ **Where do aortic dissections most often occur?**

Proximal ascending aorta (60%). Twenty percent of aortic dissections are found between the origin of the left subclavian and the ligamentum arteriosum in the descending aorta, and 10% are found in the aortic arch or the abdominal aorta. Dissection involves intimal tears propagated by hematoma formation.

○ **What aortic aneurysm diameter is generally considered to be an indication for surgery for an aneurysm in the (a) in the thorax and (b) in the abdomen?**

Those with a nondissecting thoracic aneurysm larger than 7 cm in diameter are candidates for surgery. However, surgery should be considered with smaller aneurysms for those with Marfan syndrome because of higher incidence of rupture. Nondissecting abdominal aortic aneurysms larger than 4 cm in diameter should be considered for surgical repair.

○ **Describe the Stanford classification of aortic dissections:**

Stanford type A: Always involves the ascending aorta but could include the descending aorta. Stanford type B: Involves the descending aorta only.

○ **What dissections can be treated medically?**

Patients with Stanford type B and (type III) are eligible for medical, rather than, surgical treatment. Surgical treatment may be required for those with uncontrollable pain, aortic bleeding, hemodynamic instability, increasing hematoma size, or an impending rupture.

○ **What is the prognosis of an untreated aortic dissection?**

20% of afflicted individuals die within 24 hours, 60% within 2 weeks, and 90% within 3 months. With surgical treatment, the 10-year survival rate is 40%. Redissection occurs in 25% of these patients within 10 years of the original episode.

○ **Where is the most common site of peripheral aneurysms that develop from arteriosclerosis?**

The popliteal artery. Other sites include the femoral, carotid, and subclavian arteries.

○ **What artery is usually affected by arterial occlusive disease in diabetic patients?**

The popliteal artery. Because of diabetic neuropathy and the potential for the development of a necrotizing infection in a leg with compromised circulation, it is very important that patients with diabetes are knowledgeable about pedal hygiene.

○ **What is the Budd–Chiari syndrome?**

Thrombosis in the hepatic vein resulting in abdominal pain, jaundice, and ascites.

○ **Which arteries are most commonly involved in giant cell arteritis (chronic inflammation of the large blood vessels)?**

The carotid arteries and its branches. Treatment includes high doses of corticosteroids.

○ **What is the most common source of acute mesenteric ischemia?**

Arterial embolism (40%–50%). The source is usually the heart, generally from mural thrombus. The most common point of obstruction is the superior mesenteric artery.

○ **What laboratory results strongly suggest that a patient has mesenteric ischemia?**

Leukocytosis >15,000, metabolic acidosis (sometimes with anion gap), hemoconcentration, and elevated phosphate and amylase.

○ **Describe the Trendelenburg test for varicose veins:**

Raise the leg above the heart and then quickly lower it. If the leg veins become distended immediately after this test is performed, valvular incompetency is evident.

○ **A 68-year-old male patient with diabetes and a 60 pack-year history of smoking presents with sudden, severe substernal chest discomfort, radiating through the interscapular area. His BP is 158/80 mm Hg in the right arm and 135/65 mm Hg in the left arm. He complains of right arm numbness and weakness and you hear a grade II/VI diastolic murmur along the left sternal border. EKG reveals 1.5-mm ST elevation in the inferior leads. What is the diagnosis?**

Acute proximal thoracic aortic dissection, with involvement of the right coronary artery and brachiocephalic artery, as well as acute aortic regurgitation.

○ **In the patient described in the last question, what other life-threatening complication must one look for, both on auscultation and on chest radiograph?**

Pericardial effusion with cardiac tamponade. Listen for a pericardial rub on auscultation and look for marked cardiomegaly on CXR. Pulsus paradoxus of >10 mm Hg is virtually diagnostic of cardiac tamponade in this setting.

○ **What CXR findings occur with a dissecting thoracic aortic aneurysm?**

Tortuosity of the proximal aorta with an enlarged aortic knob, mediastinal widening, pleural effusion (most common on the left), extension of the aortic shadow, displaced trachea to the right, cardiomegaly, and separation of the intimal calcification from the outer contour that is greater than 5 mm.

○ **What is the prognosis for an untreated dissecting aortic aneurysm?**

25% die within 24 hours, 50% die within 1 week, 75% die within 1 month, and 90% die within 3 months. With surgical treatment, the 10-year survival is 50%, the 5-year survival is 75% to 80%. Redissection occurs in 25% of patients within 10 years of the original dissection.

○ **What is an ABI and why is it significant?**

An ankle/brachial index is the ankle systolic pressure (numerator) compared to the brachial systolic pressure (denominator). It is used as a screening tool for determining the presence of obstructive arterial disease of the lower extremities. A positive ABI is also considered an independent risk factor for coronary artery disease.

○ **What technical factors can affect the accuracy of the ABI?**

Probe pressure, rapid deflation of the BP cuff, arterial wall calcifications, and probe placement, which should be longitudinal to the vessel and at a 30- to 60-degree angle to the skin surface.

○   **Complete the following matching:**

1.	Quinke pulse	a.	Uvular pulsation during systole
2.	Corrigan pulse	b.	Head bobbing
3.	de Musset sign	c.	Visible pulsations in nail bed capillaries
4.	Muller sign	d.	Collapsing pulse
5.	Duroziez sign	e.	Drop in the systolic blood pressure >10 mm Hg with inspiration
6.	Pulsus paradoxus	f.	Femoral artery murmurs during systole if the artery is compressed proximally and during diastole if the artery is compressed distally

(1) c, (2) d, (3) b, (4) a, (5) f, and (6) e. These are all signs pertaining to aortic insufficiency.

CONGENITAL HEART DISEASE

○   **What are the more common symptoms of a child with an atrial septal defect (ASD)?**

In most cases, the patient is asymptomatic. In later teen to adult years, the patient may complain of mild fatigue or dyspnea. In rare cases, heart failure is present.

○   **What is the typical murmur that is heard in a patient with an ASD?**

A midsystolic crescendo–decrescendo over the left upper sternal border.

○   **A 5-month-old male infant is brought to the pediatrician's office because the mother is concerned about his feeding. She notes that the child appears to be short of breath, has poor weight gain, and his feeding is about half of what it should be. On physical examination, you note that his weight is in the 35th percentile, and a gallop is present on auscultation. There is also a slight murmur detected on the intrascapular region of the back on the left side. What is the most likely diagnosis?**

Coarctation of the aorta.

○   **What is the difference between the pressures of the upper half of the body compared to the lower in a patient with a coarctation of the aorta?**

The pulse pressures in the upper arms will be strong, whereas the lower extremities will be diminished or in some cases not detected by Doppler.

○   **What is the most common extracardiac congenital anomaly found in children?**

Patent ductus arteriosus (PDA).

○   **What is the most characteristic physical examination finding in an infant with a PDA?**

The infant will have a systolic thrill that is felt over the pulmonary artery and suprasternal notch. The child will also have a machine-like continuous murmur over the left upper sternal border.

○   **Name the four defects that are characteristic of tetralogy of Fallot:**

1. Ventricular septal defect (VSD)
2. Right ventricular hypertrophy
3. RV outflow obstruction from infundibular stenosis (pulmonary valve)
4. Overriding aorta (<50%); a right-sided aortic arch is seen in 25%

○ **What is the preferred test to determine if a child has tetralogy of Fallot?**

Echocardiogram.

○ **What is the most common congenital cardiac anomaly?**

Ventricular septal defect (VSD).

○ **Describe symptoms that can present in a child with a VSD:**

The size of the defect will determine the degree of symptoms. Small defects in children may not produce any symptoms, but clinical deterioration may occur at any time. In patients with a large defect, parents may describe grunting, sweating, failure to gain weight, tachypnea, and fatigue.

○ **What are some of the physical examination characteristics found in a patient with a VSD?**

The patient may have some respiratory distress, a thrill at the left lower sternal border (common), S_2 splits, S_3 is common, and a holosystolic murmur at the apex is common. Hepatic enlargement may also be present.

○ **What percentage of VSDs will resolve with conservative medical management?**

About 70% of small defects. Larger defects will either be monitored with symptoms and close examinations, or by surgical correction early in the child's life.

○ **What murmur is expected in patients with substantial aortic stenosis?**

A prolonged, harsh, loud (IV, V, or VI) systolic murmur.

○ **What is the most common cause of aortic regurgitation in adults?**

Mild aortic regurgitation frequently develops as a result of a bicuspid aortic valve. A severe aortic valve regurgitation is induced by rheumatic heart disease, syphilis, endocarditis, trauma, an idiopathic degeneration of the aortic valve, a spontaneous rupture of the valve leaflets, or aortic dissection.

○ **What are the signs and symptoms of acute aortic regurgitation?**

Dyspnea, tachycardia, tachypnea, and chest pain.

○ **What is the most common cause of aortic stenosis in patients younger than 50 years and older than 50 years?**

- Younger than 50: Calcification of congenital bicuspid aortic valves (1% of the population has congenital bicuspid valves).
- Older than 50: Calcification of degenerating leaflets.

○ **What triad of symptoms characterizes aortic stenosis?**

Syncope, angina, and left heart failure. As the disease progresses, systolic BP decreases and pulse pressure narrows.

○ **What are the findings in a patient with aortic stenosis?**

Angina, dyspnea on exertion, syncope, sustained apical impulse, narrow pulse pressure, parvus et tardus, systolic ejection crescendo–decrescendo murmur that radiates to the neck, systolic ejection click (not heard in severe cases when the valve is so stenosed that it is immobile), paradoxically split S_1 and soft S_2, and audible S_4.

○ **How does the heart murmur reflect the severity of aortic stenosis?**

A longer duration associated with an increase in intensity indicates severe aortic stenosis. The "loudness" of the murmur is not as important in assessing its severity.

○ **A patient presents to the hospital 1 month after placement of a mechanical prosthetic valve with fever, chills, and a leukocytosis. Endocarditis is suspected. Which bacterium is most commonly encountered in this situation?**

Staphylococcus aureus or *Staphylococcus epidermidis.*

○ **What percentage of non-anticoagulated patients with mitral stenosis experience system emboli?**

About 25%. Patients with chronic atrial fibrillation or mitral stenosis should be chronically anticoagulated to prevent atrial mural thrombi.

○ **What is the most common cause of mitral stenosis?**

Rheumatic heart disease. The most common initial symptom is dyspnea.

○ **What physical findings may be associated with mitral stenosis?**

Prominent *a*-wave, early systolic left parasternal lift, loud and snapping first heart sound, and early diastolic opening snap with a low-pitched mid-diastolic rumble that crescendos into S_1.

○ **A midsystolic click with a late systolic crescendo murmur is indicative of what cardiac disease?**

Mitral valve prolapse (MVP). This is the hallmark sign of MVP.

○ **Is mitral valve prolapse more common among men or women?**

Women have a stronger genetic link to the disease. However, only 2% to 5% of the entire population has symptomatic MVP.

○ **What age group typically develops MVP syndrome?**

Patients in their twenties and thirties. Most patients with MVP are asymptomatic. MVP syndrome is symptomatic with chest pain, fatigue, palpitations, postural syncope, and dizziness.

○ **Rheumatic heart disease is the most common cause of stenosis of what three heart valves?**

Mitral, aortic (along with congenital bicuspid valve), and tricuspid.

○ **What is the most frequent cause of mitral stenosis?**

Rheumatic fever. Far less common causes include congenital, malignant carcinoid, SLE, rheumatoid arthritis, infective endocarditis with large vegetation, and the mucopolysaccharidoses of the Hunter-Hurley phenotype.

○ **What percentage of patients with rheumatic heart disease have pure mitral stenosis?**

25%. An additional 40% have combined MS and MR.

○ **What are the principal symptoms in mitral stenosis?**

Dyspnea is the most common. Patients with severe mitral stenosis can experience orthopnea, hemoptysis, chest pain, and frank pulmonary edema, often precipitated by exertion, fever, URI, sexual intercourse, pregnancy, or the onset of rapid atrial fibrillation.

○ **What are two most serious complications of mitral stenosis?**

Thromboembolism, most often occurring in the setting of atrial fibrillation, and pulmonary edema.

○ **What maneuvers can one do to differentiate the opening snap of mitral stenosis from a split S_2 sound?**

Sudden standing widens the A_2-opening snap interval, whereas a split S_2 narrows on standing. Progressive narrowing of the A_2-opening snap interval on serial examinations suggests an increase in the severity of mitral stenosis.

○ **What is the most accurate noninvasive technique for quantifying the severity of mitral stenosis?**

Doppler echocardiography.

○ **What is the medical management strategy of rheumatic mitral stenosis?**

- Penicillin prophylaxis for beta-hemolytic streptococcal infections and prophylaxis for infective endocarditis
- Aggressive and prompt treatment of anemia and infections
- Avoidance of strenuous exertion
- Oral diuretics and sodium restriction in symptomatic patients
- Beta-blockers to reduce heart rate
- Cardioversion of atrial fibrillation
- Aggressive slowing of refractory atrial fibrillation
- Anticoagulant therapy in patients who have experienced one or more thromboembolic episodes, or who have mechanical prosthetic valves

○ **What is the symptomatic period after an attack of rheumatic fever in patients with mitral stenosis?**

In temperate zones, such as the United States and Europe, about 15 to 20 years. In tropical and subtropical areas and in underdeveloped areas, about 6 to 12 years.

○ **What is the indication for mitral valve surgery or balloon valvuloplasty in patients with mitral stenosis?**

Moderate symptoms (class II) or greater in a patient with moderate to severe mitral stenosis (mitral valve orifice size of less than 1 cm^2 per square meter BSA or less than 1.5 to 1.7 cm^2 mitral valve area in normal adults).

○ **A 28-year-old Hispanic woman is referred to you for evaluation of dyspnea and palpitations. She has a diastolic murmur consistent with mitral stenosis. Echocardiography confirms severe, noncalcific mitral stenosis with trivial mitral regurgitation, with a mitral valve area of 0.8 cm^2. EKG reveals atrial fibrillation. What is the most appropriate course of therapy for this patient?**

Open mitral valvotomy (commissurotomy) followed by cardioversion to normal sinus rhythm. This is palliative, obviates the need for anticoagulation for the immediate future, and results in at least 5 to 10 years of symptom-free life for over half of the patients.

○ **What is the most common cause of mitral regurgitation?**

Rheumatic fever. It is more frequent in men than women. Other causes include infective endocarditis, mitral valve prolapse, ischemic heart disease, trauma, SLE, scleroderma, hypertrophic cardiomyopathy, dilated cardiomyopathy involving the left ventricle, and idiopathic degenerative calcification of the mitral annulus.

○ **What are the physical findings of patients with chronic mitral regurgitation?**

Harsh, pansystolic murmur heard best at the apex, radiating to the axilla or the base. The murmur is diminished by maneuvers that decrease preload or afterload, such as amyl nitrate inhalation, Valsalva, or standing, and increases with maneuvers that increase preload or afterload, such as squatting, handgrip, or phenylephrine administration.

○ **What are the most common causes of acute mitral regurgitation?**

Acute myocardial infarction with papillary muscle dysfunction (15% of acute MI results in acute mitral regurgitation) or papillary muscle rupture (3% of acute MI), infective endocarditis, chordate tendinea rupture secondary to chest trauma, rheumatic fever, mitral valve prolapsed, and hypertrophic cardiomyopathy with rupture of chordate tendinea.

○ **Which is the best test to assess the detailed anatomy of rheumatic mitral valve disease and determine whether mitral valve replacement is necessary or whether reconstruction is feasible?**

Transesophageal echocardiography.

○ **What is the appropriate medical management of mitral regurgitation?**

Vasodilator therapy with ACE inhibitors is the hallmark of therapy, even in patients who are asymptomatic. Diuretics are used in patients with severe MR. Cardiac glycosides, such as digoxin, are indicated in patients with severe MR and clinical evidence of heart failure. Endocarditis prophylaxis is indicated in all patients with MR. Anticoagulation should be given to all patients in atrial fibrillation.

○ **A 33-year-old female patient comes to you for a physical examination and you notice a harsh systolic murmur at the apex that is also heard at the base. The murmur increases on standing and Valsalva and decreases with handgrip. What is the most likely finding on echocardiography?**

Mitral valve prolapse. The murmur of pure mitral regurgitation decreases with Valsalva and standing and increases with handgrip or squatting.

○ **A 46-year-old male patient with a history of rheumatic fever at age 12 is admitted with an acute myocardial infarction. The patient's post-MI course is complicated by congestive heart failure. Echocardiogram reveals severe mitral regurgitation with rupture of one of the papillary muscles and prolapsed posterior mitral valve leaflet without apparent calcification. Systolic function by echocardiogram is mildly reduced. What is the appropriate course of action in this patient?**

Mitral valve reconstruction and repair of the papillary muscle.

○ **What is the classic triad of symptoms of aortic stenosis?**

Syncope (often exertional), angina, and heart failure.

○ **What is the most common cause of aortic stenosis in patients younger than 65 years?**

Calcification of congenitally bicuspid aortic valves (50%) followed by rheumatic heart disease (25%).

○ **What is the most common cause of aortic stenosis in patients older than 65 years?**

Calcific degeneration of the aortic leaflets.

○ **Once patients with aortic stenosis become symptomatic, what is their average survival without valve replacement?**

From the onset of syncope and/or angina, the mean survival is 2 to 3 years. From the onset of congestive heart failure, the mean survival is 1.5 years.

○ **How does the heart murmur reflect the severity of aortic stenosis?**

The longer the duration of the murmur and the greater the increase in intensity of the murmur, the more severe the aortic stenosis. The degree of loudness of the murmur is not as important in assessing severity. As the severity of an AS murmur worsens the murmur will be louder at the base of the heart.

○ **What is the best pharmacologic agent for patients with asymptomatic aortic stenosis?**

Without contraindications, beta-blockers are the best agents as they are the most useful in treating left ventricular hypertrophy and its sequelae that develop as a result of aortic stenosis.

○ **A 68-year-old female patient with severe asymptomatic aortic stenosis suddenly complains of dyspnea and palpitations. On EKG, she is found to be in atrial fibrillation with a ventricular rate of 130 bpm. What is the most appropriate action to be taken?**

Immediate DC cardioversion followed by a search for previously unrecognized mitral valve disease. Once stabilized, the patient should be referred for cardiac catheterization and aortic valve replacement.

○ **What is a mitral valve prolapsed syndrome?**

A symptom complex consisting of palpitations, chest pain, easy fatigability, exercise intolerance, dyspnea, orthostatic phenomena, and syncope or presyncope in patients with mitral valve prolapsed, predominately related to autonomic dysfunction.

○ **What disorders are seen with increased frequency in patients with MVP syndrome?**

Graves disease, asthma, migraine headaches, sleep disorders, fibromyositis, and functional gastrointestinal syndromes.

○ **What is the most common cause of isolated severe aortic regurgitation?**

Aortic root dilatation resulting from medial disease. Other common causes include congenital (bicuspid) aortic valve, previous infective endocarditis, and rheumatic heart disease.

○ **What is the survival rate of chronic aortic regurgitation after diagnosis?**

The 5-year survival, after diagnosis, is 75%. The 10-year survival is 50%. Once symptoms begin, without surgical treatment, death occurs within 4 years after the development of angina, 2 years after the development of CHG.

○ **What is the preferred pharmacologic agent in patients with asymptomatic chronic aortic regurgitation?**

Nifedipine or ACE inhibitors. Both have major improvements in LVEF and major reduction in LV end-diastolic volume and mass with significantly lower incidence of the need for aortic valve replacement at 5 years.

○ **What is the most common cause of acute tricuspid regurgitation and what is the preferred management of this situation?**

Tricuspid valve endocarditis, often as a result of intravenous drug abuse. The preferred management is complete removal of the valve with immediate or eventual replacement of the valve. Antibiotic therapy usually is futile in preventing valve surgery.

○ **A 38-year-old female patient with known mitral valve prolapse is scheduled for dental cleaning. Her dentist calls for you asking recommendations for endocarditis prophylaxis. She is not allergic to penicillin. What are your recommendations?**

No antibiotic prophylaxis is necessary for patients with only the diagnosis of mitral valve prolapse. Antibiotic prophylaxis is recommended for those with prosthetic heart valves, history of infective endocarditis, and other specific congenital heart defects or congenital heart defect repairs utilizing prosthetic material.

○ **A 55-year-old man who underwent a 4-vessel CABG 3 years ago and has mild mitral and tricuspid regurgitation is scheduled for a colonoscopy for rectal bleeding. What recommendations regarding endocarditis prophylaxis would you give this surgeon?**

No antibiotic prophylaxis is needed in this setting.

○ **Which valve is most commonly injured during blunt trauma?**

The aortic valve.

○ **What is the abnormality seen in the M-mode echocardiogram shown in Figure 2-25?**

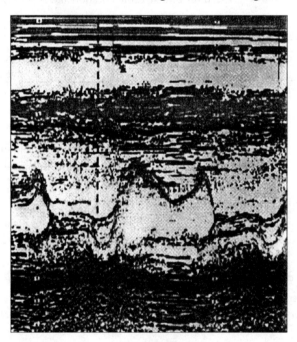

Figure 2-25

Prolapse of the posterior leaflet of the mitral valve.

OTHER HEART DISEASE AND CONDITIONS

○ **What are some adverse drug effects of lidocaine?**

Drowsiness, nausea, vertigo, confusion, ataxia, tinnitus, muscle twitching, respiratory depression, and psychosis.

○ **In CPR, what is the ventilation to compression ratio for one or two rescuers?**

One and two rescuers should perform 2 breaths to 30 compressions at a rate of 100 compressions per minute. (New guidelines emphasize compressions over ventilations during the first several minutes of a cardiac arrest.)

○ **What are the most common causes of myocarditis in the United States?**

Viruses. Other causes include post–viral myocarditis, an autoimmune response to recent viral infection, bacteria (diphtheria and tuberculosis), fungi, protozoa (Chagas disease), and spirochetes (Lyme disease).

○ **A 25-year-old patient presents with splinted breathing and sharp, precordial chest pain that radiates to the back. The pain increases with inspiration and is mildly relieved by placing the patient in a forward sitting position. What might the EKG show?**

The patient probably has pericarditis. The EKG may reveal intermittent supraventricular tachycardias, ST-segment depression in leads aVR and VI with ST segment elevation in all of the remaining leads. PR depression and T-wave inversion may also arise.

○ **What is the most common cause of pericarditis?**

Idiopathic. Viral pericarditis is a common cause and the most common infectious etiology. Other causes are myocardial infarction, post–viral syndrome, aortic dissection that has ruptured into the pericardium, malignancy, radiation, chest trauma, connective tissue disease, uremia, and drugs, that is, procainamide or hydralazine.

○ **What physical findings indicates acute pericarditis?**

Pericardial friction rub. The rub is heard best at the left sternal border or apex with the patient in a forward sitting position. Other findings include fever, tachycardia, and pleuritic chest pain.

○ **What will be the appearance of a pericardial effusion on an X-ray?**

A water bottle silhouette.

○ **What is the treatment for pericarditis without effusion?**

A 2-week treatment of 650-mg aspirin every 4 hours, if no contraindications exist. Ibuprofen, indomethacin, or colchicines are other alternatives. The use of corticosteroids is controversial because recurrent pericarditis is common as the dose is tapered.

○ **What is the 1-year recurrence rate for patients who have been resuscitated from sudden cardiac death?**

30%.

○ **Splinter hemorrhages, Osler nodes, Janeway lesions, petechiae, and Roth spots can be indications of what process?**

They are physical signs associated with infective endocarditis.

○   **True/False: Osler nodes are usually nodular and painful:**

True. In contrast, the macular Janeway lesions are painless.

○   **What percentage of patients with infective endocarditis display peripheral manifestations of the disease?**

50%.

○   **What is bacterial endocarditis?**

An infectious process where bloodborne bacteria that attach onto damaged or abnormal heart valves or on the endocardium near anatomical defects.

○   **How is bacterial endocarditis diagnosed?**

By evidence of valvular vegetations on echocardiogram combined with a positive blood culture. The Duke criteria is often utilized as a diagnostic tool for infectious endocarditis.

○   **Who is at high risk for developing endocarditis?**

People with prosthetic heart valves, persons with previous incidents of endocarditis, persons with complex congenital heart disease, intravenous drug user, and persons with surgically devised systemic pulmonary shunts.

○   **What are the risk factors for endocarditis?**

Risk factors include intravenous drug use, prosthetic valves, acquired valvular heart disease, hypertrophic cardiomyopathy, hemodialysis, peritoneal dialysis, indwelling venous catheters, post–cardiac surgery, rheumatic heart disease, and uncorrected congenital conditions. It is controversial as to whether mitral valve prolapsed with significant regurgitation is a moderate risk factor.

○   **What are the most common organisms associated with endocarditis?**

Streptococcus viridians, Staphylococcus aureus, Enterococcus, and fungal organisms. *S. aureus* is responsible for 75% of disease in IVDAs.

○   **What is more common in the general population: left-sided or right-sided endocarditis?**

Left-sided (aortic and mitral involvement).

○   **What is more common in intravenous drug abusers: left-sided or right-sided structural disease?**

Right-sided (60%) is most common.

○   **How is infective endocarditis treated?**

Intravenous antibiotics for 4 to 6 weeks. Close follow-up is necessary and the patient should have a series of two separate negative blood cultures to demonstrate resolution of the condition. If resolution of the infections does not occur promptly, embolization occurs, or fulminant CHF ensues and surgical valve replacement is indicated.

○   **What are the EKG changes associated with pericarditis?**

Concave upward ST elevation in at least seven leads except V1 and aVR. PR segment depression may also be present.

○ **What is the most frequently reported bacterial isolate in patients with myocardial abscesses?**

Staphylococcus aureus.

○ **What is the clinical picture of myocardial abscesses?**

Low-grade fevers, chills, leukocytosis, conduction system abnormalities, nonspecific EKG changes, and signs and symptoms of acute MI.

○ **What is mural endocarditis?**

Inflammation and disruption of the nonvalvular endocardial surface of the cardiac chambers.

○ **What are the risk factors for mural endocarditis?**

Usually, mural endocarditis is from seeding of an abnormal area of endocardium during bacteremia or fungemia. Infectious thrombi from pulmonary veins, ventricular aneurysms, mural thrombi, chordal friction lesions, pacemaker lead insertion sites, idiopathic hypertrophic subaortic stenosis, jet lesions from ventriculoseptal defects, and other congenital defects are other factors. Immunocompromised patients are also at increased risk.

○ **What is the clinical presentation of prosthetic vascular graft infection?**

Erythema, skin breakdown, or purulent drainage. Other symptoms may be thrombosis of the graft, fluid around the graft, or pseudoaneurysm formation.

○ **What are the complications from arterial catheterization?**

Thrombosis (19%–38%), infection (4%–23%), pseudoaneurysm, and rupture.

○ **How many deaths per year in the United States are caused by cardiovascular disease?**

864,480 in 2005 or 35.3% of all deaths. CVD death rates have declined with a 26.4% drop between 1995 and 2005.

○ **A radial pulse on examination indicates a BP of at least what level?**

80 mm Hg.

○ **A femoral pulse on examination indicates a BP of at least what level?**

70 mm Hg.

○ **A carotid pulse on examination indicates a BP of at least what level?**

60 mm Hg.

REFERENCES

Crawford MH *Current Medical Diagnosis and Treatment: Cardiology.* 3rd ed. New York, NY: McGraw-Hill; 2009.

Fauci AS, Braunwald E, Kasper DL, et al., eds. *Harrison's Principles of Internal Medicine,* 17th ed. New York, NY: McGraw-Hill; 2008.
    http://www.accessmedicine.com

Fuster Valentin OR-W. *Hurst's The Heart.* 12th ed. New York, NY: McGraw-Hill; 2008.

McPhee SJ, Papadakis MA, eds. *Current Medical Diagnosis and Treatment 2009.* New York, NY: McGraw-Hill; 2009.

McPhee SJ, Ganong WF. *Pathophysiology of Disease: An Introduction to Clinical Medicine.* 5th ed. New York, NY: McGraw-Hill; 2006.

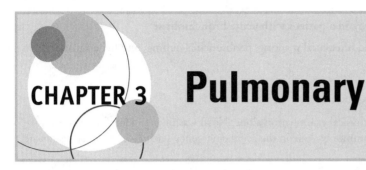

CHAPTER 3 Pulmonary

Daniel Thibodeau, MHP, PA-C, DFAAPA

INFECTIOUS DISORDERS

○ **What are the main symptoms of individuals with acute bronchitis?**

Persistent cough for more than 3 weeks, fever, and constitutional symptoms.

○ **What is the main causative agent of acute bronchitis?**

Viral pathogen. Most of the time, adenovirus, rhinovirus, and influenza are the agents. In some cases, *Haemophilus influenzae, Mycoplasma pneumoniae,* and *Chlamydophila* pneumoniae can be the causative agents.

○ **Name some diseases that can mimic acute bronchitis:**

Asthma and allergic bronchospasm can present with the same symptoms of acute bronchitis. Other causes can be congestive heart failure, bronchogenic tumors, and reflux esophagitis which can all present with respiratory symptoms similar to that of bronchitis.

○ **Is the use of antibiotics indicated for an acute case of bronchitis?**

No, it is usually a self-limiting illness.

○ **What are the treatment options for patients with acute bronchitis?**

Supportive care. If the patient presents with wheezing on examination, the use of albuterol is supported. If, however, the patient presents only with a cough, bronchodilators are not indicated. In some cases, mild analgesic agents can be of help for those with pain related to cough.

○ **What percentage of cigarette smokers develop chronic bronchitis?**

10% to 15%. Chronic bronchitis generally develops after 10 to 12 years of smoking.

○ **What are the signs and symptoms of patients with acute bronchiolitis?**

Fever, cough, rhinorrhea, wheezing, tachypnea, and respiratory distress.

○ **Describe the typical findings of a chest X-ray in a patient with acute bronchiolitis:**

They are nonspecific but can include increased interstitial marking, peribronchial cuffing, and hyperinflation, and in some cases segmental atelectasis.

○ **How do you confirm a case of bronchiolitis?**

Most cases can be diagnosed on history and physical examination alone. Nasal washings to look for respiratory syncytial virus (RSV) may be done and are commonly done in the acute emergency setting. Laboratory results are nonspecific and may show mild leukocytosis.

○ **Which is the most common type of pathogen in bronchiolitis?**

RSV. It generally affects children younger than 2 years. Bronchiolitis rarely develops in adults. Second most common pathogen is adenovirus.

○ **What is the treatment for severe RSV documented bronchiolitis?**

Ribavirin.

○ **A 24-year-old female patient has a high fever, hoarseness, and increased stridor of 3 hours duration. She also has a low fever and sore throat. Examination shows an ill-appearing woman with a temperature of 40°C, inspiratory stridor, drooling, and mild intercostal retractions. She prefers to sit up. What is the most likely diagnosis?**

Epiglottitis.

○ **What pathogen is responsible for most cases of epiglottitis?**

Group A Streptococcus. It is followed by *Streptococcus pneumoniae*, *Haemophilus parainfluenzae*, and *Staphlococcus aureus*. Usually, viruses are not the causative agents.

○ **What is the narrowest part of the adult airway?**

The glottic opening.

○ **What is the "thumb print sign"?**

It is a soft tissue inflammation of the epiglottis seen on a lateral X-ray of the neck. The epiglottis, normally long and thin, appears swollen and flat at the base of the hypopharynx in patients with epiglottitis.

○ **What is the treatment of choice for acute epiglottitis?**

Maintaining the airway is of paramount importance. If the airway is stable, treatment with a cephalosporin is indicated. Ampicillin/sulbactam is the preferred treatment for 7 to 10 days. Cefuroxime, cefotaxime, or ceftriaxone is appropriate for beta-lactam allergic patients.

○ **A 2-year-old child presents with wheezing, rhonchi, inspiratory stridor, and a sudden harsh cough similar to a barking seal, which worsens at night. What is the diagnosis?**

Croup, also known as laryngotracheitis. This condition is usually preceded by a URI and is frequently caused by the parainfluenza virus.

○ **What age group usually contracts croup?**

6 months to 3 years. Croup is characterized by cold symptoms; a sudden, barking cough; inspiratory and expiratory stridor; and a slight fever.

○ **What is the difference between the cough of croup and the cough of epiglottitis?**

Croup has a seal-like barking cough, while epiglottitis is accompanied by a minimal cough. Children with croup have a hoarse voice, while those with epiglottitis have a muffled voice.

○ **What is the most common pathogen that causes croup?**

Parainfluenza type virus. Other pathogens include influenza, RSV, adenovirus, and in some cases *Mycoplasma pneumoniae.*

○ **What is the "steeple sign"?**

Subglottic edema, which creates a symmetrically tapered configuration in the subglottic portion of the trachea when imaged in a frontal soft tissue X-ray of the neck. This is consistent with croup.

○ **A 3-year-old male child is woken in the middle of the night with a barking seal-like cough and signs and symptoms that are consistent with croup. On examination, the child's respirations are 35/min and oxygen saturation is 95% on room air. There is no evidence of stridor on examination and his lungs are clear. What is the recommended treatment for this patient?**

Supportive care, fluids, and observation at home. If oxygen saturation is down, oxygen therapy is indicated. In all cases, inhalable racemic epinephrine by nebulizer is warranted.

○ **What if the child presented with stridor on examination?**

Administer dexamethasone 0.6 mg/kg IM one-time dose along with all the other therapies mentioned above.

○ **A 34-year-old woman wakes up with a history of sudden onset of fever, body aches, malaise, chills, cough, and a sore throat. She reports that several other members at home have the same symptoms, as do some of her coworkers. On examination, her temperature is 101°F, pulse 100, respiratory rate 18, and BP 122/86. Her throat appears to be moist without any abnormalities, lungs are clear, and the rest of the examination is unremarkable. What is the most probable cause of this illness?**

Influenza.

○ **Which strain of influenza is considered to cause more pandemic outbreaks?**

Influenza A.

○ **Which syndrome can be caused by an outbreak of influenza B virus?**

Reyes syndrome.

○ **What is the main method of transmission for the influenza virus?**

It spreads via aerosol by cough and sneeze and via hand-to-hand contact.

○ **What is the most common type of pneumonia seen in influenza patients?**

Viral. A secondary bacterial pneumonia can be caused by *Streptococcus pneumoniae, Staphylococcus aureus,* and *Haemophilus influenzae.*

○ **What method is used to detect a positive influenza illness?**

Throat, nasopharyngeal, or sputum samples with a rapid influenza A or B test. The rapid nasal test is the more commonly used and more accurate of the three.

○ **What is the treatment of choice for a patient with influenza B virus?**

Oseltamivir orally or Zanamivir inhaled. However, these medications must be started within 24 to 36 hours of onset of the illness for them to be effective.

○ **Name some other therapies that are helpful in symptomatic relief of an influenza illness:**

Supportive care with fluids, analgesics such as acetaminophen for body aches, myalgias, and fever. A cough suppressant with or without codeine may be helpful also.

○ **Which patients should be vaccinated with the influenza vaccine?**

Children between the ages of 6 and 59 months, pregnant women (during flu season), children and adults with chronic disorders of the cardiovascular and pulmonary systems, nursing home and chronic care facility patients, any care workers who are at risk of exposure, and health care workers.

○ **What age group is usually afflicted by pertussis?**

Infants younger than 2 years of age.

○ **What are some of the hallmark symptoms of a patient with pertussis?**

Initially, the patient has the same types of symptoms as in common cold. Within 1 to 2 weeks of the illness progressing, the patient develops a cough that evolves into a paroxysmal phase with more frequent and spasmodic bursts of 5 to 10 at a time. This can also have the sound of a terminal audible whoop. Post-tussive vomiting may also occur.

○ **What is the main pathway for infection leading to pneumonia?**

Aspiration via the oropharynx.

○ **Describe the different presentations of bacterial and viral pneumonia:**

• Bacterial pneumonia is typified by a sudden onset of symptoms, including pleurisy, fever, chills, productive cough, tachypnea, and tachycardia. The most common bacterial pneumonia is pneumococcal pneumonia.
• Viral pneumonia is characterized by the gradual onset of symptoms, no pleurisy, chills or high fever, general malaise, and a nonproductive cough.

○ **What is the leading identifiable cause of acute community-acquired pneumonia in adults?**

Streptococcus pneumoniae.

○ **Name the risk factors for community-acquired pneumonia:**

Alcoholism, asthma, immunosuppression, ≥70 years of age.

○ **Name the risk factors for pneumococcal pneumonia:**

Dementia, seizure disorder, alcoholism, smoking, COPD, and HIV.

○ **A young infant patient who you suspect has pneumonia is ordered to have a chest X-ray performed. When you view the results, you note the presence of pneumatoceles on the film. What pathogen is likely responsible for this type of finding?**

Staphylococcus aureus.

○ **A 24-year-old male patient has had fevers, chills, and a productive cough with dark green sputum for the last week. On physical examination, his temperature is 101.3°F, P 90, R 22, and BP 124/85. There is coryza with moist mucous membranes and a regular rhythm on cardiac examination. Lung sounds reveal an area of crackles with a mild expiratory wheeze at the right lower base of the lung fields. Based on this history and physical examination, what is the treatment of choice for this patient?**

A macrolide antibiotic (clarithromycin or azithromycin) for the treatment of community-acquired pneumonia.

○ **If this patient required inpatient treatment of pneumonia but without ICU admission, what is the class of antibiotics that would be indicated? What if the patient needed to be in the ICU?**

Fluoroquinolone for non-ICU patients (moxifloxacin, levofloxacin, and gemifloxacin). For ICU patients, ceftriaxone, ampicillin-sulbactam, **plus** azithromycin or fluoroquinolone.

○ **What are some of the more common complications associated with community-acquired pneumonia?**

Respiratory failure, shock, worsening of comorbid diseases, especially metastatic infection, lung abscess, and complicated pleural effusion.

○ **Which bacterial pneumonias frequently cause frank hemoptysis?**

Pseudomonas aeruginosa, Klebsiella pneumoniae, and *Staphylococcus aureus.*

○ **What bacteria are associated with pneumonia following influenza?**

Streptococcus pneumoniae, Staphylococcus pneumoniae, and *Haemophilus influenzae.*

○ **What two underlying medical conditions are associated with *Haemophilus influenzae* pneumonia?**

Chronic obstructive lung disease and HIV infection.

○ **What is the most common etiologic agent of atypical pneumonia?**

Mycoplasma pneumoniae.

○ **What are the typical findings seen on chest X-ray for a *Mycoplasma pneumoniae* pneumonia?**

The typical pattern consists of peribronchial pneumonia with thickened bronchial markings, streaks of interstitial infiltration, and areas of subsegmental atelectasis.

○ **What is considered to be the second most common cause of atypical pneumonia?**

Chlamydia pneumoniae.

○ **Of the following organisms, which is commonly spread by person-to-person contact: *Legionella pneumoniae* or *Mycoplasma pneumoniae*?**

Mycoplasma pneumoniae.

○ **What three X-ray findings are associated with a poor outcome in patients with pneumonia?**

Multilobar involvement, a cavitary lesion, and pleural effusions.

○ **What is the most common cause of pneumonia in children?**

Viral pneumonia. Infecting viruses include influenza, parainfluenza, RSV, and adenoviruses.

○ **Match the pneumonia with the treatment:**

1. *Klebsiella pneumoniae*   a. **Erythromycin, tetracycline, or doxycycline**
2. *Streptococcal pneumoniae*   b. **Penicillin G**
3. *Legionella pneumophila*   c. **Cefuroxime and clarithromycin**
4. *Haemophilus influenzae*   d. **Erythromycin and rifampin**
5. *Mycoplasma pneumoniae*

1. (1) c, (2) b, (3) d, (4) c, and (5) a.

○ **Empyema is most often caused by what organism?**

Staphylococcus aureus, and in most cases methicillin-resistant *S. aureus* (MRSA). Gram-negative organisms and anaerobic bacteria may also cause empyema.

○ **What is the chest X-ray finding that suggests a right middle lobe pneumonia?**

Loss of the right heart border.

○ **What is the chest X-ray finding of a patient with a left upper lobe consolidation?**

Infiltrate seen on the AP to the lower lung field without obstruction of the diaphragm, with confirmation on the lateral film.

○ **What are the most common causes of staphylococcal pneumonias?**

Drug use and endocarditis. This pneumonia produces high fever, chills, and a purulent productive cough.

○ **What are the extrapulmonary manifestations of mycoplasma?**

Erythema multiforme, pericarditis, and CNS disease.

○ **What is the most frequent etiology of nosocomial pneumonia?**

Pseudomonas aeruginosa. There is a high mortality associated with pneumonia caused by *Pseudomonas.* It most frequently occurs in immunocompromised patients or patients on mechanical ventilation.

○ **A 67-year-old alcoholic man was found in an alley, covered in his own vomit and beer. Upon examination, he is shaking, has a fever of 103.5°F and is coughing up currant jelly sputum. What is the diagnosis?**

Pneumonia induced by *Klebsiella pneumoniae.* This is the most probable etiology in alcoholics, the elderly, the very young, and the immunocompromised patients. Other gram-negative bacteria, such as *Escherichia coli* and other Enterobacteriaceae, may cause pneumonia in alcoholic patients who have aspirated.

○ **Describe the classic chest X-ray finding associated with *Legionella* pneumonia:**

Dense consolidation and bulging fissures. Expect elevated liver enzymes and hypophosphatemia. The patient with *Legionella* pneumonia classically presents with a relative bradycardia.

○ **A 43-year-old man presents with pleurisy, sudden onset of fever and chills, and rust-colored sputum. What is the probable diagnosis?**

Pneumococcal pneumonia caused by *Streptococcus pneumoniae;* it is the most common community-acquired pneumonia. It is a consolidating lobar pneumonia and can be treated with penicillin G or erythromycin.

○ **A 20-year-old college student is home for winter break and presents complaining of a 10-day history of a nonproductive dry hacking cough, malaise, a mild fever, and no chills. What is a probable diagnosis?**

Mycoplasma pneumoniae, also known as walking pneumonia. Although this is the most common pneumonia that develops in teenagers and young adults, it is an atypical pneumonia and most frequently occurs in close contact populations, that is, schools and military barracks.

○ **A 56-year-old smoker with COPD presents with chills, fever, green sputum, and extreme shortness of breath. An X-ray shows a right lower lobe pneumonia. What is expected from the sputum culture?**

Haemophilus influenzae. This organism is generally found in pneumonia and bronchitis patients with underlying COPD. The next most common organism detected in this patient population is *Moraxella catarrhalis.*

Ampicillin/clavulanate (Augmentin) is the drug of choice, but patients at high risk should have yearly influenza vaccinations.

○ **If a patient has a patchy infiltrate on a chest X-ray and bullous myringitis, what antibiotic should be prescribed?**

Erythromycin which is the typical treatment for mycoplasma.

○ **In what season does *Legionella* pneumonia most commonly occur?**

Summer. *Legionella pneumophila* thrives in environments such as the water-cooling towers that are used in large buildings and hotels. Staphylococcal pneumonias also occur more frequently in summer.

○ **An older patient with GI symptoms, hyponatremia, and a relative bradycardia probably has which type of pneumonia?**

Legionella.

○ **What is the most common cause of pneumonia in sickle cell disease?**

Streptococcus pneumoniae.

○ **Which type of pneumonia is often associated with cold agglutinins?**

Mycoplasma pneumoniae.

○ **Name four antibiotics known to have in vitro activity against anaerobic bacteria in virtually all cases:**

1. Metronidazole
2. Chloramphenicol
3. Imipenem
4. Beta-lactam/beta-lactamase inhibitors

O   **What is the drug of choice for pneumonias acquired in the outpatient setting caused by anaerobic bacteria?**

Clindamycin.

O   **What is the recommended duration of antibiotic therapy for necrotizing anaerobic pneumonia, lung abscess, or empyema?**

4 to 8 weeks.

O   **Which anaerobic respiratory infection is associated with slowly enlarging pulmonary infiltrates, pleural effusions, rib destruction, and fistula formation?**

Actinomycosis.

O   **What proportion of the patients with pneumonia develop pleural effusions?**

40%.

O   **What is the definition of nosocomial pneumonia?**

Pneumonia occurring in patients who have been hospitalized for at least 72 hours.

O   **What are the two most important routes of transmission of nosocomial bacterial pneumonia?**

Person-to-person transmission via health care workers and contaminated ventilator tubing.

O   **Which type of bacterial pneumonia commonly occurs secondary to viral illness?**

Staphylococcal infection.

O   **What two types of pneumonia are often contracted during the summer months?**

Staphylococcal and *Legionella* pneumonia.

O   **Describe the chest X-ray image of *Legionella* pneumonia:**

Dense consolidation and bulging fissures. Expect elevated liver enzymes and hypophosphatemia. Relative bradycardia is evident upon physical examination.

O   **What are the potential, often rare, complications of Mycoplasma pneumonia?**

- Nonpulmonary: Hemolytic anemia, aseptic meningitis, encephalitis, Guillain–Barré syndrome, pericarditis, and myocarditis.
- Pulmonary: ARDS, atelectasis, mediastinal adenopathy, pneumothorax, pleural effusion, and abscess.

O   **Describe a patient with chlamydial pneumonia:**

Chlamydial pneumonia is usually seen in infants 2 to 6 weeks of age. The patient is afebrile and does not appear toxic.

O   **In which type of patients is staphylococcal pneumonia likely?**

Patients who are hospitalized, debilitated, or abusing drugs.

○ **What pathogen is suggested by pneumonia with a single rigor?**

Pneumococcus.

○ **Where is the most common site of aspiration pneumonitis?**

Right lower lobe.

○ **A patient with currant jelly sputum is likely to have which type of pneumonia?**

Klebsiella or type 3 pneumococcus.

○ **What conditions should staphylococcal pneumonia be considered as a possible diagnosis?**

Although staphylococcal pneumonia accounts for only 1% of bacterial pneumonias, it should be considered in patients with sudden chills, hectic fever, pleurisy, and cough (especially following a viral illness, such as measles or influenza).

○ **Where does aspiration generally occur as revealed by chest X-ray?**

The lower lobe of the right lung. This is the most direct path for foreign bodies into the lung.

○ **What three findings should be present to consider a sputum sample adequate?**

1. >25 PMNs

2. <10 squamous epithelial cells per low-powered field

3. A predominant bacterial organism

○ **What degree of leukocytosis is considered a risk factor for poor outcome among patients with bacterial pneumonia?**

Greater than 30,000 cells/mm^3.

○ **At what age should the pneumococcal vaccine be administered to healthy adults with no comorbid conditions?**

Age 65 or older.

○ **A patient has a staccato cough and a history of conjunctivitis in the first few weeks after birth. What is the most likely type of pneumonia would this patient have?**

Chlamydial pneumonia.

○ **What are the two most common ventilator associated pneumonias?**

Pseudomonas aeruginosa and MRSA.

○ **What percentage of people in the Ohio and the Mississippi valleys are infected with histoplasmosis?**

100% in endemic areas. However, only 1% of these individuals develop the active disease. The spores of *Histoplasma capsulatum* can remain active for 10 years. For unknown reasons, bird and bat feces promote the growth of the actual fungus. The disease is transmitted when the spores are released and inhaled.

○ **How is the diagnosis of histoplasmosis made?**

By bronchoalveolar lavage or by tissue biopsy and blood cultures.

○ **What does the chest X-ray of a patient with histoplasmosis look like?**

Interstitial pneumonitis, patchy alveolar infiltrates, and mediastinal adenopathy may be present.

○ **What is the treatment of choice for a histoplasmosis pneumonia?**

Itraconazole for 6 to 12 weeks duration.

○ **Where in the United States is coccidioidomycosis most prevalent?**

The southwest. In most mild to moderate cases the infection will resolve with just supportive care. If severe, treat the afflicted patient with amphotericin B.

○ **A 46-year-old man with a history of HIV has been diagnosed with coccidioidomycosis pneumonia. His examination and vital signs are stable. What is the initial treatment plan for this patient?**

Most of these immunocompromised patients do not require specific therapy. Close follow-up and monitoring of symptoms are enough to ensure that the illness is resolving. In most mild to moderate cases the infection will resolve with just supportive care. If severe, treat the afflicted patient with amphotericin B.

○ **Which type of fungal pneumonia seen in immunocompromised patients, is highly invasive into the lung parenchyma?**

Aspergillosis.

○ **What is characteristic of the chest X-ray of aspergillosis pneumonia?**

Usually a bilateral upper lobe infiltrate. In some cases, a fungal ball with a cavitary lesion can be seen on CT scan.

○ **What is the primary treatment for aspergillosis pneumonia?**

Itraconazole.

○ **What is the best method for detecting adenovirus pneumonia?**

Detecting adenovirus pneumonia is difficult because it appears quite similar to CAP; but if suspected, the PCR from respiratory secretions, blood, urine, and solid tissues is used.

○ **What is the mortality rate of adenovirus pneumonia?**

Around 30%, and up to 50% in immunocompromised patients.

○ **How does a human get infected and develop pneumonia by the hantavirus?**

This is by rodent-to-human contact or by cleaning up after a rodent. The virus enters via the respiratory epithelium.

○ **Hantavirus occurs most commonly in what geographic location?**

Southwestern United States, especially in areas with deer mice.

○ **Name the antiviral medications that are used for viral pneumonia:**

Amantadine and Flumadine for influenza A, and ribavirin for RSV, adenovirus, and hantavirus pneumonia. Oseltamivir and Zanamivir can both be used for influenza A and B pneumonia.

○ **A 67-year-old female patient presents with a 4-day history of fevers, malaise, cough, and a generalized vesicular rash that started on the scalp and then spread to arms and legs. The cough and respiratory symptoms have been correlating to the rash on the legs in timing. The chest X-ray reveals patchy diffuse infiltrates and there is also a small right pleural effusion. What is the etiology of this illness?**

Varicella pneumonia. This type of pneumonia can also be at risk for immunocompromised, pregnant, and postpartum patients.

○ **What is the treatment for varicella pneumonia?**

Acyclovir for 7 to 10 days.

○ **What secondary bacterial infection often occurs following a viral pneumonia?**

Staphylococcal pneumonia.

○ **What is the pathogen that is responsible for HIV-/AIDS-related pneumonia?**

Pneumocystis jirovecii.

○ **What is the difference between PCP pneumonia and *Pneumocystis jirovecii* pneumonia?**

PCP is transmitted through animal contact and does not transmit to humans. *P. jirovecii* is the human form.

○ **Name five HIV-related pulmonary infections:**

PCP, TB, histoplasmosis, Cryptococcus, and CMV.

○ **Describe the chest X-ray of a patient with PCP:**

A reticular or miliary pattern ranging from fine to course, ill-defined patchy areas, and segmental and subsegmental consolidation; 5% to 10% of PCP pneumonias will have a normal chest X-ray. In some instances you will note a "bat wing" appearance on X-ray.

○ **What laboratory tests aid in the diagnosis of PCP?**

A rising LDH or an LDH > 450 and an ESR > 50. A low albumin implies a poor prognosis.

○ **The initial therapy for PCP includes what antibiotic?**

Trimethoprim-sulfamethoxazole.

○ **What other medication should be prescribed to a patient with PCP?**

Corticosteroids when the P_{O_2} is <70 mm Hg or an oxygen saturation of <90%.

○ **What two drugs are used as prophylactic treatment to prevent PCP in HIV patients?**

Aerosolized pentamidine or trimethoprim/sulfamethoxazole.

○ **What is the most common cause of community-acquired bacterial pneumonia among patients infected with HIV?**

Streptococcus pneumoniae.

○ **What is the recurrence rate of PCP for those patients who do not receive prophylaxis?**

30%.

○ **What is the typical time of year that RSV has an outbreak?**

During late winter and early spring.

○ **What are the usual cases that present with an RSV infection?**

Pneumonia, tracheobronchitis, and bronchiolitis.

○ **What are some of the common presenting symptoms of RSV?**

Fever (low grade), tachypnea, and wheezing are all signs. Apnea is a common symptom. In children, RSV can also cause acute and recurrent otitis media.

○ **What is the treatment of an RSV illness?**

Supportive care, which includes hydration, humidified air, and fever reduction with acetaminophen. In very serious cases, ribavirin can be used.

○ **What are the classic signs and symptoms of TB?**

Night sweats, fever, weight loss, malaise, cough, and greenish yellow sputum most commonly observed in the mornings.

○ **What are the three stages of TB infections?**

Primary, active, and latent.

○ **What is the most common complaint of individuals with TB?**

Cough.

○ **What is the main transmission of TB to humans?**

Airborne spread through respiratory droplets that are infected with tuberculosis.

○ **Which population is at greatest risk for tuberculosis?**

Patients who have had recent infections, fibrotic lesions, and comorbidities such as HIV, silicosis, chronic renal failure, diabetes, IV drug use, immunosuppressive therapy, and gastrectomy, as well as post-transplantation patients.

○ **What age group is most affected by the tuberculosis mycobacterium? And what gender?**

Age group: 25 to 34 years; women more than men. As the age becomes older, the gender changes to men. The reasons are unknown.

○ **What do chest X-rays reveal in cases of tuberculosis?**

Cavitation of the right upper lobe. Lower lung infiltrates, hilar adenopathy, atelectasis, and pleural effusion are also common.

○ **What is a Ghon lesion?**

It is a spontaneously healed TB lesion and presents on chest X-ray as a small calcified lesion.

○ **What is the range of time that results in an immune response to occur?**

2 to 10 weeks.

○ **A positive TB test is which type of reaction?**

Type 4. Cells are mediated, hypersensitivity is delayed, and neither complements nor antibodies are involved.

○ **What laboratory test is used to detect TB microscopically?**

Acid-fast bacillus smear.

○ **What is the best method to yield a positive TB samples?**

Needle biopsy, pleural fluid analysis, and needle biopsy of the pleura together gives a 90% diagnosis rate. Individually, each test alone produces a much lower yield.

○ **Right upper lobe cavitation with parenchymal involvement is a classic indicator for what?**

TB. Lower lung infiltrates, hilar adenopathy, atelectasis, and pleural effusion are also common.

○ **Does latent TB transmit to other humans?**

No, and the disease is not active.

○ **Name the first-line treatment drugs for TB in patients who are HIV negative:**

Isoniazid, rifampin, pyrazinamide, and ethambutol for 2 months daily. After the initial 2-month regimen, INH and rifampin can be continued for 4 months.

○ **What is the treatment for HIV-positive patients with TB?**

Similar to the non-HIV class with exception to adding an additional 6 months of treatment for a total of 12 months. Resistance to isoniazid will cause a longer treatment plan with the other primary medications.

○ **What are the side effects of INH?**

Neuropathy, pyridoxine loss, lupus-like syndrome, anion-gap acidosis, and hepatitis.

○ **What percentage of tuberculosis cases are drug resistant?**

About 15%. The rate is highly dependent upon geographic location.

○ **Name some common extrapulmonary TB sites:**

The lymph nodes, bone, GI tract, GU tract, meninges, liver, and the pericardium.

○ **True/False: Patients younger than 35 years of age with positive TB skin tests should undergo at least 6 months of isoniazid chemoprophylaxis:**

True.

○ **What are the typical roentgenographic features of a tuberculous pleural effusion?**

They are usually unilateral, small to moderate, and more commonly on the right side. Two-thirds of these can be associated with coexisting parenchymal disease (which may not be apparent on chest radiograph). They are commonly associated with primary disease. The incidence of loculations may be up to 30%.

○ **Is the tuberculin skin test a reliable test for active TB?**

No. It has a low sensitivity and specificity to detect active or latent disease.

○ **In whivch patients should you reserve caution in prescribing INH, rifampin?**

Patients with renal failure or a patient who has the possibility of renal compromise.

○ **What is the relapse rate for TB?**

It is less than 5%; the main cause for this is noncompliance.

○ **Hoarseness can herald far greater problems than viral laryngitis. At what point is a more thorough work-up indicated?**

A work-up indicated if hoarseness persists for greater than 6 to 8 weeks or is accompanied by a mass, chest pain, weight loss, aspiration dyspnea, or any other signs of malignancy. Be suspicious of smokers with chronic cough or hoarseness if there is a change in either.

○ **What percent of upper respiratory infectious agents are nonbacterial?**

Nonbacterial agents account for more than 90% of pharyngitis, laryngitis, tracheal bronchitis, and bronchitis.

○ **In treating a patient with a common cold, you prescribe an oral decongestant. Is it necessary to also suggest an antitussant?**

No. Most coughs, arising from a common cold, are caused by the irritation of the tracheobronchial receptors in the posterior pharynx as a result of postnasal drip. Postnasal drip can be relieved with decongestant therapy, thus eliminating the need for cough suppressant therapy.

○ **What are the most common etiologies of a chronic cough?**

Postnasal drip (40%), asthma (25%), and gastroesophageal reflux (20%). Other etiologies include bronchitis, bronchiectasis, bronchogenic carcinoma, esophageal diverticula, sarcoidosis, viruses, and drugs.

○ **What age group is afflicted with the most colds per year?**

Kindergartners win the top billing with an average of 12 colds/year. Second place goes to preschoolers with 6 to 10 colds/year. School children contract an average of 7 colds/year. Adolescents and adults average only 2 to 4 colds/year.

○ **What is the duration of a common cold?**

3 to 10 days (self-limited).

○   **What antibiotic is the most effective for treating uncomplicated lung abscesses?**
Clindamycin.

○   **True/False: Flora of lung abscesses are usually polymicrobial:**
True.

○   **Which gram-negative aerobes are known to cause lung abscess?**
Pseudomonas and *Klebsiella.*

○   **What are the two major risk factors for the development of anaerobic lung infection?**
Periodontal disease and predisposition to aspiration.

○   **Empyema in the absence of parenchymal lung infiltrate suggests what underlying process?**
Subphrenic or other intra-abdominal abscess.

○   **What are the two most important risk factors for the development of anaerobic lung abscess?**
Poor oral hygiene and a predisposition toward aspiration.

○   **What organisms are most commonly present in a pulmonary abscess?**
Mixed anaerobes.

○   **Which general group of bacteria is most commonly found in lung abscesses?**
Anaerobic bacteria.

○   **How do retropharyngeal abscesses arise?**
Lymphatic spread of infections in the nasopharynx, oropharynx, or external auditory canal.

NEOPLASTIC DISEASE

○   **What is the most common cancer in the United States?**
Lung cancer, which accounts for 29% of all cancer deaths.

○   **What is the average age range for a patient with lung cancer?**
55 to 65 years.

○   **What are some of the symptoms that are present in patients with lung cancer?**
Cough, hemoptysis, wheeze and stridor, dyspnea, and postobstructive pneumonitis (fever and productive cough) are a few complaints.

○   **Which form of lung cancer is the most common?**
Adenocarcinoma followed by squamous cell, then small cell (oat cell) carcinoma.

○ **What percentage of effusions are associated with malignancy?**

25%. These are all exudative effusions.

○ **What routine program is recommended for screening lung cancer in the adult population?**

None. Screening programs for lung cancer have not demonstrated a decrease in morbidity or mortality. Practitioners must be aware of the signs and symptoms associated with lung cancer, including chronic nonproductive cough, increased sputum production, hemoptysis, dyspnea, recurrent pneumonia, hoarseness, pleurisy, weight loss, shoulder pain, SVC syndrome, exercise fatigue, and anemia. Incidental findings on a chest X-ray should also be investigated.

○ **Where do the following cancers most commonly develop within the lung: adenocarcinoma and large cell carcinomas and squamous and small cell carcinomas?**

Adenocarcinoma and large cell carcinomas are usually located peripherally, whereas squamous and small cell carcinomas are located centrally. These four malignancies account for 88% of all lung cancers.

○ **What type of lung cancer is commonly associated with hypercalcemia?**

Squamous cell carcinoma. The production of parathormone-related peptide can produce hypercalcemia even without bony metastases.

○ **What type of lung tumors can cause excessive ACTH production and Cushing syndrome?**

Small cell carcinoma and carcinoid tumors.

○ **Second-hand cigarette smoke exposure is a risk factor for the development of what two major lung diseases?**

Lung cancer and COPD.

○ **The incidence of lung cancer is increasing in the United States among members of which gender?**

Women.

○ **What percentage of lung cancers are a result of smoking, either active or former smokers?**

85%.

○ **What is the relative risk for first-degree family members getting lung cancer?**

Two- to three-fold risk.

○ **What accounts for this increase?**

Increased cigarette smoking prevalence.

○ **Which vitamin has been associated with a protective effect against the development of lung cancer?**

Vitamin A.

○ **Bilateral periostitis, typically affecting the long bones and associated with lung cancer, is known as what other disease?**

Hypertrophic osteoarthropathy (HPO).

○ **What myopathic syndrome is associated with lung cancer?**
Eaton–Lambert syndrome.

○ **What is the initial diagnostic test in a clinically stable patient suspected of having lung cancer?**
Sputum cytologic examination.

○ **What is the 5-year survival of all patients diagnosed with primary lung cancer?**
~15%.

○ **Which primary lung cancer is most likely to cavitate?**
Squamous cell carcinoma.

○ **Which lung cancer is the most prevalent in nonsmoking women?**
Adenocarcinoma.

○ **What percentages of patients that have lung cancer are asymptomatic?**
5% to 15%.

○ **The increase in death rate from lung cancer among smokers, as opposed to nonsmokers, is how high?**
8- to 20-fold.

○ **Do low tar cigarettes decrease the risk of lung cancer?**
No.

○ **The risk of lung cancer following smoking cessation approaches that of lifelong nonsmokers after how many years?**
15.

○ **The incidence of lung cancer among urban residents is how many times higher than among rural residents?**
About 1.5 times higher among urban residents.

○ **The most common malignancy associated with asbestos exposure is which of the following: esophageal carcinoma, primary lung cancer, mesothelioma, or gastric carcinoma?**
Primary lung cancer.

○ **What is the incidence of pleural effusion associated with malignancy?**
Malignant pleural effusions are the second most common exudative effusions after parapneumonic effusions. The most common malignancies are lung and breast cancer.

○ **What are the conditions associated with malignant transudative effusions?**
Lymphatic obstruction, endobronchial obstruction, and hypoalbuminemia caused by the primary malignancy.

○ **What type of effusions are suggestive of malignancy?**

Massive effusions, large effusions without contralateral mediastinal shift, or bilateral effusions with normal heart size suggest malignancy.

○ **What percentage of lung cancer is related to smoking?**

80%.

○ **What other exposures are also factors contributing to the development of bronchogenic carcinoma?**

Radon, uranium, nickel, arsenic, bis (chloromethyl) ether, ionizing radiation, vinyl chloride, mustard gas, polycyclic aromatic hydrocarbons, and chromium.

○ **What is the major indication for laser bronchoscopy in the treatment of bronchogenic carcinoma?**

Tumor obstruction of large airways.

○ **What is Pancoast syndrome?**

Tumor of the apex of the lung that gives rise to Horner syndrome and shoulder pain. The tumor invades the bronchial plexus.

○ **Which primary lung cancer is most frequently associated with paraneoplastic syndromes?**

Small cell undifferentiated carcinoma.

○ **What finding indicates emergent radiation therapy for superior vena cava syndrome?**

Cerebral edema.

○ **The best 5-year survival for non–small cell carcinoma of the lung is achieved by what therapy modality?**

Surgical resection.

○ **Are carcinoid tumors related to smoking?**

No.

○ **What are the clinical features of carcinoid syndrome?**

Flushing and diarrhea is the most common. Other symptoms include salivation, lacrimation, diaphoresis, diarrhea, and hypotension.

○ **What is the treatment for a nonmetastatic carcinoid tumor?**

Surgery is the only option and may improve the symptoms.

○ **What cancers generally metastasize to the lungs?**

Breast, colon, prostate, and cervical cancers.

○ **What is the description of a solitary pulmonary nodule?**

It is defined as a density that is sharply marginated and surrounded by lung tissue that ranges in size on average of 1 to 6 cm in size.

○ **What percentage of pulmonary nodules is malignant?**
35%.

○ **Radiographic stability for what period is assumed to indicate benign origin of a solitary pulmonary nodule?**
2 years.

○ **A 27-year-old female nonsmoker is found to have a 2-cm nodule found on a chest X-ray during a preoperative screening film. The patient is asymptomatic and is otherwise healthy. What is the standard of care in monitoring this nodule?**
For patients younger than 35 years of age, 3-month serial CT scans of the chest for 1 year are required. If the patient is older than 35 years of age and is a smoker, an immediate evaluation of the tissue is required.

○ **A solitary pulmonary nodule in an HIV-infected patient may represent which of the following: PCP, histoplasmosis, cryptococcosis, or bronchogenic carcinoma?**
All of the above.

OBSTRUCTIVE PULMONARY DISEASE

○ **What is the peak age of asthma?**
3 years of age.

○ **What is the gender ratio of asthmatic patients in childhood and adults?**
There is a 2:1 male-to-female ratio in childhood, but evens in numbers in adult populations.

○ **What are some categories of risk factors for those with asthma and what are some of those factors?**
There are three categories:
- **Endogenous:** Gender, atopy, hyperresponsiveness, and genetic predisposition.
- **Triggers:** Allergens, URI viral infections, exercise, cold air, beta-blockers, aspirin, stress, and irritants.
- **Environmental:** Indoor/outdoor allergens, occupational, passive smoking, and respiratory infections.

○ **What blood cell is known to cause the initial inflammatory changes that result in asthma?**
Mast cells.

○ **Which blood cell is proliferated during an allergen response?**
Eosinophils.

○ **What extrinsic allergens most commonly affect asthmatic children?**
Dust and dust mites.

○ **What are the common symptoms that present in asthma?**
Cough, shortness of breath, pain between the scapula, itching under the chin (sometimes), and a nonproductive cough especially in children (aka variant asthma cough).

○ **What is the "best" pulmonary function test for the diagnosis of asthma?**

FEV1/FVC. This test determines the amount of air exhaled in 1 minute compared to the total amount of air in the lung that can be expressed. A ratio under 80% is diagnostic of asthma. Peak flow monitors are helpful in monitoring asthma at home or during an acute exacerbation.

○ **Is wheezing an integral part of asthma?**

No; 33% of children with asthma will only have cough variant asthma with no wheezing.

○ **What X-ray markings may be observed in a patient with a long history of bronchial asthma?**

Increased bronchial wall markings and flattening of the diaphragm. The bronchial wall markings are caused by epithelial inflammation and thickening of the bronchial walls.

○ **Patients with exercise-induced asthma will most likely trigger their asthma with what kind of exercise?**

High intensity exercise for more than 5 to 6 minutes.

○ **What is the first-line treatment for asthma?**

Use of beta-2-agonist bronchodilators, specifically albuterol in either metered dose inhaler (MDI) or nebulized.

○ **Are anticholinergics medications (i.e., ipratropium bromide) alone effective for the treatment of asthma?**

No. They are effective only with the use of albuterol as the first-line treatment and if the first-line treatment is not effective on its own.

○ **What is the clinical indication for the use of theophylline?**

It is indicated for use in patients with severe asthma who require additional bronchodilators.

○ **What are some of the common side effects of theophylline?**

Nausea, vomiting, and headaches.

○ **What is the most effective medication for reduction of inflammation in the treatment of asthma?**

Inhalable corticosteroids.

○ **Is there a need to administer a tapering dose of steroids?**

No. In cases of steroid regimens of 5 to 10 days duration, a tapering dose is not needed.

○ **Is the sole use of antileukotrienes effective for the suppression of asthma symptoms?**

No, they are useful in conjunction with inhalable corticosteroids but are not effective as a stand-alone treatment.

○ **At what point do you need to consider adding more therapy above the normal albuterol regimen so as to control asthma? What is the treatment of choice when you must administer an additional medication?**

When rescue inhaler is used three or more times in a week, and inclusion of inhalable corticosteroids will be the next medication added to the regimen.

○ **Which is more effective for relieving an acute exacerbation of bronchial asthma in a conscious patient: nebulized albuterol or albuterol MDI administered via an aerosol chamber?**

They are both equally effective.

○ **What are the positive effects of administering beta-agonists in the treatment of asthma?**

Relaxation of smooth muscle, inhibition of mast cells, inhibition of airway edema, increase in mucociliary clearance, increase mucus production, and decrease in cough.

○ **What are the chances that a child born to two asthmatic parents will also have asthma?**

Up to 50%.

○ **Are there any contraindications to administering a topical beta-2-blocker for glaucoma (i.e., timolol) to a patient with asthma?**

Yes, there is evidence that even a topical beta-blocking agent may exacerbate asthma symptoms.

○ **What treatment should be initiated for an acute asthmatic patient who does not improve with humidified O2, albuterol nebulizers, steroids, or anticholinergics?**

Subcutaneous epinephrine, 0.3 cm^3 administered every 5 minutes.

○ **Asthmatic patients will most likely have a family history of what?**

Asthma, allergies, or atopic dermatitis.

○ **What are the recommended therapeutic serum theophylline levels?**

10 to 15 mg/L.

○ **What medications should be avoided for an asthmatic patient who is pregnant?**

Epinephrine and parenteral beta-adrenergic agonists.

○ **A 23-year-old woman who has a history of asthma is 29 weeks pregnant. She is having an asthma attack and is receiving treatment in the emergency room with an albuterol nebulizer. Given this scenario, is this patient a candidate for oral or parenteral steroids?**

Yes. If steroids are indicated for this condition, then one should not hold back from giving them.

○ **What is a normal peak expiratory flow rate in adults?**

Men: 550 to 600 L/minute. Women: 450 to 500 L/minute. However, this varies somewhat with body size and age.

○ **Which beta-adrenergic receptors primarily control bronchiolar and arterial smooth muscle tone?**

beta-2-adrenergic receptors.

○ **Terbutaline is administered subcutaneously for asthma in what dose?**

0.01 mL/kg of 1 mg/mL terbutaline up to 0.25 mL, that is, 0.25 mg, which may be repeated once in 20 to 30 minutes.

○ **Is theophylline useful in the emergency management of a severely asthmatic pediatric patient?**

No. It has not been shown to affect further bronchodilatation in patients fully treated with beta-adrenergic agents. However, theophylline can be used successfully for inpatient management of asthma and may be started in the hospital.

○ **If corticosteroids are prescribed for acute asthma exacerbation, how should prednisone be dosed?**

1 to 2 mg/kg/day in two divided doses. Tapering is not necessary if the duration of therapy is 5 days or less.

○ **What is the appropriate parenteral dose of methylprednisolone (Solu-Medrol) to administer to a pediatric patient with status asthmaticus?**

1 to 2 mg/kg every 6 hours.

○ **Can beta-adrenergic agonists result in tolerance?**

Yes. Repeated administration of beta-agonist bronchodilators can result in hyposensitization of the receptors, but this should not preclude their use. Glucocorticoids have been shown to restore the depressed receptor responsiveness.

○ **True/False: Cardioselective beta-blockers avoid precipitation of bronchospasm in asthmatic individuals:**

False.

○ **What is the therapeutic drug of choice for beta-blocker–induced bronchospasm?**

Inhalable ipratropium bromide. If severe, parenteral glucagon can reverse effects.

○ **How do steroids function in the treatment of asthma?**

Steroids increase cAMP, decrease inflammation, and aid in restoring the function of beta-adrenergic responsiveness to adrenergic drugs.

○ **What is the most common cause of refractory asthma?**

Medical noncompliance.

○ **What is bronchiectasis?**

Bronchiectasis is an abnormal dilatation of the proximal medium-sized bronchi greater than 2 mm in diameter. It occurs because of the destruction of the muscular and elastic components of their walls and is usually associated with chronic bacterial infection and foul-smelling sputum.

○ **Which gender is more affected by bronchiectasis?**

Women.

○ **What are the symptoms of bronchiectasis?**

Chronic cough, purulent sputum, fever, weakness, weight loss, dyspnea in some patients, and hemoptysis. Hemoptysis is generally mild, originates from bronchial arteries, and is seen in 50% to 70% of all cases.

○ **What are the main causative agents of bronchiectasis?**

Adenovirus and influenza.

○ **What are the most common complications of bronchiectasis?**

Recurrent attacks of pneumonia, empyema, pneumothorax, and lung abscess.

○ **A chest X-ray shows honeycombing, atelectasis, and increased bronchial markings. What is the diagnosis?**

Bronchiectasis, an irreversible dilation of the bronchi that is generally associated with infection. Bronchography shows dilations of the bronchial tree, but this method of diagnosis is not recommended for routine use.

○ **Bronchiectasis occurs most frequently in patients with what conditions?**

Cystic fibrosis, immunodeficiencies, lung infections, or foreign-body aspirations.

○ **Which lung segments are most frequently involved in bronchiectasis?**

Posterior basal segments of the left or right lower lobes.

○ **What are the most common causes of upper lobe bronchiectasis?**

Tuberculous endobronchitis and allergic bronchopulmonary aspergillosis (ABPA).

○ **What is the mainstay of treatment of bronchiectasis?**

Antibiotics.

○ **What are the adjunctive treatment measures that may be beneficial in patients with bronchiectasis?**

Chest physiotherapy, nutritional support, inhalable indomethacin (shown to decrease bronchial hypersecretion by inhibiting neutrophil recruitment), bronchodilators, supplemental oxygen, immunoglobulin administration for immunoglobulin deficiency, replacement treatment for patients with alpha-1-anti-trypsin deficiency, and recombinant DNAase to reduce sputum viscosity in patients with cystic fibrosis (CF).

○ **What is the definition of chronic bronchitis?**

A productive cough for 3 months out of each year for 2 years straight.

○ **What is the definition of emphysema?**

Emphysema is a pathologic diagnosis of the destruction of terminal bronchioles with air trapping and enlargement of the air spaces. Coupled with chronic bronchitis, these two diseases make up COPD.

○ **What is the hallmark symptom of COPD?**

Exertional dyspnea.

○ **What is a "blue bloater"?**

An overweight patient with COPD, bronchitis, and central cyanosis. These individuals have normal lung capacity and are hypoxic.

○ **What is a "pink puffer"?**

A patient with COPD and emphysema. These patients are generally thin and noncyanotic. They have an increased total lung capacity and a decreased FEV1.

○ **What percentage of all COPD patients have either smoked or had a significant exposure to cigarette smoke?**

80%.

○ **Other than smoking, what are the risk factors for COPD?**

Environmental pollutants, recurrent URIs (especially in infancy), eosinophilia or increased serum IgE, bronchial hyperresponsiveness, a family history of COPD, and protease deficiencies.

○ **Is there any hope for patients with COPD who quit smoking?**

Yes. Symptomatically speaking, coughing stops in up to 80% of these patients, and 54% of COPD patients find relief from coughing within a month of quitting.

○ **If a patient with chronic bronchitis suffers an acute exacerbation of illness, such as dyspnea, cough, or purulent sputum, what type of O_2 therapy should be initiated?**

In the case of acute exacerbation of bronchitis, oxygen therapy should be guided by Po_2 levels. Adequate oxygen must be maintained at a Po_2 above 60 mm Hg. This should be accomplished with the minimal amount of oxygen necessary. The Po_2 must be kept above 60 mm Hg even if the patient loses the drive to breathe.

○ **What are the more common pathogens that are found in the sputum of COPD patients?**

Streptococcus pneumoniae, Haemophilus influenzae, or *Moraxella catarrhalis.*

○ **Are there any changes to the EKG if the patient has COPD?**

Yes, there can be several. Sinus tachycardia can be seen as well as RVH and LVH. Supraventricular arrhythmias (MAT, A-fib/flutter) as well as ventricular irritability can also be present.

○ **Which pulmonary function test shows an increase in COPD?**

Residual volume. All other tests (FEV_1, FEV_1/FVC, and $FEV_{25\%-75\%}$) indicate decreases and diffusion capacity.

○ **Which part of the lung is affected by emphysema? By chronic bronchitis?**

- Emphysema: Terminal bronchi
- Chronic bronchitis: Large airways

○ **What is the typical appearance of a chest X-ray in a patient with emphysema?**

Increased inflation from cephalo to caudal, with flattening of the diaphragm. In some patients, bullae can develop.

○ **What is the risk of placing a patient with COPD on a high Fio_2?**

Suppression of the hypoxic ventilatory drive.

○ **What are some potential complications related to COPD?**

Pneumonia, cor pulmonale, bronchitis, pulmonary thromboembolism, and left-sided heart failure.

○ **What is the single most important therapy for patients with COPD?**

Smoking cessation.

○ **What pharmacologic agents are used for the initial treatment of COPD?**

Bronchodilators are the mainstay treatment.

○ **Are there any other therapies in addition to bronchodilators?**

Yes, corticosteroids (usually inhaled) are a second-line treatment. This is followed by theophylline as a third-line therapy.

○ **Are there any changes to therapy for COPD patients who require admission to the hospital?**

Yes, the addition of ipratropium as well as of broad-spectrum antibiotic and oxygen is indicated. Chest PT is also helpful in clearing secretions for those patients who may be developing mucous plugging.

○ **What parameters should make you consider initiating "home oxygen" therapy for a patient with COPD?**

If the patient has a resting Po_2 less than 55 mm Hg, or if the patient has a Po_2 less than 60 mm Hg with evidence of tissue hypoxia. O_2 desaturation with exercise may also require home O_2. Home O_2 therapy, 18 h/day, may increase the life span of a patient with COPD by 6 to 7 years.

○ **What nonpharmacologic therapies are indicated for the treatment of COPD?**

Aside from smoking cessation, respiratory therapy to increase the clearing of secretions is helpful. Aerobic exercise is also helpful to increase exercise capacity.

○ **What are some late-stage diseases that are caused by COPD?**

Cor pulmonale, pulmonary hypertension, pneumonia, and chronic respiratory failure.

○ **What is the most common lethal, inheritable disease among the Caucasian population?**

Cystic fibrosis, an autosomal recessive disease that occurs in 1 in 3200 births, and 1 in 25 is a carrier.

○ **A newborn presents with poor weight gain, steatorrhea, and a GI obstruction arising from thick meconium ileus. What test should be performed?**

The sweat test, which detects electrolyte concentrations in the sweat. The infant may have cystic fibrosis, an autosomal recessive defect that affects the exocrine glands, producing higher electrolyte concentrations in the sweat glands.

○ **What condition must be ruled out when childhood nasal polyps are found?**

Cystic fibrosis (CF).

○ **What is the classic triad of cystic fibrosis?**

- COPD
- Pancreatic enzyme deficiency
- Abnormally high concentration of sweat electrolytes

○ **What are the diagnostic criteria for cystic fibrosis?**

Primary Criteria:

- Characteristic pulmonary manifestations and/or
- Characteristic gastrointestinal manifestations and/or
- A family history of CF

Plus

- Sweat Cl (concentration >60 mEq/L) [repeat measurement if sweat Cl is 50–60 mEq/L].

Secondary Criteria:

- Documentation of dual CFTR mutations and
- Evidence of one or more characteristic manifestations

○ **What are the immunological defects in cystic fibrosis?**

Patients with have low levels of serum IgG in the first decade of life, which increase dramatically once chronic infection is established. T-lymphocyte numbers are adequate. With advancing severity of pulmonary disease, lymphocytes proliferate less briskly in response to *Pseudomonas aeruginosa* and other gram-negative organisms. Deficient opsonic activity of alveolar macrophages is seen in patients with established *P. aeruginosa* infection. Major IgG subclass in serum and lungs in CF patients is IgG.

○ **Pathology in cystic fibrosis is confined predominantly to what part of the lung?**

The conducting airways.

○ **What is the most common site of nonpulmonary pathology in cystic fibrosis?**

The GI tract, with striking changes seen in the exocrine pancreas. Islets of Langerhans are spared.

○ **What are the reproductive abnormalities in cystic fibrosis?**

- *In men:* The vas deferens, tail and body of the epididymis, and the seminal vesicles are either absent or rudimentary.
- *In women:* Uterine cervical glands are distended. The mucous and cervical canals are plugged with tenacious mucous secretions. Endocervicitis also seen.

○ **What are the most frequent respiratory pathogens in patients with cystic fibrosis?**

Staphylococcus aureus and *Pseudomonas aeruginosa.*

○ **What are the various radiographic manifestations of cystic fibrosis?**

Hyperinflation, peribronchial cuffing, mucous impaction in airways seen as branching finger-like shadows, bronchiectasis, subpleural blebs, (most prominent along the mediastinal border), and prominent pulmonary artery segments with advanced disease.

○ **What is the immediate mortality with massive hemoptysis?**

~10%.

○ **What are the conditions associated with an elevated sweat chloride?**

CF, hypothyroidism, pseudohypoaldosteronism, hypoparathyroidism, nephrogenic diabetes insipidus, type I glycogen storage disease, mucopolysaccharidosis, malnutrition, PGE administration, hypogammaglobulinemia, and pancreatitis.

○ **What are some of the more common pulmonary complications of Cystic Fibrosis? How do you manage them?**

Pulmonary Complication	Management
Right-sided heart failure	Improve oxygenation through intensive pulmonary therapy.
Respiratory failure	Vigorous medical therapy of the underlying lung disease and infection.
Atelectasis Pneumothorax	Aggressive antibiotic therapy and frequent chest physiotherapy. Conservative if <10% and patient asymptomatic. Pleurodesis to avoid recurrence.
Small-volume hemoptysis	Aggressive treatment of lung infection.
Persistent massive hemoptysis	Bronchial artery embolization along with aggressive treatment of the lung infection.

○ **What two vaccinations should be given to all cystic fibrosis patients?**

Pneumococcal and influenza vaccines.

○ **What is the only definitive treatment for advanced cystic fibrosis?**

Double lung transplant.

○ **What is the life expectancy of a patient with cystic fibrosis?**

The median survival age is over 35 years of age.

○ **Prior steroid administration can precipitate adrenal insufficiency under conditions of stress. How long can these effects last?**

Up to 1 year.

PLEURAL DISEASES

○ **Differentiate between transudate and exudate:**

- *Transudate:* Systemic factors that influence the formation and shift of fluid into the pleural space.
  Pleural: Serum protein <0.5
  Pleural: Serum LDH is <0.6
  Most common with heart failure from LV dysfunction, renal disease, and liver disease.
- *Exudate:* Local factors that influence the formation and absorption of fluid into the pleural space.
  Pleural: Serum protein >0.5
  Pleural: Serum LDH >0.6
  Most common with pneumonia, malignancy, pulmonary embolism, and trauma.

○ **What are the clinical features associated with pleural effusion?**

A pleural rub (may be the only finding in the early stages), pleuritic chest pain because of the involvement and inflammation of parietal pleura, cough (distortion of lung), dyspnea (mechanical inefficiency of respiratory muscles stretched by outward movement of chest wall and downward movement of diaphragm), diminished chest wall movements, dull percussion, decreased tactile and vocal fremitus, decreased breath sounds, and whispering pectoriloquy. With large amounts, there may be contralateral shift of the mediastinum.

○ **Where does pain from pleurisy radiate?**

The shoulder, as a result of diaphragmatic irritation.

○ **What is the minimum amount of pleural liquid that can be detected roentgenographically?**

Approximately 250 mL in upright views of the chest. A lateral decubitus film taken with the patient lying on the affected side can detect as little as 50 mL of liquid.

○ **What are the indications for the chest tube placement in parapneumonic effusion?**

Presence of a complicated parapneumonic effusion, as evidenced by presence of fever, presence of loculations, gross appearance of fluid purulent (pus), increased WBC count and low glucose (usually <40 mg/dL), a decreased pH (<7 or 0.15 < arterial pH), and elevated LDH (>1000 IU/L) are usually considered indications for placement of chest tube for drainage.

○ **What are the characteristic features of a tuberculous pleural effusion?**

Pleural fluid is exudative with a protein content >0.5 g/L, >90% to 95% lymphocytes (in the acute phase, there may be a polymorphonuclear response).

○ **What is the treatment of tuberculous pleural effusion?**

A 9-month course of isoniazid 300 mg and rifampin 600 mg, daily. A therapeutic thoracentesis is recommended only to relieve dyspnea. Corticosteroids can decrease the duration of fever and the time required for fluid absorption, but do not decrease the amount of pleural thickening at 12 months after treatment is initiated. They are therefore recommended only for patients who are markedly symptomatic and only after institution of appropriate antimicrobial therapy.

○ **What are the common features of pleural effusions associated with congestive heart failure?**

Bilateral effusion, more commonly right-sided, associated with cardiomegaly. Fluid is transudate, serous, <1000 mononuclear cells, pH >7.4, and pleural fluid glucose levels same as serum.

○ **What are the radiological features of pleural effusion associated with cirrhosis?**

They are small to massive right-sided effusion in 70%, left-sided effusion in 15%, and bilateral effusions in 15% with normal heart size.

○ **What is the mechanism of pleural effusions associated with atelectasis?**

Atelectasis leads to decreased perimicrovascular pressure, resulting in a pressure gradient. Fluid moves from the parietal pleural interstitium into the pleural space due to decreased perimicrovascular pressure.

○ **What is the primary mechanism of pleural effusion in nephritic syndrome?**

Decreased plasma oncotic pressure caused by hypoalbuminemia.

○ **What factors play a role in the pathogenesis of pleural effusions associated with pulmonary embolism?**

Effusions are present in 40% to 50% of cases of pulmonary embolism. Increased capillary permeability, because of ischemia and leak of protein rich fluid into pleural space, are the main factors. Atelectasis may contribute to transudate and lung necrosis can lead to hemorrhage.

○ **What are the characteristics of a pleural effusion associated with chronic pancreatitis?**

Pleural effusions associated with chronic pancreatitis are usually large or massive unilateral effusions that occur rapidly after thoracentesis. The pleural fluid can have very high amylase content (>200,000 IU/L). Direct fistulous communications from the pancreatic bed are responsible. Failure of conservative treatment is an indication for the surgical intervention, such as drainage (up to 50%).

○ **What are the characteristic features of pleural fluid in patients with lupus?**

LE cells in the pleural fluid. A ratio of pleural fluid/serum ANA of >1 is suggestive of lupus.

○ **What are some drugs reported to be associated with pleural effusion?**

Procainamide, nitrofurantoin, Dantrolene, Methysergide, procarbazine, methotrexate, Amiodarone, mitomycin, and Bleomycin.

○ **What pathological process is suggested by an air–fluid level in the pleural space?**

Bronchopleural fistula.

○ **What is the profile of a classic patient with a spontaneous pneumothorax?**

Male, athletic, tall, slim, and 15 to 35 years of age.

○ **What is the recurrence rate of spontaneous pneumothorax?**

50%.

○ **What is the main cause for a patient to develop a pneumothorax?**

The most common reason is rupture of a bleb.

○ **A 20-year-old male patient presents with pleuritic chest pain with shortness of breath that has worsened over the last 24 hours after he had a violent cough. In general, the patient is healthy and has no medical problems. On examination, he is afebrile, has a pulse of 100, respirations of 22, and blood pressure is 122/83. Head and neck is normal, and the patient has decreased breath sounds on the right with hyperresonant percussion. What is the likely diagnosis?**

Primary spontaneous pneumothorax.

○ **Which types of pneumonia are commonly associated with pneumothorax?**

Staphylococcal, TB, Klebsiella, and PCP.

○ **What therapy may increase the body's absorption of a pneumothorax or pneumomediastinum?**

A high FIO_2.

○ **Do all pneumothoraces need to have a chest tube or surgical intervention?**

No. A small pneumothorax that is <25% with mild to minimal symptoms can be observed as an outpatient with serial chest X-rays to observe reinflation.

○ **A 26-year-old man has been diagnosed with a primary spontaneous pneumothorax, which has been treated and now has a reoccurrence. What is the treatment for this patient?**

Surgical pleurodesis. This procedure should completely resolve the condition.

○ **What is the definition of a secondary pneumothorax?**

It is a pneumothorax that is caused by COPD, typically by an emphysematous bleb. This tends to be more life-threatening because of the underlying lung disease present.

○ **Is therapy for secondary pneumothorax different from a primary pneumothorax?**

Yes, the initial treatment is with a chest tube to re-inflate the lung, then surgical intervention with pleurodesis. If required, a blebectomy or stapling is indicated.

○ **What are some of the more common techniques for pleurodesis?**

Mechanical abrasion of the chest wall, chemical application with multiple agents (tetracycline, urea, mechlorethamine, iodoform, and hypertonic glucose), or pleural staple ling are used. Talc has been implemented in the past but is a controversial technique. It is still used in some places.

○ **What is the indication for a chest tube in a patient with a pneumothorax?**

Over 20% to 25% pneumothorax or a clinical indication, such as respiratory distress or enlarging pneumothorax.

○ **What are the most common reasons for a traumatic pneumothorax?**

Insertion of a transthoracic needle, thoracentesis, and central line placement.

○ **What is the most important cause of hypoxia in a patient with flail chest?**

Underlying lung contusion.

○ **Signs of tension pneumothorax on a physical examination include:**

Tachypnea, unilateral absent breath sounds, tachycardia, pallor, diaphoresis, cyanosis, hyperresonant percussion on affected side, tracheal deviation, hypotension, and neck vein distention.

○ **What is the most significant finding on a chest X-ray in a patient with a tension pneumothorax?**

Shift of the mediastinum away from the effected side.

○ **What is the initial treatment for a tension pneumothorax?**

Large-bore IV catheter placed in the anterior second intercostal space (not a chest tube).

○ **What are the risk factors of pneumothorax? Pneumothorax (risk factors):**

Tall stature

Thin body mass

Twenties of age

Tobacco smoking

Trauma

Tumors

PULMONARY CIRCULATION

○ **What does normal ventilation with decreased lung perfusion suggest?**

Pulmonary embolus.

○ **What are the most common signs and symptoms of PE?**

In order from most to least common: tachypnea, CP, dyspnea, anxiety tachycardia, fever, DVT, hypotension, and syncope.

○ **What percentage of patients with a symptomatic PE will also have a DVT present in the lower extremities?**

50% to 70%.

○ **What is the most common type of substance that forms a pulmonary embolus?**

A thrombus.

○ **Are there any other substances that can cause the formation of an embolus?**

Yes, there are several which include air from a surgery or a central venous line, amniotic fluid, fat embolus, foreign bodies, parasites, septic emboli, and tumor cells.

○ **Name some risk factors that can predispose a patient to a PE:**

Venous stasis (immobility, obesity, stroke), injury to the vascular wall (prior embolus, trauma, and orthopedic surgery), and hypercoagulability (Virchow triad).

○ **What is Virchow triad?**

- Injury to the endothelium of the vessels
- Hypercoagulable state
- Stasis. These represent risk factors for pulmonary embolus.

○ **Most pulmonary embolisms arise from what veins?**

The iliac and femoral veins.

○ **What is the most common hypercoagulability genetic disorder in White patients?**

Factor V Leiden, which is a resistance to protein C.

○ **Name some other hypercoagulable states predisposing individuals to thrombosis and pulmonary embolism:**

Deficiencies of protein S and antithrombin III, antiphospholipid syndrome, malignancy particularly adenocarcinoma, nephritic syndrome, protein losing enteropathy, extensive burns, paroxysmal nocturnal hemoglobinuria, and oral contraceptives.

○ **What historical findings suggest an embolus as opposed to a thrombosis in a lower extremity?**

- *Embolus:* Associated with a history of arrhythmia, valvular disease, MI, no skin changes from chronic arterial insufficiency, and no symptoms in the opposite extremity.
- *Thrombosis:* Opposite extremity shows evidence of chronic arterial occlusive disease with history of rest pain, claudication, etc.

○ **What three syndromes are associated with the various degrees of pulmonary embolism?**

1. Acute cor pulmonale: Occurs with massive embolism that obstructs over 60% of the pulmonary circulation.

2. Pulmonary infarction: Occurs with embolization to the distal branches of the pulmonary circulation.

3. Acute dyspnea: Milder obstruction not enough to warrant infarction.

○ **What is the equation for the A–a gradient?**

A–a = (713 mm Hg $\times$ FIO$_2$) − PCO$_2$ − PO$_2$/0.8)

The normal A–a gradient is 5 to 15 mm Hg (though it increases with age). The A–a gradient increases with PE and diffusion defects (i.e., pulmonary edema and right to left cardiac shunts).

○ **Can a patient with a PE have a PO$_2$ greater than 90 mm Hg?**

Yes, but this is rarely seen (only about 5% of the time).

○ **What are the most common CXR findings in PE?**

Pleural effusions, atelectasis, and pulmonary infiltrates.

○ **What are two relatively specific CXR findings in PE?**

1. Hampton hump: Area of lung consolidation with a rounded border facing the hilus.

2. Westermark sign: Dilated pulmonary outflow tract proximal to the emboli with decreased perfusion distal to the lesion.

While both of these findings are specific to PE, they are rarely identified.

○ **What test is considered the gold standard for the diagnosis of DVT? For the diagnosis of PE?**

- DVT: venography.
- PE: pulmonary angiography.

○ **What changes to an EKG are commonly seen in patients with a PE?**

Sinus tachycardia is the most common, followed by nonspecific ST-T changes. These will be seen in about 40% of patients.

○   **When treating DVT/PE, when should warfarin therapy be initiated?**

On the first or second day after initiation of heparin therapy. Although heparin should be administered immediately, it can be discontinued when the PTT is 1.5 to 1.8 times normal for at least 3 days.

○   **How long should chronic warfarin therapy, as a prophylaxis for DVT, be given?**

Warfarin should be administered for at least 3 to 6 months after a DVT to maintain an INR at two to three times the normal.

○   **What is the anticoagulant treatment schedule for a PE?**

IV heparin until PTT is 2 to 2.5 times normal. After 1 day of treatment, warfarin is added until the INR is greater than 2. If clots recur, consider a Greenfield filter in the IVC. Pulmonary embolectomy is only necessary in cases of massive embolisms. Lovenox may also be used instead of heparin.

○   **What is the risk factor for PE in a patient with an axillary or subclavian vein thrombus?**

About 15%.

○   **What test is most sensitive for evaluating a PE?**

Ventilation–perfusion scan is the most sensitive test. However, it is not as specific as a pulmonary angiogram; 5% of normal volunteers will have an abnormal scan and virtually any pulmonary pathology will produce an abnormal scan (i.e., pneumonia).

○   **What is the preferred test to detect a PE in a pregnant patient?**

V/Q scan. The IV dye load during pregnancy is not ideal. When performing a V/Q scan, make sure to insert a Foley catheter in the bladder to remove the radioactive material from the bladder so that it does not expose the fetus.

○   **What is the major etiology of pulmonary hypertension?**

Chronic hypoxia, most commonly from COPD.

○   **What are the major mechanisms that cause pulmonary hypertension to occur?**

- **Reduction of the cross section of the pulmonary bed,** such as in hypoxemia, emphysema, interstitial lung disease, parasitic infections, and sickle cell disease.
- **Increase in pulmonary venous pressure** as in LV failure, mitral stenosis, restrictive pericarditis, or left atrial myxoma.
- **Increase in pulmonary venous flow** such as a congenital left to right shunt.
- **Increase in blood viscosity** (polycythemia).
- **Other conditions** such as HIV, and HTN related to cirrhosis, and portal hypertension.

○   **What are the common symptoms related to pulmonary hypertension?**

Dyspnea, fatigue, chest pain, and syncope on exertion.

○   **Primary pulmonary hypertension is most common in what population?**

Young women. PPH is rapidly fatal within a few years.

○ **What heart sounds accompany pulmonary hypertension?**

A splitting of the second heart sound and a louder P2.

○ **What could you expect to see on an ECG in a patient with pulmonary HTN?**

Right ventricular strain or hypertrophy, and right atrial enlargement.

○ **What is the most effective method in measuring pulmonary venous pressures in cases of suspected pulmonary hypertension?**

Right-sided heart catheterization.

○ **Which noninvasive method can be done to measure pressures?**

Echocardiography with Doppler flow.

○ **What is the main treatment plan for patients with secondary pulmonary hypertension?**

Treat the underlying disorder that is causing the hypertension.

○ **What is the 2-year survival rate in patients with pulmonary hypertension?**

50%.

○ **What is cor pulmonale?**

It is the dilation and hypertrophy of the right ventricle in response to changes within the pulmonary vascular and parenchymal system.

○ **What are the two leading conditions that predispose a patient to developing cor pulmonale?**

COPD and chronic bronchitis, which leads to pulmonary hypertension.

○ **What is the most common symptom of patients with cor pulmonale?**

Dyspnea.

○ **What is the effect of brain natriuretic peptide (BNP) levels in patients with cor pulmonale?**

They are usually markedly elevated chronically.

○ **What is the treatment for cor pulmonale?**

There is no direct treatment for cor pulmonale. You need to treat the underlying cause for the disease being present.

○ **What are the pulmonary manifestations in Paget disease?**

High output cardiac failure with pulmonary edema, impaired respiratory control from bony involvement at base of skull, vertebral fractures leading to kyphosis, and restrictive lung disease.

○ **What are the pulmonary manifestations of polycythemia?**

Pulmonary embolism related to hyperviscosity and pulmonary hemorrhage related to an increased bleeding tendency.

○   **What is the classic presentation of venous air embolism?**

Sudden hypotension with a mill wheel murmur audible over the precordium.

○   **What is the preferred patient position in suspected venous air embolism?**

Left lateral decubitus and Trendelenburg.

RESTRICTIVE PULMONARY DISEASE

○   **What are some of the signs and symptoms of idiopathic pulmonary fibrosis (IPF)?**

Exertional dyspnea, nonproductive cough, inspiratory crackles, and digital clubbing on examination.

○   **What are some expected findings on chest X-rays and lung scans in patients with IPF?**

Basilar, and subpleural reticular opacities. These are associated with bronchiectasis and honeycombing.

○   **Name some illnesses that can accelerate the disease and overall prognosis of patients with IPF:**

Infections (pneumonia, bronchitis), pulmonary embolism, pneumothorax, and heart failure.

○   **What is the survival rate of a patient with IPF who is intubated?**

Only 25% of patients make it off the vent and survive.

○   **Is there a recommended therapy for patients with an exacerbation of IPF?**

No. There is no one therapy that is recommended. Symptomatic treatment is done. The only other option is lung transplantation for those patients who qualify.

○   **Name the four major groups of pneumoconiosis and the more common types within those groups:**

1. Metal dusts: siderosis, stannosis, and baritosis.
2. Coal dusts: coal dust from mining.
3. Inorganic dusts: free silica from mining
4. Silicate dusts: asbestosis, talcosis, kaolin (sands), and Shaver disease (from aluminum production).

○   **What is the major mechanism that these dusts are routed into the lungs?**

By inhalation.

○   **How do these products injure the lungs?**

They cause an initial inflammatory reaction and then over time create a fibrosis to the lung tissue.

○   **Upper lobe nodules and eggshell hilar node calcification are displayed on X-rays of an individual with what disease?**

Silicosis.

○ **What is the average exposure time necessary for the development of silicosis following silicon dioxide inhalation?**

20 to 30 years. Employees in mining, pottery, soap production, and granite quarrying are at risk. This population also has a higher chance of acquiring TB.

○ **A 14-year-old adolescent boy was exposed to asbestos for 3 days has a nonproductive cough and chest pain. Does this boy have asbestosis?**

No. Although a nonproductive cough and pleurisy are symptoms of asbestosis, other signs, such as exertional dyspnea, malaise, clubbed fingers, crackles, cyanosis, pleural effusion, and pulmonary hypertension, should be displayed before making a diagnosis of asbestosis. In addition, asbestosis does not develop until 10 to 15 years after regular exposure to asbestos.

○ **Asbestosis increases the risk of what two diseases?**

Lung cancer and malignant mesothelioma.

○ **Exposure to what mineral, used as insulation, greatly enhances the carcinogenic potential of exposure to cigarette smoke?**

Asbestos.

○ **What parts of the pulmonary system are affected by asbestosis?**

The pleura and peritoneum. Asbestosis increases the risk of mesothelioma. It also causes pneumoconiosis that invade the lungs.

○ **What age population and race is the most prevalent in the United States for sarcoidosis?**

Patients in the age groups of 30 to 40 years, black, women more than men.

○ **What are the usual presenting symptoms in patients with sarcoidosis?**

They are usually nonpulmonary. They include symptoms of the skin, eyes, and peripheral nerves. Some patients will have quick onset of malaise, fever, and dyspnea. Erythema nodosum, parotid enlargement, lymphadenopathy, and hepatomegaly are also common findings.

○ **What are the three stages of findings in the chest X-ray of a sarcoidosis patient?**

- Stage I: bilateral hilar adenopathy alone
- Stage II: hilar adenopathy and parenchymal involvement
- Stage III: parenchymal involvement alone

○ **What is the best method of test to determine pulmonary sarcoidosis?**

Transbronchial biopsy.

○ **What is the treatment for patients with sarcoidosis?**

Oral steroids (prednisone) 0.5 to 1 mg/kg/day to suppress the symptoms.

○ **What are some advanced pulmonary disease complications related to sarcoidosis?**

Advanced fibrosis, bronchiectasis, cavitation, pneumothorax, hemoptysis, and respiratory failure.

OTHER PULMONARY DISEASES AND CONDITIONS

○ **What is ARDS?**

Acute respiratory distress syndrome is a syndrome of rapid dyspnea, hypoxia, and pulmonary infiltrates, which lead to respiratory failure. This can be a result of a direct or indirect insult on the lungs.

○ **What are some direct and indirect illnesses that can cause ARDS?**

- Direct: Pneumonia, near drowning, toxic inhalation
- Indirect: Sepsis, trauma, drug overdose, pancreatitis

○ **What is the most common cause of ARDS?**

Sepsis and pneumonia.

○ **What are the three phases of ARDS progression?**

Exudative, proliferative, and fibrotic phase.

○ **What is the goal of management in patients with ARDS?**

There is little that can be done for these patients. However, by maintaining a low left atrial filling pressure, higher pressures can be prevented from developing into the pulmonary system, thus reducing the chance of increased permeability of fluid into the extravascular space. Mechanical ventilation is helpful in patients whose respiratory drive is failing and can no longer oxygenate themselves.

○ **What is the mortality range in patients with ARDS?**

Anywhere from 41% to 65%.

○ **A preterm infant is breathing rapidly and grunting. Intercostal retractions, nasal flaring, and cyanosis are noted. Auscultation shows decreased breath sounds and crackles. What is the diagnosis?**

Newborn respiratory distress syndrome, also known as hyaline membrane disease. X-rays show diffuse atelectasis. Treatment involves artificial surfactant and O_2 administration through CPAP.

○ **At what age is the preterm infant more likely to have hyaline membrane disease?**

When the infant is around 26 to 28 weeks old.

○ **How is fetal lung maturity assessed?**

By measuring the ratio of lecithin to sphingomyelin (L/S). An L/S ratio greater than 2 and the presence of phosphatidyl glycerol confirm that the fetal lungs are mature.

○ **Other than avoiding prematurity, what can be done to prevent newborn respiratory distress syndrome?**

If the fetus is older than 32 weeks, administer betamethasone 48 to 72 hours before delivery to augment surfactant production.

○ **If newborn hyaline membrane disease is present, what is the treatment for these patients?**

In addition to intravenous surfactant, oxygen with or without nasal CPAP long term is indicated. This is done until the lung maturity has reached an acceptable level.

○ **What factor determines the magnitude of injury in gastric acid aspiration?**

The gastric pH. A pH less than 3 produces the most severe injury.

○ **Under what circumstances is aspiration of vomitus, oral secretions, or foreign material likely?**

Anything producing an altered level of consciousness (e.g., alcohol, overdose, general anesthesia, stroke), impaired swallowing or abnormal gastrointestinal motility, or disruption of the esophageal sphincters predisposes to aspiration.

○ **What are the signs of a large obstructing foreign body in the larynx or trachea?**

Respiratory distress, stridor, inability to speak, cyanosis, loss of consciousness, and death.

○ **What are the symptoms of a smaller (distally lodged) foreign body?**

Cough, dyspnea, wheezing, chest pain, and fever.

○ **What is the procedure of choice for foreign-body removal?**

Rigid bronchoscopy. Fiberoptic bronchoscopy is an alternate procedure in adults, not in children. If bronchoscopy fails, thoracotomy may be required.

○ **What are the common radiographic findings in foreign-body aspiration?**

Normal film, atelectasis, pneumonia, contralateral mediastinal shift (more marked during expiration), and visualization of the foreign body.

○ **What are the common directly toxic (noninfectious) respiratory tract aspirates?**

Gastric contents, alcohol, hydrocarbons, mineral oil, and animal and vegetable fats. All of these produce an inflammatory response and pneumonia. Gastric contents are the most common offender.

○ **What are the consequences of aspirating acid?**

The response is rapid, with near-immediate bronchitis, bronchiolitis, atelectasis, shunting, and hypoxemia. Pulmonary edema may occur within 4 hours. The clinical manifestations are dyspnea, wheezing, cough, cyanosis, fever, and shock.

○ **Under what circumstances are antibiotics used in aspiration?**

Aspiration of infected material, intestinal obstruction, immune compromised host, and evidence of bacterial superinfection after a noninfected aspirate (new fever, infiltrates, or purulence after the initial 2 to 3 days).

○ **What are the radiographic manifestations of acid aspiration?**

Varied, may be bilateral diffuse infiltrates, irregular "patchy" infiltrates, or lobar infiltrates.

○ **What outcomes occur in patients who do not rapidly resolve gastric acid aspiration pneumonitis?**

ARDS (adult respiratory distress syndrome), progressive respiratory failure, and death; bacterial superinfection.

○ **At what percentage of an airway obstruction will inspiratory stridor become evident?**

70% occlusion.

○ **A foreign body is suspected in the lower airways. What will plain films show?**

Air trapping on the affected side. Inspiration and expiration views demonstrate mediastinal shift away from the affected side.

○ **What is the most common cause of death among infants 1 to 12 months old?**

Sudden infant death syndrome.

○ **Where in the airway are foreign bodies usually lodged in children older than 1 year?**

In the lower airway.

○ **Stridor is observed in what phase of respiration?**

Inspiratory.

○ **What is stridor caused by?**

With extrathoracic airway obstruction, the pressure inside the extrathoracic part of the airway is much more negative relative to atmospheric pressure. This results in further narrowing of the larynx during inspiration and therefore, stridor.

○ **Grunting is observed during what phase of respiration?**

Expiratory, as exhalation occurs against a closed glottis.

○ **In the diagnosis of a radiolucent foreign body lodged in the right mainstem bronchus, producing incomplete obstruction, inspiratory and expiratory films will show air trapping and increased lucency of the lung on the involved side. This phenomenon is because of:**

Ball-valve air trapping. Air enters around the foreign body during inspiration, but is trapped as the airway closes around the foreign body during expiration, preventing emptying of that side.

○ **You are at a restaurant and the person at the table next to you begins coughing loudly. She stands up and begins wheezing between coughs, but she is still able to eke out a "Help! I'm choking." How should you help?**

Encourage her to cough deeper and keep breathing. Do not interrupt her spontaneous attempts at expulsion if she still has good air exchange, as evidenced by her state of consciousness and the degree of coughing and wheezing. Should she display severe respiratory difficulty with a weakening cough and the inability to talk, perform the Heimlich maneuver.

○ **What should be done if this patient above is markedly obese and in severe respiratory distress?**

The normal Heimlich maneuver will not be as effective. Instead of positioning your fists above the patient's navel, place your cupped fist on the patient's chest and deliver swift thrusts. This is also the method of choice for pregnant women.

○ **True/False: Pulse oximetry is a reliable method for estimating oxyhemoglobin saturation in a patient suffering from CO poisoning:**

False. COHb has light absorbance that can lead to a falsely elevated pulse oximeter transduced saturation level. The calculated value from a standard ABG may also be falsely elevated. The oxygen saturation should be determined by using a co-oximeter that measures the amounts of unsaturated O_2Hb, COHb, and metHb.

○ **What is the indication for long-term tracheostomy?**

When intubation is expected to exceed 3 weeks.

○ **What are the potential mechanisms of cardiorespiratory collapse?**

Mechanical obstruction of pulmonary vasculature, alveolar capillary leak, pulmonary edema from LV failure, and anaphylaxis.

○ **What are the indications for intubation and ventilation after near drowning?**

Apnea, pulselessness, altered mental status, severe hypoxemia, and respiratory acidosis.

○ **Calculate the alveolar–arterial oxygen (A-aO_2) gradient given the following arterial blood gas obtained at sea level: pH 7.24, PaCO_2 60, PaO_2 45:**

30 mm Hg.

To calculate the alveolar–arterial oxygen gradient, first calculate the expected alveolar partial pressure of oxygen (PAO_2) using the alveolar gas equation: $PAO_2 = PIO_2 - PaCO_2/R$, where PIO_2 is the partial pressure of oxygen in the inspired gas and R is the respiratory exchange ratio, commonly estimated at 0.8. PIO_2 is calculated as follows: $PIO_2 = FIO_2 (PB - PH_2O)$, where F$IO_2$ is the inspired concentration of oxygen (0.21 at sea level), P_B is the atmospheric pressure (760 mm Hg at sea level), and PH_2O is the partial pressure of water (47 mm Hg). At sea level, PIO_2 is equal to 150 mm Hg. Thus, for this example, $PAO_2 = 150 - 60/0.8$ or 75 mm Hg. The A-aO_2 gradient is PAO_2 – PaO_2. Therefore, in this example, the A-aO_2 gradient is 75 – 45 or 30 mm Hg.

○ **What is the age-related decline in PaO_2?**

The PaO_2 declines by 2.5 mm Hg per decade. Given that a PaO_2 of 95 to 100 mm Hg is normal for a 20-year-old, a PaO_2 of 75–80 would be normal for an 80-year-old.

○ **What are the four principal mechanisms that lead to hypoxemia?**

Hypoventilation, diffusion limitation, shunt, and ventilation–perfusion inequality. A fifth mechanism, low inspired oxygen concentration, is important only at altitudes above 8000 feet.

○ **Which of the four above mechanisms is the most common?**

Ventilation–perfusion inequality.

○ **What are the three major mechanisms of hypoventilation and what clinical conditions are associated with each?**

1. Failure of the central nervous system ventilatory centers: drugs (narcotics, barbiturates) and stroke.
2. Failure of the chest bellows: chest wall diseases (kyphoscoliosis), neuromuscular diseases (amyotrophic lateral sclerosis), and diaphragm weakness.
3. Obstruction of the airways: asthma and chronic obstructive pulmonary disease.

○ **How can hypoxemia secondary to hypoventilation alone be distinguished from the other causes of hypoxemia?**

If the hypoxemia is from hypoventilation alone, the A-aO_2 gradient is normal. It is elevated in all other causes.

○ **What are the most common clinical conditions in which shunt is the primary mechanism for hypoxemia?**

Alveolar filling with fluid (pulmonary edema) and pus (pneumonia) are the most commonly seen clinically. Any condition that fills or closes the alveoli preventing gas exchange can lead to shunt.

○ **How can shunt be distinguished from the other causes of hypoxemia?**

If given 100% oxygen, the hypoxemic patient with shunt will not have a significant increase in their PaO_2. There will be a significant increase in PaO_2 when 100% oxygen is given to patients with hypoventilation or ventilation–perfusion inequality.

○ **A leftward shift in the oxyhemoglobin dissociation curve indicates an increased or decreased hemoglobin affinity for oxygen?**

Ventilation-increased.

○ **Changes in temperature, $PaCO_2$ or pH, or the level of 2,3-diphosphoglycerate (2,3-DPG) cause a shift in the oxyhemoglobin dissociation curve. To cause a rightward shift, what are the changes that must occur?**

Increased temperature, increased $PaCO_2$, decreased pH, and increased 2,3-DPG level. An easy way to remember this is that these conditions are often associated with decreased tissue oxygen levels. By right shifting the curve, more oxygen is released from the hemoglobin to the tissues.

○ **How does the shape of the oxyhemoglobin dissociation curve effect the oxygen content of blood?**

Since SaO_2 does not increase significantly if the PaO_2 >60 mm Hg, the oxygen content of blood will increase significantly above this level only by increasing the hemoglobin concentration.

○ **What are the determinants of oxygen delivery to the peripheral tissues?**

Oxygen content of the blood (CaO_2) and cardiac output. An increase in either will increase oxygen delivery to the tissues.

○ **What is the difference between anatomic and physiologic dead space?**

Dead space refers to areas of lung that are ventilated but not perfused. Anatomic dead space refers to the conducting airways (trachea, bronchi, and bronchioles) where there is no gas exchange because there are no alveoli. Physiologic dead space includes the anatomic dead space and any diseased lung in which there is ventilation but no perfusion.

○ **What is the normal dead space in an average 70 kg subject?**

150 mL.

○ **Which pulmonary diseases are most associated with an increased physiologic dead space?**

Asthma and chronic obstructive pulmonary disease (COPD).

○ **How is the minute ventilation related to alveolar and dead space ventilation?**

Minute ventilation (V_E) is the product of tidal volume multiplied by breathing frequency ($V_E = V_T \times f$). Alveolar ventilation (V_A) is that portion of the minute ventilation that contributes to gas exchange, whereas dead space ventilation (V_D) is that portion that does not contribute to gas exchange. Thus, $V_E = V_A + V_D$.

○ **What is the effect of increased alveolar ventilation (V_A) on $Paco_2$?**

$Paco_2$ will decrease as V_A increases.

○ **Why do asthmatic patients eventually have an increased $Paco_2$ if untreated?**

As the asthma attack continues untreated, the work of breathing will continue to increase. Eventually, the diaphragm fatigues and the patient hypoventilates. The hypoventilation, in association with the increased dead space and increased Co_2 production, increases the $Paco_2$.

○ **What is the normal $Paco_2$ and does it vary with age?**

Normal $Paco_2$ is 35 to 45 mm Hg and does not vary with age.

○ **What is the normal expected change in pH if there is an acute change in the $Paco_2$?**

The pH will increase or decrease 0.8 U for every 10 mm Hg decrease or increase (respectively) in $Paco_2$.

○ **What are the consequences of hypercapnia?**

Acute hypercapnia has physiologic consequences because of the increased $Paco_2$ itself and the decreased pH. Physiologic effects of the $Paco_2$ increase include:

- increases in cerebral blood flow.
- confusion, headache ($Paco_2$ >60 mm Hg), obtundation and seizures ($Paco_2$ >70 mm Hg).
- depression of diaphragmatic contractility.

The primary consequences of the decreased pH are on the cardiovascular system with changes in cardiac contractility (decreased), the fibrillation threshold (decreased), and vascular tone (predominantly vasodilatation).

○ **What are the consequences of hypocapnia?**

Acute hypocapnia has physiologic consequences because of the decreased $Paco_2$ itself and the increased pH. Physiologic effects of the $Paco_2$ decrease include:

- decreases in cerebral blood flow. This reflex is used in the management of neurologic disorders with high intracranial pressures as a short-term measure to decrease the increased intracranial pressure.
- confusion, myoclonus, asterixis, loss of consciousness, and seizures.

The primary consequences of the increased pH are, again, primarily on the cardiovascular system with increased cardiac contractility and vasodilatation.

○ **What is the cause of the hypoxemia?**

Hypoventilation is one cause. However, since the A-ao_2 gradient is elevated, there is another cause in addition to the hypoventilation. In an obese patient, both ventilation–perfusion inequality and shunt (secondary to atelectasis) can contribute to the development of hypoxemia.

○ **A 50-year-old woman presents with a pneumonia in the right lower and middle lobes. On 50% oxygen by facemask, her Pao_2 is 75 mm Hg. Should the patient be positioned right side down or up?**

Right side up. Blood flow is gravity dependent. If the patient is positioned right side down, blood flow will preferentially go to the right side. However, because of the pneumonia, this will increase the amount of shunt, lowering the Pao_2 further.

○ **True/False: If a patient presents with a Pa_{CO_2} of 75, he/she should be emergently intubated:**

False. There is no Pa_{CO_2} level at which a patient must be intubated. Intubation is based upon the total clinical condition of a patient, not just upon a blood gas result.

○ **A 45-year-old patient presents to the emergency department after being rescued from a fire. The patient is dyspneic and cyanotic. Sa_{O_2} on 50% mask is 84%. The blood gas, however, reveals a Pa_{O_2} of 125 mm Hg. Why the discrepancy?**

A fire victim is likely to have carbon monoxide poisoning. The carbon monoxide has converted the hemoglobin to carboxyhemoglobin, which decreases the binding of oxygen to hemoglobin and prevents an accurate pulse oximetry reading. However, carbon monoxide does not affect dissolved oxygen, which is what is measured in the arterial blood gas.

○ **What is the treatment for carbon monoxide poisoning?**

100% oxygen, which increases carbon monoxide clearance by competing for binding to hemoglobin. If there is no significant response to 100% oxygen, hyperbaric oxygen (oxygen provided at higher than atmospheric pressure) is an alternative therapy.

○ **A 25-year-old woman with a history of mitral valve prolapse presents with "nervousness," chest tightness, hand numbness, and mild confusion. Arterial blood gas reveals pH 7.52, Pa_{CO_2} 25 mm Hg, and Pa_{O_2} 108 mm Hg. What is the diagnosis?**

Acute anxiety attack. She is hyperventilating.

○ **Why is the Pa_{O_2} elevated?**

Because the lower Pa_{CO_2} means a higher Pa_{O_2} (see alveolar gas equation above).

○ **What is the treatment?**

The acute hyperventilation can be terminated by having the patient breathe in and out of a bag. Anxiolytics can also be provided.

○ **True/False: Oxygen should never be given to a hypoxemic patient with COPD who has chronic CO_2 retention:**

False. Oxygen should always be given to a patient who is hypoxemic.

○ **Adequacy of alveolar ventilation is reflected by which component of arterial blood gas analysis?**

Pa_{CO_2}.

○ **Patients on mechanical ventilation can develop hypoventilation based on what factors?**

Increased dead space (including length of ventilator circuit proximal to the "Y" piece separating the inspiratory and expiratory limbs), decreased tidal volume, overdistention of lung, air leaks, and massive pulmonary embolism.

○ **What is the principal mechanism of increased Pa_{CO_2} with increased $F_{I_{O_2}}$?**

Worsening V/Q mismatch and the Haldane effect.

○ **How does malnutrition contribute to respiratory failure?**

Increase in the oxygen cost of breathing and respiratory muscle weakness.

○ **How can the work of breathing with mechanical ventilation associated with intrinsic PEEP be reduced?**

Add CPAP, reduce tidal volume, reduce inspiratory time, and increase expiratory time.

○ **Through what mechanism does PEEP decrease cardiac output?**

Reduced preload.

○ **Through what mechanism does positive pressure ventilation increase cardiac output?**

Decreased afterload.

○ **How can compliance of the lung/chest wall be approximated from airway pressure measurements during mechanical ventilation?**

Compliance = tidal volume/(inspiratory plateau pressure − end expiratory pressure)

○ **What are the primary determinants of the work of breathing?**

Minute ventilation, lung/chest wall compliance, and presence of intrinsic PEEP.

○ **When may end-tidal carbon dioxide detectors prove inaccurate?**

In patients with very low blood flow to the lungs, or in those with a large dead space (i.e., following a pulmonary embolism).

○ **What is the most common complication of endotracheal intubation?**

Intubation of a bronchus. Other complications include lacerations of the lip, tongue, pharyngeal, or tracheal mucosa resulting in bleeding, hematoma, or abscess. Tracheal rupture, avulsion of an arytenoid cartilage, vocal cord injury, pharyngeal–esophageal perforation, intubation of the pyriform sinus, aspiration of vomitus, hypertension, tachycardia, or arrhythmias can also occur.

○ **What oxygen concentration will be supplied by nasal cannula with a flow rate of 1 L/min?**

24%. For each 1 L/min increase in flow, a 4% increase in oxygen concentration will occur; 6 L/min produces a 44% oxygen concentration.

○ **What oxygen flow rate is recommended for face mask ventilation?**

At least 5 L/min. Recommended flow is 8 to 10 L/min, which will produce oxygen concentrations as high as 40% to 60%.

○ **What oxygen concentration can be supplied with a face mask and oxygen reservoir?**

6 L/min provides approximately 60% oxygen concentration, and each liter increases the concentration by 10%; 10 L/min is almost 100%.

○ **A pulmonary embolism causes which type of cyanosis?**

Central cyanosis. However, secondary shock and right-sided heart failure can lead to peripheral cyanosis.

○ **What are the two most common errors made in the intubation of a neonate?**

- Placing the neck in hyperextension; this moves the cords even more anteriorly.
- Inserting the laryngoscope too far.

○ **Name the two primary causes of peripheral cyanosis with a normal Sao_2:**

Decreased cardiac output and redistribution (may be secondary to shock, DIC, hypothermia, vascular obstruction).

○ **As Pco_2 increases, pH will decrease. How much is the pH expected to decrease for every 10 mm Hg increase in Pco_2?**

pH decreases by 0.08 U for each 10 mm Hg increase in Pco_2.

○ **Describe Kerley A and B lines:**

Kerley A lines are straight, nonbranching lines in the upper lung fields. Kerley B lines are horizontal, nonbranching lines at the periphery of the lower lung fields.

○ **A patient presents with cough, lethargy, dyspnea, conjunctivitis, glomerulonephritis, fever, and purulent sinusitis. What is the probable diagnosis?**

Wegener granulomatosis. This is a necrotizing vasculitis and pulmonary granulomatosis that attacks the small artery and veins. Treat the patient with corticosteroids and cyclophosphamide.

○ **What serological test is diagnostic for Wegener granulomatosis?**

c-ANCA in association with appropriate clinical evidence. A renal, lung, or sinus biopsy may also be helpful in making the diagnosis.

○ **What is the typical time period during which acute radiation pneumonitis develops?**

Within the first eight weeks postradiation treatment.

○ **What laboratory finding distinguishes patients with primary SLE and drug-induced lupus?**

Drug-induced lupus has a positive ANA, but a *negative* ds-DN

○ **The chest X-ray reveals no pulmonary parenchymal lesions but does show prominent hila and an enlarged right ventricle. What diagnostic test should be performed?**

The patient has no pulmonary parenchymal lesions to cause a shunt; therefore, she most likely has an intracardiac right-to-left shunt (most likely a previously undiagnosed atrial septal defect). An echocardiogram should be performed.

○ **Of the following, which pattern of calcification of a solitary pulmonary nodule is most likely to be associated with a malignant lesion: lamellar (onion skin), popcorn, eccentric, or central?**

Eccentric.

○ **What happens to minute ventilation at submaximal work rates in interstitial lung disease?**

It increases because of increased dead space ventilation. As the respiratory rate increases, tidal volume decreases.

○ **What is the incidence of postoperative respiratory complications in patients with COPD?**

50% or more.

○ **Which neuromuscular diseases and spinal diseases can lead to ventilatory insufficiency?**

Muscular dystrophy, polymyositis, myotonic dystrophy, polyneuritis, Eaton–Lambert syndrome, myasthenia gravis, amyotrophic lateral sclerosis, injury, Guillain–Barré syndrome, multiple sclerosis, Parkinson disease, and stroke.

○ **What are some clinical disorders associated with increased capillary permeability causing exudative pleural effusion?**

Pleuropulmonary infections, circulating toxins, systemic lupus erythematosus, rheumatoid arthritis, sarcoidosis, tumor, pulmonary infarction, and viral hepatitis.

○ **What is the incidence of pleural involvement in systemic lupus erythematosus?**

50% to 75% of patients with systemic lupus erythematosus develop pleural effusion or pleuritic pain during the course of their disease.

○ **What are the clinical features of lupus pleuritis?**

Pleuritic chest pain is the most common presentation. Other features are cough, dyspnea, pleural rub, and fever. An episode of pleuritis usually indicates exacerbation of lupus.

○ **What percentage of elderly have sleep apnea?**

40%.

○ **What is the most common cause of sleep apnea in adults?**

An upper airway obstruction, generally by the tongue or enlarged tonsils. A medulla that is not responsive to CO_2 buildup is the most common cause in children. Obstruction by the tongue or enlarged tonsils also induces sleep apnea.

○ **What is a complication of central sleep apnea in children?**

SIDS. Affected children develop morning cyanosis. However, children can be treated with theophylline.

○ **Under what conditions does neurogenic pulmonary edema occur?**

Neurogenic pulmonary edema is commonly associated with increased intracranial pressure. It is commonly seen with head trauma, subarachnoid hemorrhage, and even with seizures.

○ **Is a nonsmoker who has lived with a smoker for 25 years at greater risk of lung cancer than a nonsmoker who has not lived with a smoker?**

Of course. The risk is 1.34 times as great as a person living in a smoke-free environment.

○ **What percentage of smokers who quit lapse back into their smoking habits?**

85%.

REFERENCES

Brunton LL, Lazo JS, Parker KL, eds. *Goodman and Gilman's the Pharmacological Basis of Therapeutics.* 11th ed. New York, NY: McGraw-Hill; 2006.

Fauci AS, Braunwald E, Kasper DL, et al. *Harrison's Principles of Internal Medicine* [Online]. New York, NY: McGraw-Hill; 2008, 7 1.

Hall JB, Schmidt G, Wood LD. *Principles of Critical Care,* 3rd ed. New York, NY: McGraw-Hill; 2005.

McPhee SJ, Papadakis MA. *Current Medical Diagnosis and Treatment 2009.* New York, NY: McGraw-Hill; 2009.

McPhee SJ, Ganong WF. *Pathophysiology of Disease—An Introduction to Clinical Medicine.* 5th ed. New York, NY: McGraw-Hill; 2006.

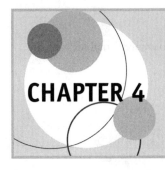

CHAPTER 4 **Endocrine**

Jacqueline Jordan Spiegel, MS, PA-C

DISEASES OF THE THYROID GLAND

○ **What level of the cervical vertebra is the thyroid located?**

Fourth cervical vertebra (C4).

○ **What is a goiter?**

An enlarged thyroid gland that may be diffuse or nodular.

○ **What are the etiologies associated with goiter?**

- Autoimmune thyroiditis (Graves, Hashimoto, or postpartum thyroiditis)
- Iodine deficiency
- Infection (bacterial, viral, mycobacterial, fungal, parasitic)
- Inflammatory or malignant cells
- Neoplastic changes (benign or malignant)
- Thyroid hormone resistance
- Goitrogens

○ **What medications are commonly associated with causing simple goiters?**

Amiodarone, lithium, or aminoglutethimide.

○ **What is thyrotoxicosis?**

Clinical manifestations associated with excessive serum levels of T4 or T3 (hyperthyroidism).

○ **What are the etiologies for thyrotoxicosis?**

- Graves disease
- Toxic multinodular goiter and thyroid adenomas
- Thyroiditis (subacute, postpartum, silent)
- Amiodarone-induced
- Iodine-induced
- Pregnancy and hCG-secreting trophoblastic tumors

○   **What are the clinical findings of thyrotoxicosis due to any cause?**

Symptoms: Sweating, weight loss or gain, anxiety, palpitations, loose stools, heat intolerance, irritability, fatigue, weakness, and menstrual irregularity.

Signs: Tachycardia, warm and moist skin, stare, and tremor.

○   **What imaging study is useful in determining the cause of hyperthyroidism?**

Radioactive iodine (RAI) scanning and uptake.

○   **What causes of hyperthyroidism are indicated by RAI results?**

High RAI uptake:

- Graves disease and
- toxic nodular goiter.

Low RAI:

- subacute thyroiditis (de Quervain or granulomatous) and
- iodine-induced hyperthyroidism.

○   **What are the laboratory findings associated with thyrotoxicosis (hyperthyroidism)?**

Decreased or suppressed TSH and increased T4, FT4, T3, and FT3.

○   **What is the most common cause of hyperthyroidism?**

Graves disease (toxic diffuse goiter).

○   **What is the etiology of Graves disease?**

Autoantibodies bind to TSH receptors in thyroid cell membranes and stimulate the gland to hyperfunction.

○   **Which human leukocyte antigen (HLA) group is associated with Graves disease?**

HLA-DR3 and HLA-B8.

○   **Which gender and age group is Graves disease more commonly found?**

More common in women than men (8:1) with an onset between the ages of 20 and 40 years.

○   **What are the classic clinical findings associated with Graves disease?**

Symptoms typical of thyrotoxicosis include:

- weight loss,
- heat intolerance
- sweating
- nervousness
- diarrhea
- palpitations
- and tremors.

Possible physical examination findings:

- Goiter often with bruit,
- upper eyelid retraction (Dalrymple sign),
- lid lag with downward gaze (von Graefe sign)
- staring appearance (Kocher sign)
- exophthalmos
- and pretibial myxedema.

○ **What laboratory findings are diagnostic for Graves disease?**

Serum thyroid stimulating immunoglobulin (TSI) or thyroid stimulating hormone receptor antibodies (TSHrAb) are present.

○ **What are the treatment options for Graves disease?**

Thiourea drugs: Methimazole or propylthiouracil (PTU)
Iodinated contrast agents: Iopanoic acid or ipodate sodium
Radioactive iodine: ^{131}I, RAI
Thyroid surgery: Total and/or subtotal thyroidectomy

○ **What morbidities may occur with surgical management of Graves disease?**

- Vocal cord paralysis (recurrent laryngeal nerve damage)
- Hypoparathyroidism
- Hyperthyroidism recurrence (bilateral subtotal thyroidectomy)
- Post-treatment hypothyroidism

○ **What are the precipitants for thyroid storm?**

- Stressful illness (trauma, infection)
- Thyroid or nonthyroidal surgery
- RAI administration
- Parturition

○ **What are the clinical manifestations of thyroid storm?**

- Marked delirium
- Severe tachycardia (>140 bpm)
- Vomiting, diarrhea, and dehydration
- Very high fever (104–106°F)

○ **How is thyroid storm managed?**

- Beta blocker (propranolol) for symptom control
- Thiourea drug (methimazole or PTU) to block new hormone synthesis
- Iodine solution (Lugol solution) to block release of thyroid hormone
- Iodinated radiocontrast (ipodate sodium 1 hour after first dose of thiourea) agent to inhibit peripheral conversion of T4 and T3
- Glucocorticoids (hydrocortisone) to reduce T4 to T3 conversion, promote vasomotor stability, and treat any associated relative adrenal insufficiency

○ **What is the most common cause of primary hypothyroidism in iodine-sufficient areas of the world?**

Chronic autoimmune (Hashimoto) thyroiditis.

○ **What are the common clinical manifestations of hypothyroidism?**

Weakness, fatigue, cold intolerance, constipation, weight change, depression, menorrhagia, hoarseness, dry skin, bradycardia, and delayed return of deep tendon reflexes.

○ **What laboratory findings distinguish primary, secondary, and subclinical hypothyroidism?**

Primary (due to thyroid disease): High serum TSH with low serum free T4.

Secondary (due to causes of hypopituitarism): Low or normal serum TSH and low serum free T4.

Subclinical: Elevated serum TSH with normal free T4.

○ **What medications and substances may interfere with medical treatment of hypothyroidism?**

Medications that increase the hepatic metabolism of levothyroxine include:

- carbamazepine
- phenobarbital
- primidone,
- phenytoin
- rifabutin
- rifampin
- sunitinib
- and imatinib.

Those that cause malabsorption of thyroxine through binding substances:

- iron in multivitamins
- fiber
- raloxifene
- sucralfate
- aluminum hydroxide antacids
- orlistat,
- calcium and magnesium supplements
- soy milk, and soy protein supplements

○ **What is the recommended treatment for hypothyroidism?**

Replacement of thyroxine (T4) hormone with the medication levothyroxine.

○ **What is the initial dosing for thyroid replacement therapy with the medication levothyroxine?**

Approximately 1.7 µg/kg/day. In otherwise healthy young and middle aged adults begin initial oral doses of 25 to 75 µg daily. In patients with known ischemic heart disease or over age 60 begin smaller initial doses of 25 to 50 µg daily. Levothyroxine dose may be increased according to clinical response and serum TSH levels.

○ **What is the recommended monitoring of thyroid hormone replacement therapy?**

For patients receiving treatment for primary hypothyroidism with levothyroxine, dosing changes should be made every 6 to 8 weeks until TSH is in target range. For patients with secondary hypothyroidism, free T4 levels are monitored rather than TSH.

○ **What are the hallmark clinical features of severe, life-threatening hypothyroidism (myxedema crisis)?**

Altered mental status, severe hypothermia, bradycardia, coma, and hyponatremia.

○ **What is the treatment for myxedema crisis?**

Levothyroxine sodium 400 µg is given IV as a loading dose, followed by 50 to 100 µg intravenously daily. Supportive measures with correction of hypothermia, ventilatory support, and hydration as indicated.

○ **What are the classifications of thyroiditis?**

1. Chronic lymphocytic thyroiditis (Hashimoto thyroiditis)
2. Subacute thyroiditis (de Quervain thyroiditis)
3. Suppurative thyroiditis
4. Riedel thyroiditis

○ **What is de Quervain thyroiditis?**

A self-limited thyroid condition associated with a triphasic clinical course of hyperthyroidism, hypothyroidism, and a return to normal function.

○ **What is the etiology of de Quervain thyroiditis?**

Most likely caused by viral illness since episodes often follow upper respiratory infections and are associated with various viruses including influenza, adenovirus, mumps, and coxsackievirus.

○ **What is the diagnostic approach to evaluating thyroid nodules?**

Evaluation is primarily related to the need to exclude thyroid cancer.

History: Increased risk of malignancy with rapid growth of a neck mass, childhood head and neck irradiation, total-body irradiation for bone marrow transplantation, family history of thyroid cancer, or thyroid cancer syndromes.

Physical: Fixed hard mass, obstructive symptoms, cervical lymphadenopathy, or vocal cord paralysis suggest possibility of cancer.

Diagnostic testing:

- If TSH is low, there is an increased possibility that the nodule is hyperfunctioning and thyroid scintigraphy should be performed next.
- If TSH is normal or elevated, then fine needle aspiration (FNA) biopsy is indicated.
- Thyroid scintigraphy determines the functional status of a nodule. It can be used to select nodules for FNA, but not for surgical resection.
- Ultrasound assesses nodule size, thyroid gland anatomy, and adjacent structures in the neck and is superior to thyroid scintigraphy.
- FNA biopsy with cytologic examination is the procedure of choice and most accurate method for evaluating thyroid nodules and candidates for resection.

○ **How are thyroid scintigraphy findings interpreted?**

Nonfunctioning: Appear cold (uptake is less than surrounding thyroid tissue) and are associated with higher index of suspicion of cancer.

Autonomous: Appear hot (uptake is greater than surrounding thyroid tissue) and are associated with lower index of suspicion of cancer.

Indeterminate: Should be evaluated by FNA.

○ **What is the most common thyroid carcinoma?**

- Papillary (80%)
- Follicular (14%)
- Medullary (3%)
- Anaplastic (2%)

○ **What is sick euthyroid syndrome?**

Abnormal thyroid function tests without thyroid disease associated with conditions such as severe illness, caloric deprivation, or major surgery.

○ **What is the diagnosis of sick euthyroid syndrome based on?**

Diagnosis is based on excluding secondary hypothyroidism.

DISEASES OF THE PARATHYROID GLAND

○ **What is primary hyperparathyroidism the most common cause of?**

Hypercalcemia.

○ **What determines the regulation of the parathyroid gland?**

Serum calcium levels.

○ **What are the main effects of parathyroid hormone (PTH)?**

Causes a net increase in serum calcium by

- increasing osteoclastic activity in bone.
- increasing the renal tubular reabsorption of calcium.
- stimulating the synthesis of 1,25-dihydroxycholecalciferol by the kidney.
- inhibiting absorption of phosphate and bicarbonate by the renal tubule.

○ **What is pseudohypoparathyroidism?**

Characterized by renal tubular resistance to PTH causing hypercalciuria with resultant hypocalcemia, hyperphosphatemia, and additional features known as Albright heredity osteodystrophy including mental retardation, short stature, obesity, round face, short fourth metacarpals, hypothyroidism, ectopic bone formation, and hyogonadism.

○ **What are the etiologies of hyperparathyroidism?**

Primary hyperparathyroidism:

- Single parathyroid adenoma (80%)
- Hyperplasia by two or more parathyroid glands (20%)
- Carcinoma (<1%)

Secondary hyperparathyroidism:

- Physiologic response to low calcium level usually as a result of renal disease

○ **What are the clinical manifestations of hyperparathyroidism?**

Skeletal: Low bone density

Associated with hypercalcemia: "Bones, stones, abdominal groans, psychic moans, with fatigue overtones."

- Bone pain and arthralgias
- Kidney stones (calcium)
- Abdominal pain, nausea, vomiting, heartburn
- Depression, irritability, cognitive impairment, insomnia
- Fatigue

○ **What are the diagnostic laboratory findings seen in hyperparathyroidism?**

The hallmark of primary hyperparathyroidism is hypercalcemia along with an elevated serum level of intact PTH which confirms the diagnosis.

○ **What are the indications for surgical treatment of hyperparathyroidism?**

- 1 mg/dL above the upper limit of the reference range for serum calcium
- 24-hour urinary calcium excretion >400 mg
- A 30% reduction in creatinine clearance
- Bone mineral density T-score below −2.5 at any site
- Age younger than 50 years

○ **What are the etiologies of hypoparathyroidism?**

- Following thyroidectomy or parathyroidectomy
- Autoimmune
- Damage from heavy metals (copper or iron)
- Magnesium deficiency
- Congenital

○ **What are the clinical manifestations of hypoparathyroidism?**

Symptoms: Tetany, muscle cramps, carpopedal spasm, irritability, altered mental status, convulsions, tingling of the circumoral area, hands, and feet.

Signs: Positive Chvostek sign (facial muscle contraction on tapping the facial nerve in front of the ear), and positive Trousseau sign (carpal spasm after application of a sphygmomanometer cuff).

○ **What are the laboratory findings associated with hypoparathyroidism?**

Diagnostic triad: Low serum calcium, high serum phosphate, and low PTH; low magnesium, low urinary calcium, and normal alkaline phosphatase.

○ **What are the treatment options for hyperparathyroidism?**

Surgical: Parathyroidectomy.

Medical: Large fluid intake unless contraindicated, Vitamin D and vitamin D analogs.

○ **What is the maintenance treatment for hypoparathyroidism?**

Goals of management:

- Maintain serum calcium in a slightly low, but asymptomatic range of 8 to 8.6 mg/dL (2–2.15 mmol/L) to minimize hypercalciuria,
- prevent damage to kidney function.
- Calcium supplementation (1 g/day) is given along with a vitamin D preparation (e.g., calcitriol, ergocalciferol, teriparatide).
- Monitoring serum calcium at regular intervals (at least every 3 months) is mandatory.

DISEASES OF THE ADRENAL GLAND

○ **What are the components of adrenals glands?**

Adrenal cortex (outer layer):

- Largest part of the gland.
- Divided into three zones from exterior to interior are the zona glomerulosa, zona fasciculata, and zona reticularis.
- Secretes three types of hormones including mineralocorticoids (most important is aldosterone) by zona glomerulosa, glucocorticoids (mainly cortisol) predominately by the zona fasciculata, and adrenal androgen (mainly DHEA) predominately by the zona reticularis.

Adrenal medulla (inner layer):

- Composed of chromaffin cells.
- Produce epinephrine and norepinephrine.

○ **How are the adrenal gland hormones regulated?**

- Aldosterone, cortisol, and dehydroepiandrosterone (DHEA) are regulated by adrenocorticotropic hormone (ACTH) from the pituitary.
- Aldosterone is also regulated by the renin–angiotensin system.
- DHEA is also regulated by circulating levels of testosterone and estrogens.

○ **What are the effects of the adrenal cortex hormones aldosterone, cortisol, and DHEA?**

- Aldosterone is a major regulator of sodium, potassium, and fluid balance.
- Cortisol majorly affects protein, glucose, and fat metabolism.
- DHEA is a precursor steroid to testosterone and estradiol.

○ **What is acute and chronic adrenocortical insufficiency?**

- Acute adrenocortical insufficiency (adrenal crisis) is an emergency caused by insufficient cortisol.
- Chronic adrenocortical insufficiency or primary adrenal insufficiency (Addison disease) is caused by dysfunction or absence of the adrenal cortices.

○ **What are the etiologies of primary adrenal insufficiency?**

- Autoimmune destruction (most common as Addison disease)
- Tuberculosis (leading cause where TB is prevalent)
- Adrenal hemorrhage (i.e., sepsis, anticoagulation therapy, antiphospholipid antibody syndrome)
- Congenital

○ **What are causes of adrenal crisis?**

- Stress (e.g., trauma, surgery, infection, hyperthyroidism, or prolonged fasting) in a patient with latent or treated adrenal insufficiency.
- Sudden withdrawal of adrenocortical hormone in a patient with chronic insufficiency or temporary insufficiency (suppression by exogenous corticosteroids).
- Bilateral adrenalectomy or removal of a functioning adrenal tumor that suppressed the other adrenal.
- Sudden destruction of the pituitary gland (pituitary necrosis).
- Injury to both adrenals (e.g., trauma, hemorrhage, anticoagulant therapy, thrombosis, infection, or metastatic carcinoma).
- Administration of etomidate (rapid anesthesia induction or intubation).

○ **What is secondary adrenal insufficiency?**

Deficient secretion of ACTH by the pituitary gland which may be isolated or occur in conjunction with other pituitary hormone deficiencies.

○ **What are the clinical manifestations of adrenal insufficiency?**

- Muscle weakness, fatigue, fever, anorexia, nausea, vomiting, weight loss, hypotension, salt craving, orthostasis, anxiety, mental irritability, and depression.

Significant pain:

- Arthralgias, myalgias, chest pain, abdominal pain, back pain, leg pain, or headache.
- Changes in skin pigmentation from none at all to dark diffuse tanning over nonexposed as well as exposed areas. Hyperpigmentation is prominent over the knuckles, elbows, knees, posterior neck, palmar creases, and gingival mucosa.

○ **What are causes of secondary adrenal insufficiency?**

- Iatrogenic (adrenal suppression from prolonged steroid use)
- Pituitary or hypothalamic tumors
- Long-term glucocorticoid therapy
- Sheehan syndrome
- Traumatic brain injury
- Subarachnoid hemorrhage

○ **What are common laboratory findings associated with adrenocortical insufficiency?**

- WBC count with moderate neutropenia, lymphocytosis, and total eosinophil count over 300/µL
- Low serum Na^+
- Elevated K^+
- Low fasting blood glucose

○ **What laboratory findings are diagnostic for adrenocortical insufficiency?**

- Low plasma cortisol (<3 µg/dL or <83 nmol/L) in the morning (8 AM).
- Elevation of plasma ACTH level (>200 pg/mL or >44 pmol/L).
- Cortisol levels are low or fail to rise after giving cosyntropin (ACTH1-24) stimulation test (confirmatory).

○ **What is the management for primary adrenal insufficiency (Addison disease)?**

Replacement therapy with a combination of corticosteroids and mineralocorticoids. Hydrocortisone is the drug of choice. Adjustments in dosage are made according to the clinical response. A proper dose usually results in a normal WBC count differential.

○ **What is Cushing syndrome and its causes?**

Manifestations of prolonged exposure to elevated levels of endogenous or exogenous glucocorticoids. Endogenous glucocorticoid overproduction (hypercortisolism) that is independent of ACTH is usually caused by primary adrenocortical neoplasm (usually adenoma, but rarely carcinoma).

○ **How does Cushing syndrome differ from Cushing disease?**

Cushing disease accounts for about 40% of Cushing syndrome cases in which manifestations of hypercortisolism are caused by ACTH hypersecretion by the pituitary as a result of a benign pituitary adenoma.

○ **What are the clinical manifestations of Cushing syndrome?**

Central obesity, moon facies, buffalo hump, supraclavicular fat pads, thin extremities, purple striae (thighs, breasts, abdomen), easy bruisability psychologic changes, osteoporosis, hypertension, poor wound healing, growth retardation (children), oligomenorrhea or amenorrhea (women).

○ **What laboratory findings are diagnostic for Cushing syndrome (hypercortisolism)?**

Administer high dose overnight dexamethasone suppression test. Results are normal if cortisol is suppressed (no Cushing syndrome). If results are abnormal, administer a 24-hour urine free cortisol (UFC) test. UFC results will reflect a high ACTH level if there is a pituitary tumor (Cushing disease resulting in Cushing syndrome) or ectopic tumor (e.g., small cell lung cancer) or low ACTH for a probable adrenal tumor.

○ **What is the best treatment for Cushing syndrome?**

Transsphenoidal selective resection of the pituitary adenoma.

○ **What is primary hyperaldosteronism and its clinical manifestations?**

Inappropriately high aldosterone secretion that does not suppress adequately with sodium loading and contributes to hypertension, resistant hypertension, hypokalemia, muscular weakness, paresthesias with frank tetany, headache, polyuria, and polydipsia.

○ **What are the laboratory findings associated with hyperaldosteronism?**

- Low plasma potassium
- Low plasma renin activity (PRA)
- Aldosterone: PRA ratio >67
- High plasma and urine aldosterone levels with low urine PRA (confirmatory)

○ **What are the treatment options for hyperaldosteronism?**

Major goals of therapy include normalization of blood pressure, serum potassium levels and other electrolytes, and serum aldosterone levels. Treatment options include:

- Surgical intervention for apparent adrenal adenoma.
- Medical therapy is indicated for idiopathic adrenal hyperplasia, preoperatively for persistent hypertension postoperatively, poor surgical candidates, and those who refuse surgery. Treatment includes antihypertensive medication and correction of electrolyte abnormalities. Spironolactone and eplerenone can achieve blood pressure control and normalization of electrolytes.

○ **What is a pheochromocytoma?**

Rare fatal tumor of the sympathetic nervous system that arises from the adrenal medulla and usually secretes both epinephrine and norepinephrine. Extra-adrenal pheochromocytomas (i.e., paragangliomas) arise from sympathetic paraganglia, often metastasize, and secrete norepinephrine or are nonsecretory. Tumors that secrete catecholamines have an affinity for chromium salts and are known as "chromaffin" tumors.

○ **What are the most common clinical manifestations of pheochromocytomas?**

Paroxysmal episodes produce hypertension, severe headache, perspiration, palpitations, anxiety, a sense of impending doom, or tremor.

○ **What is the etiology and incidence of pheochromocytoma?**

- Majority are sporadic and approximately 30% result from inherited mutations (e.g., MEN 2A and 2B, neurofibromatosis, VHL disease).
- Incidence is rare (0.05%–0.2% of hypertensive individuals) and may occur in people of all races and any age. Peak incidence is the third to fifth decades of life.

○ **What laboratory findings are diagnostic for pheochromocytoma?**

- Plasma fractionated free metanephrines is the single most sensitive test for secretory pheochromocytomas and paragangliomas.
- Urinary assay for total metanephrines is confirmatory.

○ **What are the treatment options for pheochromocytoma?**

Surgical: Resection of pheochromocytomas or abdominal paragangliomas is the treatment of choice.

Medical: Antihypertensive medications.

- Long-acting nonselective alpha blocker phenoxybenazmine and alpha-1-blockers such as doxazosin, terazosin, or prazosin (preparatory to surgery and maintenance).
- Calcium channel blockers nifedipine ER or nicardipine ER (long-term use and acute hypertensive crisis).
- Beta blockers like metoprolol XR are often required after institution of alpha blockade or calcium channel blockade.

DISEASES OF THE PITUITARY GLAND

○ **What are the effects of the anterior and posterior pituitary hormones?**

Anterior pituitary:

- Adrenocorticotropic hormone (ACTH) stimulates production of adrenal gland hormones which regulate water and sodium balance, inflammation, and metabolism.
- Growth hormone (GH) exerts direct and indirect effects on tissue growth and differentiation.
- Prolactin (PRL) stimulates breast development and milk production.
- Thyroid stimulating hormone (TSH) stimulates thyroid gland hormone production which regulate growth, differentiation, and energy balance.
- Luteinizing hormone (LH) and follicle stimulating hormone (FSH) stimulate gonadal production of sex steroids which mediate reproductive function and behavior.

Posterior pituitary:

- Arginine vasopressin (AVP) (i.e., antidiuretic hormone) increases water reabsorption by the kidneys and increases vascular resistance.
- Oxytocin stimulates milk ejection and uterine contraction.

○ **What are the characteristics of pituitary tumors?**

- Usually in the anterior pituitary
- Usually benign (adenoma)
- Functioning (majority) or nonfunctioning (secreting inactive hormones)
- Most common functioning pituitary adenomas include PRL-producing or prolactinoma (majority), GH-producing, ACTH-producing, and TSH-producing
- Size classification: Microadenoma (<1 cm) or macroadenoma (>1 cm)

○ **What symptoms are commonly associated with pituitary tumors?**

- Mass effects
- Hypersecretion of one of the pituitary gland products

○ **What are the most common clinical manifestations of a prolactinoma?**

Hormonal effects of excess PRL:

- Menstrual cycle disturbances (e.g., oligomenorrhea, amenorrhea, irregularities) and/or infertility
- Galactorrhea (women)
- Hypogonadism in men (e.g., decreased libido, erectile dysfunction, infertility)

Space occupying (mass) effects:

- Headache
- Visual field defects (bitemporal hemianopsia) to total vision loss and ophthalmoplegia
- Other hormone deficiencies (compression of hormone secreting pituitary cells)

○ **What diagnostic testing is indicated for evaluation of prolactinoma?**

Laboratory studies: Serum PRL, serum hCG (pregnancy), serum TSH and free T4 (hypothyroidism), BUN and serum creatinine (kidney disease), liver function tests (cirrhosis), serum calcium (hyperparathyroidism), LH, FSH, and serum total and free testosterone (men).

Imaging: If other causes are ruled out, evaluate with MRI of the pituitary hypothalamic area with gadolinium enhancement (soft tissue delineation and small lesions) or CT scan with contrast (bone destruction or distortion).

○ **What are the treatment options for prolactinomas?**

Surgical: Transsphenoidal pituitary adenomectomy (preferred surgical treatment)

Medical: Bromocriptine or cabergoline (bromocriptine not well tolerated or unresponsive to bromocriptine)

○ **What is diabetes insipidus?**

An uncommon disease caused by deficiency of (central) or resistance to (nephrogenic) AVP which results in increased thirst and passage of large quantities of urine with low specific gravity.

○ **What is the most common cause of acromegaly?**

Growth hormone secreting pituitary adenoma or hyperplasia.

○ **What is the difference between gigantism and acromegaly?**

- Gigantism refers to abnormally high linear growth originating from primary GH excess released from the pituitary while the epiphyseal plates are open during childhood.
- Acromegaly is the same disorder, but occurs after the growth plate cartilage fuses in adulthood.

○ **What are the clinical manifestations of gigantism and acromegaly?**

- Tall stature, excessive growth of hands, feet, jaw, and internal organs
- Soft, doughy, sweaty handshake
- Amenorrhea, headaches, visual field loss, weakness
- Macroglossia
- Insulin resistance
- Hypertension, cardiomegaly

○ **What are the most common etiologies of central diabetes insipidus (DI)?**

- Idiopathic (autoimmune)
- Malignant or benign tumors of the brain or pituitary
- Cranial surgery
- Head trauma
- Hereditary

○ **What are the clinical manifestations of diabetes insipidus?**

- Intense thirst (especially with a craving for ice water)
- Ingesting large volumes of fluid (2 to 20 L daily)
- Polyuria (corresponds to ingested fluid)
- Hypernatremia and dehydration (if no access to water)

○ **What diagnostic testing should be done to evaluate for diabetes insipidus (DI)?**

24-hour urine collection:
- Volume (volume of <2L/24 hours in the absence of hypernatremia rules out DI)
- Urinary specific gravity (1.005 or less is hallmark for DI)
- Urinary osmolality (<200 mOsm/kg is hallmark for DI)

Vasopressin challenge test:
- Administer desmopressin acetate usually intranasally
- Measure urine volume for 12 hours before and 12 hours after administration
- Patients with central DI notice distinct reduction in thirst and polyuria

MRI of the pituitary and hypothalamus:
- Mass lesions
- Pituitary stalk thickening (Langerhans cell histiocytosis, sarcoidosis, lymphocytic hypophysitis)
- Absence of hyperintense signal (bright spot) in the posterior pituitary with central DI

○ **What is the treatment for central diabetes insipidus (DI)?**

Desmopressin (intranasal, oral, IM, SC) is the treatment of choice.

○ **What is anterior hypopituitarism?**

Partial or complete deficiency of one or any combination of anterior pituitary hormones.

○ **What are causes of anterior hypopituitarism?**

- Lesions (e.g., adenomas, pituitary tumors, granulomas, apoplexy, metastatic carcinomas, aneurysms) in the hypothalamus, pituitary stalk, or pituitary
- Congenital
- Iatrogenic (e.g., cranial radiation, pituitary surgery, CABG)
- Infection (i.e., encephalitis)
- Autoimmunity
- Injury (e.g., traumatic brain injury, subarachnoid hemorrhage, stroke)

○ **What is the presentation and effects of growth hormone (GH) deficiency?**

- **Childhood** (congenital or acquired): Hypoglycemia, hypogonadism, growth failure (infancy); short stature, low growth velocity for age, and delayed puberty or no sexual development (childhood).
- **Adulthood** (between fourth and fifth decades often with discovery of pituitary tumors): Mild to moderate central obesity, increased systolic blood pressure, increased low density lipoprotein, reduced cardiac output, reduced muscle and bone mass, physical and mental energy, impaired concentration and memory, depression.

○ **What is the etiology and clinical manifestations of congenital growth hormone (GH) deficiency?**

- Pituitary dwarfism (few cases) with normal body proportions because of the affected overall growth and normal mental development.
- Laron syndrome (Laron-type dwarfism) is an autosomal recessive disorder mainly associated with mutations in GH receptor gene. This causes resistance to GH and severe insulin-like growth factor-I (IGF-I) deficiency which results in short stature. Present with features of prominent forehead, depressed nasal bridge, small mandible, and central obesity.

○ **What diagnostic studies are indicated for diagnosis of GH deficiency?**

- Difficult to diagnose since GH secretion is normally pulsatile and nearly undetectable most of the day; as well as, adults produce less GH with age. GH deficiency may be inferred by symptoms or history (e.g., pituitary surgery or treatment, other pituitary hormone deficiencies).
- GH stimulation (provocative) testing: Insulin tolerance test (ITT) and growth hormone-releasing hormone (GHRH) with or without arginine. There is a high frequency of false negative results with GH stimulation testing which may require two provocative tests that meet certain criteria.

○ **What are the treatment options for GH deficiency?**

- **Surgical:** Resection of pituitary tumors
- **Medical:** Subcutaneous recombinant human growth hormone (rhGH, somatropin)

○ **What are the clinical manifestations of gonadotropin deficiency (central hypogonadism)?**

Childhood (congenital):
- Partial or lack of pubertal development
- Kallmann syndrome, Prader–Willi syndrome

Adulthood (acquired):
- Loss of secondary sexual characteristics (axillary, pubic, and body hair)
- Infertility
- Hypogonadism (decreased libido and impotence)
- Amenorrhea
- Predisposition to osteopenia and muscle atrophy

○ **What diagnostic studies are indicated to determine gonadotropin deficiency?**

Men: Serum total testosterone and free testosterone (older men). Serum FSH and LH if serum testosterone is low to distinguish primary hypogonadism from pituitary dysfunction.
Women: Serum FSH and LH.

○ **What is the treatment for gonadotropin deficiency?**

Replace end-organ hormones (estrogen, progesterone, testosterone).

DIABETES MELLITUS

○ **What is the most common cause of hypoglycemia in patients with diabetes mellitus (DM)?**

Reaction to insulin injection, skipping a meal, or overdosing insulin.

○ **What are the two principal types of spontaneous hypoglycemia and their clinical manifestations?**

- Fasting hypoglycemia that is often subacute or chronic and usually presents with neuroglycopenia including symptoms of weakness, tiredness, dizziness, inappropriate behavior, difficulty with concentration, confusion, blurred vision, and coma or death if extreme.
- Postprandial hypoglycemia is acute with neurogenic (adrenergic) symptoms of sweating, palpitations, anxiety, tremulousness, and sensation of hunger.

○ **What is the management for hypoglycemia?**

- Mainstay of therapy is glucose as well as other medications based on the underlying cause and symptoms. Common medications used include glucose supplements (e.g., dextrose), glucose-elevating agents (e.g., glucagon), inhibitors of insulin secretion (e.g., diazoxide, octreotide), and antineoplastic agents (e.g., streptozocin).
- Dietary therapy with restriction of refined carbohydrates, avoidance of simple sugars, increased meal frequency, and increased protein and fiber.

○ **What is the criteria for pre-diabetes according to the National Health Institutes National Diabetes Education Program?**

1. Fasting plasma glucose (FPG) 100 to 125 mg/dL (impaired fasting glucose) or

2. 2-hour post 75 g oral glucose challenge 140 to 199 mg/dL (impaired glucose tolerance) or

3. A1c 5.7% to 6.4%

For all tests, risk of diabetes is continuous, extending below the lower limit of the range and becoming disproportionately greater at higher ends of the range.

○ **How is the etiology of type 1 DM different from type 2 DM?**

- Type 1 DM is associated with human leukocyte antigens (HLA), autoimmunity, and or islet cell antibodies.
- Type 2 DM usually involves a genetic mutation resulting in inactive pancreatic and liver enzymes as well as insulin receptor defects leading to resistance.

○ **What is the most important environmental factor contributing to insulin resistance?**

Obesity.

○ **What are the common clinical manifestations associated with diabetes mellitus?**

- Common features of type 1 and 2 diabetes mellitus include: Polyuria, polydipsia, weakness or fatigue, recurrent blurred vision, vulvovaginitis or pruritus, and peripheral neuropathy.
- Type 1 diabetes mellitus also includes polyphagia with weight loss and nocturnal enuresis. While with type 2 diabetes mellitus, obesity is common, chronic skin infections, and many patients having few or no symptoms.

○ **What is the current criteria for diagnosis of diabetes according to the National Institutes of Health National Diabetes Education Program?**

1. A1c >6.5% or

2. Fasting plasma glucose >126 mg/dL or

3. 2-hour plasma glucose >200 mg/dL post 75 g oral glucose challenge or

4. Random plasma glucose >200 mg/dL with symptoms (polyuria, polydypsia, and unexplained weight loss)

For criteria 1 to 3: Repeat test to confirm unless symptoms are present. It is preferable that the same test be repeated for confirmation. If two different tests are used (e.g., FPG and A1c) and both indicate diabetes, consider the diagnosis confirmed. If the two different tests are discordant, repeat the test above the diagnostic cut point.

○ **What is hemoglobin A1c and its utilization for diagnosis of diabetes mellitus?**

Hemoglobin A1c is the fraction of nonenzymatic irreversible glycation of hemoglobin by plasma glucose. It is abnormally elevated in diabetic persons with chronic hyperglycemia. Since glycohemoglobins circulate within red blood cells whose life span lasts up to 120 days, they generally reflect the state of glycemia over the preceding 8 to 12 weeks and provide a method to assess diabetic control.

○ **What are the common complications or late manifestations associated with uncontrolled or chronic diabetes mellitus?**

Hypertension, end-stage chronic kidney disease, blindness, autonomic and peripheral neuropathy, amputations of the lower extremities, myocardial infarction, and cerebrovascular accidents.

○ **What are the ocular complications associated with uncontrolled or chronic diabetes?**

Cataracts, retinopathy (proliferative is leading cause of blindness), and glaucoma (uncommon).

○ **What are the common peripheral and autonomic neuropathy complications associated with uncontrolled or chronic diabetes?**

Peripheral: Distal symmetric polyneuropathy with loss of function in a stocking-glove pattern (most common), neuropathic plantar ulcers, and painful diabetic neuropathy with hypersensitivity to light touch and occasionally severe "burning" pain.

Autonomic: Gastroparesis, incomplete emptying of the bladder, and erectile dysfunction.

○ **What are the associated renal complications with uncontrolled or chronic diabetes mellitus? What can be done to prevent or slow its progression?**

Diabetic nephropathy. Prevention includes glycemic control and angiotensin inhibition with antihypertensive agents such as an angiotensin converting enzyme inhibitor (ACE-I) or an angiotensin receptor blocker (ARB).

○ **What is the initial manifestation of diabetic nephropathy?**

Proteinuria.

○ **What are the factors that contribute to the increased incidence of gangrene of the feet in diabetics?**

Peripheral vascular and small vessel disease, peripheral neuropathy with loss of both pain sensation and neurogenic inflammatory responses, and secondary infection.

○ **What is the Somogyi effect?**

A hyperglycemic event that results from an overzealous response by counter regulatory hormones during a period of hypoglycemia.

○ **What is the Dawn phenomenon?**

A term used to describe an abnormal early-morning (usually between 4 and 8 AM) increase in blood sugar in patients with diabetes. The dawn phenomenon is more common in people with type 1 diabetes than with type 2 diabetes.

○ **What are the current treatment recommendations made by the American Diabetes Association for diabetes mellitus?**

- Weight loss + exercise + metformin
- If HgA1c target not reached after almost 3 months: Metformin + another agent
- If HgA1c target not reached after almost 3 months: Metformin + 2 other agents
- If HgA1c target not reached after almost 3 months: Metformin + more complex insulin regimen ± other noninsulin agent

○ **What are the main classes of medications for treatment of type 2 diabetes mellitus?**

- Biguanides (metformin)
- Sulfonylureas (glimepiride, glipizide, glyburide)
- Meglitinide analogs and D-phenylalanine derivative (nateglinide, repaglinide)
- Thiazolidinediones (pioglitazone)
- GLP-1 receptor agonists (exenatide)
- DPP-4 inhibitors (sitagliptin)
- Insulins

○ **What are the available insulin preparations in the United States?**

Short-acting insulin: Regular insulin has an onset of 30 minutes, peaks at 2.5 to 5 hours, and a duration of 4 to 12 hours.

Rapid acting insulin analogs: Insulin lispro (Humulog), aspart (Novolog), and glulisine (Apidra) have an onset of 5 to 10 minutes, peak at 45 to 75 minutes, and a duration of 2 to 4 hours.

Intermediate-acting insulin: NPH insulin has an onset of 1 to 2 hours, peaks at 4 to 12 hours, and a duration of 14 to 24 hours.

Long-acting insulin: Insulins glargine lasts for about 24 hours without any peaks. Insulin detemir lasts about 17 hours without any peaks.

○ **What elements need to be monitored in the management of diabetes mellitus at routine visits?**

- Weight
- Blood pressure
- Foot examination
- Self-monitoring glucose record
- Review or adjust medications to control glucose, blood pressure, and lipids
- Review self-management skills, dietary needs, and physical activity
- Assess for depression or other mood disorder
- Counsel on smoking cessation and alcohol use

○ **What elements need to be monitored annually in the management of diabetes mellitus?**

- Quarterly hemoglobin A1c in patients whose therapy has changed or who are not meeting glycemic goals or twice a year if at goal with stable glycemia.
- Fasting lipid profile (every 2 years if low risk).
- Serum creatinine to estimate glomerular filtration rate and estimate the level of chronic kidney disease.
- Urine test for albumin-to-creatinine ratio in patients with type 1 diabetes >5 years and in all patients with type 2 diabetes.
- Dilated eye examination.
- Comprehensive foot examination.
- Dental/oral examination at least once a year.
- Administer influenza vaccination.
- Administer pneumococcal vaccination.

○ **What are the treatment goals for diabetes mellitus according to the National Health Institutes National Diabetic Education Program?**

A1c <7% for many people

- Preprandial capillary plasma glucose 70 to 130 mg/dL
- Peak postprandial capillary plasma glucose <180 mg/dL usually 1 to 2 hours after the start of a meal

Blood pressure (mm Hg)

- Systolic <130 for most people
- Diastolic <80

Cholesterol-lipid profile (mg/L)

- LDL cholesterol <100
- HDL cholesterol men >40, women >50
- Triglycerides <150

Individualize target levels based on patient characteristics, response to therapy, and hypoglycemia.

○ **What are the common causes of abdominal pain, nausea, and vomiting in a diabetic patient?**

Diabetic gastroparesis, gallbladder disease, pancreatitis, and, perhaps, ischemia bowel.

○ **What are some agents used to treat severe diabetic gastroparesis?**

Cisapride and metoclopramide are the key agents. Erythromycin has also been tried in very severe cases.

○ **What are the signs and symptoms of diabetic ketoacidosis (DKA)?**

- Nausea/vomiting with abdominal pain
- Hyperventilation (Kussmaul respirations)
- Hypotension/shock
- Polyuria, polydipsia, and weight loss

○ **What laboratory findings are expected with DKA?**

- Hyperglycemia >250 mg/dL (13.9 mmol/L)
- Acidosis with blood pH <7.3
- Serum bicarbonate <15 mEq/L
- Serum positive for ketones (acetone)
- Ketonuria and glucosuria

○ **What is the most important initial step in treating DKA?**

Volume replacement, with the first liter administered over about 60 minutes.

○ **What major insults are likely to lead to DKA in an otherwise controlled diabetic patient?**

Always look for infection (even a minor one), cardiac ischemia, medications, and lack of compliance with insulin and diet.

REFERENCES

ADA clinical practice recommendations. American Diabetes Association Website. http://professional.diabetes.org/ResourcesFor Professionals.aspx?cid=84160. Updated January 2013. Accessed August 2013, September 2013.

Arlt W. Chapter 342. Disorders of the adrenal cortex. In: Longo DL, Fauci AS, Kasper DL, Hauser SL, Jameson JL, Loscalzo J, eds. *Harrison's Principles of Internal Medicine.* 18th ed. New York, NY: McGraw-Hill; 2012. http://www.accessmedicine.com/content. aspx?aID=9140931. Accessed August 2013, September 2013.

Diabetes numbers at-a-glance. National Diabetes Education Program Website. http://ndep.nih.gov/publications/PublicationDetail. aspx? PubId=114. Updated March 2012. Accessed September 2013.

Dynamed [database online]. Ipswich (MA): EBSCO Information Services. http://www.ebscohost.com.evms.idm.oclc.org/DynaMed/. Accessed July 2013 to September 2013.

Fitzgerald PA. Chapter 26. Endocrine disorders. In: Papadakis MA, McPhee SJ, Rabow MW, Berger TG, eds. *CURRENT Medical Diagnosis & Treatment 2014.* New York, NY: McGraw-Hill; 2013. http://www.accessmedicine.com/content.aspx?aID=14198. Accessed July 2013, August 2013, September 2013.

Gonzalez-Campoy JM, Hypoparathyroidism. In: Griffing GT, ed. *Medscape Family Medicine Reference.* New York, NY: Medscape; 2013.

Jameson JL. Chapter 338. Principles of endocrinology. In: Longo DL, Fauci AS, Kasper DL, Hauser SL, Jameson JL, Loscalzo J, eds. *Harrison's Principles of Internal Medicine.* 18th ed. New York, NY: McGraw-Hill; 2012. http://www.accessmedicine.com/content. aspx?aID=9139719. Accessed July 2013, August 2013.

Khardori R, Type 1 diabetes mellitus. In: Griffing GT, ed. *Medscape Reference.* New York, NY: Medscape; 2013.

Kim L, Hyperparathyroidism. In: Griffing GT, ed. *Medscape Family Medicine Reference.*, New York, NY: Medscape; 2012.

Masharani U. Chapter 27. Diabetes mellitus & hypoglycemia. In: Papadakis MA, McPhee SJ, Rabow MW, Berger TG, eds. *CURRENT Medical Diagnosis & Treatment 2014.* New York, NY: McGraw-Hill; 2013. http://www.accessmedicine.com/content. aspx?aID=15524. Accessed August 2013, September 2013.

Melmed S, Jameson JL. Chapter 339. Disorders of the anterior pituitary and hypothalamus. In: Longo DL, Fauci AS, Kasper DL, Hauser SL, Jameson JL, Loscalzo J, eds. *Harrison's Principles of Internal Medicine.* 18th ed. New York, NY: McGraw-Hill; 2012. http://www.accessmedicine.com/content.aspx?aID=9139876. Accessed August 2013, September 2013.

Melmed S, Polonsky K, Larsen PR, Kronenber HM. *Williams Textbook of Endocrinology.* 12th ed. Philadelphia, PA: Elsevier Saunders. 2011.

Molina, PE, Ashman, R. E*ndocrine Physiology.* 4th ed. New York, NY: McGraw-Hill Companies, Inc.; 2013.

Mulinda JR, Goiter. In: Griffing GT, ed. *Medscape Reference.* New York, NY: Medscape; 2013.

Ross DS, Diagnostic approach to and treatment of thyroid nodules. In: Cooper DS, ed. *UpToDate.* Waltham, MA: UpToDate; 2013.

Ross DS, Diagnosis of and screening for hypothyroidism. In: Cooper DS, ed. *UpToDate.* Waltham, MA: UpToDate; 2013.

Weetman AP, Jameson JL. Chapter 341. Disorders of the thyroid gland. In: Longo DL, Fauci AS, Kasper DL, Hauser SL, Jameson JL, Loscalzo J, eds. *Harrison's Principles of Internal Medicine.* 18th ed. New York, NY: McGraw-Hill; 2012. http://www. accessmedicine. com/content.aspx?aID=9140510. Accessed August 2013, September 2013.

CHAPTER 5

EENT (Eyes, Ears, Nose, Throat)

David J. Klocko, MPAS, PA-C

EYE

O **What is a hordeolum?**

A meibomian gland infection, usually of the upper lid.

O **What is a pinguecula?**

It is a yellowish nodule, particularly on the nasal aspect of the eye, but it may be lateral. It is often caused by wind and dust.

O **What is a pterygium?**

It is a chronic growth over the medial or lateral aspect of the cornea approaching the pupil. It is much thicker than pingueculae.

O **What is the most common cause of orbital cellulitis?**

Staphylococcus aureus.

O **What is a chalazion?**

This is a meibomian gland granuloma. A painless localized swelling that develops over the course of a few weeks.

O **An elderly patient presents with bilateral eye irritation. He states this persists despite using eye-lubricating drops. On physical examination you notice his lower eyelid margins are rolled in and his eyelashes appear to be rubbing against the conjunctiva and cornea. What is this condition called?**

Entropion. This is an inward turning of the eyelid margin from a degeneration of the eyelid fascia. For cases that involve continual irritation of the cornea from the eyelashes, surgery is indicated. **Ectropion** also occurs at an advanced age, and creates and outward turning or drooping of the lower eyelid. Complications from this are excessive tearing, exposure keratitis and bad cosmetic appearance.

O **What are the clinical history and physical examination findings of a Central Retinal Vein Occlusion?**

Sudden painless vision loss. Physical findings can range from a few hemorrhages and cotton wool spots to a massive superficial and deep hemorrhage with vitreous involvement.

○ **A patient presents with a painful reddened area over the tear duct at the nasal side of his right eye. A small amount of pus is draining from the tear duct. What is this condition called?**

Dacryocystitis. The most common pathogens for acute dacryocystitis are *Staphylococcus aureus*, and beta-hemolytic streptococci. In chronic dacryocystitis, candida albicans, anaerobic streptococci, and *Staphylococcus epidermidis* can be causative pathogens. Treatment is with systemic antibiotics.

○ **An elderly patient complains of decreasing central vision clarity. He has long smoking history. Upon physical examination you notice Drusen formations and retinal atrophy when you do the direct ophthalmoscopic examination. What condition is likely?**

Age-related macular degeneration.

○ **What medications are likely to exacerbate angle closure glaucoma?**

Anticholinergics, antihistamines, antidepressants, benzodiazepine, carbonic anhydrase inhibitors, CNS stimulants, phenothiazine, sympathomimetics, theophylline, and vasodilators.

○ **A child with blurry vision has an abnormal pupillary reflex and a white reflex upon funduscopic examination. What is the likely diagnosis?**

This is a retinoblastoma that can grow to other sites in the brain or body. Surgical removal is indicated. This condition is inheritable and thus the parents should be counseled about the risks.

○ **How should a chalazion be treated?**

Surgical curettage.

○ **A patient presents with eye pain. She has a constricted pupil, ciliary flush, and pain to the affected eye when the penlight is shined in the unaffected eye. Diagnosis?**

Acute iritis.

○ **A patient presents with loss of central vision. What is the most likely diagnosis?**

A retrobulbar neuritis is likely. MS is associated with about 25% of retrobulbar neuritis cases. Macular degeneration and central retinal vein occlusion can also lead to loss of central vision.

○ **What is the most common cause of periorbital and orbital infections?**

Staphylococcus aureus, Streptococcus pneumoniae, and Haemophilus influenzae.

○ **What organisms are typically responsible for causing bacterial conjunctivitis?**

Staphylococcus aureus, Streptococcus pneumoniae, Haemophilus influenzae.

○ **A patient presents with a painful eye, blurred vision, and conjunctivitis. Upon slit-lamp examination, you detect a dendritic ulcer. What is the most likely cause of this patient's symptoms?**

Herpes simplex keratitis. Treat with topical antivirals. Immediate ophthalmology consult is warranted. Corticosteroids are not to be used unless under direction of an ophthalmologist. If the eye has a bacterial superinfection, prescribe topical antibiotics.

○   **What are cotton wool spots?**

White patches on the retina that are observed upon funduscopic examination. These patches are because of the ischemia of the superficial nerve layer of the retina. They are most commonly associated with hypertension but also occur in patients with diabetes, anemia, collagen vascular disease, leukemia, endocarditis, and AIDS.

○   **Do visual changes in chronic open-angle glaucoma patients begin centrally or peripherally?**

Peripherally. Patients with chronic glaucoma experience a gradual and painless loss of vision. Those with acute or subacute angle glaucoma will have either dull or severe pain, blurry vision, lacrimation, and even nausea and vomiting. The pain may be more severe in the dark.

○   **Which is more common, chronic open-angle glaucoma or acute closed-angle glaucoma?**

Chronic open-angle glaucoma (90%). Four percent of the population over age 40 has glaucoma.

○   **What is the most common cause of chronic open-angle glaucoma?**

Outflow obstruction through the trabecular meshwork. Other causes are obstruction of Schlemm canal and excess secretion of aqueous fluid.

○   **What is the normal range of intraocular pressure?**

10 to 23 mm Hg. Patients with acute angle-closure glaucoma generally have pressures elevated to 40 to 80 mm Hg.

○   **Topical steroids for the eyes are absolutely contraindicated in what cases?**

If the patient has a herpetic infection. Herpetic lesion in the eye is often seen as dendritic patterns of fluorescein uptake upon slit-lamp examination.

○   **What is the most common finding upon funduscopic examination of a patient with AIDS?**

Cotton wool spots caused by disease of the microvasculature. Other findings are hemorrhage, exudate, or retinal necrosis.

○   **What findings are most commonly associated with orbital floor fractures?**

Diplopia, globe lowering, and numbness over the cheek (second division of the trigeminal nerve).

○   **What radiographic findings might suggest an orbital blowout fracture?**

1. Fracture lines or bony fragments in the maxillary sinus
2. Subcutaneous or orbital emphysema
3. Air–fluid level in the maxillary sinus
4. A "teardrop" sign where a soft tissue mass protrudes into the maxillary sinus

○   **A patient presents with an itching, tearing, right eye. Upon examination large cobblestone papillae are found under the upper lid. What is the probable diagnosis?**

Allergic conjunctivitis.

○ **A patient is seen with herpetic lesions on the tip of the nose. Why is this a problem?**

The tip of the nose and the cornea are both supplied by the nasociliary nerve. Thus, the cornea may also be involved. This is an ophthalmological emergency.

○ **A patient presents with conjunctiva and lid margin inflammation. Slit-lamp examination reveals a "greasy" appearance of the lid margins with scaling, especially around the base of the lashes. Diagnosis?**

Blepharitis. This is often caused by a staphylococcal infection of the oil glands and skin next to the lash follicles. Treatment consists of scrubbing with baby shampoo and, after consultation with an ophthalmologist, sulfacetamide drops and steroids.

○ **A patient presents with a painful red eye. Slit-lamp examination reveals a localized, white, flocculent infiltrate in the anterior chamber. What is this?**

Hypopyon, which is an accumulation of white inflammatory exudate in the anterior chamber.

○ **A welder presents with severe eye pain. What is the expected finding upon slit-lamp examination?**

Diffuse punctate keratopathy (welder's flash) which presents as a multiple pinpoint area of fluorescein uptake representing ruptured corneal epithelial cells.

○ **A patient presents with a painful pustular vesicle at the lid margin. What is the diagnosis and treatment?**

A hordeolum (sty) is a painful, red, swelling occurring on the upper or lower eyelids. An internal hordeolum is an abscess of the meibomian gland and "points" toward the conjunctival side of the eyelid. An external hordeolum is a painful swelling at the eyelid margin which "points" outward.

○ **A patient presents with a chronic, nontender, uninflamed nodule of the upper lid. What is the diagnosis?**

Chalazion. Treat with surgical curettage.

○ **A patient presents with the sensation of a foreign body in the eye. Slit lamp reveals a dendritic (branch-like) lesion on the cornea. What is the treatment?**

Antiviral agents and cycloplegics. This is most probably a herpes simplex keratitis. Steroids are contraindicated because they allow for viral replication. Emergent ophthalmology consultation is indicated.

○ **A patient presents with sudden onset of vision loss in one eye that quickly returns. This should be diagnosed as?**

Amaurosis fugax. Usually caused by central retinal artery emboli from extracranial atherosclerosis.

○ **A patient presents with painless vision loss in one eye described as a wall slowly developing in the visual field. What finding do you expect upon examination?**

A gray, detached retina. The patient may also complain of flashing lights in the peripheral visual field or spider webs in the visual field. Inferior detachment is treated with the patient sitting up. Superior detachment is treated with the patient lying flat.

○ **A patient was hit in the eye during a fight. He presents 8 hours after the incident with proptosis and visual loss. Examination reveals an intact globe and an afferent pupillary defect. What is the problem?**

Retro orbital hematoma with ischemia of the optic nerve or retina. The pressure of the blood in the orbit exceeds the perfusion pressure resulting in a lack of blood flow and loss of function. Treatment is to release the pressure by lateral canthotomy. A similar situation can occur with orbital emphysema.

○ **What five lid lacerations should be referred to an ophthalmologist?**

1. Near the lacrimal canaliculi (between the medial canthus and the punctum).
2. Near the levator (transverse lacerations of the upper lid).
3. Near the orbital septum (upper lid deep wounds, between the tarsus and the superior orbital rim).
4. Canthal tendons (wounds penetrating the lateral and medial canthi).
5. Lid margins (wounds through the tarsal plate and lid margins).

○ **What are complications of a hyphema?**

The four Ss are:

1. **Staining** of the cornea because of hemosiderin deposits.
2. **Synechiae,** which interfere with iris function.
3. **Secondary rebleeds,** which usually occur between the second and fifth day after the injury (since this is the time of clot retraction) and tend to be worse than the initial bleed.
4. **Significantly increased intraocular pressure,** which can lead to acute glaucoma, chronic late glaucoma, and optic atrophy.

○ **Why do patients with sickle cell anemia and a hyphema require special consideration when presenting with ophthalmologic concerns?**

Increased intraocular pressure can occur if the cells sickle in the trabecular network, preventing aqueous humor from leaving the anterior chamber. Some medications, such as hyperosmotics and Diamox, increase the likelihood of sickling.

○ **A patient presents with a history of trauma to the orbit with dull ocular pain, decreased visual acuity, and photophobia. An examination reveals a constricted pupil and ciliary flush. What will be found on a slit-lamp examination?**

Flare and cells in the anterior chamber are present with traumatic iritis.

○ **What are causes of a subluxed or dislocated lens?**

Trauma, Marfan syndrome, homocystinuria, and Weill-Marchesani syndrome.

○ **Physiologically, what causes flare?**

Flare is caused by inflammatory proteins resulting in the "dust in the movie projector lights" or "fog in the headlights" phenomena in slit-lamp examination.

○ **Which is worse, acid or alkaline burns of the cornea?**

Alkaline, because of deeper penetration than acid burns. A barrier is formed from precipitated proteins with acid burns. The exception is hydrofluoric acid and heavy metal containing acids which can penetrate the cornea.

○ **When should an eye not be dilated?**

With known narrow angle glaucoma and with an iris-supported intraocular lens.

○ **Why shouldn't topical ophthalmologic anesthetics be prescribed?**

The anesthetics inhibit healing and decrease the patient's ability to protect his eye because of the lack of sensation.

○ **What is the most common organism in contact lens associated corneal ulcers?**

Pseudomonas.

○ **How can Krazy-Glue (cyanoacrylate) be removed if a patient has stuck their eyelids together?**

Copious irrigation immediately and then mineral oil. Acetone and ethanol are unacceptable in the eyes. Surgical separation must be done with extreme care to prevent laceration of the lids or globe. Often the patient will have a corneal abrasion, which should be treated in the usual manner.

○ **Three hours ago, a patient experienced sudden, painless visual loss in her right eye. Central retinal artery occlusion (CRAO) is suspected. What findings are expected upon eye examination? What is the prognosis?**

Afferent pupillary defect, pale gray retina, and a small cherry red dot near the fovea. This dot is the choroidal vasculature being seen at the macula where the retina is the thinnest. After 2 hours the prognosis is extremely poor for visual recovery. Digital massage or anterior chamber paracentesis may dislodge the clot. Immediate ophthalmic consultation is necessary.

○ **What conditions have been associated with central retinal vein occlusion?**

Hyperviscosity syndromes, diabetes, and hypertension. Funduscopic examination shows a chaotically streaked retina with congested dilated veins. There are superficial and deep retinal hemorrhages, cotton wool spots, and macular edema.

○ **A patient presents with atraumatic pain behind the left eye, a left pupil afferent defect, central visual loss, and a left swollen disc. Diagnosis and potential causes?**

Optic neuritis. This may be idiopathic or may be associated with multiple sclerosis, Lyme disease, neurosyphilis, lupus, sarcoid, alcoholism, toxins, or drug abuse.

○ **A patient developed eye pain, nausea, vomiting, blurred vision, and sees halos around lights. Why would this patient be given mannitol, pilocarpine, and acetazolamide?**

This patient has acute narrow angle glaucoma. The goal of treatment is to decrease intraocular pressure.

1. Decrease the production of aqueous humor with carbonic anhydrase inhibitor.
2. Decrease intraocular volume by making the plasma hypertonic to the aqueous humor with glycerol or mannitol.
3. Constrict the pupil with pilocarpine, allowing increased flow of the aqueous humor out through the previously blocked canals of Schlemm.

○ **A patient presents with multiple vertical linear corneal abrasions. What should be suspected?**

A foreign body under the upper lid. This pattern is sometimes called an "ice rink" sign.

○ **What technique can be used to identify and narrow anterior chamber?**

Tangential light (from a penlight) is shone perpendicular to the line of vision across the anterior chamber. If the entire iris is in the light then the chamber is most likely a normal depth. If part of the iris is in a shadow, the chamber is narrow. This can occur with narrow angle glaucoma and with perforating corneal injuries.

○ **What is the difference between a sympathomimetic and a cycloplegic medication when dilating the eye?**

A sympathomimetic simulates the iris's dilator muscle. The cycloplegic inhibits the parasympathetic stimulation which constricts the iris and inhibits the ciliary muscle. Thus, cycloplegics will cause blurred near vision.

○ **A patient felt something fly into his eye while mowing the lawn. On examination, there is a brown foreign body on the cornea and a tear drop iris pointing toward the foreign body. What is the diagnosis?**

Perforated cornea with extruded iris. A similar foreign body may appear black on the sclera with scleral perforation.

○ **A patient's cornea fluoresces prior to instillation of fluorescein. What should be considered?**

Pseudomonal infection. Several species are fluorescent.

Which anesthetic is faster acting? Proparacaine or tetracaine?

Proparacaine has a rapid onset and a duration of 20 minutes. Tetracaine has a delayed onset, and a duration of 1 hour.

○ **Place the following mydriatic–cycloplegic medications in order of duration of activity: tropicamide, homatropine, atropine, and cyclopentolate.**

1. Tropicamide (onset 15 to 20 minutes, brief duration)
2. Cyclopentolate (onset 30 to 60 minutes, duration <24 hours)
3. Homatropine (long lasting, 2 to 3 days)
4. Atropine (very long lasting, 2 weeks)

○ **What condition should be suspected in a patient with vision loss and a pale fundus?**

Central retinal artery occlusion. Vision loss is usually acute and painless.

○ **Describe the symptoms of optic neuritis.**

Variable loss of central visual acuity with a central scotoma and change in color perception. The disk margins are blurred from hemorrhage, the blind spot is increased, and the eye is painful, especially with movement.

○ **Describe a patient with acute narrow angle closure glaucoma.**

Symptoms include nausea, vomiting, and abdominal pain. Visual acuity is markedly diminished. The pupil is semi-dilated and nonreactive. There is usually a glassy haze over the cornea, and the eye is red and very painful. Intraocular pressure may be as high as 50 to 60 mm Hg.

○ **Describe the treatment of acute narrow angle glaucoma.**

Intravenous acetazolamide (a carbonic anhydrase inhibitor to minimize aqueous humor production), miotics (such as pilocarpine) to open the angle, topical beta-blocker, alpha-adrenergic receptor agonist and if necessary, intravenous hyperosmotic agent like mannitol to reduce intraocular pressure. After the ocular pressure is stabilized and iridectomy is eventually performed to provide aqueous outflow.

○ **What is the appropriate treatment of hyphema?**

Rest, elevation of the head and topical steroids. Avoid aspirin and NSAIDs. Rebleeding can occur in up to 20% at 3 days. Complications include glaucoma and corneal staining.

○ **What is the differential diagnosis of a red eye with decreased visual acuity?**

Conjunctivitis, keratitis, iritis, glaucoma, and central corneal lesions.

○   **What disease is associated with retrobulbar optic neuritis?**

Multiple sclerosis.

○   **What are the signs and symptoms of an ophthalmoplegic migraine?**

Unilateral headache with palsies of the extraocular muscles served by cranial nerves III, IV, and VI may also occur. Ptosis is usually seen. The palsies outlast the pain in most cases. After numerous episodes, mydriasis and ophthalmoplegia can be a complication.

○   **Define strabismus, esotropia, and exotropia.**

- Strabismus: Lack of parallelism of the visual axis of the eyes.
- Esotropia: Medial deviation.
- Exotropia: Lateral deviation.

○   **A patient presents with a painful eye, blurred vision, and conjunctivitis. Upon slit-lamp examination, you detect a dendritic ulcer. What is the most likely cause of this patient's symptoms?**

Herpes simplex keratitis. Treat with topical antivirals. Immediate ophthalmology consult is warranted. Corticosteroids are not to be used unless under direction of an ophthalmologist. If the eye has a bacterial superinfection, prescribe topical antibiotics.

○   **An elderly patient presents with the complaint of seeing halos around lights. What diagnosis is suspected?**

Glaucoma. Another presenting complaint of glaucoma is blurred vision. Also, consider digitalis toxicity.

○   **What diseases are commonly associated with central retinal vein occlusion?**

Hypertension and glaucoma.

○   **What are common eye findings in patients with AIDS?**

Cotton wool spots and hemorrhages are most commonly caused by cytomegalovirus (CMV) retinitis.

○   **What is a frequent complication of ethmoid sinusitis?**

Orbital cellulitis.

○   **A patient presents with a painful, red eye and a decrease in visual acuity. What is the differential?**

Central corneal lesions, glaucoma, and iritis.

○   **On funduscopic examination, microaneurysms and soft exudates are typical of:**

Hypertension.

○   **On funduscopic examination, macular microaneurysms and hard exudates are typical of:**

Diabetes.

○   **What is the most common cause of retrobulbar optic neuritis?**

Multiple sclerosis.

○ **Describe a patient presenting with Sjögren syndrome.**

Sjögren syndrome usually occurs in women older than 50 years of age. Symptoms often include diminished lacrimal and salivary gland secretions, salivary gland enlargement, and arthritis. Sjögren syndrome predisposes a patient to corneal irritation, ulceration, and superimposed infection. It may complicate many rheumatic diseases or may occur independently. The most probable cause of Sjögren syndrome is lymphatic infiltration of the lacrimal and salivary glands, which results in dry eyes and a dry mouth.

○ **What are the medications used in treating glaucoma and what is their mechanism of action?**

Medication Example	Drug Class	MOA
Timolol	Beta-blocker	Suppression of aqueous humor
Acetazolamide (Topical or oral)	Carbonic anhydrase inhibitor	Suppression of aqueous humor
Brimonidine	Alpha-adrenergic agonist	Decrease aqueous humor and increase outflow
Latanaprost	Prostaglandin analog	Increase aqueous outflow
Pilocarpine (rarely used with the development of the prostaglandin analogs)	Parasympathomimetic	Ciliary muscle contraction to increase aqueous outflow of the canal of Schlemm
Oral glycerine, IV mannitol	Hyperosmotic agents	Diuresis causing decrease in aqueous fluid

○ **A 28-year-old female presents with eye pain and acute vision blurriness, upon examination the eye is not red. She denies injury. What is the most common cause of PAINFUL vision loss without redness of the eye?**

Acute optic neuritis. Causes include multiple sclerosis, lupus, sarcoid, post viral infection, sphenoidal sinusitis, and encephalomyelitis. Anterior redness is not seen because of the inflammation being confined to the retrobulbar portion of the eye.

○ **What is the evaluation and treatment for an acute optic neuritis?**

IV or oral steroids. Antibiotics if a suspected bacterial infection. MRI if the patient is stable, and CT if the patient is unstable.

○ **What condition is known as "nearsightedness"?**

Myopia. The vision rays come into focus in front of the retina. Corrective lenses adjust the focal point of the light rays posteriorly to the retina.

○ **What condition is known as "farsightedness"**

Hyperopia. The vision rays come into focus behind the retina. Corrective lenses adjust the focal point of light rays anteriorly to the retina.

○ **What conditions may cause an afferent pupillary defect?**

Ischemic optic neuropathy, glaucoma, optic neuritis.

○ **What types of tonometry are there? And how do they work?**

Applanation tonometry	This is attached to a slit lamp and pressure is measured when the device is pressed against the cornea
Schiotz	Hand help device with a weighted gauge that is placed over the cornea
Tono-pen	Hand held pen applied to the corneal surface
Noncontact "air puff"	Pressure sensing device measures the rebound from the air puff (not as accurate as applanation tonometry).

○ **What are the three most common causes of preventable vision loss?**

Amblyopia, diabetic retinopathy, glaucoma.

○ **Compare and contrast indirect ophthalmoscopy and direct ophthalmoscopy.**

The direct ophthalmoscopic examination is done with the hand help ophthalmoscope with the variable strength diopters. It's field of vision is 10 degrees and magnification is 15 times. The indirect ophthalmoscope is a binocular that is worn by the examiner with a light show through variable strength hand held lenses. The field of vision is 37 degrees, and the entire retina can be examined with the indirect ophthalmoscope.

○ **A patient presents with a post-traumatic iritis. What signs and symptoms would you expect?**

Severe eye pain, severe photophobia, eye redness, blurred vision. On physical examination, pain to the affected eye when shining a penlight into the unaffected eye (consensual pain), ciliary flush and a nonreactive pupil.

○ **Compare and contrast the signs and symptoms of herpes keratitis and herpes zoster ophthalmicus.**

Herpes keratitis. The patient will have eye pain, foreign body sensation and a red eye. Upon physical examination with the slit lamp and dendritic corneal defect will be see with fluorescein staining. There is no skin involvement.

Herpes zoster ophthalmicus. The patient will complain of headache, facial discomfort, tingling or burning pain a day or two before a vesicular, pustular, and crusting rash develops in a dermatomal distribution on the face. If the tip of the nose develops the characteristic lesions, the eye will be involved. This involves the ophthalmic branch of the trigeminal nerve.

Treatment of both conditions described above include topical antiviral eyedrops (trifluridine) and oral antivirals (acyclovir, famcyclovir, valacyclovir).

○ **What conditions are associated with bilateral optic disk swelling?**

Raised intracranial pressure and malignant hypertension.

○ **What conditions are associated with unilateral optic disk swelling?**

Optic neuritis, ischemic optic neuropathy, central retinal vein occlusion, intracranial optic nerve compression, posterior scleritis.

○ A patient presents with severe eye pain after being scratched by a tree branch while hiking. His vision in the affected eye is 20/100. Your examination on slit lamp with fluorescein stain reveals a large corneal abrasion. He is in obvious pain. What pain controlling medications can you apply or prescribe in this case?

Medication	Mechanism of Action
Cycloplegic	Reduces pain by preventing ciliary muscle spasm
Topical NSAID	Reduces pain by direct antiprostaglandin effect on the cornea
Topical antibiotic	Prevention of secondary infection
Oral analgesics and sedatives	Allows for patient to sleep, with eyes closed which promotes healing

○ A patient complains of repeated corneal abrasions occurring in the mornings upon awakening and chronic dry eyes, what should you consider?

Sjögren syndrome. This condition causes dysfunction in tear production and is predominantly seen in females.

○ What cranial nerves innervate ocular function and what is their function?

Cranial Nerve	Function
II. Optic	Vision
III. Oculomotor	Pupillary constriction, opening the eyelid, most extra ocular motions
IV. Trochlear	Downward internal rotation
VI. Abducens	Lateral deviation

EAR DISORDERS

○ The Weber test is performed on a patient complaining of hearing loss. The patient hears sounds more loudly in his right ear. Which types of hearing loss may this patient have?

Conductive hearing loss on the right or sensory hearing loss on the left.

○ Describe Rinne test and explain the normal findings.

Rinne test is performed by placing the tip of the tuning fork on the mastoid process until the patient can no longer hear the tone. The fork is then relocated to just in front of the pinna until the patient can no longer hear the tone. In normal patients, the ratio is 1:2 of the duration of time the patient can hear the fork.

○ A 35-year-old woman with a history of flu-like symptoms (URI) 1 week ago presents with vertigo, nausea, and vomiting. No auditory impairment or focal deficits are noted. What is the likely diagnosis?

Labyrinthitis or vestibular neuronitis.

○ **Describe the key features of Ménière disease, also known as endolymphatic hydrops.**

Vertigo, hearing loss, and tinnitus. Ménière disease typically presents with the rapid onset of vertigo, nausea, and vomiting that lasts for hours to 1 day. Nystagmus may be spontaneous during the critical stage. Tinnitus may be present and is louder during attacks, and sensorineural hearing loss may occur. There also may be an aura with a sensation of fullness in the ear during an attack. Symptoms are unilateral in over 90% of patients, and recurring attacks are typical.

○ **What are the distinguishing characteristics of benign positional vertigo?**

Positional vertigo is usually provoked by certain head positions or movement. Nystagmus is always positional, of brief duration, and with fatigability.

○ **What are the key features of viral labyrinthitis or vestibular neuritis?**

Severe vertigo (usually lasting 3 to 5 days), with nausea and vomiting. Symptoms generally regress over 3 to 6 weeks. Nystagmus may be spontaneous during the severe stage.

○ **A 50-year-old female with acute vertigo, nausea, and vomiting reports similar episodes over the last 20 years that are sometimes associated with hearing change, hearing loss, and tinnitus. She has permanent right > left sensorineural hearing loss. What is the diagnosis?**

Ménière disease.

○ **For the following clinical presentations, identify which are associated with peripheral vertigo or with central vertigo.**

1. Intense spinning, nausea, hearing loss, diaphoresis.

2. Swaying or impulsion, worse with movement, tinnitus, acute onset.

3. Unidirectional nystagmus inhibited by ocular fixation, fatigable.

4. Mild vertigo, diplopia, and ataxia.

5. Multidirectional nystagmus not inhibited by ocular fixation, nonfatigable.

peripheral vertigo: (1), (2), and (3); central vertigo: (4) and (5).

○ **What are the common features of central vertigo?**

Symptoms are gradual and continuous. They include focal signs, nausea, and vomiting. Hearing loss is rare.

○ **What are the signs and symptoms of peripheral vertigo?**

Symptoms are usually acute and intermittent. Hearing loss is common; nausea and vomiting are severe.

○ **What is the significance of bilateral nystagmus with cold caloric testing?**

It signifies that an intact cortex, midbrain, and brainstem are present.

○ **What is a mnemonic for remembering the drugs that cause nystagmus?**

MALES TIP. Methanol, Alcohol, Lithium, Ethylene glycol, Sedative hypnotics, and Solvents, Thiamine depletion and Tegretol (carbamazepine), Isopropanol, PCP, and phenytoin.

○ **Describe the clinical presentation and treatment for Ménière Disease.**

A patient will complain of aural pressure, episodic vertigo that lasts for hours, tinnitus and hearing loss. The treatment includes a sodium-restricted diet, limiting caffeine, alcohol, and prescribing diuretics like hydrochlorothiazide. Acute episodes can be managed with vestibular suppressant benzodiazepines and antiemetics.

○ **Describe the signs and symptoms in a patient with vestibular neuronitis (labyrinthitis).**

The patient with have a rapid onset of severe vertigo (but some may have a gradual prodromal period) accompanied by nausea, vomiting, and imbalance. This is usually preceded by an upper respiratory infection. Rapid phase nystagmus and the feeling of body motion are toward the opposite ear with falling and past pointing toward the affected ear.

○ **What is a vestibular schwannoma?**

An acoustic neuroma or a tumor of the eighth cranial nerve. In addition to hearing loss and vertigo, patients also present with tinnitus. Surgical removal is the treatment of choice because this tumor may spread to the cerebellum and the brainstem.

○ **What are the most common initial symptoms of an acoustic neuroma?**

Tinnitus, hearing loss, and unsteadiness.

○ **Describe the signs and symptoms of acoustic neuroma.**

Unilateral high tone sensorineural hearing loss and tinnitus. Decreased corneal sensitivity, diplopia, headache, facial weakness, and positive radiographic findings may also be displayed. Vertigo usually appears late, is more often exhibited as a progressive feeling of imbalance, and can be provoked by changes in head movement. Nystagmus is frequently present and is usually spontaneous. The CSF may have elevated protein.

○ **A 17-year-old female presents to clinic with a history of ear discharge and pain, fever, and swelling and redness over the mastoid bone. She was treated for an otitis media 2 weeks ago. What is your clinical suspicion?**

Mastoiditis is a complication of otitis media and is caused by bacterial invasion into the mastoid air cells. The most common causative pathogens are *Streptococcus pneumoniae*, *Haemophilus influenzae*, *Staphylococcus* aureus. If a subperiosteal abscess develops, surgical drainage is indicated.

○ **Which medications put patients at risk for hearing loss?**

Aminoglycoside, antineoplastic agents, loop diuretics, and salicylates.

○ **What is the most common causative organism of otitis externa?**

Pseudomonas species.

○ **A patient presents with hearing loss, nystagmus, facial weakness, and diplopia. Vertigo is provoked with sudden movement. A lumbar puncture reveals elevated CNS protein. What diagnosis is suspected?**

An acoustic neuroma.

○ **What is the most common complication of acute otitis media?**

Tympanic membrane perforation. Other complications include mastoiditis, cholesteatoma, and intracranial infections.

○ **A 44-year-old man has lost sensorineural hearing in his left ear. What ear will the Weber test lateralize to?**

The right or normal ear. The damaged ear is less prone to detect sound waves via vibration.

○ **A patient presents with ear pain and fluid-filled blisters on the tympanic membrane. What is the diagnosis?**

Bullous myringitis, commonly caused by Mycoplasma or a virus. Treat with erythromycin.

○ **A 16-year-old boxer presents with a hematoma of the external right ear after receiving a blow to the ear. What is the treatment?**

The hematoma should be aseptically drained by incision or aspiration and a mastoid conforming dressing should be applied. ENT follow-up is mandatory. If the ear is not treated appropriately, a cauliflower deformity may result.

○ **A patient presents with a swollen, tender, red left auricle. What is the diagnosis?**

Perichondritis. This is most often caused by Pseudomonas.

○ **What is the most common cause of hearing loss?**

Cerumen impaction.

○ **Describe the physical finding of unilateral sensory hearing loss.**

The patient will lateralize and have air conduction greater than bone conduction (i.e., normal Rinne test) indicating no conductive loss. The Weber test will lateralize to the normal ear. The most common cause of unilateral sensory hearing loss is viral neuritis.

○ **Which causes should be suspected in a patient with bilateral sensory hearing loss?**

Noise or ototoxins (e.g., aminoglycosides, loop diuretics, or antineoplastics).

○ **What is the most common neuropathy associated with acoustic neuroma?**

The corneal reflex may be lost because of the trigeminal nucleus involvement.

○ **Name some causes of tympanic membrane perforation.**

Air or water blast injuries, foreign bodies in the ear (particularly cotton tip swabs), lightning strikes, otitis media, and associated temporal bone fractures.

○ **A young man who was involved in a bar room brawl complains of ear pain, significantly decreased hearing, and vertigo. A tympanic membrane rupture is determined by examination. What is the concern?**

Injury to the ossicles, temporal bone, or labyrinth. An urgent ENT consult is necessary.

○ **A diver on vacation decided to go scuba diving despite having an upper respiratory infection. While descending, she had acute ear pain followed by vertiginous symptoms and vomiting. What happened?**

Middle ear squeeze. Pressure from the middle ear could not be equalized because of abnormal eustachian tube function resulting from the illness. The middle ear volume decreased until the tympanic membrane retracted to the point of rupture. The inrush of cold water caused vestibular stimulation. This is the most common form of barotrauma in amateur scuba divers. Similar problems may occur while flying on aircraft.

O **What organism usually causes pediatric acute otitis media?**

Streptococcus pneumoniae, followed by *Haemophilus influenzae* and *Moraxella catarrhalis.*

O **Why are preschool children more susceptible to acute otitis media?**

Children have shorter, more horizontal eustachian tubes, which may prevent adequate drainage and allow aspiration of nasopharyngeal bacteria into the middle ear, particularly with URIs.

O **What is the most common type of hearing loss in the elderly?**

Presbycusis. This is an idiopathic, insidious, symmetrical decline in hearing that is associated with aging.

O **What systemic sexually transmitted disease is associated with sensorineural hearing loss?**

Syphilis. Seven percent of patients with idiopathic hearing loss test positive for treponemal antibodies.

O **Acute tinnitus is associated with toxicity of what medications?**

Salicylates, loop diuretics, and aminoglycosides. Other causes of tinnitus are vascular abnormalities, mechanical abnormalities, and damaged cochlear hair cells. Unilateral tinnitus is associated with chronic suppurative otitis, Ménière disease, and trauma.

O **What is the most common cause of otitis media?**

Streptococcus pneumoniae.

O **What is the bone seen behind the tympanic membrane?**

The malleus.

O **What is the first-line medication for otitis media?**

Amoxicillin (80–90 mg/kg/day divided in two doses, Erythromycin (50 mg/kg/day), Erythromycin + sulfisoxazole (50 mg/kg/day based on erythromycin component, Amoxicillin-clavulanate (20–40 mg/kg/day based on amoxicillin component).

O **When using the pneumatic insufflation bulb on the otoscope, what physical findings would you expect with an otitis media?**

Tympanic hypomobility.

O **A patient has a chronically draining ear with purulent discharge. Your physical examination identifies a small perforation in the tympanic membrane, what is your diagnosis?**

Chronic otitis media.

O **What is the treatment for a chronic otitis media?**

Keeping the canal clear of debris, avoidance of water in the ear, topical antibiotic drops, an example would be ciprofloxacin + dexamethasone. Ciprofloxacin has anti-pseudomonal activity.

O **What must be suspected in an adult with recurrent unilateral serous otitis media?**

Oropharyngeal cancer.

○   **A 75-year-old patient presents with a complaint of vertigo, especially with turning her head or looking upward. It is transient. What is the most likely diagnosis?**

Vertebrobasilar insufficiency.

○   **What is the indicated diagnostic test for suspected vertebrobasilar insufficiency?**

Magnetic resonance angiography.

○   **What is a cholesteatoma?**

As a result of chronic eustachian tube dysfunction, negative pressure forms in the middle ear which causes a squamous epithelium membrane to form that accumulates keratinized debris and becomes chronically infected. A major complication is erosion of the mastoid bone. Treatment includes intravenous antibiotics such as cefazolin (1g every 6–8 hours) and surgery.

○   **What is the diagnostic test of choice when evaluating a suspected case of mastoiditis? What findings would you expect?**

Computerized Tomography (CT scan). Radiographic findings would be destruction of the mastoid air cell septa with accumulation of pus.

MOUTH/THROAT

○   **What nutritional deficiencies may lead to aphthous ulcers?**

B12, folate, and iron deficiencies.

○   **Name the most likely pathogens to cause acute parotitis.**

The most likely causes of acute parotitis are paramyxovirus (mumps), influenza A virus, coxsackie A virus, cytomegalovirus, and echovirus.

○   **List the criteria that would be helpful to diagnose Group A hemolytic strep:**

Tonsillar exudate, tender anterior cervical adenopathy, absence of cough, and history of fever.

○   **What is the first-line drug of choice for treating Streptococcus pyogenes?**

The first-line treatment for Group A beta-hemolytic strep is penicillin. Clindamycin or Erythromycin is recommended for patients with a penicillin allergy.

○   **A patient presents with a history of sore throat, fever, "hot potato" voice, and difficulty swallowing. What must you be clinically suspicious of?**

Peritonsillar abscess.

○   **A patient presents with a history of sudden pain and swelling over the submandibular gland. He states this occurred while eating lunch. What is your diagnosis?**

Sialolithiasis. Salivary duct stones develop in the submandibular gland 80% of the time with 10% to 20% occurring in the parotid gland. If the stone doesn't pass spontaneously, ENT referral for endoscopic extraction is indicated.

○ **A patient presents to you with a dental abscess. What antibiotic is indicated for this condition?**

Clindamycin or amoxicillin-clavulanate will provide good coverage for the oral flora and anaerobes such as *Bacteroides fragilis.*

○ **A patient presents with a painful cluster of vesicles on the lower lip. What is your diagnosis?**

Herpes simplex type 1 causes lesions to develop on the lips and mouth. HSV-1 can also cause genital lesions transmitted by oral–genital contact. Herpes simplex type 2 causes genital herpes. Approximately 25% of the population has serologic evidence of HSV-2.

○ **What anatomic abnormalities exist when a patient presents with stridor?**

Swelling or obstruction in the larynx or trachea. Inspiratory stridor indicates obstruction at glottis or supraglottis. Expiratory stridor is created in the trachea. Biphasic stridor is created at the subglottis.

○ **In the evaluation of retropharyngeal abscess, what is the usual age of the patients, how do they present, what diagnostic tests are used in their evaluation, and what treatment modalities are recommended?**

Retropharyngeal abscess is most commonly seen in children less than 3 years old. Usual presentation is with dysphagia, a muffled voice, stridor, and drooling. Patients usually prefer to lie supine. Diagnosis is made with a soft tissue lateral neck film which may demonstrate edema with the retropharyngeal space being wider than the body of C4, and air/fluid levels. CT may be useful. Treatment includes careful airway monitoring, IV antibiotics, and admission to the ICU.

○ **The causes of epiglottitis include:**

Haemophilus influenzae is by far most common. Pneumococcus, Staphylococcus, and Branhamella may also be causes. Presentation is most common among children around age 5.

○ **What is Ludwig angina?**

An odontogenic abscess of the submandibular and sublingual space caused by infection of the lower molars. The most common pathogen is Streptococcus, Staphylococcus, and Bacteroides.

○ **What is the presentation of a patient with post-extraction alveolitis?**

"Dry socket" pain occurs on the second or third day after the extraction.

○ **Ludwig angina typically involves what spaces in the head?**

The submental, sublingual, and submandibular spaces.

○ **What are the signs and symptoms of a peritonsillar abscess?**

Sore throat, dysarthria (hot potato voice), odynophagia, ipsilateral otalgia, low-grade fever, trismus, and uvular displacement.

○ **What is the presentation of a patient with diphtheria?**

Sore throat, dysphagia, fever, and tachycardia. A dirty, tough gray fibrinous membrane so firmly adherent that removal causes bleeding may be present in the oropharynx. Corynebacterium diphtheriae exotoxin acts directly on cardiac, renal, and nervous systems. It can cause ocular bulbar paralysis that may suggest botulism or myasthenia gravis. The exotoxin may also cause flaccid limb weakness. Of note, such weakness may also include decreased or absent DTRs, a finding suggestive of Guillain–Barré or tick paralysis.

○   **How does a patient present with a retropharyngeal abscess?**

Patients typically prefer a supine position. Retropharyngeal abscesses are common under 3 years of age. On examination, the uvula and tonsil are displaced away from the abscess. Soft tissue swelling and forward displacement of the larynx are present. Soft tissue X-ray films of the neck may show the retropharyngeal space to be wider that the vertebral body of C4.

○   **How does an adult with epiglottitis present?**

Sore throat and severe dysphagia, drooling, muffled voice are prominent symptoms. Adults have and indolent course preceded by a viral URI. Pain is out of proportion to objective findings.

○   **What is the initial antibiotic treatment for a child with epiglottitis?**

Treat with a second- or third-generation cephalosporin. The most likely cause of this condition is *Haemophilus Influenzae* B. This pathogen is seen in patients who lack Hib vaccination or have had vaccination failure. Other pathogens are Group A Streptococcus, *and Streptococcus pneumoniae.*

○   **What viral agent most commonly induces laryngotracheitis?**

Parainfluenza virus type I, II, and III are most common, but can be Influenza A and B or RSV (respiratory syncytial virus). *Staphylococcus aureus* and *Streptococcus pneumoniae* are the most common bacterial pathogens.

○   **Herpangina is caused by what virus?**

Coxsackievirus group A. A sore throat, fever, malaise, and vesicular lesions on the posterior pharynx or the soft palate are prevalent with this disease.

○   **What is the IM treatment for adult streptococcal pharyngitis?**

1.2 million units of benzathine penicillin G. Use 0.6 million units of benzathine penicillin G for children under 27 kg.

○   **Can a parapharyngeal abscess present with an associated finding of edema in the area of the parotid gland?**

Yes.

○   **Retropharyngeal abscess is most common in what age group?**

Children less than 4 years old. Symptoms include difficulty breathing, fever, enlarged cervical nodes, difficulty swallowing, and a stiff neck. Examination may reveal a mass or fullness in the posterior pharyngeal area.

○   **Peritonsillar abscess is most common in what age group?**

Adolescents and young adults. Symptoms may include ear pain, trismus, drooling, and alteration of voice.

○   **What is the most common cause of sialadenitis?**

Stasis of the flow of saliva. The most common bacterial pathogens are *Staphylococcus aureus, Streptococcus pneumoniae, Escherichia coli, Haemophilus influenzae* and viruses. Signs and symptoms include, fever, pain, swelling of the salivary glands, which may include the parotid gland.

○ **A patient presents with trismus, fever, and an erythematous, tender parotid gland. Pus is expressed from Stensen duct. What conditions predisposes the patient to bacterial parotitis?**

Any situation which decreases salivary flow including irradiation, phenothiazines, antihistamines, parasympathetic inhibitors, dehydration and debilitation. Up to 30% of cases occur postoperatively.

○ **A patient presents with well-demarcated swelling of the lips and tongue. She was started on an antihypertensive agent 3 weeks ago. What is the most likely agent?**

Angiotensin-converting enzyme inhibitor (ACEI). Although angioneurotic edema may occur anytime during therapy, it is most likely to occur within in first month when using an ACE inhibitor.

○ **Retropharyngeal abscesses are most common in what age group? Why?**

6 months to 3 years of age. Retropharyngeal lymph nodes regress in size after age 3.

○ **Describe the overall appearance of a child with a retropharyngeal abscess.**

These children are often ill appearing, febrile, stridorous, drooling, and in an opisthotonic position. They may complain of difficulty swallowing or may refuse to eat.

○ **What radiographic sign indicates a retropharyngeal abscess?**

A widening of the retropharyngeal space which is normally 3 to 4 mm, or less than half the width of the vertebral bodies. False widening may occur if the X-ray is not taken during inspiration and with the patient's neck extended. Occasionally, an air–fluid level may be noted in the retropharyngeal space.

○ **Retropharyngeal abscesses are most commonly caused by which organisms?**

Beta-hemolytic streptococcus.

○ **A 48-year-old male presents with a high fever, trismus, dysphagia, and swelling inferior to the mandible in the lateral neck. What is the diagnosis?**

Parapharyngeal abscess.

○ **Where is the most common origin of Ludwig angina?**

The lower second and third molar. Ludwig angina is a swelling in the region of the submandibular, sublingual, and submental spaces, which may cause upward and posterior displacement of the tongue. It is most commonly caused by hemolytic streptococci, staphylococci, and mixed anaerobic/aerobic bacteria.

○ **What are the signs and symptoms of a mandibular fracture?**

Malocclusion, pain, opening deviation or abnormal movement, decreased range of motion, bony deformity, swelling, ecchymosis, and lower lip (mental nerve) anesthesia.

○ **A bilateral mental fracture can lead to what acute complication?**

Acute airway obstruction caused by the tongue because of a loss of anterior support.

○ **A patient was yawning in lecture and is now unable to close his mouth. He is having difficulty talking and swallowing. What is the diagnosis?**

Bilateral dislocation of the mandibular condyles. This can occur if the mouth is opened excessively wide. X-rays can rule out bilateral condyle fractures, which may have a similar clinical appearance.

○ **What are the major sequelae of untreated streptococcal infections?**

Post-streptococcal glomerulonephritis and rheumatic heart disease.

○ **A 42-year-old female presents with dull pain in her right ear and jaw, and a burning sensation in the roof of her mouth. The pain is worse in the evening. She also hears a "popping" sound when opening and closing her mouth. Further examination reveals tenderness of the joint capsule. What is the diagnosis and treatment?**

TMJ syndrome. Treat with physiotherapy, analgesia, a soft diet, muscle relaxants, and occlusive therapy. Apply warm, moist compresses four to five times daily for 15 minutes for 7 to 10 days.

○ **What plain radiographic view best reveals a zygomatic arch fracture?**

The modified basal view of the skull. Synonyms include jug-handle view, submental occipital view, or submental vertical view.

○ **What are the signs and symptoms of a fracture of the zygomaticomaxillary complex?**

Subcutaneous emphysema, edema, ecchymosis, facial flattening, subconjunctival hemorrhage, ecchymosis around the orbit, unilateral epistaxis, anesthesia of the cheek upper, lip and gum from infraorbital nerve injury, step deformity, decreased mandibular movement, and diplopia.

○ **Hairy leukoplakia is characteristic of which two viruses?**

HIV and Epstein–Barr virus. Hairy leukoplakia is usually found on the lateral aspect of the tongue. Oral thrush may also be associated with HIV infection.

○ **A child presents after falling and knocking out his front tooth. How would the management differ if the child were 3 versus 13?**

With primary teeth no reimplantation should be attempted because of the risk of ankylosis or fusion to the bone. However, with permanent teeth, reimplantation should occur as soon as possible. Remaining periodontal ligament fibers are a key to success. Thus, the tooth should not be wiped dry since this may disrupt the fibers still attached.

○ **How can Ellis class II and III fractures be differentiated?**

Class II fractures involve the dentin and enamel. The exposed dentin will be pinkish. Class III fractures involve the enamel, dentin, and pulp. A drop of blood is frequently noted in the center of the pink dentin.

○ **A patient presents 3 days after tooth extraction with severe pain and a foul mouth odor and taste. What is the appropriate diagnosis and treatment?**

Alveolar osteitis (dry socket) results from loss of the blood clot and local osteomyelitis. Treat by irrigation of the socket and application of a medicated dental packing or iodoform gauze moistened with Campho-Phenique or eugenol.

○ **A patient presents with gingival pain and a foul mouth odor and taste. On examination, fever and lymphadenopathy are present. The gingiva is bright red, and the papillae are ulcerated and covered with a gray membrane. What is the diagnosis and treatment?**

Acute necrotizing ulcerative gingivitis. Treat with antibiotics (tetracycline or penicillin) and a topical anesthetic. A possible complication of this disease is the destruction of alveolar bone.

○ **What is the most common oral manifestation of AIDS?**

Oropharyngeal thrush. Some other AIDS-related oropharyngeal diseases are Kaposi sarcoma, hairy leukoplakia, and non-Hodgkin lymphoma. Thrush and be differentiated from leukoplakia if it can be scraped from the mucosa with a tongue blade. Hairy leukoplakia cannot be removed.

○ **What are the key features of Ellis type I, II, and III dental fractures?**

Type I: Enamel, dentin, and pulp.
Type II: Enamel, dentin, and pulp.
Type III: Pulp bleeds.

○ **What risk factors create a higher incidence of oral thrush?**

Immunocompromised patients, dentures, diabetes, inhalers, oral or inhaled steroids and patients taking broad-spectrum antibiotics.

○ **When doing an oral examination, what differentiates oral thrush from leukoplakia?**

Thrush can be scraped off with a tongue depressor revealing inflamed mucosa underneath. Leukoplakia will remain intact when attempting to remove with a tongue depressor.

○ **What are the oral medications of choice for suspected Group A Strep?**

Penicillin V potassium 500 mg twice daily for 10 days. Cefuroxim axetil 250 mg twice daily for 5 to 10 days. Azithromycin 500 mg once daily for 3 days.

○ **Upon physical examination what are the identifying characteristics of an aphthous ulcer?**

Small round erosions in freely moving mucosa, not on the gingiva or palate. They will have whitish-yellow centers with surrounding erythema.

○ **What medical conditions are associated with ulcerative stomatitis?**

Erythema multiforme (drug reaction), herpes, pemphigus, Behçet disease, and inflammatory bowel disease.

○ **What time period is most common for post-tonsillectomy bleeding?**

1 week.

○ **List the "Centor Criteria" for clinical diagnosis of strep throat.**

Fever over 38°C, lack of cough, tonsillar exudate, and tender anterior cervical adenopathy. When three out of four are present there is 90% sensitivity for a positive Group A beta-hemolytic strep rapid antigen test.

NASAL DISORDERS

○ **What are the two common pathogens in adult acute sinusitis?**

Streptococcus pneumoniae and *Haemophilus influenzae*.

○ **A 3-year-old child presents with a unilateral purulent rhinorrhea. What is the probable diagnosis?**

Nasal foreign body.

○ **What potential complications of nasal fracture should always be considered on physical examination?**

Septal hematoma and cribriform plate fractures. A septal hematoma appears as a bluish mass on the nasal septum. If not drained, aseptic necrosis of the septal cartilage and septal abnormalities may occur. A cribriform plate fracture should be considered in a patient who has a clear rhinorrhea after trauma.

○ **What four physical examination findings would make posterior epistaxis more likely than anterior epistaxis?**

  1. Inability to see the site of bleeding. Anterior nosebleeds usually originate at Kiesselbach plexus, and are easily visualized on the nasal septum.

  2. Blood from both sides of the nose. In a posterior nosebleed, the blood can more easily pass to the other side because of the proximity of the choanae.

  3. Blood trickling down the oropharynx.

  4. Inability to control bleeding by direct pressure.

○ **Where is the most common site of bleeding in posterior nosebleeds?**

The sphenopalatine artery's lateral nasal branch.

○ **A patient returns to the emergency department with fever, nausea, vomiting, and hypotension 2 days after having nasal packing placed for an anterior nosebleed. What potential complication of nasal packing should be considered?**

Toxic shock syndrome. Toxic shock syndrome is caused by toxin releasing *Staphylococcus aureus*.

○ **A child with a sinus infection presents with proptosis; a red, swollen eyelid; and an inferolaterally displaced globe. What is the diagnosis?**

Orbital cellulitis and abscess associated with ethmoid sinusitis.

○ **A patient with frontal sinusitis presents with a large forehead abscess. What is the diagnosis?**

Pott puffy tumor. This is a complication of frontal sinusitis in which the anterior table of the skull is destroyed, allowing the formation of the abscess.

○ **An ill-appearing patient presents with a fever of 103°F, bilateral chemosis, third nerve palsies, and untreated sinusitis. What is the diagnosis?**

Cavernous sinus thrombosis. This life-threatening complication occurs from direct extension through the valveless veins. Complications of sinusitis may be local (osteomyelitis), orbital (cellulitis), or within the central nervous system (meningitis or brain abscess).

○ **Boggy blue turbinates and a nasal swab slide showing eosinophils indicate what condition?**

Allergic rhinitis.

○ **Which type of rhinitis is associated with anxious patients?**

Vasomotor rhinitis. This is a nonallergic rhinitis of unknown etiology that involves nasal vascular congestion.

○ **In a patient with nasal polyps and asthma, what medication should be avoided?**

Patients with these findings may also have an immunologic sensitivity to aspirin. Aspirin may precipitate acute bronchospasm (Samter triad).

○ **What diagnosis should be considered for children with nasal polyps?**

Cystic fibrosis.

○ **When evaluating a patient with an acute uncomplicated sinusitis, what imaging diagnostic test is indicated?**

None. Acute bacterial rhinosinusitis is a clinical diagnosis. Plain X-ray films are not cost effective and not recommended.

○ **What is the imaging diagnostic test indicated for evaluation of a patient with chronic sinusitis that is not responding to conventional medical therapy?**

Noncontrast computed tomography (CT) of the paranasal sinuses reveals much more accurate images of the sinuses.

○ **What is the medication of choice for bacterial sinusitis?**

Antibiotic use in sinusitis is controversial in uncomplicated cases. Nasal steroids may reduce facial pain. Nonsteroidal anti-inflammatory drugs also reduce pain. If an antibiotic is indicated, amoxicillin, trimethoprim/sulfamethoxazole or amoxicillin/clavulanate can be used.

○ **What medications can be used for the treatment of allergic rhinitis? What are examples of each medication?**

Medication	Medication Example
Intranasal, oral, or IM steroids	N-Mometasone, fluticasone
	O-Prednisone, methylprednisolone
	IM-Dexamethasone, solu medrol
Antihistamines	loratadine, fexofenadine
Leukotriene inhibitor	montelukast
H1 histamine inhibitor nasal spray	azelastine

○ **What is the most common form of nasopharyngeal cancer?**

Squamous cell carcinoma.

○ **Describe the complications of an untreated septal hematoma.**

Loss of septal cartilage and a "saddle nose deformity"

○ **A patient presents with large amount of bleeding from both nares, and also has posterior pharyngeal drainage of blood, anterior nasal pressure has been ineffective. What do you suspect and what is the treatment?**

Posterior epistaxis. A posterior–anterior packing or balloon tamponade device is needed. Patients with these types of packing usually need to be admitted for pain control and observation for recurrent bleeding.

CHAPTER 6

Gastrointestinal/ Nutritional

Travis Kirby, MPAS, PA-C

○ **A patient presents with chronic, progressive dysphagia of solids and liquids. A barium study shows a dilated esophagus with a distal "bird beak" appearance. What is the likely diagnosis?**

Achalasia.

○ **What study is the gold standard for diagnosing achalasia?**

Esophageal manometry.

○ **What infectious disease closely mimics idiopathic achalasia?**

Chagas disease. It is caused by *Trypanosoma cruzi*, a parasite that damages the myenteric plexus.

○ **What is the most common symptom of esophageal disease?**

Heartburn (pyrosis).

○ **What is the single, best diagnostic study for evaluating a patient with GERD?**

Esophagogastroduodenoscopy (EGD).

○ **Is odynophagia (painful swallowing) a common symptom of GERD?**

No, odynophagia rarely results from GERD. It is normally associated with infectious or eosinophilic esophagitis, malignancy, or ingestion of corrosive agents.

○ **Name four common symptoms of Gastroesophageal reflux disease:**

1. Heartburn
2. Regurgitation of gastric juices
3. Dysphagia (difficulty swallowing)
4. Water brash (overproduction of saliva as a response to acid reflux)

○ **List four atypical symptoms associated with GERD:**
1. Cough
2. Hiccups
3. Throat clearing
4. Wheezing

○ **A hypotensive lower esophageal sphincter (LES) pressure is just one pathophysiological cause of GERD. Provide four dietary examples that can lower LES pressure:**
1. Fatty foods
2. Alcohol
3. Caffeine (coffee, tea, chocolate)
4. Peppermint

○ **List five medicines that can lower LES pressures, thus leading to GERD:**
1. Calcium channel blockers
2. Theophylline
3. Diazepam (Valium)
4. Meperidine (Demerol)
5. Morphine

○ **Do all patients with GERD need esophageal function testing?**
No, any additional testing beyond an EGD should be reserved for patients who either fail medical therapy and lifestyle modification or in whom the correlation of reflux symptoms are in doubt.

○ **Provide five extraesophageal manifestations of GERD:**
1. Asthma
2. Laryngitis/pharyngitis
3. Dental decay
4. Recurrent sinusitis
5. Recurrent otitis media

○ **What are the most serious complications from chronic GERD (gastroesophageal reflux disease)?**
Esophageal stricture and Barrett esophagitis.

○ **Barrett esophagitis is associated with which type of cancer?**
Esophageal adenocarcinoma.

○ **How often should patients with Barrett esophagitis have routine endoscopic surveillance?**
Every 2 to 3 years.

○ **Name four risk factors for the development of esophageal cancer:**

   1. Smoking

   2. Alcohol

   3. Uncontrolled, chronic GERD

   4. Obesity

○ **What is the most predominant type of cancer of the <u>proximal</u> esophagus?**

   Squamous cell carcinoma usually involves the proximal esophagus, whereas adenocarcinoma is predominantly of distal esophageal origin.

○ **What percentage of patients with esophageal cancer is also afflicted with distant metastasis?**

   80%. The 5-year survival rate is 5%.

○ **What is the most common benign esophageal neoplasm?**

   Leiomyoma.

○ **What is the most common cause of infectious esophagitis?**

   Candida albicans.

○ **Name three medications that may predispose a patient to fungal esophagitis:**

   1. Antibiotics

   2. Steroids (both systemic and inhaled)

   3. H2 blockers/PPIs (acid suppression therapy)

○ **List four medical conditions that are strongly associated with fungal esophagitis:**

   1. HIV

   2. Diabetes mellitus

   3. Cushing disease

   4. Alcoholism

○ **A <u>globus sensation</u> is a feeling of a "lump in the throat." Name three potential causes of this symptom:**

   1. GERD

   2. Anxiety disorder

   3. Goiter (causing external compression on the hypopharyngeal area)

○ **What is the most common viral cause of infectious esophagitis?**

   Herpes simplex virus (HSV).

○ **The most common cause of oropharyngeal dysphagia in the elderly is of neuromuscular etiology. Give three examples:**

   1. Cerebrovascular accident (CVA)

   2. Parkinson disease

   3. Motor neuron disorders

O **What is a Zenker diverticulum?**

It is a diverticular outpouching usually located posteriorly in the hypopharynx.

O **List the common symptoms associated with a Zenker diverticulum:**

- Halitosis
- Regurgitation of undigested foods
- Lower neck dysphagia

O **A 24-year-old female patient with dysphagia is found to have an esophageal web on barium studies. What blood disorder should be considered?**

Iron deficiency anemia (related to Plummer–Vinson syndrome).

O **Repeated violent bouts of vomiting can result in both Mallory–Weiss tears and Boerhaave syndrome. Differentiate between the two:**

Mallory–Weiss tears involve the submucosa and mucosa, typically in the right posterolateral wall of the gastroesophageal junction.

Boerhaave syndrome is a full-thickness tear, usually in the unsupported left posterolateral wall of the distal esophagus.

O **What are the signs and symptoms of Boerhaave syndrome?**

Substernal and left-sided chest pain with a history of forceful vomiting, leading to spontaneous esophageal rupture. The abdomen can become rigid and shock may follow.

O **What is the test of choice to confirm the diagnosis of Boerhaave syndrome?**

An esophagram. A water-soluble contrast medium should be used in place of barium to confirm the diagnosis.

O **What is Hamman sign?**

It is air in the mediastinum following an esophageal perforation. This condition produces a "crunching" sound over the heart during systole.

O **What is the best way to remove a meat bolus causing esophageal obstruction?**

Upper endoscopy.

O **What test must be performed after a food bolus is cleared or passes through spontaneously?**

Either a barium study or preferably an endoscopy to check for underlying pathology (e.g., strictures, masses).

O **What are the most common symptoms of gastritis?**

- Dyspepsia (epigastric discomfort or burning)
- Postprandial fullness or bloating
- Nausea
- Vomiting

○ **List three common causes of <u>acute gastritis</u>:**

1. NSAIDs

2. Alcohol

3. Bisphosphonates

○ **What etiologies are more commonly associated with <u>chronic gastritis</u>?**

- *Helicobacter pylori* infection
- Alcohol
- NSAIDs
- Bile acid reflux

○ **What are potential risk factors for exposure to *Helicobacter pylori* infection?**

Crowded living conditions, suboptimal sanitation, and low socioeconomic status.

○ **List the various methods in which *Helicobacter pylori* can be diagnosed:**

- <u>Invasively</u> via endoscopic gastroduodenal biopsies
- <u>Noninvasively</u> via:
  - serology (*H. pylori* antibody)
  - urea breath test
  - stool antigen test

○ **Does *Helicobacter pylori* play a role in either gastric or duodenal ulcers?**

Yes, most gastric ulcers occur in the setting of *H. pylori* gastritis (~60%–80%). The association is quite strong with duodenal ulcers as well.

○ **Can *Helicobacter pylori* be considered a "potential suspect" in causing gastric cancer?**

Yes, gastric cancer is the second most common cancer in the world and is classified as a group I carcinogen by the World Health Organization (WHO). Patients with *H. pylori* have a fivefold higher incidence of gastric cancer.

○ **What continents and countries have the highest prevalence of gastric cancer?**

Asia and South America have the highest rate of gastric cancer. Japan, Chile, and Costa Rica have the greatest risk.

○ **What lifestyle or dietary factors are suspected to be linked to gastric cancer?**

- Highly salted meats or fish
- Smoked meats
- Tobacco smoking

○ **What is the most common type of gastric carcinoma? What percent of these are ulcerative, polypoid, or linitis plastica?**

Adenocarcinomas account for 90% of gastric cancers. Of these, 75% are ulcerative, 10% are polypoid, and 15% are diffuse infiltrative (linitis plastica).

○ **What percentage of gastric carcinomas produces a positive hemoccult test?**

50%.

○ **What percentage of gastric carcinomas is associated with a palpable mass?**

25%.

○ **What is a Krukenberg tumor?**

It is a gastric carcinoma that has metastasized to the ovary.

○ **Stomach cancer is associated with the enlargement of what lymph nodes?**

Supraclavicular nodes (sentinel nodes).

○ **Is peptic ulcer disease (PUD) more common in men or women?**

Men (a 3:1 male-to-female ratio).

○ **Are patients with duodenal PUD usually younger or older?**

Younger. Duodenal PUD is more often associated with *Helicobacter pylori*. Older people tend to develop gastric ulcers as a result of NSAID use.

○ **Do gastric or duodenal ulcers heal faster?**

Duodenal.

○ **What medical conditions are associated with an increased incidence of peptic ulcer disease?**

- COPD
- Cirrhosis
- Chronic renal failure

○ **Are gastric and duodenal <u>perforations</u> more commonly associated with malignant or benign ulcerations?**

Benign ulcers.

○ **Is gastrointestinal bleeding common with a perforated ulcer?**

No.

○ **After the fluid and blood resuscitation of a bleeding ulcer, what is the most useful diagnostic test?**

Upper endoscopy is the most useful test because it can also be therapeutic via cryo- or electrocautery of an arterial bleeder.

○ **What are some indications for surgery in a bleeding ulcer?**

- A visible vessel in the ulcer bed
- More than 6 units of blood transfused in 24 hours
- More than 3 to 4 units transfused per day for 3 days

○ **Name two endocrine problems that can cause PUD:**

Zollinger–Ellison syndrome and hyperparathyroidism (hypercalcemia).

○ **What anatomic location do most gastric ulcers occur?**

The lesser curvature of the stomach.

○   **A 48-year-old female diabetic patient presents with a multimonth history of chronic nausea, early satiety, and postprandial bloating. What is the most likely diagnosis?**

Diabetic gastroparesis.

○   **Define gastroparesis:**

It is a motility disorder of the stomach that results in impairment of the normal gastric emptying mechanism. "Delayed gastric emptying."

○   **What is the most common etiology of gastroparesis?**

Idiopathic. Other associated factors may include diabetes, gastric cancer, prior gastric bypass surgery, chronic gastritis, or exposure to viral gastroenteritis.

○   **How prevalent are gallstones in the Western population?**

Approximately 10% to 15% of adults have gallstones, with women being twice as likely. Approximately 20% of those adults will develop symptoms.

○   **List the ultrasound findings that are suggestive of acute cholecystitis:**

- Formation of gallstones or sludge
- Thickening of the gallbladder wall by more than 5 mm
- Presence of pericholecystic fluid
- A dilated common bile duct (>10 mm may suggest common bile duct obstruction).

○   **A patient with a history of gallstones presents with acute, postprandial RUQ pain. What is the KUB likely to show?**

Nothing specific. Only about 10% to 15% of gallstones are radiopaque.

○   **Gallbladder stones are made predominantly of what two materials?**

Cholesterol (80%) and bile pigments (20%).

○   **What is the diagnostic test of choice to evaluate a patient suspected to have gallstones?**

Abdominal ultrasound has a 95% detection rate for gallstones.

○   **If the abdominal ultrasound is nondiagnostic for gallstones, could the patient still have gallbladder disease? If so, what additional tests can be ordered?**

Yes, although structurally things may look normal, a patient may still exhibit symptoms from a functional disorder of the gallbladder. Biliary dyskinesia and acalculous cholecystitis are two examples. The test of choice would be a HIDA scan (radionuclide biliary scan) with cholecystokinin to calculate a gallbladder ejection fraction and to gauge if CCK administration reproduces the patient's episodic symptoms.

○   **What drugs can impair gallbladder emptying?**

1. Anticholinergic agents
2. Narcotic medications

○ **A 54-year-old man, 2 days postop for a right knee replacement, presents with RUQ abdominal pain, nausea, and low-grade fevers. His ultrasound fails to reveal any gallstones or other obvious GB abnormality. What is the probable diagnosis?**

<u>Acalculous cholecystitis</u>: This is a condition most often seen in postoperative, posttraumatic, and burn patients secondary to dehydration.

○ **Which types of patients are at greatest risk for gallbladder perforation?**

The elderly patients, diabetic patients, and those with recurrent cholecystitis.

○ **What dietary history would be suspicious for underlying biliary disease?**

The ingestion of fried, fatty, greasy, oily or rich foods within 20 minutes to 2 hours prior to symptom onset. Patients may describe any of the following: epigastric or RUQ abdominal pain accompanied by nausea and/or vomiting, bloating, belching, and heartburn.

○ **What clinical sign can assist in the diagnosis of cholecystitis?**

Murphy sign is pain on inspiration with palpation of the RUQ. As the patient breathes in, the gallbladder is lowered in the abdomen and comes in contact with the peritoneum just below the examiner's hand. This will aggravate an inflamed gallbladder, causing the patient to abruptly discontinue breathing deeply.

○ **Which ethnic group has the largest proportion of people with symptomatic gallstones?**

<u>Native Americans</u>. By the age of 60 years, 80% of native Americans with previously asymptomatic gallstones will develop symptoms as compared to only 30% of Caucasian Americans and 20% of African Americans.

○ **Eight years after cholecystectomy, a woman develops RUQ pain and jaundice. What is the chance of recurrent biliary tract stones developing?**

At least 10%; the recurrence may be because of either retained stones or in situ formation by the biliary epithelium.

○ **What is the significance of a porcelain gallbladder?**

Defined as intramural calcification of the gallbladder wall that is normally seen on CT or plain radiographs. It has a 20% association with gallbladder carcinoma, and if discovered, cholecystectomy is recommended.

○ **Should the presence of gallbladder polyps necessitate cholecystectomy?**

Yes, all lesions >1 cm in size should be removed to rule out malignancy. Smaller lesions should be followed closely with ultrasound every 6 months.

○ **An 11-year-old child with sickle cell anemia presents with fever, RUQ abdominal pain, and jaundice. What is the most likely diagnosis?**

Charcot triad suggests ascending cholangitis. The precipitating cause in this case is probably pigment stones resulting from chronic hemolysis.

○ **What is the difference between cholelithiasis, cholangitis, cholecystitis, and choledocholithiasis?**

Cholelithiasis: Gallstones within the gallbladder sac.

Cholangitis: Inflammation of the common bile duct, often caused by infection or choledocholithiasis.

Cholecystitis: Inflammation of the gallbladder.

Choledocholithiasis: Gallstones that have migrated from the gallbladder sac into the common bile duct.

○ **What is the most frequent complication of choledocholithiasis?**

Cholangitis (60%). Other complications include bile duct obstruction, pancreatitis, biliary enteric fistula, and hemobilia. Cholangitis is a medical emergency when fever exceeds 101°F or is associated with sepsis, hypotension, peritoneal signs, or a bilirubin level >10 mg/dL. CT or abdominal ultrasonography is supportive of the diagnosis.

○ **What is the most likely diagnosis for a patient who presents with epigastric pain that radiates to the back and is partially relieved by sitting up?**

Pancreatitis.

○ **What are the major causes of acute pancreatitis?**

Alcoholism (40%) and gallstone disease (40%). The other causes of acute pancreatitis are familial inheritance, hyperparathyroidism, infection, hypertriglyceridemia, drugs, trauma, and protein deficiency.

○ **Name two metabolic causes of acute pancreatitis:**

Hypertriglyceridemia and hypercalcemia.

○ **What are some of the drugs known to cause pancreatitis?**

Sulfonamides, estrogens, tetracyclines, thiazides, furosemide, and valproic acid.

○ **What are some of the infectious causes of pancreatitis?**

Mumps, viral hepatitis, Coxsackie virus group B, and mycoplasma.

○ **What is the most common cause of <u>chronic</u> pancreatitis in Western society?**

Chronic alcohol abuse.

○ **Does acute pancreatitis <u>commonly</u> progress to chronic pancreatitis?**

No, only rarely.

○ **What are the laboratory abnormalities associated with pancreatitis?**

Leukocytosis, hyperglycemia, elevated amylase, elevated lipase, hepatic enzyme elevation, hypoxemia, and prerenal azotemia.

○ **What are some abdominal X-ray findings associated with acute pancreatitis?**

- A sentinel loop (either of the jejunum, transverse colon, or duodenum)
- A colon cutoff sign (an abrupt cessation of gas in the mid or left transverse colon)
- Calcification of the pancreas

○ **Serum amylase is frequently elevated in acute pancreatitis. What other conditions can cause a similar rise in amylase?**

Salivary stones, renal failure, mumps, cholecystitis, bowel infarction, perforated ulcer, ovarian disorders, pancreatic cancer, and macroamylasemia.

○ **When is surgery indicated in pancreatitis?**

When a patient has an infected pancreatic necrosis or an abscess that cannot be adequately drained and treated.

○ **Should immediate surgery be performed in gallstone-induced pancreatitis?**

NO, it should be performed after the pancreatitis has subsided.

○ **What is <u>Cullen sign</u>?**

Periumbilical ecchymosis indicative of <u>pancreatitis</u>, severe upper GI bleeding, or ruptured ectopic pregnancy.

○ **What is <u>Courvoisier sign</u>?**

It is a palpable, distended gallbladder in the RUQ of patients with jaundice. It is usually the result of a malignant bile duct.

○ **Where is the most common site of pancreatic cancer?**

The pancreatic duct system (~80%) found in the <u>head of the pancreas.</u>

○ **With regard to pancreatic cancer, distinguish between periampullary lesions and lesions of the body and tail.**

Periampullary lesions most commonly develop at the head of the pancreas. These lesions are usually adenocarcinomas and are associated with jaundice, weight loss, and abdominal pain.

Lesions in the body and tail tend to be much larger at presentation because of their retroperitoneal location and their distance from the common bile duct. Weight loss and pain are typical.

○ **What are the risk factors for pancreatic cancer?**

- Smoking
- High-fat diet
- Chronic pancreatitis

○ **What are the associated symptoms of pancreatic cancer?**

- Weight loss
- Abdominal pain
- Nausea and anorexia
- Easy fatigability
- Painless jaundice

○ **What is the tumor marker that can assist in diagnosing pancreatic cancer?**

CA 19-9.

○ **What is the survival rate for pancreatic cancer?**

Less than 20% survive beyond 1 year from their initial diagnosis and less than 30% survive longer than 5 years.

○ **What are the two most common causes of ascites?**

- Chronic liver disease
- Peritoneal carcinomatosis

○ **What are the two main mechanisms of liver injury?**

Hepatocellular injury indicates damage or destruction of the liver cells; most often caused by viral hepatitis, autoimmune hepatitis, and drugs/toxins.

Cholestatic injury indicates impaired transport of bile. This may be caused by:

- Extrahepatic obstruction (gallstones)
- Intrahepatic duct narrowing (primary sclerosing cholangitis)
- Bile duct damage (primary biliary cirrhosis)

○ **How is cholestatic injury best detected?**

By an elevated alkaline phosphatase (AP) level. However, keep in mind that alkaline phosphatase can be derived from other body tissue (e.g., bone, intestine), so a concurrent elevation of GGT or 5′-nucleosidase helps to support a cholestatic mechanism.

○ **What is the test of choice to assess for hepatocellular injury?**

ALT level. The AST level may also be elevated but is not as specific.

○ **Name the two most common causes of drug-induced liver disease:**

Alcohol and acetaminophen.

○ **What recreational drugs are associated with hepatotoxicity?**

Cocaine and ecstasy.

○ **How are hepatitis viruses transmitted?**

- A and E = fecal, oral route
- B, C, D = blood borne

○ **Name four other viruses, other than Hepatitis A through E, which can affect the liver:**

1. Cytomegalovirus
2. Herpes simplex virus
3. Epstein–Barr virus
4. Arthropod-borne flaviviruses (e.g., dengue, yellow fever)

○ **What are the predominant characteristics of <u>autoimmune hepatitis</u>?**

This condition affects mostly women (~70%) and is typically diagnosed in the fourth to fifth decade of life. It is essentially an idiopathic, unresolving inflammation of the liver, which can lead to cirrhosis, portal hypertension, liver failure, or even death.

○ **Differentiate primary biliary cirrhosis (PBC) with primary sclerosing cholangitis (PSC):**

- Primary biliary cirrhosis mainly affects women in their fifties and is characterized by destruction of the septal bile ducts.
- Primary sclerosing cholangitis mainly affects men in their forties and involves diffuse inflammation and fibrosis of the entire biliary tree.

Both are chronic cholestatic liver diseases of unknown etiology that can eventually progress to end-stage liver disease.

○ **What other gastrointestinal condition is strongly associated with primary sclerosing cholangitis?**

Inflammatory bowel disease.

○ **What is hemochromatosis?**

It is a disease of <u>iron overload</u> in the liver and other organs with the most likely defect occurring in a regulatory mechanism for iron absorption in the small intestine.

○ **What is the most common screening test for hemochromatosis?**

Serum ferritin—an elevated level >400 mg/dL suggests the possibility of iron overload, but unfortunately serum ferritin can be an acute phase reactant. Thus, supportive testing (e.g., iron saturation, genetic testing, or liver biopsy) is needed to confirm the diagnosis.

○ **What is the treatment for genetic hemochromatosis?**

Phlebotomy, with the removal of 1 to 2 units per week.

○ **A 52-year-old patient presents with tremor, ataxia, dementia, cirrhosis, and gray-green rings around the edge of the cornea. What is the diagnosis?**

Wilson disease—this is a disorder of <u>copper storage</u> and is associated with deficiency of an enzyme derived from hepatic cells. Deposition of copper may be seen in the eye (*Kayser–Fleischer rings*) and in parts of the brain.

○ **How is Wilson disease accurately diagnosed?**

A <u>diminished serum ceruloplasmin level</u> is strongly suggestive of Wilson disease. A quantitative copper level in liver tissue from liver biopsy should provide a definitive diagnosis.

○ **The development of acute liver failure would be indicated by what hallmark diagnostic signs?**

1. Coagulopathy (INR > 1.5)
2. Encephalopathy (that occurs within 8 weeks of illness onset)

○ **List six extra hepatic manifestations of alcoholic liver disease:**

1. Ascites
2. Spider angiomata
3. Asterixis
4. Palmar erythema
5. Korsakoff syndrome
6. Wernicke encephalopathy

○ **In the United States, what is the percentage of patients with chronic alcohol abuse that will evolve to develop cirrhosis of the liver?**

Approximately 25%.

○ **What are the most common vascular tumors of the liver?**

Hemangiomas.

○ **What is the most common cause of jaundice in pregnancy?**

Viral hepatitis.

○ **What is the most common liver disorder related to pregnancy?**

Intrahepatic cholestasis.

○ **What is the most common clinical symptom of intrahepatic cholestasis of pregnancy?**

Severe pruritus in the third trimester.

○ **Nonalcoholic steatohepatitis (NASH) is becoming a growing concern in the United States. What other clinical conditions are associated with primary NASH?**

- Morbid obesity
- Non-insulin–dependent diabetes
- Hyperlipidemia

○ **What is the most common laboratory abnormality in patients with NASH?**

A two- to threefold increase in the serum AST and ALT.

○ **What is the most specific imaging technique used to evaluate NASH?**

Hepatic ultrasound.

○ **Patients with cirrhosis or chronic active hepatitis should have what routine testing performed to screen for hepatomas?**

Alpha-fetoprotein levels and a hepatic ultrasound should be performed every 6 months. These patients have a higher risk for developing hepatic cancer.

○ **List four common symptoms of cirrhosis:**

1. Fatigue
2. Generalized weakness
3. Poor appetite
4. Weight loss

○ **A 43-year-old patient presents with a 6-week history of frequent, malodorous diarrhea that leaves an oily sheen to the surface of the toilet water. You suspect a malabsorption disorder. What is the best study to screen for fat malabsorption?**

A microscopic stool examination using Sudan stain; it has 100% sensitivity and 96% specificity.

○ **What is the best test to differentiate malabsorption caused by small bowel versus pancreatic etiology?**

d-Xylose test.

○ **What is the most sensitive and specific serum marker for celiac disease?**

Tissue transglutaminase (tTG).

○ **What condition should be considered in a celiac patient who had previously responded well to a gluten-free diet, but now has developed refractory symptoms?**

Small bowel lymphoma.

○ **What are the signs and symptoms of <u>Whipple disease</u>?**

- Weight loss
- Diarrhea
- Arthralgias
- Cardiac involvement

○ **What gastrointestinal disease is most commonly associated with _Dermatitis Herpetiformis_?**

Celiac disease (gluten enteropathy).

○ **List the signs and symptoms of Crohn disease:**

- Abdominal pain (especially RLQ)
- Weight loss
- Diarrhea
- Fever
- Perianal fistulas
- Arthritis
- Hematochezia

○ **What other diseases can mimic Crohn disease?**

- Ischemic colitis
- Diverticulitis
- Colorectal cancer
- Infection with _Yersinia_ species

○ **Name five potential treatment options for Crohn disease:**

1. 5-Aminosalicylic acid (5ASA) agents
2. Immunosuppressant therapy (azathioprine, 6-mercaptopurine)
3. Steroids (prednisone)
4. Biologic therapy
5. Surgery

○ **What effect does smoking have on Crohn disease and ulcerative colitis?**

- Crohn disease: <u>detrimental effect</u>; cigarette smokers are more likely to develop Crohn, have a worse prognosis, and have an increased number of recurrent flares.
- Ulcerative colitis: <u>protective effect</u>; the incidence of ulcerative colitis is higher in non- and exsmokers than in current smokers.

○ **What is the greatest risk factor for ulcerative colitis?**

Family history. Approximately 15% of patients with ulcerative colitis have a first-degree relative with the disease.

○ **What are the signs and symptoms of ulcerative colitis?**

- Diarrhea
- Rectal bleeding (hematochezia)
- Tenesmus
- Passage of mucus

○ **Name five extraintestinal manifestations of ulcerative colitis:**

1. Arthritis
2. Erythema nodosum
3. Uveitis
4. Ankylosing spondylitis
5. Primary Sclerosing cholangitis

○ **What are the two histologic types of microscopic colitis?**

1. Lymphocytic
2. Collagenous

○ **What class of medication is commonly associated with the development of microscopic colitis?**

Nonsteroidal anti-inflammatory drugs (NSAIDs)

○ **What is the least common site of primary gastrointestinal cancer?**

Small bowel. Although it contains 75% of the length and 90% of the mucosal surface area, the small bowel only accounts for 1% to 2% of GI cancers. Adenocarcinoma remains the most prevalent type followed by lymphoma.

○ **Define carcinoid syndrome:**

Carcinoid syndrome refers to systemic symptoms resulting from the secretion of humoral factors by the Carcinoid (neuroendocrine) tumor. These symptoms may include:

- Episodic flushing of the face and upper trunk
- Watery diarrhea
- Bronchospasm

○ **What is the most likely distribution of carcinoid tumors?**

Carcinoid tumors are slow growing and can occur anywhere along the GI tract. Most are found incidentally, thus at the time of discovery, most patients are asymptomatic. Only 5% of patients with carcinoid tumors have carcinoid syndrome (see above). Common sites for carcinoid growth include the appendix (most common), followed by the ileum, then stomach, rectum, colon, and pancreas.

○ **If carcinoid syndrome is strongly suspected, what is the best initial diagnostic study to pursue?**

A urine analysis for 5-HIAA (hydroxyindoleacetic acid) will be increased. If the urine for 5-HIAA is increased then a CT of the abdomen and pelvis or an Octreoscan (Octreotide scintigraphy) should identify the primary site of the tumor in 80% of cases.

○ **What is the most common cancer arising in the colon?**
Adenocarcinoma.

○ **How does colorectal cancer rank in mortality for the population of the United States?**
Second, behind lung cancer.

○ **Considering those within the United States population who do not have a significant family history of colorectal cancer, at what age should general screening begin?**
Caucasians and other races = age 50 years African
Americans = age 45 years

○ **What two clinical conditions should raise the suspicion for the presence of colon cancer?**
1. An unexplained iron deficiency anemia
2. Sepsis with *Streptococcus bovis*

○ **What is the "gold standard" for identifying colorectal cancer?**
Colonoscopy.

○ **What endocrine disorder has the highest incidence of colorectal cancer?**
Acromegaly.

○ **Name two endocrine disorders that can cause constipation:**
1. Hypothyroidism
2. Diabetes mellitus

○ **What is melanosis coli ?**
It is a benign disorder of pigmentation that develops within the walls of the colon. The most common cause of the brownish pigment (Lipofuscin) is the prolonged use of laxatives. Although it does not lead to any colonic dysfunction, the hyperpigmentation can present greater challenges to the gastroenterologist when trying to locate polyps for colorectal cancer screening.

○ **What laxatives are most commonly associated with melanosis coli?**
Anthraquinones, including aloe, cascara, and senna.

○ **A 72-year-old female patient presents with a 2-day history of progressively worsening LLQ abdominal pain associated with constipation and "chills." What is the most likely diagnosis?**
Diverticulitis.

○ **What are potential complications of diverticulitis?**
• Abscess formation
• Perforation leading to peritonitis
• Diverticular bleeding
• Obstruction from diverticular strictures or luminal narrowing

○ **List three risk factors for diverticulosis:**

1. Increasing age
2. Chronic constipation that leads to increased luminal pressures
3. Westernized diet—low in fiber and high in refined carbohydrates

○ **What groups are most at risk for perforation of appendicitis?**

- Children younger than 5 years of age
- Elderly patients
- Diabetic patients
- Immunosuppressed patients

○ **What is the most common tumor of the appendix?**

Carcinoid tumor.

○ **What antibiotics are commonly associated with *Clostridium difficile* colitis?**

C. difficile colitis can occur with any antibiotic, even a single-dose preop. But the most likely suspects remain clindamycin, ampicillin, and third-generation cephalosporins.

○ **What is the first-line treatment of *C. difficile* colitis?**

Metronidazole (Flagyl). Improvement should begin with 2 to 4 days and resolution of diarrhea by 2 weeks. If the patient does not respond to metronidazole, then vancomycin should be considered.

○ **List the most common sources of upper gastrointestinal bleeding:**

- Duodenal ulcers
- Gastric erosions
- Gastric ulcers
- Esophagitis

○ **What is the most likely source of acute hematemesis in a 43-year-old male patient with a history of cirrhosis?**

Esophageal varices (50%).

○ **What is the most common cause of hematochezia (bright red rectal bleeding) or lower GI bleeding in adults?**

Internal hemorrhoids.

○ **List four other causes of lower GI bleeding:**

1. Diverticulitis
2. Vascular ectasias
3. Neoplasms
4. Ischemic colitis

○ **What is the most common cause of lower GI bleeding in children?**

Meckel diverticulum—located in the ileum, it is the most common congenital abnormality of the gut.

O **What is the most common complication of a Meckel diverticulum?**

Bleeding. It presents with painless melena or hematochezia described as "currant jelly" like stools. Diagnosis is established via a Meckel scan (technetium-99m scintiscan).

O **An 82-year-old male patient presents with an acute onset of crampy LLQ abdominal pain with the urge to defecate and expulsion of bloody diarrhea. Associated symptoms include nausea, fever, and tachycardia. Plain film abdominal X-rays reveal "thumbprinting" changes. What is the most likely diagnosis?**

Ischemic colitis.

O **A differential diagnosis for <u>bloody diarrhea</u> would include:**

- Ischemic colitis
- Infectious colitis
- Radiation proctitis
- Inflammatory bowel disease (UC or Crohn disease)
- Meckel diverticulum

O **How much blood is needed to produce a positive hemoccult (fecal occult blood test)?**

As little as 2 mL.

O **What is the test of choice to accurately diagnose celiac sprue (gluten enteropathy)?**

Upper endoscopy with biopsies obtained from the duodenum that demonstrates <u>flattened small bowel villi in association with increased epithelial lymphocytes.</u>

O **Name two methods used to diagnose lactose intolerance:**

1. Dietary history and response to empiric therapy
2. Hydrogen breath test

O **What are the four types of stimuli for abdominal pain?**

1. Stretching or tension
2. Inflammation
3. Ischemia
4. Neoplasms

O **What is the single best test to evaluate HIV-infected patients who present with abdominal pain?**

CT of the abdomen and pelvis.

O **What gastrointestinal symptoms may occur in patients with pheochromocytoma?**

- Weight loss
- Anorexia
- Abdominal pain caused by cholelithiasis

O **What is the significance of <u>Sister Mary Joseph node</u>?**

It is an umbilical metastasis manifesting as periumbilical lymphadenopathy from an internal malignancy. It usually indicates advanced disease with an average survival time of up to 10 months.

○ **What other type of <u>node</u> may represent an intra-abdominal malignancy?**

Virchow node, presenting as a supraclavicular mass, may indicate a bowel carcinoma.

○ **What is a common cause of acute abdominal pain in illicit drug users?**

<u>Acute mesenteric ischemia</u> ("crack belly") can be seen in cocaine abusers.

○ **What is the differential diagnosis of yellowish discoloration of the skin?**

- Jaundice
- Hypercarotenemia (overingestion of carotene, e.g., carrots, squash)
- Lycopenodermia (overingestion of lycopenes, e.g., red veggies, tomatoes)
- Profound hypothyroidism

○ **What type of gastroenteritis is closely associated with the consumption of seafood?**

Vibrio parahaemolyticus.

○ **What is the most common cause of gastroenteritis in the United States?**

Viruses.

○ **What is the most common cause of childhood diarrhea?**

Rotavirus.

○ **Ordering stool cultures is appropriate in patients presenting with what characteristics?**

- Bloody diarrhea
- High fever
- Presence of fecal leukocytes
- Immunocompromised patients
- Diarrhea persisting longer than 72 hours

○ **Name the most common bacterial causes of infectious diarrhea in the United States:**

Remember C, C, S, S, Y, and sometimes E:

Campylobacter
Clostridium
Salmonella
Shigella
Yersinia
Escherichia coli O157:H7

○ **What is the most common bacterial source to infectious diarrhea in the United States?**

Campylobacter jejuni.

○ **What is the most common parasitic diarrhea infection in the United States? In the world?**

<u>Giardia lamblia</u> is the most common in the United States.
<u>Amebiasis</u> (*Entamoeba histolytica*) is the most common in the world.

○ **Deficiency of what two vitamins can cause a macrocytic anemia?**

Folate and B12.

○ **What is the leading cause of death in bulimia nervosa?**

Cardiac arrhythmia.

○ **What proportion of adults in the United States is obese?**

Approximately one-third.

○ **What vitamin deficiency does the Schilling test evaluate?**

Vitamin B12.

○ **Pellagra is caused primarily by a deficiency of what nutrient?**

Niacin.

○ **What are the three D's of pellagra?**

Dermatitis

Diarrhea

Dementia

○ **What is the most common dermatologic finding in patients with hemochromatosis?**

Bronze pigmentation of the skin.

○ **What two dermatologic signs may assist in the diagnosis of acute pancreatitis?**

1. Cullen sign (periumbilical bruising)

2. Grey Turner sign (flank bruising)

○ **What is a possible finding on an upper GI series from a woman with telangiectasias, tight knuckles, and acid indigestion?**

Aperistalsis. The defective peristalsis can be associated with connective tissue disorders such as scleroderma, or in this clinical scenario, a CREST syndrome:

Calcinosis cutis

Raynaud phenomenon

Esophageal dysfunction

Sclerodactyly

Telangiectasias

○ **Rickets is associated with a deficiency of what vitamin?**

Vitamin D.

○ **A 38-year-old male patient presents with anorexia, lethargy, arthralgias, and swollen gums. What vitamin deficiency may be present?**

Vitamin C (scurvy).

○ **Deficiencies in either of these two micronutrients may cause paresthesias, tetany, seizures, or arrhythmia:**

Calcium or magnesium.

○ **Night blindness may be associated with what vitamin deficiency?**

Vitamin A.

○ **What is the most common risk factor for hepatitis C?**

Intravenous drug abuse accounts for 43% of cases.

○ **List four factors that increase the risk for colorectal cancer:**

1. Increasing age
2. Family history of polyps or CRC
3. Inflammatory bowel disease
4. Diets high in fat and low in fiber

○ **What are three basic mechanisms of weight loss?**

1. Decreased food intake (e.g., esophageal stricture)
2. Increased metabolism (e.g., hyperthyroidism)
3. Increased loss of energy (e.g., intestinal malabsorption with steatorrhea)

○ **What are the leading causes of unexplained weight loss in the elderly?**

- Psychiatric
- Malignancy
- Gastrointestinal disorders

○ **What is the most common digestive complaint in the United States?**

Constipation.

○ **List four common causes of acute abdominal pain in the elderly from most to least prevalent:**

1. Biliary tract disease
2. Bowel obstruction
3. Incarcerated hernias
4. Appendicitis

○   **Identify six causes of chronic hiccups:**
   1. Abdominal distention
   2. Brain stem lesion
   3. Gastric malignancy
   4. Pleural irritation
   5. Pancreatitis
   6. Chronic renal failure

CHAPTER 7

Genitourinary/ Nephrology

Courtney C. Anderson, MPA, PA-C

CONDITIONS OF THE GU TRACT

○ **What is the most common benign tumor found in men?**

Benign prostatic hyperplasia (BPH).

○ **A 56-year-old male reports that his urinary stream has weakened. He also complains of nocturia, hesitancy, and postvoid dribbling. On the basis of this patient's history, what do you expect to find on his physical examination?**

In most cases of suspected BPH, the prostate will have a smooth, symmetric, firm, and elastic consistency. If you detect an irregular, harder nodule or lesion, cancer must be suspected.

○ **How well does the size of the prostate in BPH correlate with the symptoms?**

Not well. Symptoms can arise because of a small fibrous prostate as well as a large one. Additional symptoms can also develop as a result of median lobe hypertrophy, detrusor muscle decompensation, or instability.

○ **What percentage of men with BPH are afflicted with occult prostate cancer?**

10% to 30%.

○ **What classes of drugs are used in the first-line treatment of BPH?**

1. Alpha-blockers—reduce muscle tone in the prostate/bladder neck (i.e., Terazosin, Doxazosin, Tamsulosin, Alfuzosin, Silodosin)
2. 5-alpha reductase inhibitors—block intracellular DHT conversion; generally best for larger glands; may take 6 to 12 months for improvement in symptoms (i.e., Finasteride, Dutasteride)
3. Antimuscarinic agents—may help with bladder overactivity

○ **What are the absolute surgical indications for BPH?**

Refractory urinary retention (failing at least one attempt at catheter removal), recurring urinary tract infection from BPH, recurrent gross hematuria from BPH, bladder stones from BPH, renal insufficiency from BPH, or large bladder diverticula.

○ **Cryptorchidism places a patient at increased risk for what issues later in life?**

The undescended testis is considered a developmental defect and places the affected testis at higher risk for developing cancer. The relative risk is approximately 40 times greater in men with a history of cryptorchidism regardless of whether orchiopexy is performed or not. These patients also have an increased risk of infertility because of the deterioration in germ cell numbers.

○ **Which children are at higher risk for having cryptorchidism?**

Premature births (<37 weeks) have up to 30% prevalence.

○ **What is the most common systemic cause of erectile dysfunction?**

Diabetes. Erectile dysfunction in men with diabetes occurs approximately threefold more often than that of the general population.

○ **Name some systemic conditions that can cause erectile dysfunction:**

Diabetes, hypercholesterolemia, heart disease, depression, renal failure, adrenal and thyroid dysfunction.

○ **What are the most common treatment options for improving erectile dysfunction:**

Hormonal replacement (in young hypogonadal men without contraindications), oral phosphodiesterase (PDE) inhibitors, vacuum constriction device (VED), vascular surgery, intracavernosal injection, transurethral therapy, and penile prosthesis.

○ **A 4-year-old boy presents with a painless mass in his scrotum that fluctuates in size with palpation. The mass transilluminates. What is the probable diagnosis?**

A communicating hydrocele (also called congenital hydrocele). A transscrotal ultrasound should distinguish hydrocele from bowel and rule out tumor. A testicular nuclear scan or Doppler ultrasound should rule out testicular torsion.

○ **When do congenital hydroceles need repair?**

Most resolve in first year of life. Persistence suggests the presence of a patent indirect hernia sac that should be repaired. So, if after 1 year to 18 months they do not reduce in size or become larger, surgery is indicated.

○ **Varicoceles are most common on which side of the scrotum?**

The left. The left internal spermatic vein is longer than the right; in addition, it joins the left renal vein at right angles, resulting in higher venous pressures and retrograde reflux of blood. Varicoceles are a collection of dilated and tortuous veins within the pampiniform plexus in the scrotum. These patients have a higher incidence of infertility. Hernias are also more common on the left side, too.

○ **Are varicoceles commonly treated surgically?**

No, most are left alone. Treatment is reserved for cases of suspicion of infertility.

○ **What is the postvoid residual volume that suggests urinary retention?**

A volume greater than 150 mL would constitute an inability to properly empty the urinary bladder. Normal PVR is <30 mL but can vary.

○ **Name the most common classifications (types) of urinary incontinence:**

Stress incontinence—associated with increased intra-abdominal pressure such as coughing, sneezing, or exertion.

Urge incontinence—sudden uncontrollable urgency, leading to leakage of urine (aka overactive bladder)

Overflow incontinence—high residual or chronic urinary retention results in leakage because of overdistention

Mixed incontinence—loss of urine from a combination of stress and urge incontinence

Functional—loss of urine because of the deficits of cognition and mobility

Total incontinence—continuous leakage of urine

○ **Which type of incontinence is most common?**

Stress urinary incontinence (SUI) is most common (49%), followed by mixed (29%), and urge (21%) incontinence.

○ **What is the mnemonic that refers to the correctable causes of urinary incontinence?**

"DIAPPERS"

Delirium

Infection—urinary

Atrophic urethritis and atrophic vaginitis

Pharmaceuticals: sedatives, hypnotics, alcohol, diuretics, and anticholinergics

Psychological disorders: depression, psychosis

Excessive urinary output—for example, heart failure, hyperglycemia

Restricted mobility

Stool impaction

○ **What is the most common underlying etiology of urge incontinence?**

Detrusor instability. (Sphincteric instability is less common.)

○ **What is the anatomic feature of genuine stress incontinence?**

Hypermobility or a lowering of the position of the vesicourethral segment. (The intrinsic structure of the sphincter itself is intact and normal; however, it loses efficiency because of the excessive mobility and/or loss of support.)

○ **What are some examples of stress incontinence?**

Incontinence after laughing, coughing, sneezing, exercising, or lifting heavy objects.

○ **What are Kegel exercises?**

First described by Arnold Kegel in 1948, these are pelvic floor muscle exercises. The usual regimen consists of multiple contractions of the pubococcygeus muscle. If properly performed, they can help improve the symptoms of urinary incontinence. Average improvement rates are 50% to 80%.

○ **What is the most effective treatment for stress incontinence (in terms of patient satisfaction and sustained outcome)?**

Surgery, which can include periurethral injection of bulking agents, vesicourethral suspension procedures for females (MMK, Burch), slings (male and female), or artificial urinary sphincter for males. As always, surgery should only be considered after attempts at nonsurgical management have occurred.

○   **A 33-year-old male patient presents with a history of sudden onset right flank pain that was sharp and doubled the patient over. It radiated from the right flank around to the lower quadrant of the abdomen and into the scrotum. This was also associated with nausea and vomiting. On the basis of this history, what is the most likely diagnosis?**

Kidney stone/Urolithiasis.

○   **Which gender is more prone to typical calcium oxalate kidney stones?**

Men (a 3:1 male-to-female ratio). Of note, males = females in pediatric patients.

○   **What is the most sensitive imaging option for ruling out a kidney stone?**

Spiral CT scan.

○   **What percentage of urinary calculi are radiopaque?**

85% to 90%.

○   **Differentiate between radiolucent and radiopaque renal calculi:**

90% of all stones are radiopaque and are composed of calcium oxalate, cysteine, calcium phosphate, or magnesium ammonium phosphate. Radiolucent stones consist of pure uric acid.

○   **What is the one greatest factor in the prevention of kidney stones?**

The amount of fluid intake by the patient. The more fluid a patient is able to take in, the less likely he or she will develop a stone. If a patient has a history of a stone, the recommendation is to consume 1.6 L/24 hrs.

○   **What are the admission criteria for patients with renal calculi?**

Infection with concurrent obstruction; a solitary kidney and complete obstruction; uncontrolled pain; intractable emesis; or large stones. (Only 10%–15% of stones >6 mm pass spontaneously.) Other indications include renal insufficiency and complete obstruction or urinary extravasation as demonstrated by imaging.

○   **A urinary pH of 7.3 is conducive to the formation of what type of stones?**

Struvite and phosphate stones. Normal urine pH is approximately 5.85. Alkalotic urine actually inhibits the formation of uric acid and cystine stones. Conversely, struvite and phosphate stones are inhibited by more acidic urine.

○   **Which type of stone formation is caused by a genetic error?**

Cysteine stones. These stones are produced because there is an error in the transport of amino acids that results in cystinuria.

○   **What is the 5-year recurrence rate for kidney stones?**

50%.

○   **What percentage of patients spontaneously pass kidney stones?**

80%. This is largely dependent on size. 75% of stones <4 mm pass spontaneously, while only 10% of those >6 mm pass spontaneously. Analgesics and increased fluid intake aid in outpatient passage of kidney stones.

○ **Name the three most common anatomical sites where kidney stones are likely to obstruct the genitourinary tract:**

1. Ureteropelvic junction (UPJ)

2. Crossing over the iliac vessels

3. Entering the bladder at the ureterovesical junction (UVJ)

○ **Which bacterium is associated with magnesium ammonium phosphate urolithiasis?**

Stones that are composed of magnesium, ammonium, and phosphate are termed <u>struvite stones</u> and are considered infection stones associated with urea-splitting organisms, including *Proteus, Pseudomonas, Providencia, Klebsiella, Staphylococci, and Mycoplasma.* Antibiotics will help treat the UTI and will generally cease stone formation and urinary acidification.

○ **What is phimosis?**

A condition in which the foreskin cannot be retracted posterior to the glans. Chronic infection from poor local hygiene is the most common cause.

○ **What is the treatment for phimosis?**

Manual reduction should be attempted. If unsuccessful, a dorsal slit or circumcision should be performed.

○ **What is paraphimosis?**

A condition in which the foreskin, once retracted over the glans, cannot be replaced to its normal position.

○ **What is a nonsurgical method used to reduce paraphimosis?**

Firmly squeeze the glans for 5 minutes to reduce the tissue edema and size of glans, then place thumbs on the glans while stabilizing the foreskin in between the second and third fingers. Apply pressure on the thumbs while attempting to pull the foreskin over the glans.

○ **Testicular torsion is most common in which age group?**

12 to 18-year olds. Two-thirds of the cases occur in this age group. The next most common group is newborns.

○ **True/False: Testicular torsion is always preceded by a history of trauma, exercise, or sexual activity:**

False. Although testicular torsion frequently follows a history of strenuous physical activity, it can also occur during sleep.

○ **How can testicular torsion be distinguished from epididymitis by history?**

By the rate of the pain onset. Torsional pain typically begins instantaneously at maximum intensity (often associated with nausea or vomiting), whereas epididymal pain grows steadily over hours or days.

○ **How can testicular torsion be distinguished from epididymitis by physical examination?**

In torsion, you classically have a loss of the cremasteric reflex and a swollen, firm, high riding testicle with an abnormal transverse lie. Clinically, elevation of the scrotum may relieve pain related to epididymitis but is not effective with torsional pain (Prehn sign). This test is not, however, considered diagnostic.

○ **What does a blue dot sign suggest?**

Torsion of the appendix testis. The appendix testis is a remnant of the mullerian duct and is located on the upper pole of the testis. The clinical significance of torsion of this appendage is that it must be distinguished from testicular torsion. The testicle with a torsed appendix testis features a distinct, tender, indurated mass near the upper pole. The classic blue dot sign over the point of tenderness is pathognomonic but found infrequently. Torsion of the appendix testis can be treated conservatively with anti-inflammatory agents and scrotal support if the clinician is CERTAIN that the testicle itself is not torsed. Most appendages will calcify or degenerate within 10 to 14 days without harm to the patient.

○ **How is testicular torsion diagnosed?**

Doppler US is the diagnostic imaging study of choice. However, emergent surgical exploration by a urologist should never be delayed in order to obtain diagnostic imaging.

○ **True/False: The left testicle torses more often than the right:**

True.

○ **How do you manually attempt to reduce a testicular torsion?**

Standing in front of the patient, you manually twist simultaneously the patient's right testicle counterclockwise and the left testicle clockwise. Remember: "open the book" to reduce the testicles.

○ **What is the definitive treatment for testicular torsion?**

Surgical exploration, including bilateral orchiopexy in which both the testes are surgically attached to the scrotum (vs. orchiectomy if the torsed testicle is nonviable + orchiopexy of the contralateral testis).

○ **What is the testicular viability at 6, 12, and 24 hours of ischemia?**

The time elapsed between onset of pain and performance of detorsion, and the corresponding salvage rate, is as follows:

<6 hours: 90% to 100% salvage rate
12–24 hours: 20% to 50%
>24 hours: 0% to 10%

○ **What causes priapism?**

60% of cases are idiopathic and the other 40% are associated with diseases (i.e., leukemia, sickle cell disease, pelvic tumors, and pelvic infections), penile trauma, spinal cord trauma, or use of medications. Currently, intracavernous injection therapy for impotence may be the most common cause.

○ **What is the initial treatment for priapism?**

Terbutaline, 0.25 to 0.5 mg subcutaneously in the deltoid area, repeated in 30 minutes, if needed.

INFECTIOUS/INFLAMMATORY CONDITIONS

○ **What is the most common pathogen of urinary tract infections (UTIs)?**

Escherichia coli (80%). *E. coli* is also the most common cause of pyelonephritis because of its ascension from the lower urinary tract. Other less common uropathogens include *Klebsiella, Proteus,* and *Enterobacter* spp. and enterococci. In hospital-acquired UTIs, a wider variety of causative organisms is found, including *Pseudomonas* and *Staphylococcus* spp. Group B beta-hemolytic streptococci can cause UTIs in pregnant women.

O **What are some clinical complaints of patients with cystitis?**

Irritative voiding symptoms, such as urinary frequency, dysuria, and urgency. Low back pain and suprapubic pain, cloudy/foul-smelling urine, and hematuria are also common symptoms.

O **Name three commonly used antibiotics for the treatment of uncomplicated cystitis:**

1. Trimethoprim-sulfamethoxazole (TMP-SMX)
2. Fluoroquinolones (Ciprofloxacin)
3. Nitrofurantoin

O **What is the drug of choice for treating urinary tract infection caused by *Proteus mirabilis*?**

Ampicillin.

O **What is the most common anatomical abnormality associated with chronic urinary tract infections?**

Vesicoureteral reflux.

O **A 23-year-old female presents with 5-day history of fever, right flank pain, dysuria, and nausea with vomiting. On examination, there is right-sided CVA tenderness but the abdomen and pelvic examinations are benign. What is the likely diagnosis?**

Acute pyelonephritis.

O **What are the most common pathogens for acute, uncomplicated pyelonephritis?**

Gram-negative rods: *Escherichia coli* (80% of cases in women, 70% in men), *Klebsiella pneumoniae* (5%–10% of cases).

O **In making a correct diagnosis of pyelonephritis, what are some differentials to consider?**

Any intra-abdominal inflammatory process, such as acute cholecystitis, appendicitis, diverticulitis, and pancreatitis. Gynecologic conditions such as PID, ectopic pregnancy, ruptured ovarian cysts. Other urologic conditions such as renal colic with fever (infected stone) or renal/perinephric abscess. Lower lobe pneumonia. Musculoskeletal pain.

O **What is the treatment for an uncomplicated case of pyelonephritis?**

Empiric antibiotics that are active against the possible organisms, often intravenous ampicillin and Gentamicin, or IV Ceftriaxone, or an IV fluoroquinolone. As an outpatient treatment, oral fluoroquinolones or TMP-SMZ are used. Most patients continue to have fever or flank pain for several days after appropriate therapy has been started. Supportive care should also be instituted: hydration, antipyretics, and analgesics.

O **What is the course for a pregnant patient with pyelonephritis?**

This requires inpatient care with aggressive fluids and IV antibiotics. In some early cases of pregnancy, outpatient therapy can be attempted with very close follow-up. All pregnant patients with pyelonephritis should be placed on suppressive antibiotics (i.e., nitrofurantoin 100 mg/day PO or cephalexin 250 mg/day PO) after initial treatment until delivery because of a relapse rate of up to 60% in nonsuppressed patients.

O **Outpatient management of pyelonephritis should be reserved for what patients?**

Reliable, otherwise healthy patients who tolerate oral intake and do not have signs of sepsis may be treated as an outpatient with close follow-up.

○ **What are the risk factors for pyelonephritis?**

Anatomic or functional abnormalities of the GU tract that cause incomplete emptying of the bladder (vesicoureteral reflux, neurogenic bladder); foreign body which allows bacterial colonization (i.e., stone disease, indwelling catheters); certain medical conditions such as diabetes mellitus, immunosuppression, and alcohol abuse; patients with poor perineal hygiene or those with multiple sexual partners.

○ **Acute testicular pain and relief of pain with elevation of the scrotum (Prehn sign) is classically associated with:**

Epididymitis.

○ **What is the most common cause of epididymitis in the following age groups: prepubertal boys, men younger than 35 years, and men older than 35 years?**

Prepubertal boys: *Escherichia coli* and other *Coliform* bacteria

Men younger than 35: *Chlamydia* or *Neisseria gonorrhoeae*

Men older than 35: *E. coli* and other *Coliform* bacteria

Epididymitis is also frequently caused by urinary reflux, prostatitis, or urethral instrumentation.

○ **What percentage of patients with epididymitis will also have pyuria?**

50%.

○ **How does the pain associated with epididymitis differ from that produced by prostatitis?**

Epididymitis: Pain begins in the scrotum or groin and radiates along the spermatic cord. It intensifies rapidly, is associated with dysuria, and can be relieved with scrotal elevation (Prehn sign).

Prostatitis: Patients have frequency, dysuria, urgency, bladder outlet obstruction, and/or retention. They may have low back pain and perineal pain associated with fever, chills, arthralgias, and myalgias.

○ **Aside from antibiotics, what other instructions do you give a patient with acute epididymitis?**

Rest with scrotal elevation/scrotal support. NSAIDs for pain and inflammation are often helpful. For a sexually transmitted bacterium, the sexual partner must also be treated.

○ **What are risk factors for acute orchitis:**

Not being vaccinated against mumps virus; STD infection; epididymitis; immunocompromised patients; history of intravesical BCG for bladder cancer.

○ **What is the basic treatment for uncomplicated orchitis?**

Supportive care, bed rest, hot or cold packs for analgesia, and scrotal elevation and support. Bacterial orchitis requires coverage with an appropriate antibiotic for the suspected organism.

○ **A 35-year-old male patient has a 4-day history of dysuria, perineal pain, and subjective fevers. On examination, you note a tender, boggy prostate. What is the likely diagnosis?**

Acute prostatitis.

○ **What is the most common causative organism of acute bacterial prostatitis?**

Escherichia coli (80%). Other gram-negative bacteria (Proteus, Klebsiella, Enterobacter, Pseudomonas, and Serratia spp.) and enterococci are less frequent pathogens. Anaerobic and other gram-positive bacteria are rarely a cause of acute prostatitis.

○ **What is the outpatient treatment for acute bacterial prostatitis?**

TMP-SMX, double strength PO BID × 4 to 6 weeks; or ciprofloxacin, 500 mg PO BID for 4 to 6 weeks; Anti-inflammatory agents are often helpful in improving patient's symptoms.

○ **What is the most common cause of urethritis in men?**

Neisseria gonorrhoeae (gonococcal urethritis) or *Chlamydia trachomatis* (nongonococcal urethritis) are the most common causes. Nongonococcal urethritis may also be caused by *Ureaplasma* or *Mycoplasma* in up to 40% of patients.

○ **How can you differentiate gonococcal urethritis from chlamydial urethritis on examination?**

Gonorrhea presents with a purulent discharge from the urethra, whereas chlamydia is generally associated with a thinner, white mucous discharge.

○ **How do you treat urethritis?**

Treatment should cover both gonorrhea and chlamydia because there is a high incidence of coinfection. Ceftriaxone 125 mg IM once for gonorrhea and azithromycin 1 gm PO once or doxycycline 100 mg PO BID × 10 to 14 days for nongonococcal urethritis are the drugs of choice.

○ **What are the symptoms of disseminated gonococcal infection?**

Arthritis, dermatitis, meningitis, and endocarditis. Systemic manifestations of gonococcal dissemination are rare today.

○ **A 62-year-old diabetic male presents to the emergency department with fever, dysuria, pain, and swelling of the scrotum for the past several days. On examination, his scrotum is erythematous, swollen, and malodorous, with pain and crepitus on palpation. What is the diagnosis and treatment?**

Fournier gangrene. This is a form of necrotizing fasciitis that usually presents in immunocompromised patients in their 5th to 6th decade of life (but can occur at any age) and is because of the infection or trauma of the perianal area.

○ **What causes Fournier gangrene?**

Bacteroides fragilis, Enterococcus, and *Escherichia coli* predominate.

○ **How is Fournier gangrene treated?**

This condition is considered a urologic emergency requiring immediate, wide surgical debridement of the involved skin and subcutaneous tissue. Triple antibiotic coverage should also occur, using broad-based agents that are effective against anaerobes and gram-negative enteric organisms. Modern mortality rates are approximately 20%.

○ **What is the inflammation of the foreskin called?**

Balanitis or balanoposthitis.

NEOPLASTIC DISEASES

○ **A 66-year-old male patient presents with a 3-day history of painless gross hematuria. There are no other complaints and his examination is normal with exception of mild bloody discharge from the urethral meatus. There is no history of trauma. What is the most likely etiology?**

Bladder cancer.

○ **What is the number one risk factor for bladder cancer?**

Tobacco smoking, which increases risk two to four times compared to those who have never smoked. Other risk factors include occupational exposure (dye, textile, rubber, leather, and aromatic amines) and male gender.

○ **How is bladder cancer confirmed as a diagnosis?**

By cystoscopy and bladder biopsy.

○ **What is the most common histologic type of bladder cancer?**

Transitional (urothelial) cell carcinoma.

○ **How often do prostate cancers present with voiding problems?**

Infrequently, they normally are asymptomatic and are found by the PSA and/or digital rectal examination (DRE). Larger growths can cause voiding issues, but these are usually later stage cancers.

○ **What percentage of men with PSAs greater than 10 ng/mL will have prostate cancer?**

Between 50% and 70%.

○ **What is the standard method for diagnosing prostate cancer?**

Transrectal ultrasound-guided biopsy.

○ **Which is the most common type of prostate cancer?**

Adenocarcinoma (95%). The next most common type is transitional cell which constitutes <5%.

○ **Which zone of the prostate is prostate cancer most commonly found?**

In the peripheral region of the prostate (60%–70% of prostate cancers originate here). 10% to 20% of prostate cancers originate in the transition zone, and 5% to 10% in the central zone. Of note, benign prostatic hyperplasia (BPH) uniformly originates in the transition zone.

○ **What is the biggest risk factor for prostate cancer?**

Age. The median age for diagnosis of prostate cancer is 72 years. The probability of prostate cancer developing in a man under the age of 40 is 1 in 10,000; for men 40 to 59 it is 1 in 103, and for men 60 to 79 it is 1 in 8.

○ **What is the most common site for distant metastases of prostate cancer?**

The axial skeleton, with the lumbar spine being most frequently involved. The next most common sites (in decreasing order) are proximal femur, pelvis, thoracic spine, ribs, sternum, skull, and humerus.

○ **What is the most common grading system used for prostate cancer?**

The Gleason grading system. In this grading system, pathologists assign a primary grade to the pattern of cancer that is most commonly observed and a secondary grade to the second most commonly observed pattern in the specimen. Grades range from 1 to 5. The Gleason score or Gleason sum is obtained by adding the primary and secondary grades together. Because Gleason grades range from 1 to 5, Gleason scores or sums thus range from 2 to 10. Well-differentiated tumors have a Gleason sum of 2–4, moderately differentiated tumors have a Gleason sum of 5–6, and poorly differentiated tumors have a Gleason sum of 8–10.

○ **What is the definitive surgical treatment for prostate cancer?**

Radical prostatectomy. Patients with organ-confined cancer have 10-year disease-free survival rates ranging from 70% to 85% following radical prostatectomy. In some localized tumors, radiation therapy may be indicated as an alternative.

○ **What is the single most important factor in preventing post-prostatectomy incontinence?**

Surgical technique. Intraoperative preservation of as much urethral length as possible is essential to preserve the external urethral sphincter. A careful vesicourethral anastomosis is also important.

○ **A 61-year-old male patient presents to the emergency department with a 1-month history of right-sided abdominal pain, intermittent gross hematuria, weight loss, and subjective fever. On examination, you palpate a firm small mass inferior to the liver edge. The prostate examination is normal. What is the likely diagnosis in this patient?**

Renal cell carcinoma. RCC can present in a variety of ways. The classic triad of pain, hematuria, and flank mass is considered pathognomonic but it is rarely found in patients and, if present, usually indicate an advanced disease. Hematuria is the most common presenting sign.

○ **What percentage of patients with renal cell carcinoma present with hematuria (gross or microscopic)?**
60%.

○ **What are the most common risk factors for developing renal cell carcinoma?**

Smoking, positive family history in first- or second-degree relative, hypertension.

○ **What is the best method for detecting renal cell carcinoma?**

CT scan is the preferred test. Most tumors are found incidentally.

○ **While considering the work-up for a patient with a suspected renal cell carcinoma, what other tests should be ordered?**

LFTs, creatinine, electrolytes, CBC, and urinalysis are standard initial labs. Any renal mass that enhances with IV contrast on CT or MRI should be considered RCC until proven otherwise. CT or MRI is adequate for metastatic evaluation of the abdomen. Chest X-ray is sufficient to rule out pulmonary mets. Nuclear bone scan should be performed to rule out bony metastases in patients with elevated alkaline phosphatase or bone pain.

○ **What is the definitive treatment for a patient with renal cell carcinoma?**

Radical nephrectomy. In some cases where the tumor is isolated, a partial nephrectomy can be performed.

○   **Is chemotherapy an effective treatment option for renal cell carcinoma?**

No, the general lack of active agents and the excessive toxicity of many of the agents that exhibit some activity have contributed to the absence of adjuvant or neoadjuvant chemotherapy for renal cell cancer.

○   **What is the most common cancer in young adult males?**

Testicular cancer is the most common malignancy in males 15 to 35 years old.

○   **A 27-year-old male patient presents with a painless nodular growth on his right testicle that has been present for the last 3 months. There is no history of pain, urinary symptoms, or difficulty with ejaculation. What is the most likely diagnosis for this patient?**

Testicular cancer until proven otherwise.

○   **Which testicle is more likely to have a cancer, the right or the left?**

The right. This parallels the increased incidence of cryptorchidism on that side.

○   **What are the risk factors for testicular cancer?**

The only known risk factors for testicular cancer are age, race, and cryptorchidism. Caucasians have four times the incidence of testicular cancer as opposed to African American males.

○   **What tumor markers should be drawn during the work-up for testicular cancer?**

Alpha-fetoprotein (AFP), human chorionic gonadotropin (hCG), and lactate dehydrogenase (LDH). AFP is present in nonseminomatous germ cell tumors (NSGCT), but is never found in seminomas. HCG is classically elevated in choriocarcinoma (a type of NSGCT) but may be elevated in seminomas 7% of the time. LDH may be elevated in both NSGCTs and seminomas.

○   **What imaging technique is used to confirm a testicular mass?**

Testicular ultrasound (95% sensitivity and specificity in identifying intratesticular lesions).

○   **How is the diagnosis of testicular cancer confirmed?**

By pathological interpretation at the time of radical orchiectomy.

○   **What are the treatments for testicular cancer?**

Orchiectomy (with high ligation of the spermatic cord at the level of the inguinal ring), chemotherapy, and retroperitoneal radiation, depending on histology (seminoma vs. NSGCT) and clinical stage.

○   **What is an important difference between testicular teratomas in children and adults?**

Teratomas are a type of NSGCT. In children (prepubertal boys), teratomas have not been reported to metastasize. In adults, they metastasize in 60% of cases.

○   **A mother brings in her 3-year-old son because she has noticed that his abdomen has increased in size. In addition, the child has been having subjective fever. On examination, the child is found to be hypertensive and has a palpable mass on the left side of the abdomen. There is also microscopic hematuria and mild anemia on laboratory reports. Given this history, what is the likely diagnosis of the child?**

Wilms tumor (nephroblastoma).

○　**What is the most common primary malignant renal tumor in children?**

Wilms tumor: It represents 6% of all childhood cancers and is a highly malignant tumor of mixed histology. A suspected hereditary form of Wilms tumor that is transmitted as an autosomal dominant disorder accounts for about 40% of all tumors. 80% of all cases occur prior to the age of 5 years old.

○　**What is the most common sign of Wilms tumor?**

An abdominal mass.

○　**What is the most common site for metastases of Wilms tumor?**

Metastatic disease is present at diagnosis in 10% to 15% of patients, with the lungs (85%–95%) and liver (10%–15%) the most common sites of involvement. Metastases to the bone and brain are uncommon.

○　**What is the treatment for a patient with a Wilms tumor?**

Surgical resection, if possible. Wilms tumor has also been long recognized as a chemosensitive and radiosensitive tumor (though radiation therapy is infrequently used because of cardiac, pulmonary, and hepatic toxicities).

○　**What is the prognosis for a Wilms tumor?**

The 4-year survival of patients with favorable histology Wilms tumor now approaches 90%.

RENAL DISEASES

○　**What are some causes of false-positive hematuria?**

Foods such as rhubarb, beets, paprika, fava beans, and artificial food colorings can cause urine to change color and be mistaken for blood. In addition, drugs such as rifampin, phenytoin, phenazopyridine, chloroquine, and methyldopa can cause false-positives. Menstruation history should also be considered.

○　**If a urine dipstick is positive for blood, but the urine sediment has no red blood cells, what is the probable disease?**

Rhabdomyolysis. Severe muscle damage can result in free myoglobin in the blood. Very high levels can lead to acute renal failure. The "blood" seen on dipstick is actually myoglobin (false-positive).

○　**A urinalysis reveals RBC casts and dysmorphic RBCs. What is the probable origin of hematuria?**

Glomerulus.

○　**What is the most common cause of hemolytic uremic syndrome?**

Epidemic HUS is usually caused by infection with *Escherichia coli* O157:H7, an organism associated with ingestion of undercooked meat, unpasteurized milk, and contaminated vegetables and fruits. HUS is the most common cause of acute renal failure in young children, typically occurs in children less than 10 years of age (two-thirds of cases are in children <5 years).

○　**The laboratory reports from a patient with hematuria show depressed levels of C3. What etiologies should you suspect?**

Chronic infection, lupus, poststreptococcal glomerulonephritis, or membranoproliferative glomerulonephritis.

○ **What is the definition of oliguria? Of anuria?**

Oliguria: Urine output < 400 mL/24 hrs in adults

Anuria: Urine output < 100 mL/24 hrs in adults

○ **Total and persistent anuria with renal failure should prompt a work-up for what?**

Urinary obstruction. These patients are presumed to be obstructed until proven otherwise.

○ **What are the different types of acute renal failure (ARF)?**

ARF can be divided into three broad categories: <u>prerenal</u> causes (kidney hypoperfusion leading to lower glomerular filtration rate [GFR]), <u>intrinsic kidney disease</u>, and <u>postrenal</u> causes. Intrinsic kidney disease includes acute tubular necrosis, acute glomerulonephritis, and acute interstitial nephritis.

○ **What are some common causes of <u>prerenal</u> acute renal failure?**

The term prerenal denotes inadequate renal perfusion or lowered effective arterial circulation. The most common cause of this form of acute renal failure is dehydration because of renal or extrarenal fluid losses from diarrhea, vomiting, excessive use of diuretics, etc. Less common causes are septic shock, "third spacing" with extravascular fluid pooling (e.g., pancreatitis), and excessive use of antihypertensive drugs. Heart failure with reduced cardiac output also can reduce effective renal blood flow.

○ **What is the most common cause of <u>intrinsic</u> renal failure?**

Acute tubular necrosis (80%–90% of intrinsic renal failure), resulting from an ischemic injury (the most common cause of ATN) or from a nephrotoxic agent. Less frequent causes of intrinsic renal failure (10%–20%) include vasculitis, malignant hypertension, acute glomerulonephritis, or allergic interstitial nephritis.

○ **Name some common nephrotoxic agents:**

The most common causes of drug-induced acute nephrotoxicity include NSAIDs, penicillins and cephalosporins, rifampin, sulfonamides (including medications that include sulfa components such as furosemide, bumetanide, and thiazide-type diuretics), cimetidine, allopurinol, ciprofloxacin, 5-aminosalicylates (e.g., mesalamine), and, to a lesser degree, other quinolone antibiotics. Contrast dye is also a common source of drug-induced nephropathy.

○ **What comorbid factors are likely to increase the risk of contrast-induced renal failure?**

Azotemia, diabetic nephropathy, CHF, multiple myeloma, and dehydration.

○ **What is the major therapy used to treat allergic interstitial nephritis not responding to discontinuation of the culprit medication?**

Short course of corticosteroids.

○ **What are the causes of <u>postrenal</u> acute renal failure?**

Ureteral and urethral obstruction.

○ **What is the most common cause of acute renal failure (including prerenal, intrinsic, and postrenal causes)?**

Acute tubular necrosis (ATN) constitutes 45% of cases of ARF.

○ **What does acute renal failure in a patient with alcoholic cirrhosis and a urine sodium of less than 10 suggest?**

Prerenal azotemia or hepatorenal syndrome.

○ **Sudden ARF, seen after initiation of ACE inhibitors, should prompt a work-up for what condition?**

ACE inhibitors are likely to cause ARF in patients with bilateral <u>renal artery stenosis</u> or renal artery stenosis in a solitary kidney. This can lead to acute tubular necrosis.

○ **Acute renal failure seen after use of cocaine may be due to what?**

Rhabdomyolysis.

○ **What type of ARF is usually seen with rhabdomyolysis?**

Acute tubular necrosis. Rhabdomyolysis is a syndrome characterized by injury to skeletal muscle with subsequent effects from the release of intracellular contents. Renal tubular obstruction occurs secondary to precipitation of uric acid and myoglobin.

○ **What factors predispose one to acute papillary necrosis?**

Analgesics, sickle cell disease, diabetes mellitus, prolonged NSAID use, and alcoholism are usual predisposing factors.

○ **What continuous modes of renal replacement therapy are used in ARF?**

The principal methods of <u>continuous</u> renal replacement therapy are continuous venovenous hemodiafiltration (CVVH) and peritoneal dialysis. Hemodialysis may be used but it is an **intermittent** therapy, not continuous.

○ **When should renal replacement therapy be instituted for ARF?**

Renal replacement therapy in ARF is considered necessary when a patient has uncontrolled hyperkalemia, intractable fluid overload, uremic pericarditis or encephalopathy, bleeding dyscrasia, life-threatening poisoning, or excessive BUN/Cr levels.

○ **What are some common physical examination findings in patients with chronic renal disease?**

In general, the patients appear ill and complain of fatigue, weakness, and malaise. Hypertension is frequently seen. Skin may exhibit pallor (because of anemia) and is often easy to bruise (because of platelet dysfunction). Cardiovascular examination may have cardiomegaly with a displaced PMI, rales, and edema. Extremities may also have edema.

○ **What is the most common cause of chronic renal failure (CRF)?**

Diabetes mellitus.

○ **What type of anemia is characteristic of chronic renal failure?**

Normochromic, normocytic anemia.

○ **Describe abnormal ultrasound findings that suggests chronic renal failure:**

Kidneys <9 cm in length are abnormal. A difference of >1.5 cm in length between the two kidneys suggests unilateral kidney disease. Kidneys with a small or absent renal cortex are also indicative of chronic renal failure. An ultrasound may also show hydronephrosis of an obstructive cause.

○   **What is the most common cause of death in patients with end-stage renal disease (ESRD)?**

Cardiac dysfunction (50%), followed by infection (14%), and then cerebrovascular disease (6%).

○   **What is the most common cause of cardiac arrest in a uremic patient?**

Hyperkalemia.

○   **What treatments are used to ameliorate bleeding in a uremic patient?**

The bleeding diathesis seen in ESRD patients produces increased risks of GI tract bleeding, subdural hematomas, subcapsular liver hematomas, and intraocular bleeding. Several mechanisms are contributors to uremic bleeding. Dialysis may lessen bleeding as may desmopressin (DDAVP), cryoprecipitate, conjugated estrogens, or erythropoietin.

○   **What is the life expectancy of chronic renal patients after the disease has progressed to dialysis?**

Patients between the ages of 55 and 64 years have an average 22-year life expectancy. Patients older than 60 and with end-stage renal disease have a 5-year life expectancy.

○   **At what glomerular filtration rate (GFR) will patients with CRF need to start dialysis?**

Dialysis initiation should be considered when GFR is 10 mL/min. Studies suggest that the well-selected patient without overt uremic symptoms may wait to initiate dialysis until GFR is closer to 7 mL/min. Other indications for dialysis, which may occur when GFR is 10 to 15 mL/min, include uremic symptoms, fluid overload unresponsive to diuresis, and refractory hyperkalemia.

○   **What is the most common acute complication of hemodialysis?**

Hypotension.

○   **What are the causes of high levels of parathyroid hormone (PTH) in CRF?**

Decline in glomerular filtration rate (GFR) and loss of renal mass lead directly to increased serum phosphorus (hyperphosphatemia) and deficiency of vitamin D. Both of these abnormalities result in hypocalcemia and hyperparathyroidism.

○   **What are the first-line oral phosphate binders used to control hyperphosphatemia in CRF?**

Calcium carbonate (650 mg/tablet) and calcium acetate (667 mg/capsule)—both block absorption of dietary phosphorus in the gut and are given three times daily with meals. If elevated calcium levels prevent the use of these medications, sevelamer and lanthanum can be used, as they are phosphorous binding agents that do not contain calcium. Aluminum-containing agents (such as aluminum hydroxide) are best avoided because of osteomalacia and neurologic complications when used long term.

○   **What are the possible causes of advanced chronic renal failure and enlarged kidneys?**

Typically, the finding of small echogenic kidneys bilaterally (<9–10 cm) by ultrasonography supports a diagnosis of chronic kidney disease, although normal or even large kidneys can be seen with amyloidosis, adult polycystic kidney disease, diabetic nephropathy, HIV-associated nephropathy, multiple myeloma, and obstructive uropathy.

○   **Chronic renal failure with hypertension, small shrunken kidneys, and gout at an early age should suggest what?**

Lead nephropathy should be considered.

○ **What is the most common cause of proteinuria?**

Pathology of the glomerulus. Other causes include tubular pathology or overproduction of protein.

○ **A renal biopsy in a patient with acute renal failure, hematuria, and red cell casts will most likely reveal what lesion?**

A proliferative glomerulonephritis, usually with crescents. GN is caused by an immune complex deposition in glomeruli.

○ **What four clinical findings are indicative of acute glomerulonephritis (GN)?**

1. Hypertension
2. Edema—usually begins in body parts with low tissue tension, such as the periorbital and scrotal regions
3. Urine sediment containing RBCs (hematuria), protein, and RBC casts
4. Oliguria—present in half of patients

○ **Acute renal failure caused by Wegener granulomatosis may respond best to what treatments?**

This is usually rapidly progressive GN and responds to high-dose steroids and cyclophosphamide.

○ **What is the most common cause of postinfectious glomerulonephritis?**

Poststreptococcal group A beta-hemolytic. However, other infections may also produce GN-related infections. Most patients recover renal function spontaneously within a few weeks.

○ **What is the classic presentation of poststreptococcal glomerulonephritis (PSGN)?**

Sudden development of gross hematuria (can be cola-colored), hypertension, edema, and renal insufficiency following a throat or skin infection with group A beta-hemolytic streptococcus (usually symptoms develop 1–3 weeks after infection). Patients frequently also have generalized complaints of fever, malaise, lethargy, abdominal pain, etc.

○ **How early in the development of "strep throat" will antibiotic therapy decrease the risk for PSGN?**

Although antibiotic therapy has efficacy for primary prevention of acute rheumatic fever following strep infection, the role of antibiotics in the setting of GAS tonsillopharyngitis for the prevention of poststreptococcal glomerulonephritis is not certain.

○ **What laboratory test best confirms PSGN as the diagnosis?**

Anti-DNAse B antibody titer.

○ **What syndrome is characterized by a rapidly progressive, antiglomerular basement membrane antibody-induced GN that is preceded by pulmonary hemorrhage and hemoptysis?**

Goodpasture syndrome.

○ **What is the most common manifestation of Goodpasture syndrome?**

Hemoptysis. These patients usually develop pulmonary hemorrhage before any signs of renal failure develop.

○ **A kidney biopsy from a 24-year-old male patient with nephrotic syndrome shows increased mesangial cells and, on immunofluorescence, C3 deposits in the mesangium. What is the man's diagnosis and prognosis?**

This man has membranoproliferative glomerulonephritis (a type of chronic glomerulonephritis). Prognosis is poor, with many patients progressing to end-stage renal failure.

○ **What is the most common histologic pattern of acute renal failure seen on kidney biopsy in a patient with systemic lupus erythematosus (SLE)?**

SLE is associated with five histologic patterns of kidney damage, the most common of which is diffuse proliferative glomerulonephritis (Class IV). Common clinical findings include renal failure, nephrotic syndrome, hematuria, and cylindruria.

○ **How is diffuse proliferative glomerulonephritis caused by SLE generally treated?**

Steroids and IV cyclophosphamide.

○ **What is the most common cause of nephrotic syndrome in children? In adults?**

Children: Minimal change disease.
Adults: Idiopathic glomerulonephritis.

○ **What is the diagnostic triad of the nephrotic syndrome?**

Edema, hyperlipidemia, and proteinuria with hypoproteinemia.

○ **What is the main goal of treatment in nephrotic syndrome?**

Treat the underlying cause of the syndrome. One of the most important aspects in treatment is to reduce protein losses—this can be accomplished to some extent by increasing dietary protein. In addition, ACE inhibitors and ARBs can be used to lower urine protein excretion. Dietary salt restriction is essential for managing edema; most patients also require diuretic therapy (usually loop and thiazide diuretics in combination). Antilipidemic agents are used to control hyperlipidemia.

○ **Why are many nephrotic patients on warfarin?**

Nephrotic patients have urinary losses of antithrombin, protein C, and protein S and increased platelet activation; thus patients are prone to renal vein thrombosis, pulmonary embolus, and other venous thromboemboli, particularly with membranous nephropathy. Anticoagulation therapy with warfarin is warranted for at least 3 to 6 months in patients with evidence of thrombosis in any location.

○ **What pathology is usually seen in patients with CRF, nephrotic syndrome, and AIDS?**

Usually focal segmental glomerulosclerosis is seen at biopsy.

○ **What is the antihypertensive of choice in patient with chronic diabetic nephropathy?**

Angiotensin-converting enzyme inhibitors are preferred.

○ **What are some extrarenal manifestations of autosomal dominant polycystic kidney disease?**

Hepatic and pancreatic cysts, colonic diverticula, cardiac valvular abnormalities (mitral valve prolapse, aortic regurgitation, tricuspid prolapse), intracranial aneurysms, and rare cysts (arachnoid, splenic, testicular, ovarian).

○ **What is the best imaging study to detect polycystic kidney disease?**

Ultrasound (CT may be used to further evaluate inhomogeneity of cysts).

○ **What percentage of kidney transplants donated from a relative (usually a parent) are still functional after 3 years?**

75% to 80%.

○ **Patients born with what disease are more likely to have horseshoe kidneys?**

Turner syndrome.

ELECTROLYTE AND ACID/BASE DISORDERS

○ **What are some reasons for volume contraction?**

Extracellular fluid (ECF) volume contraction is caused by loss of sodium or water in excess of intake. These losses may be a result of renal or extrarenal losses or what is known as third spacing. The gastrointestinal tract is the most common extrarenal source of fluid loss (vomiting, nasogastric suctioning, diarrhea). Third-space sequestration, excessive sweating, or loss of skin barrier from burns may also result in ECF volume depletion. Renal losses are caused by diuretics, tubular disorders, mineralocorticoid deficiency (Addison disease, hypoaldosteronism), and diabetes.

○ **What is the most common electrolyte abnormality in hospitalized patients?**

Hyponatremia (defined as a plasma sodium level of <135 mEq/L [135 mmol/L]).

○ **What are the two main reasons for hyponatremia?**

Either an increase in intracellular volume and water gain, or because of a primary sodium loss.

○ **What is the most common drug that can induce hyponatremia?**

Thiazide diuretics.

○ **At what plasma sodium level do symptoms of hyponatremia generally manifest?**

Symptoms of hyponatremia do not usually appear until the plasma sodium level drops below 120 mEq/L (120 mmol/L) and usually are nonspecific (e.g., headache, lethargy, nausea). In cases of severe hyponatremia, neurologic and gastrointestinal symptoms predominate.

○ **Name three medical conditions that can commonly cause hypervolemic hyponatremia to occur:**

1. Congestive heart failure
2. Cirrhosis of the liver
3. Renal disease (nephrotic syndrome or renal failure)

○ **What disorder causes hyponatremia, euvolemia, and has a large release of arginine vasopressin (AVP) in the setting of increased water intake?**

Syndrome of inappropriate antidiuretic hormone (SIADH). Some of the causes for this are central nervous system disorders, certain pulmonary lesions, malignant tumors, surgery, and some medications.

○ **What is *beer potomania*?**

These are patients who drink excessive amounts of beer and have poor protein intake in their diet, which results in an overload of volume (free water excretion is decreased because of decreased solute consumption and production), thus causing hyponatremia.

○ **What are the two main goals in the treatment of hyponatremia?**

1. Water restriction to lower the overall water volume. (Free water intake from oral intake and intravenous fluids should generally be <1–1.5 L/day.)
2. Treatment of the underlying cause of the hyponatremia.

○ **A 93-year-old female patient is admitted for severe malnutrition and hyponatremia with a serum level of 121 mmol/L. She has mental status changes that are related to the hyponatremic state. What is the main therapy for this severely ill patient?**

In severely symptomatic patients, the clinician should calculate the sodium deficit and deliver 3% hypertonic saline. The sodium deficit can be calculated by the following formula:

Sodium deficit = Total body water (TBW) × (Desired serum Na – Actual serum Na)

where TBW is typically 50% of total mass in women and 55% of total mass in men. The goal is to correct the serum sodium by no more than 10 to 12 mEq/L over the first 24 hours. (The rise in sodium should be no greater than 0.5–1.0 mEq/L per hour; in the face of seizures, this can be increased to 1 to 2 mEq/L per hour but still should not exceed 10–12 mEq/L in a 24-hour period.) Hypertonic saline in hypervolemic patients can be hazardous, resulting in worsening volume overload, pulmonary edema, and ascites.

○ **What is the risk of treating hyponatremia too fast?**

Central pontine myelinolysis. This is an osmotic demyelination syndrome of the brain, which will cause altered levels of consciousness, paralysis, dysarthria, and dysphagia.

○ **What is the most common etiology of hypernatremia?**

Loss of overall water in the body.

○ **What are some causes for hypernatremia?**

The most common cause is when a patient does not have adequate water intake and has continuing water losses, which occurs especially in debilitated or demented individuals with brain dysfunction and impaired thirst, or hospitalized, incapacitated patients under the influence of central nervous system depressants. Additional causes include insensible skin losses (burns, perspiration), respiratory losses (fever, increased respiration, hot dry environments), diabetes insipidus (central [hypothalamic] and nephrogenic), as well as GI losses such as diarrhea and protracted vomiting.

○ **Name physical examination features that may be present in a patient with hypernatremia:**

Contracted volume with hypotension, dry mucous membranes, and neurological symptoms of altered mental status, weakness, irritability, focal deficits, coma, and seizures.

○ **What is the main goal of treatment of hypernatremia?**

Treatment of hypernatremia includes: (1) correcting the cause of the fluid loss, (2) replacing water, and (3) replacing electrolytes (as needed).

○ **How would geophagia/pica (eating clay) affect an individual's electrolytes?**

This is an uncommon cause of <u>hypokalemia</u> related to the potassium-binding properties of some clay.

○ **What effect does diabetic ketoacidosis have on potassium?**

It will cause a depletion of potassium by way of the Na+ K+-ATPase pump stimulation. Hypokalemia can be masked until insulin and fluids are administered, which leads to a rapid influx of potassium into cells.

○ **What are some gastrointestinal problems which can cause hypokalemia?**

Vomiting, diarrhea, excessive use of laxatives, and volume depletion. The potassium concentration in intestinal secretion is 10 times higher than in gastric secretions. The most common cause of hypokalemia, especially in developing countries, is gastrointestinal loss from infectious diarrhea.

○ **A 46-year-old female patient is evaluated for hypokalemia (serum potassium level of 2.9 mEq/L). She is given potassium supplements and is rechecked a week later only to find that her potassium is still at a low level of 3 mEq/L despite taking 40 mEq daily. She is not on any other medications. What disorder could be causing the hypokalemia?**

Primary hyperaldosteronism, which is sometimes caused by a primary tumor of the adrenal gland resulting in hypokalemia. Other possibilities include renal cell carcinoma, ovarian carcinoma, and Wilms tumors in children. These other possibilities are a result of hyperreninemia, which will draw off potassium.

○ **Does Cushing disease present with hypokalemia or hyperkalemia?**

Cushing's causes increased levels of cortisol. Cortisol, at high levels, acts like a mineralocorticoid (aldosterone), stimulating absorption of sodium and excretion of potassium at the collecting tubules. Hence, any disorder involving an excess of mineralocorticoids will cause hypokalemia.

○ **Name some physical examination features in patients with hypokalemia:**

Muscle weakness, fatigue, myalgias, and in more serious cases hyporeflexia, hypercapnia, and flaccid paralysis can occur. The presence of hypertension may be a clue to the diagnosis of hypokalemia from aldosterone or mineralocorticoid excess.

○ **What electrophysiological effects can be seen on an EKG in a patient with hypokalemia?**

The electrocardiogram shows flattening of T waves, prominent U waves, premature ventricular contractions, and depressed ST segments.

○ **Name some causes of hyperkalemia:**

The most common cause is factitious hyperkalemia because of the release of intracellular potassium caused by hemolysis during phlebotomy. Other causes include renal failure, decreased volume circulation (severe heart failure), hypoaldosteronism (since aldosterone is the primary hormone that facilitates urinary potassium excretion), and drugs such as ACE inhibitors, potassium sparing diuretics, and NSAIDs. A less common cause is excessive potassium intake in patients with impaired kidney function (potassium replacement therapy, high potassium diet).

○ **What are some physical symptoms of patients with hyperkalemia?**

Hyperkalemia impairs neuromuscular transmission, causing muscle weakness, flaccid paralysis, and ileus.

○ **What electrophysiological effects can be seen on an EKG in a patient with hyperkalemia?**

EKG changes in hyperkalemia include bradycardia, PR interval prolongation, peaked T waves, QRS widening, and biphasic QRS–T complexes. This can eventually lead to ventricular fibrillation or asystole.

○ **A 66-year-old male patient presents to the emergency department with an arrhythmia, which is determined to be a widened QRS complex that has resulted in the patient going in and out of ventricular fibrillation. His potassium on initial evaluation is 7.6 mEq/L and the patient's renal function is intact. What would be the treatment of choice for this life-threatening illness?**

Calcium gluconate. (Note: In severe hyperkalemia, administration of $[Ca^{2+}]$ is warranted, but should be avoided in patients taking digitalis because of the potential cardiac glycoside toxicity.)

○ **What are the treatment options for non–life-threatening hyperkalemia?**

Regular insulin and glucose or inhaled albuterol can draw potassium into the cells expeditiously. Another alternative is administration of a thiazide loop diuretic to waste potassium. In addition, hemodialysis or peritoneal dialysis can promote potassium removal.

○ **What are the most common reasons for hypocalcemia?**

Impaired vitamin D production and impaired parathyroid hormone production.

○ **Name some physical examination characteristics in patients with hypocalcemia:**

Paresthesias of the fingers and toes and circumoral regions are associated with moderate to severe hypocalcemia. Chvostek sign (twitching of the circumoral muscles in response to gentle tapping of the facial nerve just anterior to the ear) is present in approximately 10% of patients. Trousseau sign (carpal spasm induced by inflation of a blood pressure cuff to 20 mm Hg above the patient's systolic blood pressure for 3 minutes) can also be present. Severe hypocalcemia can present with seizures, bronchospasm, laryngospasm, and prolonged QT interval on EKG.

○ **What is the treatment for a patient with acute, symptomatic hypocalcemia?**

Calcium gluconate (usually 10 mL 10% wt/vol [90 mg or 2.2 mmol] intravenously, diluted in 50 mL of 5% dextrose or 0.9% sodium chloride, given intravenously over 5 minutes).

○ **For patients with chronic hypocalcemia caused by hypoparathyroidism, what is the long-term management?**

Elemental calcium supplements, 1 to 1.5 g/day usually in divided doses, and vitamin D2 or D3 (25,000–100,000 U daily) or calcitriol.

○ **What are some presenting symptoms in patients with mild hypercalcemia? Severe cases?**

In general, most patients are asymptomatic. Some will experience trouble concentrating, depression, and personality changes. Some other symptoms will be nausea, constipation, pancreatitis, peptic ulcer disease, or anorexia.

In severe hypercalcemia, the symptoms will be lethargy, coma, and stupor.

○ **What are the most common causes of hypercalcemia?**

Primary hyperparathyroidism and malignancy account for 90% of cases.

○ **What is the treatment of choice for hypercalcemia?**

Mild, asymptomatic hypercalcemia does not require immediate therapy, and management should be dictated by the underlying diagnosis. However, significant, symptomatic hypercalcemia usually requires therapeutic intervention independent of the etiology of hypercalcemia. Initial therapy begins with volume expansion since hypercalcemia invariably leads to dehydration; 4 to 6 L of intravenous saline may be required over the first 24 hours, keeping in mind that underlying comorbidities (e.g., CHF) may require loop diuretics to enhance sodium and calcium excretion. If there is increased calcium mobilization from bone (as in malignancy or severe hyperparathyroidism), drugs that inhibit bone resorption (<u>bisphosphonates</u>) should be considered.

○ **What is one factor that could mislead you in a correct diagnosis of hyper- or hypocalcemia?**

Serum albumin levels, which bind to calcium. If this level is either high or low, it can impact the serum levels of calcium. Thus, it is generally preferable to measure total calcium and albumin to "correct" the serum calcium.

○ **What are some physical examination findings in patients with hypomagnesemia?**

Common symptoms include weakness and muscle cramps. Marked neuromuscular and central nervous system hyperirritability may produce tremors, slow and writhing movements, jerking, nystagmus, a Babinski response, confusion, and disorientation. Cardiovascular manifestations include hypertension, tachycardia, and ventricular arrhythmias.

○ **What are some EKG findings in patients with hypomagnesemia?**

Prolonged PR or QT intervals, T-wave flattening or inversion, and ST straightening. Digitalis toxicity may be enhanced with low magnesium levels.

○ **What is the most common cause of hypermagnesemia in a patient with renal failure?**

Patient use of compounds high in magnesium, such as antacids. This can result in neuromuscular paralysis.

○ **How is hypermagnesemia in a patient with renal failure treated?**

Saline and furosemide-assisted diuresis may not help a patient with renal failure, so consider hemodialysis as well. Calcium, administered IV in doses of 100 to 200 mg over 1 to 2 hours, has been reported to provide temporary improvement in signs and symptoms of hypermagnesemia.

○ **How are metabolic acidoses classified?**

By the anion gap—either normal or increased.

○ **What are some common causes of increased anion gap (AG)?**

The four most common causes of a high AG metabolic acidosis are lactic acidosis, ketoacidosis, ingested toxins, and renal failure. Lactic acidosis almost always indicates the presence of impaired tissue perfusion, most commonly caused by hypotension, arterial disease, or sepsis. Rarely, an unsuspected neoplasm produces lactic acid and is the causative factor. Salicylate, ethylene glycol (found in antifreeze), and methanol are among the most common drugs/toxins that cause a high AG acidosis. Uremic acidosis is characterized by inadequate net acid excretion caused by impaired ammonia and titratable acid excretion.

Recall some pearls for sorting out the differential diagnosis of an elevated anion gap (MUDPILES):

1. Methanol—Visual disturbances and headache are common. May produce wide gaps because each 2.6 mg/dL of methanol contributes 1 mOsm/L to gap. Compare this with alcohol: each 4.3 mg/dL adds 1 mOsm/L to gap.

2. Uremia (chronic renal failure)—Must be quite advanced before it causes an anion gap.

3. Diabetic ketoacidosis—Both hyperglycemia and glucosuria typically occur. Alcoholic ketoacidosis (AKA) is often associated with low blood sugar and mild or absent glucosuria.

4. Propylene glycol

5. Infection, Iron, Isoniazid, Inborn errors of metabolism

6. Lactic acidosis—Check serum level. This condition also has broad differential, including shock, seizures, acute hypoxemia, INH, cyanide, ritodrine, inhaled acetylene and carbon monoxide, and ethanol.

7. Ethylene glycol—Also causes calcium oxalate or hippurate crystals in urine. Each 5.0 mg/dL contributes 1 mOsm/L to gap.

8. Salicylates—High levels contribute to gap.

○ **How is renal tubular acidosis (RTA) classified?**

Hyperchloremic acidosis with a normal anion gap and normal (or near normal) GFR, and in the absence of diarrhea, defines RTA. The defect is either inability to excrete H^+ (inadequate generation of new HCO_3^-) or inappropriate reabsorption of HCO_3^-. RTA is classified into one of the three types: type I (distal RTA), type II (proximal RTA), or type IV (hypoaldosteronism RTA). Type III is no longer referenced, as it is now considered a combination of Type I and Type II RTA.

○ **What are the mechanisms for the different types of RTA?**

In type I, there is a deficiency in the secretion of the hydrogen ion by the distal tubule and collecting duct. In type II, there is a decrease in the bicarbonate reabsorption in the proximal tubule. For type IV (most common type), there is aldosterone deficiency, which leads to impairment of sodium reabsorption as well as potassium and hydrogen excretion.

○ **Which form of RTA is associated with renal calculi?**

Distal (type I) RTA.

○ **What are the characteristic acid–base electrolyte abnormalities associated with type I and type II RTA?**

Hypokalemic, hyperchloremic metabolic acidosis.

○ **What are the characteristic acid–base/electrolyte abnormalities associated with type IV RTA?**

Hyperkalemic, hyperchloremic metabolic acidosis.

○ **What diseases are associated with type IV RTA?**

It is most common in diabetic nephropathy, tubulointerstitial renal diseases, AIDS, and hypertensive nephrosclerosis.

○ **What is the treatment of acute metabolic acidosis with a pH <7.10?**

Sodium bicarbonate IV. Whether metabolic acidosis should be treated with alkali depends in large part on whether acute or chronic metabolic acidosis is present. For chronic metabolic acidosis, the benefit of alkali treatment is clear-cut. For acute metabolic acidosis, the benefit of alkali treatment is less certain. Clinical trials have shown no clinically significant effect of alkali treatment of acute metabolic acidosis on either mortality or on cardiovascular performance. However, treating acute metabolic acidosis with alkali might be considered if arterial pH is less than 7.1. Slow IV administration of 50 to 100 mEq of $NaHCO_3$, over 30 to 45 minutes, during the initial 1 to 2 hours of therapy can be used. It is essential to monitor plasma electrolytes during the course of therapy, since the K^+ may decline as pH rises. Normalization of values is not recommended, and may potentially be deleterious. If alkali treatment is used, a target pH of 7.2 is reasonable. Administration of large amounts of concentrated $NaHCO_3$ in the form of multiple "ampules" can cause acute hypernatremia because of the associated sodium load.

○ **Name some causes for a patient to have metabolic alkalosis:**

Exogenous bicarbonate loads such as alkali ingestion; extracellular volume contraction in the setting of potassium deficiency such as GI problems (vomiting, aspiration) or renal disorders (diuretics, lactic acidosis recovery, hypercalcemia, or magnesium deficiency); and extracellular volume expansion with high renin (renal artery stenosis, accelerated hypertension) or low renin (licorice ingestion, primary aldosteronism, or Cushings).

○ **What are some causes of respiratory acidosis?**

Respiratory acidosis results from hypoventilation and subsequent hypercapnia. It is defined as a pH of 7.35 or less and a P_{CO_2} of 35 or more. Common causes of respiratory acidosis include drugs, CVA, infection, asthma, lung disease (such as emphysema, bronchitis, ARDS, etc.), and neuromuscular disorders (such as poliomyelitis, kyphoscoliosis, myasthenia, and muscular dystrophy). Obesity and hypoventilation are other etiologies.

○ **What is the expected change in serum bicarbonate in chronic respiratory acidosis?**

In acute respiratory acidosis, there is an immediate compensatory elevation (because of cellular buffering mechanisms) in bicarbonate, which increases 1 mmol/L for every 10-mm Hg increase in Pa_{CO_2}. In chronic respiratory acidosis (>24 hours), renal adaptation increases the bicarbonate by 4 mmol/L for every 10-mm Hg increase in Pa_{CO_2}. The serum bicarbonate usually does not increase above 38 mmol/L.

○ **A 45-year-old obese man presents with dyspnea, peripheral edema, snoring, and excessive daytime sleepiness. A room air arterial blood gas is drawn—the pH is 7.34, the Pa_{CO_2} is 60 mm Hg, the Pa_{O_2} is 58 mm Hg, and the calculated HCO_3 is 28 mEq/L. What is the acid–base disturbance?**

Chronic, compensated respiratory acidosis. If this was acute respiratory acidosis, the pH would be 7.24 with a normal HCO_3^-.

○ **What are some common causes of respiratory alkalosis?**

Respiratory alkalosis is defined as a pH greater than 7.45 and a P_{CO_2} less than 35. Common causes of respiratory alkalosis include any process that may induce hyperventilation: shock, sepsis, trauma, asthma, stroke, anemia, hepatic failure, heat stroke, exhaustion, anxiety, pregnancy, salicylate poisoning, hypoxemia, and mechanical overventilation.

○   **What are the signs and symptoms of respiratory alkalosis?**

Hyperventilation, perioral and extremity paresthesias, muscle cramps, tachypnea, hyperreflexia, seizures, and cardiac arrhythmias

○   **What medications can induce nephrogenic diabetes insipidus?**

Lithium, Foscarnet, and Amphotericin B.

○   **A patient with nephrogenic diabetes insipidus has a serum sodium level of 117 mEq/L. How do you determine how much NaCl to administer to keep the risk of cerebral edema at a minimum?**

Amount of NaCl to add in mEq/L = $0.6 \times$ wt (in kg) $\times$ (140 – serum sodium).

REFERENCES

Gomella LG, ed. *The 5-Minute Urology Consult.* 2nd ed. New York, NY: Lippincott Williams & Wilkins; 2010.

Longo DL, Fauci AS, Kasper DL, Hauser SL, Jameson JL, Loscalzo J, eds. *Harrison's Principles of Internal Medicine.* 18th ed. New York, NY: McGraw-Hill; 2012.

Papadakis MA, McPhee SJ, Rabow MW, Berger TG, eds. *CURRENT Medical Diagnosis & Treatment 2014.* New York, NY: McGraw-Hill; 2013.

Resnick MI, Schaeffer AJ, eds. *Urology Pearls.* Philadelphia, NY: Hanley & Belfus; 2000.

Tanagho EA, McAninch JW, eds. *Smith's General Urology.* 17th ed. New York, NY: McGraw-Hill; 2008.

Tintinalli JE, Stapczynski JS, Cline DM, Ma OJ, Cydulka RK, Meckler GD, eds. *Tintinalli's Emergency Medicine: A Comprehensive Study Guide.* 7th ed. New York, NY: McGraw-Hill; 2011.

CHAPTER 8 Reproductive

Jacqueline Jordan Spiegel, MS, PA-C

REPRODUCTIVE PHYSIOLOGY

○ **What are the three events that occur in the normal course of female puberty (in order of occurrence and with definition of each)?**

1. Thelarche—the development of breasts
2. Pubarche—the development of axillary and pubic hair
3. Menarche—the first menstrual cycle

○ **What is the classification system commonly used to define the progression of breast and pubic hair development in puberty, and how many stages does the system have?**

Tanner classification. There are five stages.

○ **What defines the normal menstrual cycle in terms of frequency, length, and phases?**

The normal menstrual cycle is 28 days, with a flow lasting 2 to 7 days. The variation in cycle length is set at 24 to 35 days. The luteal phase of the cycle is normally 14 days with the follicular phase being 14 to 21 days.

○ **In the normal menstrual cycle, when does ovulation typically occur?**

Ovulation in a 28-day cycle typically occurs on day 14 and is triggered by a surge of luteinizing hormone (LH) from the pituitary.

○ **What are the hormones, and their source, that are involved in maintaining a normal menstrual cycle?**

From the ovary: Estrogen and progesterone

From the pituitary: Follicle-stimulating hormone (FSH) and luteinizing hormone (LH). In addition, prolactin- and thyroid-stimulating hormones are also vital in maintaining a normal menstrual cycle.

From the hypothalamus: Gonadotropin-releasing hormone (GnRH).

○ **What is the effect of estrogen on the endometrium, when it peaks, and the effect of declining estrogen?**

Estrogen causes growth of the endometrium. The endometrial glands lengthen and the glandular epithelium becomes pseudostratified. Mitotic activity is present in both the glands and the stroma.

Serum estradiol levels are at their peak approximately 1 day prior to ovulation.

When estrogen levels begin to decline, there is a loss of endometrial blood supply, endometrial sloughing, and onset of menses.

○ **What is the function of FSH?**

It stimulates maturation of the follicle(s) and the production of estradiol from the follicles.

○ **What is the function of LH?**

It causes follicular rupture, ovulation, and establishment of the corpus luteum.

○ **What is the function of prolactin?**

It initiates and sustains lactation by the breast glands and it may influence synthesis and release of progesterone by the ovary and testosterone by the testis.

○ **What is the main physiological stimulus for prolactin release?**

Suckling of the breast.

○ **What is the purpose of the corpus luteum and its lifespan in the absence of pregnancy?**

After ovulation, the expelled follicle is called the corpus luteum. The corpus luteum secretes estradiol and progesterone, which cause secretory ducts to develop in the endometrial lining in anticipation of implantation. In the absence of pregnancy, the lifespan is approximately 14 days.

○ **What does a <u>biphasic</u> curve on a basal body temperature (BBT) chart of a 25-year-old woman indicate?**

Normal ovulation caused by the effects of progesterone. A monophasic BBT curve indicates an anovulatory cycle. A temperature remaining elevated following a normal biphasic curve would indicate pregnancy.

○ **What is the cause of midcycle spotting or light bleeding?**

A low or declined estradiol that occurs immediately prior to the LH surge.

○ **The decline in which hormone heralds the onset of menses?**

Endometrial shedding (onset of menses) occurs because of progesterone withdrawal.

○ **What is the definition of Mittelschmerz?**

The cyclic abdominal pain located on either side of the abdomen, which can be felt during ovulation and may persist for approximately 2 days after.

○ **What pelvic type is the most common in women?**

Gynecoid. It is estimated that approximately 50% of women have gynecoid pelvis. (It should be noted that in reality most women have intermediate pelvic shapes rather than true gynecoid, anthropoid, android, or platypelloid.)

MENSTRUAL DISORDERS

○ **Define the following: menorrhagia, metrorrhagia, menometrorrhagia, polymenorrhea, and oligomenorrhea**

Menorrhagia—excessive amount of vaginal bleeding or duration of bleeding during menses

Metrorrhagia—bleeding between menstrual periods

Menometrorrhagia—excessive amount of blood at irregular frequencies

Polymenorrhea—menstrual periods less than 21 days apart

Oligomenorrhea—menstrual periods greater than 35 days apart

○ **What is primary amenorrhea?**

Absence of spontaneous menstruation by age 16.

○ **What is secondary amenorrhea?**

No menstruation for 6 months or more in a woman who previously had regular menses.

○ **What is the most common cause of secondary amenorrhea?**

Pregnancy. The second most common cause is hypothalamic hypogonadism, which can be because of weight loss, anorexia nervosa, stress, excessive exercise, or hypothalamic disease.

○ **A 27-year-old woman presents with secondary amenorrhea for 6 months. What is the appropriate initial evaluation?**

Pelvic examination, pap smear, pregnancy test. If pregnancy test is negative, additional laboratory studies to include prolactin, FSH, LH, and TSH.

○ **A 26-year-old woman with secondary amenorrhea and an essentially normal work-up is given progestin 10 mg for 7 days (or an IM injection of progesterone 100 mg). She responds with a normal menstrual period. What does this tell you?**

She has a functional endometrium and a normal production of estrogen to proliferate the endometrial lining. This test is called the progesterone challenge.

○ **What are the two major differential diagnoses in a patient with secondary amenorrhea who fails a progestin challenge?**

Premature ovarian failure and hypothalamic dysfunction. Premature ovarian failure can be diagnosed if the serum FSH level is high; hypothalamic dysfunction can be diagnosed in setting of low FSH and LH.

○ **List the differential diagnosis of persistent vaginal bleeding in a preadolescent woman:**

- Neoplasia
- Precocious puberty
- Ureteral prolapse
- Trauma (including sexual assault)
- Vulvovaginitis
- Exposure to excessive estrogen
- Foreign body in vagina
- Infection

○ **What blood tests would be appropriate in the evaluation of a female child with precocious puberty?**

Serum levels of FSH, LH, prolactin, TSH, estradiol, testosterone, dehydroepiandrosterone sulfate (DHEAS), and HCG.

○ **When is the typical onset of primary dysmenorrhea?**

Onset is usually within 3 to 6 months of menarche.

○ **What is the definition of secondary dysmenorrhea?**

Painful menstruation caused by an identifiable clinical condition, usually a disease of the uterus or pelvis. It usually affects women older than 25 years.

○ **What are the four main etiologies of secondary dysmenorrhea?**

1. Endometriosis
2. Pelvic inflammatory disease
3. Uterine fibroids
4. Pelvic congestion (typically occurs in multiparous women with pelvic vein varicosities and congested pelvic organs OR s/p C-section)

○ **What diagnostic tests in the evaluation of secondary dysmenorrhea can be both diagnostic and therapeutic?**

Hysteroscopy, dilation and curettage (D&C), and laparoscopy.

○ **What are the recommended pharmacotherapeutic interventions for primary dysmenorrhea?**

NSAIDs or combined oral contraceptive agents

If nonresponsive to the above interventions, tocolytic agents (salbutamol) or calcium channel blockers (nifedipine) or progestins (medroxyprogesterone) have been shown to be effective

○ **What percentage of women with premenstrual syndrome meet the criteria for premenstrual dysphoric disorder?**

Approximately 4%. The difference between PMS and PDD is the severity of symptoms causing dysfunction in daily living.

○ **What are the most common presenting complaints in premenstrual syndrome?**

Mood alteration and psychological effects including irritability, anxiety, depression, sleep, appetite changes, poor concentration, fatigue, and insomnia.

○ **What are the most common physical symptoms of premenstrual syndrome?**

Fluid retention, breast pain, bloating, constipation, backache.

○ **What are the recommended lifestyle modifications in the treatment of premenstrual syndrome?**

Caffeine reduction, salt restriction, low-fat and high-complex carbohydrate intake, emphasis on fresh/nonprocessed foods, increased exercise, relaxation measures, and stress reduction.

UTERUS

○ **In a woman of reproductive age, what is the first step in the evaluation of abnormal uterine bleeding following the history and physical examination?**

A pregnancy test.

○ **What is the standard laboratory work-up for a perimenopausal woman presenting with dysfunctional uterine bleeding?**

CBC, PT, PTT, hCG, TSH, progesterone, prolactin, FSH, LFTs.

○ **What are the pharmaceutical treatment options for dysfunctional uterine bleeding?**

Treatment depends on severity of bleeding. Options include observation, iron therapy, volume replacement, oral contraceptives, and cyclic progestins.

○ **What is the recommended treatment for massive intractable dysfunctional uterine bleeding?**

25-mg IV conjugated estrogens.

○ **What percentage of the female population has endometriosis?**

More than 15% and 7% of women during their reproductive years.

○ **What is thought to be the most common etiology for endometriosis?**

Retrograde menstruation.

○ **Where is the most common site of endometriosis?**

The ovaries (60%). Other sites include the cul-de-sac, uterosacral ligaments, broad ligaments, fallopian tubes, uterovesical fold, round ligaments, vermiform appendix, vagina, rectosigmoid colon, cecum, and ileum.

○ **What are chocolate cysts?**

Endometriomas (cystic forms of endometriosis on the ovary).

○ **What percentage of women with endometriosis also have infertility?**

25% to 35%.

○ **What is considered the preferred means of establishing a diagnosis of endometriosis?**

Direct visualization during diagnostic laparoscopy or laparotomy. Clinical presentation, laboratory evaluation, and/or pelvic ultrasound are considered inadequate to make a definitive diagnosis.

○ **What are the pharmacotherapeutic options for treating endometriosis?**

Treatment is based on severity of symptoms, location, and desire for child bearing. Pharmacotherapeutic options include NSAIDs, prostaglandin synthetase inhibitors, combined oral contraceptive agents, progestin-only contraceptives, GnRH agonists, danazol (a 17-alpha-ethinyl testosterone derivative).

○ **What are the common side effects of danazol (Danocrine)?**

Hirsutism, amenorrhea, deepening of the voice, acne, weight gain, hot flashes, labile emotions, and decreased vaginal secretions.

○ **What is the most common gynecologic malignancy and fourth most common malignancy in women in the United States?**

Endometrial carcinoma.

○ **What percentage of postmenopausal woman presenting with vaginal bleeding have endometrial cancer?**

15%. The cardinal symptom of endometrial cancer is inappropriate uterine bleeding (90%).

○ **What are the most common etiologies of endometrial cancer?**

30% of these tumors are caused by exogenous estrogens, 30% are caused by atrophic endometriosis or vaginitis, 10% are caused by cervical polyps, and 5% are caused by endometrial hyperplasia.

○ **What are the risk factors for endometrial cancer?**

- Obesity
- Nulliparity
- Early menarche
- Late menopause
- Unopposed estrogen stimulation
- Hypertension
- Gallbladder disease
- Diabetes mellitus
- Prior ovarian, endometrial, or breast cancer.

○ **What is the gold standard test for definitive diagnosis of endometrial cancer?**

Endometrial biopsy.

○ **What percentage of women with endometrial cancer will have an abnormal Papanicolaou smear?**

Approximately 50%.

○ **What is the most common clinical condition associated with the development of endometrial hyperplasia?**

Polycystic ovarian syndrome.

○ **What is the most common type of benign gynecologic pelvic neoplasm?**

Uterine leiomyoma (or uterine fibroids).

○ **What type of leiomyoma is symptomatic?**

Submucosal myomas, though small, can cause profuse bleeding. Most other myomas are asymptomatic until grown large enough to cause obstruction or significantly distort the endometrial cavity.

○ **What is the recommended treatment for leiomyoma?**

Observation in most cases. GnRH agonists and mifepristone may reduce tumor size. Surgical intervention (myomectomy, hysterectomy). Arterial embolization is becoming increasingly popular.

○ **A 37-year-old woman, G2 P2 presents with a history of lengthening menses and secondary dysmenorrhea. This problem had been subtly going on for 2 years and now is a quality-of-life issue. Examination reveals an irregular, globular-shaped uterus. What is the most likely diagnosis?**

Adenomyosis.

○ **What is the definitive treatment for adenomyosis?**

Hysterectomy.

○ **Compare and contrast the types of hysterectomy.**

Type	Definition
Total vs. Subtotal	Total = Removal of the entire uterus and cervix. Subtotal = Uterus removal while the cervix remains intact.
Vaginal vs. Abdominal	Specifies the route of removal. Abdominal hysterectomy can be further clarified as either a laparoscopic or a cesarean (open) approach.
Simple vs. Radical	Simple = Used to denote whether vaginal tissue and pelvic lymph nodes are removed. Radical = Includes the removal of uterus, cervix, vaginal, and pelvic lymph nodes.
Oophorectomy	The removal of the ovaries and is separated from hysterectomy. Oophorectomy can be unilateral or bilateral.

○ **What is the most frequent complication of hysterectomy?**

Infection. The most common organisms are those found in normal vaginal flora. Because the vagina is difficult to cleanse, most experts recommend antibiotic prophylaxis for all patients undergoing vaginal hysterectomy.

○ **A woman presenting with pelvic pain and pressure when standing, the feeling of something protruding from the vaginal opening, and occasional urinary incontinence or constipation is likely to have what?**

Pelvic organ prolapse.

○   **Compare and contrast different types of pelvic organ prolapse.**

Type	Definition	Associated Etiology
Cystocele	Downward displacement of the bladder into the vagina along the anterior wall	Delivery of a large baby Multiple deliveries Prolonged labor
Rectocele	Displacement of the rectum into the posterior wall of the vagina	Multiparous women with a history of long end-stage labor Women who undergo midline episiotomy
Uterine Prolapse	Descent of the uterus and cervix down the vaginal canal toward the introitus secondary to broken uterosacral ligaments or relaxation of the musculature of the pelvic floor	More likely to occur in women with a retroverted uterus
Vaginal Prolapse	Downward displacement of the vaginal apex also caused by loss of muscle and ligamental support	Typically follows a hysterectomy

○   **What are the indications for performing a dilation and curettage?**

- Relief of profuse uterine hemorrhage
- Removal of endometrial polyp or hydatid mole
- Termination of pregnancy/incomplete abortion
- Removal of retained placental tissue

○   **What major complication is associated with the performance of a dilation and curettage?**

Perforation of the uterus.

○   **What is the most useful preventive measure for pelvic organ prolapse?**

Kegel exercises.

OVARY

○   **What is the most common cause of pelvic pain in an adolescent girl?**

Ovarian cysts.

○   **What is the most common type of ovarian cyst?**

Follicular. The other types are corpus luteum and theca lutein cysts.

○   **What is the most common complication of ovarian cysts?**

Torsion of the ovary. Torsion is more common in small-to-medium–sized cysts and tumors. Emergency surgery is required.

○ **What is the recommended treatment for uncomplicated follicular cysts?**

Most resolve spontaneously within a few menstrual cycles (60 days) without treatment. Combined oral contraceptive agents can be used if recurrent.

○ **By how much is the incidence of functional cysts reduced by OCP use?**

80% to 90%. Oral contraceptives suppress FSH and LH ovarian stimulation.

○ **What are the clinical manifestations of polycystic ovarian disease (PCO)? Explain using the mnemonic OVARIAN:**

O—Obesity
V—Virilization
A—Anovulation
R—Resistance to insulin
I—Increased hair growth
A—Androgen excess
N—No period/Amenorrhea

○ **What are the laboratory findings seen with polycystic ovarian syndrome?**

Increased LH/FSH ratio (2:1)
Elevated serum glucose
Elevated fasting insulin
Elevated sex androgens (DHEA-S and/or testosterone)

○ **What is the first-line treatment for polycystic ovarian syndrome?**

Weight loss.

○ **What are the other treatment options for polycystic ovarian syndrome?**

Combined oral contraceptive pills for menstrual regulation and ovarian suppression; Biguanides (metformin) for menstrual regulation, weight reduction, and to reestablish fertility; anti-androgen (spironolactone) for sex androgen suppression and hirsutism.

○ **If a woman has ascites, what is the most likely tumor to be found?**

Ovarian carcinoma.

○ **What serum marker is associated with ovarian cancer?**

CA-125.
BRCA1 gene is associated with 5% of cases.

○ **What are considered protective factors for the risk of ovarian cancer?**

Multiparity, combined oral contraceptive use, and breast-feeding.

○ **What is the treatment for ovarian cancer?**

Stage 1A or 1B—Surgical excision alone (abdominal hysterectomy and bilateral salpingo-oophorectomy).

Other stages—Surgical resection followed by adjuvant chemotherapy or radiation.

○ **What is Meigs syndrome?**

Ascites and hydrothorax in the presence of an ovarian tumor.

CERVIX

○ **What is a nabothian cyst?**

A mucous inclusion cyst of the cervix (usually asymptomatic and benign).

○ **What is the squamocolumnar junction? Describe its importance and how it changes.**

It is the junction between the columnar epithelium and the squamous epithelium of the cervix. This is also known as the transformation zone. Throughout a woman's life, the squamous epithelium of the ectocervix (and vagina) invades the columnar epithelium of the endocervix. It is important because it is the squamous epithelium in this transformation zone that is most likely to become dysplastic.

○ **What are the American College of Obstetricians and Gynecologists (ACOG) recommendations for Pap smear screening?**

Pap smear screening should be initiated at age 21. Plus at the time of initial intercourse for women under 21 who have HIV infection or who are on chronic immunosuppressive therapy for systemic lupus erythematosus or post organ transplantation.

All guidelines recommend only cytology screening for women aged 21 to 29 years every 3 years.

For women 30 years and older, combination of cytology plus HPV testing is recommended every 5 years.

Annual screening is recommended for any high-risk groups (HIV infection, immunosuppression, or in utero DES exposure) or women who have treated in the past for CIN 2, CIN 3, or cervical cancer.

○ **What are the ACOG recommendations for discontinuation of Pap smear screening?**

No cytology screening after total hysterectomy if surgery for benign condition. If surgery for CIN I, II, or III, then annually three times before discontinuing.

Discontinue screening at age 65 for women who have had adequate recent screening. Adequate screening is defined as three consecutive negative cytology tests or two consecutive negative HPV/Pap co-tests in the 10 years before stopping, with the most recent test within 5 years.

○ **What do ASC-US, LSIL, HSIL on a Pap screening pathology report represent?**

ASC-US: Atypical squamous cells of undetermined significance.

LSIL: Low-grade squamous intraepithelial lesion, that is, mild dysplasia, CIN I.

HSIL: High-grade squamous intraepithelial lesion, that is, moderate to severe dysplasia, CIN II-III, carcinoma in situ.

○ **What is the recommended management of a woman with negative cytology results and HPV positive?**

Both tests should be repeated in 12 months.

○ **What is the recommended management of a 25+ y/o woman with ASC-US Pap result and HPV positive?**

Colposcopy.

○ **What is the definition of CIN and how is it categorized?**

Cervical intraepithelial neoplasia (CIN) refers to preinvasive dysplasia of cervical epithelial cells, the precursor of malignant disease. CIN is categorized according to the depth of involvement and the atypicality of the cell.

- CIN 1—Considered a low-grade lesion, with mildly atypical cellular changes in the lower third of the epithelium.
- CIN 2—Considered a high-grade lesion, with changes affecting the basal two-thirds of the epithelium. This is equivalent to moderate dysplasia.
- CIN 3—Also a high-grade lesion, with cellular changes affecting more than two-thirds of the epithelium, including full-thickness lesions. This was formerly called severe dysplasia or carcinoma in situ.

○ **What are the known subtypes of HPV associated with cervical cancer?**

HPV types 16, 18, and 31 are risk factors for cervical dysplasia, which can lead to cervical cancer.

○ **How many times more likely is a woman with condyloma acuminatum (genital warts) to develop cervical cancer than a woman without this lesion?**

Four times more likely.

○ **What is the most common type of cervical cancer?**

80% are squamous cells and arise from the squamocolumnar junction of the cervix.

○ **What are the risk factors for carcinoma of the cervix?**

Multiple sexual partners, early age at first intercourse, early first pregnancy, and HPV positive.

○ **What is the most common presenting symptom for patients with cervical cancer?**

Up to 80% of patients present with abnormal vaginal bleeding, most commonly postmenopausal. Only 10% note postcoital bleeding. Less frequent symptoms include vaginal discharge and pain.

○ **What clinical triad is strongly indicative of cervical cancer extension to the pelvic wall?**

Unilateral leg edema, sciatic pain, ureteral obstruction.

○ **What are the advantages of radical hysterectomy relative to radiation therapy for stage I cervical cancer?**

Ovarian preservation is possible.
Unimpaired vaginal function.
Extent of disease can be established by pathology.

○ **At what age is the HPV vaccine recommended?**

Girls aged 11 to 12.

VAGINA/VULVA

○ **What is the normal pH of the vagina?**

3.8 to 4.4 (a vaginal pH > 4.9 indicates a bacterial or protozoal infection).

○ **What is the predominant organism in a healthy woman's vaginal discharge?**

Lactobacilli (95%).

○ **What is the treatment of choice for a Bartholin gland abscess?**

Marsupialization with the placement of a Word catheter. This prevents recurrences.

○ **What causes condylomata acuminata?**

Human papilloma virus types 6 and 11.

○ **What other sexually transmitted infection is commonly seen in combination with condylomata acuminata?**

Trichomonas.

○ **What are the recommended treatment options for condylomata acuminata (genital warts)?**

Liquid nitrogen, podophyllin resin, Aldara (topical imiquimod); not necessarily curative but treatment is focused on destruction of warts.

○ **What is the most frequent gynecologic disease of children?**

Vulvovaginitis, the cause of which is poor perineal hygiene.

○ **What is the most common cause of vaginitis?**

Candida albicans.

○ **What predisposes a woman to vaginal candidiasis infections?**

Diabetes, oral contraceptives, and antibiotics.

○ **What are the recommended forms of treatment for vaginal candidiasis infections?**

Topical clotrimazole (Gyne-Lotrimin).
Topical tioconazole (Monistat).
Oral fluconazole (Diflucan). It has been reported that a one-time dose of fluconazole (Diflucan) is 90% effective.
In severe infections (generally in hospitalized patients), amphotericin B, caspofungin, or voriconazole may be used.

○ **What is the causative agent in bacterial vaginosis (BV)?**

Gardnerella.

○ **What are the signs and symptoms typical for BV?**

On physical examination, a frothy, grayish white, fishy smelling vaginal discharge is noted.

○ **What would you expect on microscopic evaluation with saline and with 10% KOH on a patient with BV?**

"Clue cells," which are epithelial cells with bacilli attached to their surfaces. On saline wet mount adding 10% KOH to the discharge produces a fishy odor.

○ **What is the recommended treatment for BV?**

Metronidazole (Flagyl) either orally or vaginally.

○ **A patient presents with pain in her eyes, canker sores in her mouth, and sores and scars in her genital area. What is the diagnosis?**

Behçet disease. This is a rare disease involving ocular inflammation, oral aphthous ulcers, and destructive genital ulcers (generally on the vulva). No cure is known, but remission may occur with high estrogen levels.

○ **What are the known risk factors for the development of toxic shock syndrome (TSS)?**

Tampons, IUDs, septic abortions, sponges, soft tissue abscesses, osteomyelitis, nasal packing, and postpartum infections can all house these organisms.

○ **What causes toxic shock syndrome (TSS)?**

An exotoxin composed of certain strains of *Staphylococcus aureus*. Other organisms that cause toxic shock syndrome are group A streptococci, *Pseudomonas aeruginosa*, and *Streptococcus pneumoniae*.

○ **What criteria are necessary for the diagnosis of TSS?**

All of the following must be present:

- Temperature >38.9°C (102°F).
- Rash (blanching erythematous rash × 3 days), followed by full-thickness desquamation of the palms and soles.
- Systolic BP <90 mm Hg with orthostasis.
- Involvement of three organ systems (GI, renal, musculoskeletal, mucosal, hepatic, hematologic, or CNS).
- The patient must also have negative serologic tests for diseases such as RMSF, hepatitis B, measles, leptospirosis, and VDRL.

○ **What is the most common cell type in vulvar and/or vaginal carcinoma?**

Squamous cell (90% in vulvar carcinoma; 85% in vaginal carcinoma).

○ **What is the most common location for vaginal carcinoma?**

Upper one-third of the posterior vaginal wall.

○ **What are the known risk factors for vulvar/vaginal carcinoma?**

HPV infection
Smoking
Coexisting cervical carcinoma
In utero exposure to DES

○ **What laboratory study can be useful in the evaluation of suspicious vulvar lesions?**

Application of acetic acid or staining with toluidine blue may help direct optimal biopsy location.

SEXUALLY TRANSMITTED INFECTIONS

○ **A 22-year-old patient presents with a complaint of painful blisters on the vulva and vaginal introitus. She admits to a prodrome of burning, tingling, and/or pruritus prior to the appearance of lesions. Upon examination, you note vesicles on an erythematous base. What is the probable diagnosis?**

Herpes simplex virus.

○ **What is the causative bacterium in syphilis?**

Treponema pallidum.

○ **What is the hallmark presenting sign of primary syphilis?**

Painless ulcer (chancre).

○ **What are the presenting signs associated with secondary syphilis?**

Nonpruritus maculopapular rash that includes the palms and soles (Condyloma latum), lymphadenopathy, and constitutional symptoms (fatigue/malaise). These symptoms present 4 to 6 weeks after the hallmark syphilitic chancre and persist for 2 to 6 weeks before the infection enters the latent phase.

○ **What is the presenting feature of tertiary syphilis?**

Neurosyphilis (neuro deficits including difficulty with coordination, memory loss, paralysis, gradual blindness, or dementia).

○ **What is the treatment for syphilis?**

Benzathine PCN G, 2.4 million units IM × 1 dose. Additional doses if infection has been for >1 year or if the patient is pregnant. If the patient is penicillin-allergic, treat with doxycycline.

○ **What causes a greenish gray frothy vaginal discharge with mild itching?**

Trichomonas vaginitis.

○ **What is considered the hallmark pelvic examination finding in 20% of trichomonas infections?**

Petechiae on the cervix (also known as a "strawberry cervix").

○ **What microscopic findings are indicative of trichomonas infections?**

The presence of mobile and pear-shaped protozoa with flagella is indicative of trichomonas.

○ **A 30-year-old woman complains of a <u>painful</u> sore on her vulva that first resembled a pimple. On examination, you find an ulcer with vague borders, gray base, and foul-smelling discharge. What is the probable diagnosis and causative agent?**

Chancroid. Gram stain, culture, and biopsy (used in combination because of the high false-negative rates) show the causative agent *Haemophilus ducreyi.*

○ **What is considered the most appropriate treatment for chancroid?**

Ceftriaxone 250 mg IM × 1 dose **or** azithromycin 1 g PO × 1 dose.

○ **What is the typical clinical presentation of lymphogranuloma venereum (LGV)? Causative agent?**

Vesicopustular eruption, unilateral inguinal bubo, possible anal discharge, and rectal bleeding. The causative organism is a serotype of *Chlamydia trachomatis*.

○ **What is the most common sexually transmitted infection in the United States and sometimes asymptomatic in women?**

Chlamydia trachomatis.

○ **What finding on Gram stain is indicative of *Neisseria gonorrhoeae*?**

Gram-negative diplococci.

○ **What is the treatment for *Neisseria gonorrhoeae*?**

Ceftriaxone 125 to 250 mg IM × 1 dose **or** cefixime 400 mg PO × 1 dose **or** cefpodoxime 400 mg PO × 1 dose.

Plus include either azithromycin 1 g × 1 dose **or** doxycycline 100 mg BID × 7 days since 50% of patients are also infected with *Chlamydia trachomatis*.

PELVIC INFLAMMATORY DISEASE

○ **Which two organisms cause most cases of pelvic inflammatory disease?**

Neisseria gonorrhoeae and *Chlamydia trachomatis*.

○ **What are the risk factors for pelvic inflammatory disease?**

- Age <25 years (cervix not fully matured)
- Early onset of sexual activity
- Frequent sexual intercourse especially during menses
- Nonbarrier contraception
- New, multiple or symptomatic sexual partners
- Douching
- Presence of IUD
- Bacterial vaginosis
- Women with one episode are at increased risk for a second episode

○ **What are the criteria for diagnosis of pelvic inflammatory disease (PID)?**

All of the following must be present:

- Adnexal tenderness
- Cervical and uterine tenderness
- Abdominal tenderness

In addition, one of the following must be present:

- Temperature > 38°C
- Endocervix Gram stain positive for gram-negative intracellular diplococcic
- Leukocytosis > 10,000/mm^3
- Inflammatory mass on ultrasound or pelvic examination
- WBCs and bacteria in the peritoneal fluid

○   **Which patients with PID should be admitted?**

Admit patients who are pregnant, have a temperature >38°C (100.4°F), are nauseated or vomiting (which prohibits oral antibiotics), have pyosalpinx or tubo-ovarian abscess, have peritoneal signs, have an IUD, show no response to oral antibiotics, or for whom diagnosis is uncertain.

○   **A patient with suspected PID presents with marked tenderness in the right upper quadrant, what condition is most likely present?**

Fitz-Hughes Curtis syndrome.

○   **Cervical Motion Tenderness on physical examination in the presence of PID is known as:?**

Chandelier sign.

○   **What percentage of patients with pelvic inflammatory disease become infertile?**

10%.

INFERTILITY

○   **What is the accepted definition of infertility?**

It is defined as a failure of a couple to conceive after 12 months of regular intercourse without the use of contraception in women less than 35 years of age; and after 6 months of regular intercourse without the use of contraception in women 35 years or older.

○   **What percentage of American couples are infertile?**

12% to 18%.

○   **What is the difference between primary infertility and secondary infertility?**

Primary—no conception or history of conception.
Secondary—at least one prior episode of conception (even if it did not result in term pregnancy or birth).

○   **What are the known causes of infertility?**

- Male factor (hypogonadism, post-testicular defects, seminiferous tubule dysfunction)
- Ovulatory dysfunction
- Tubal damage
- Endometriosis
- Coital problems
- Cervical factor

○   **What percentage of infertility is due to the male factor?**

26%.

○   **What percentage of infertility is unexplained?**

25% to 30%.

◯ **What is the optimal timing of intercourse to achieve pregnancy?**

Days 11 to 16 of a women's menstrual cycle.

◯ **Besides thorough history and physical examination, what initial diagnostic evaluation should be implemented in the work-up of infertility?**

- Semen analysis
- Assessment of LH surge in urine prior to ovulation and/or luteal phase progesterone level
- Day 3 serum FSH and estradiol levels
- Hysterosalpingography

◯ **What are the values for a normal semen analysis?**

1 mL in volume (>20,000,000 sperm) with >50% motility.

◯ **How long do sperm stay in the vagina and internal reproductive organs postcoitus?**

At least 72 hours; however, sperm are motile only for 6 hours.

◯ **In the evaluation of infertility, what procedure can be both diagnostic and therapeutic?**

Hysterosalpingogram (typically performed between days 6 and 10 of cycle).

◯ **What is the greatest risk associated with in vitro fertilization (IVF) treatment?**

Multiple gestation.

◯ **What pharmaceutical agent is most often used to encourage follicular development and promote ovulation?**

Clomiphene citrate, 50 to 100 mg for 5 days beginning on day 3, 4, or 5 of cycle.

BREAST

◯ **Breast hyperplasia is a normal physiologic phenomenon in the neonatal period. How many months does this typically last?**

Up to 6 months of age.

◯ **What is the most common cause for gynecomastia in adult males?**

Persistent pubertal gynecomastia (25%). Enlargement of the breast tissue can be common in adolescent boys and typically resolves spontaneously 6 months to 2 years after onset.

◯ **What is the second most common cause of gynecomastia in adult males?**

Both prescription and abused drugs (15%–20%). Prescription drugs with the greatest association include spironolactone, cimetidine, ketoconazole, recombinant HGH, GnRH agonists, and 5-alpha reductase inhibitors. Abused drugs with the greatest association include anabolic steroids, testosterone, alcohol, amphetamines, heroin, marijuana, and methadone.

◯ **What is the most common type of benign breast tumor?**

Fibroadenomas. These are usually solitary, mobile masses with distinct borders. They are more prevalent in women younger than 30 years.

○ **What is the recommended work-up for suspected fibroadenoma?**

Diagnostic mammogram with ultrasound. If indeterminant, fine-needle aspiration of the mass with pathology. In women younger than 25 years, fibroadenomatous mass should be biopsied.

○ **What distinguishes fibrocystic breast changes from carcinoma?**

Pain, size fluctuation, and multiple lesions distinguish fibrocystic changes from carcinoma.

○ **After the establishment of fibrocystic breast disease, what is the recommended treatment?**

Avoiding trauma and by wearing a bra with adequate support.

Combined oral contraceptive agents limit the severity of the cyclical changes in the breast tissue.

Many patients report relief of symptoms after abstinence from coffee, tea, and chocolate.

○ **What is the most common causative organism in mastitis, breast infection, or breast abscess?**

Staphylococcus aureus.

○ **What is the treatment for acute mastitis?**

Warm compresses to breast, analgesics, dicloxacillin, or a cephalosporin.

○ **Can a nursing mother with mastitis continue to nurse?**

Yes, as long as there is no abscess formation. Nursing facilitates the drainage of the infection and the infant will not be harmed because he/she is already colonized.

○ **What is the most common cause of unilateral bloody nipple discharge?**

Benign intraductal papilloma. Growths usually develop just before or during menopause and they are rarely palpable. They are typically mobile and painless.

○ **What pattern of nipple discharge would one expect with benign galactorrhea?**

Bilateral, induced, clear/white/yellow color.

○ **What diagnosis must be considered in a patient presenting with crusty, eczematous erosion of the nipple without nipple discharge?**

Paget disease. This rare cancer occurs in 3% of breast cancer patients. It involves the excretory ducts of the breast.

○ **What is Peau d'orange?**

French for skin of the orange. It describes the dimpling and thickening of the skin of the breast seen with breast cancer.

○   **What are the risk factors for breast cancer?**

- Family history
- Age over 40
- High fat intake
- Nulliparity
- Early menarche
- Late menopause
- Cellular atypia in fibrocystic disease
- Radiation exposure to breast(s)
- Prior ovarian, endometrial, or breast cancer.

○   **What are the two genetic markers known to be linked to breast cancer?**

BRCA-1 and BRCA-2.

○   **What is the most common histologic type of breast cancer?**

Infiltrating ductal carcinoma (70%–80%). Subtypes are colloid, medullary, papillary, and tubular.

○   **Which two types of breast cancer are typically estrogen-receptor positive?**

All invasive lobular carcinomas and two-thirds of ductal carcinomas are estrogen-receptor positive.

○   **Are the majority of breast cancers in the ducts or in the lobes?**

Invasive ductal tumors account for 90% of all breast cancers. Only 10% are lobular.

○   **What is the gold standard screening tool for breast carcinoma?**

Mammography.

○   **What does a high cathepsin D level indicate in a woman with breast cancer?**

A high risk of metastasis.

○   **A hard mass in the upper outer quadrant of the right breast of a 45-year-old woman is detected. What are the next steps?**

Mammogram followed by a fine-needle or stereotactic core-needle biopsy. A negative-needle aspiration alone cannot rule out malignancy. False-negative rates for fine-needle biopsy are 3% to 30%.

○   **What is the recommended pharmacologic treatment for estrogen-receptor–positive breast cancer?**

Tamoxifen.

○   **What is the surgical treatment of choice for breast cancer?**

For small primary tumors, a partial mastectomy (i.e., local lumpectomy with axillary node dissection) and postoperative irradiation.

Modified radical mastectomy: The removal of the breast tissue, pectoralis minor, and axilla. (A radical mastectomy includes the pectoralis major and postoperative irradiation.)

○ **What is the most accurate prognostic indicator of breast cancer mortality?**

Axillary node involvement, which is related to the size of the tumor, not the location; 40% to 50% of patients have axillary node involvement when diagnosed.

○ **When does breast milk production typically begin?**

Colostrum secretion usually persists for 3 to 4 days after delivery. Day 5 the fluid begins to change in composition. Mature milk is usually present by 1 to 2 weeks postpartum.

○ **How does colostrum differ from breast milk?**

Colostrum is more cellular and has more minerals, but is lower in calories. True milk has more fat and carbohydrate (especially lactose), but less protein.

○ **How many extra calories above baseline does a woman need when breast-feeding?**

About 500 per day.

○ **How much daily dietary of calcium is recommended for lactating women?**

1200 to 1500 mg per day.

○ **Which vitamin is not found in human breast milk?**

Vitamin K. It is administered to newborns at birth. Formula is also deficient in vitamin K.

MENOPAUSE

○ **What are some risks factors for premature menopause?**

Smoking, radiation, chemotherapy, and anything else that limits the ovarian blood supply.

○ **What is the median age for menopause?**

51 years.

○ **What is the most common cause of postmenopausal bleeding?**

Atrophic endometrium and/or atrophic vaginitis.

○ **What are the common changes associated with estrogen depletion?**

Menstrual cycle changes, cardiovascular disease, osteoporosis, genitourinary atrophy, vasomotor, and psychological symptoms.

○ **What are the expected changes in gonadotropin levels after menopause?**

FSH increases 10- to 20-fold and LH increases 3-fold, reaching a maximum 1 to 3 years after menopause.

○ **Which hormones decline as a result of menopause?**

Estrogen and androstenedione (DHEA). Progesterone to a lesser degree.

○ **Which hormone is secreted more by the postmenopausal ovary versus the premenopausal ovary?**

Testosterone. Prior to menopause, the ovary contributes 25% of circulating testosterone, and in menopause the ovary contributes 40% of circulating testosterone.

○ **What is the cause of mild hirsutism in menopausal women?**

Increased free androgen to estrogen ratio as a result of decreased SHBG and estrogen.

○ **Why does vaginitis and vaginal atrophy increase during the postmenopausal years?**

Because of estrogen deficiency, the vaginal pH increases from 3.5–4.5 to 6–8, predisposing it to colonization of bacterial pathogens.

○ **After menopause, what is the percentage of bone loss per year?**

2.5% for the first 4 years, and then 1% to 1.5% annually.

○ **What risk factors are associated with bone loss and osteoporosis?**

- Advanced age (postmenopausal)
- Previous facture
- Family history
- Low body weight (<58 kg or 127 lbs)
- Sedentary lifestyle
- Smoking
- Excessive alcohol intake
- Coexisting endocrine disease
- Long-term steroid use

○ **According to the United States Preventive Services Task Force (USPSTF), what are the recommendations for bone mineral density screening?**

All postmenopausal women 65 years and older regardless of risk factors.
All men 70 years and older.
Men and women younger than 65 years if known risk factors.

○ **What two skeletal sites are recommended for screening bone mineral density with dual-energy x-ray absorptiomentry (DEXA)?**

Hip and spine.

○ **How does estrogen replacement therapy help maintain bone mass?**

Estrogen has a direct effect on osteoblasts, improves intestinal absorption of calcium, and decreases renal excretion of calcium.

○ **What is the mainstay pharmacologic treatment for postmenopausal osteoporosis?**

Bisphosphonates.

○   **What are the contraindications to estrogen replacement therapy?**

- Estrogen-sensitive cancers (especially breast, endometrial)
- Chronically impaired live function
- Undiagnosed genital bleeding
- Acute vascular thrombosis
- Neuro-ophthalmologic vascular disease
- Coronary heart disease
- Known or suspected pregnancy

○   **You have identified a 56-year-old postmenopausal female with decreased bone mass and symptoms of menopause. She has no contraindications to estrogen replacement therapy. She has an intact uterus. What is the most appropriate initial treatment?**

Conjugated estrogen with medroxyprogesterone acetate (MPA). Endometrial hyperplasia and cancer can occur after as little as 6 months of unopposed estrogen therapy; as a result, a progestin should be added in women who have an intact uterus.

○   **What effect does estrogen replacement therapy have on colorectal cancer?**

It significantly decreases the risk of colon cancer (50%).

○   **What effect does estrogen have on Alzheimer disease?**

Alzheimer disease is less frequent among HRT users, and those with decreases in cognitive function show improvement on HRT.

CONTRACEPTIVE METHODS

○   **What are the absolute contraindications to the use of hormonal-based contraceptive agents? Explain using the mnemonic CONTRACEPTIVES:**

C—Coronary or valvular heart disease

O—Obesity (or other risk factors for arterial cardiovascular disease)

N—Neoplasm of liver or breast

T—Thromboembolism/thrombogenic mutations

R—Regular migraines with aura at any age

A—Age ≥35 years and smoking ≥15 cigarettes per day

C—Cirrhosis or increasing liver enzymes

E—Estrogen-receptor–positive tumors

P—Pregnancy

T—TIA/Stroke

I—Ischemic heart disease

V—Vaginal bleeding (abnormal and undiagnosed)

E—Elevated blood pressure (systolic ≥ 160 mm Hg or diastolic ≥ 100 mm Hg)

S—Systemic lupus erythematosus (positive or known antiphospholipid antibodies)

○   **How much is menstrual blood flow decreased by OCP use?**

On average 60%.

○ **What is the most common side effect of OCP use?**

Breakthrough bleeding. Its occurrence does not necessarily indicate decrease in efficacy but reflects tissue breakdown as the endometrium adjusts to the new thinner, more fragile, atrophic state.

○ **What are the estrogen-mediated side effects of combined oral contraceptives?**

Headache, nausea, breast enlargement or tenderness, fluid retention, telangiectasia.

○ **What are the progesterone-mediated side effects of combined oral contraceptives?**

Decreased mood, fatigue, acne, oily skin, and increased appetite.

○ **What are the noncontraceptive benefits of OCP use?**

Less benign breast disease, iron-deficiency anemia, and PID as well as fewer ovarian cysts. In addition, protection again ectopic pregnancy, reduced dysmenorrhea and menorrhagia; and improvements in androgen-mediated symptoms (i.e., hirsutism, acne).

○ **In the setting of what autoimmune disease, does OCP use seem to have a protective side effect?**

Rheumatoid arthritis.

○ **In a 36-year-old female who smokes 1 to 1.5 packs of cigarettes per day, what is the most concerning side effect of combined oral contraceptive use?**

Deep vein thrombosis.

○ **What is the known risk ratio for venous thromboembolic disease in women taking OCPs?**

1% to 5%. Much higher in women who are obese, smokers, or over 35 years of age.

○ **What effect does oral contraceptive use have on the risk of developing cervical cancer?**

Oral contraceptive users as a group are at higher risk for cervical neoplasia. This increased risk may be secondary to sexual habits rather than the pill itself.

○ **What effect does oral contraceptive use have on the risk of endometrial cancer?**

OCP use for at least 2 years can reduce risk of endometrial cancer by up to 40%. Use for 4 years or more can reduce risk by >60%.

○ **What effect does oral contraceptive use have on the risk of ovarian cancer?**

OCP use for at least 4 years can reduce risk for ovarian cancer by 30%. Use for 12 or more years reduces risk by >80%.

○ **How effective is lactational amenorrhea as a form of birth control?**

Can be effective in delaying conception for 6 months after birth if the woman breast-feeds exclusively and amenorrhea is maintained.

○ **How does Depot medroxyprogesterone acetate (DMPA or brand name DepoProvera) work?**

High levels of progestin suppressing FSH and LH levels and eliminating the LH surge. This inhibits ovulation.

○ **What vehicle and how often is DMPA administered?**

Intramuscular injection dosed every 90 days.

○ **What is the recommended "grace period" if a woman returns late for repeat DMPA injection?**

14 days.

○ **One concern of long-term DMPA use is reduction in bone mineral density, what is the recommendation for bone mineral density (BMD) testing in women taking DMPA?**

Use of DMPA is not an indication for BMD testing either before, during, or in follow-up of its administration. Providers, however, should advise DMPA users to have adequate intake of calcium/vitamin D, engage in regular exercise, and avoid cigarette smoking and excessive alcohol consumption, to maintain optimal bone health.

○ **What is the delay in return to fertility after DepoProvera use?**

18 months after the last injection.

○ **How long after the removal of Norplant capsules must patients wait to become pregnant?**

Ovulation usually resumes within 3 months.

○ **What are the two types of IUD contraceptive devices available on the market, and how long is their duration of use?**

Progesterone (usable for 1 year)

Copper T (usable for 10 years)

○ **What is the risk of ectopic pregnancy in women with an IUD in place?**

5%. Hormone-based IUD users have a 6- to 10-fold increase in ectopic rates compared with copper IUD users.

○ **What are the absolute contraindications to placement of an IUD?**

- Current pregnancy
- Undiagnosed vaginal bleeding
- Acute infection
- Past salpingitis
- Suspected gynecologic malignancy

○ **How long after exposure can emergency oral contraceptives be given?**

Up to 72 hours. It is most effective if initiated in 12 to 24 hours. Emergency contraception provides a 75% reduction in the risk of pregnancy. Patients should have a negative pregnancy test prior to treatment.

○ **What is the total dose of estrogen that should be used in <u>combined</u> emergency oral contraceptive pills?**

200/g of ethinyl estradiol—2 doses of 100/g taken 12 hours apart.

○ **Besides emergency contraceptive pills, what other contraceptive method can be used to prevent pregnancy after unprotected intercourse?**

IUD.

○ **How long after vaginal delivery should a postpartum tubal ligation be performed?**

It is common practice to wait 8 to 12 hours postpartum before inducing anesthesia for tubal ligation. This time interval is useful to allow the patient to reach cardiovascular stability and increase the likelihood of gastric emptying.

○ **What is the most common complication of postpartum tubal ligation regardless of type of procedure?**

Bleeding. Second most common is infection.

UNCOMPLICATED PREGNANCY

○ **What percentage of pregnant women get "morning sickness"?**

50% to 70%. It generally occurs in the first trimester (up to week 14–16).

○ **How should morning sickness be treated?**

Frequent small meals, carbohydrates, IV hydration, and antiemetics as last resort.

○ **What is hyperemesis gravidarum?**

Excessive vomiting during pregnancy that results in starvation (ketonuria), dehydration, and acidosis.

○ **What is pica?**

This is a craving for eating nonfoods, such as laundry starch and clay, during pregnancy. If severe, it can result in nutritional deficiencies and anemia. It is also possible that the agent ingested may be toxic to the developing fetus.

○ **What foods put a pregnant woman at risk for mercury poisoning?**

All fish and shellfish contain some levels of mercury. However, the following contain the highest levels: Predatory fish (shark, swordfish, mackerel, tilefish) and to a lesser extent albacore tuna, pike, bass.

○ **What is the recommended fish consumption for a pregnant woman to avoid mercury poisoning?**

Limit fish consumption to 350 g per week.

○ **Does the presence of a thick endometrial stripe on ultrasound indicate an intrauterine pregnancy?**

The endometrium can be thickened because of the hormonal stimulation associated with either an ectopic or intrauterine pregnancy, so this is not a consistent sign of a normal pregnancy.

○ **When can an intrauterine gestational sac be identified by an abdominal ultrasound?**

In the fifth week. A fetal pole can be identified in the sixth week and an embryonic mass with cardiac motion in the seventh week.

○ **For a gestational sac to be visible on ultrasound, what must the β-hCG level be?**

At least 6500 mIU/mL for a transabdominal ultrasound, and 2000 mIU/mL for a transvaginal ultrasound.

○ **What secretes β-hCG? Why?**

Placental trophoblasts secrete β-hCG to maintain the corpus luteum, which in turn maintains the uterine lining. The corpus luteum is maintained through the sixth to eighth week of pregnancy, by which time the placenta begins to produce its own progesterone to maintain the endometrium.

○ **How soon after implantation can β-hCG be detected?**

2 to 3 days.

○ **At what rate do β-hCG levels rise?**

They double every 48 hours.

○ **At what gestational age does β-hCG peak?**

8 to 10 weeks.

○ **Name four physiologic actions of hCG:**

1. Maintenance of corpus luteum and continued progesterone production
2. Stimulation of fetal testicular testosterone secretion promoting male sexual differentiation
3. Stimulation of the maternal thyroid by binding to TSH receptors
4. Promotes relaxin secretion by the corpus luteum

○ **What does a progesterone level of 25 ng/mL or higher indicates about a pregnancy?**

A viable, uterine pregnancy. Serum progesterone is produced by the corpus luteum in the pregnant patient and remains constant for the first 8 to 10 weeks of pregnancy.

○ **Which routine screenings should be performed at the first prenatal visit?**

CBC, blood type and Rh, Coombs' test, Rubella titer, Hepatitis B and C, urine DNA probe for chlamydia and gonorrhea, serologic testing for syphilis, pap smear, and urinalysis.

All offer all women HIV testing and couple screening for cystic fibrosis, sickle cell, other conditions per maternal/paternal history.

○ **When is an amniocentesis usually performed?**

15 to 18 weeks, gestation.

○ **When should the Glucose challenge test for screening of gestational diabetes be performed?**

24 to 28 weeks. In women at high risk can screen during first prenatal visit and repeat at 24 to 28 weeks.

○ **When should a vaginal–rectal culture for group B streptococci be conducted during pregnancy?**

35 weeks.

○ **What are the risk factors for elevated maternal serum alpha-fetoprotein? Explain using the mnemonic MSAFP:**

M—Multiple gestation

S—Spina bifida (or other neural tube defect)

A—Abdominal wall defects (omphalocele, gastroschisis)

F—Fetal death

P—Placental anomalies

○ **What condition is indicated by a low alpha-fetoprotein?**

Down syndrome.

○ **Which week of gestation can the fetal heart be auscultated or detected by the following: Ultrasound, Doppler, Stethoscope?**

Ultrasound—6 weeks

Doppler—10 to 12 weeks

Stethoscope—18 to 20 weeks

○ **What is the normal fetal heart rate by Doppler?**

120 to 160 bpm.

○ **By which week of gestation can a mother feel fetal movement? What is the term used to describe this?**

18 to 20 weeks in primigravida and as early as 14 to 18 weeks in a multigravida. Termed "quickening."

○ **By which week of gestation is the fundus at the umbilicus?**

20 weeks.

○ **What immunizations are contraindicated during pregnancy?**

In general, live viruses are contraindicated. Including MMR, Oral Polio, Varicella.

○ **What is the known effect of folic acid deficiency in pregnancy?**

Folate deficiency is associated with neural tube defects (i.e., spinal bifida, anencephaly).

○ **In general, at what time during pregnancy is the fetus most susceptible to teratogens?**

During embryonic period which lasts from 2 to 8 weeks postconception. This is the time of organogenesis.

○ **Define the five drug-labeling categories for use during pregnancy?**

Category A—Safe for use in pregnancy.

Category B—Animal studies have demonstrated the drug's safety and human studies do not reveal any adverse fetal effects.

Category C—The drug is a known animal teratogen, but no data are available about human use; or there is no date on humans or animals.

Category D—There is positive evidence of human fetal toxicity, but the benefits in selected situations make use of the drug acceptable despite the risks.

Category X—The drug is a definite human and animal teratogen and should NOT be used in pregnancy.

○ **What is a safe anticoagulant to use in pregnancy?**

Heparin. Warfarin is contraindicated.

○ **What antibiotics are safe to use in pregnancy?**

Nitrofurantoin
Amoxicillin
Amoxicillin—Clavulanate
Third-generation cephalosporins (i.e., Cephalexin, Ceftriaxone, Cefpodoxime)
Macrolides (i.e., Erythromycin, Azithromycin)
Trimethoprim-sulfamethaxazole (avoid in first trimester or near term)

○ **What is the average weight gain in pregnancy?**

11 kg (25 lbs). 30% attributed to placenta and fetus. 30% attributed to blood, amniotic fluid, and extravascular fluid. 30% to maternal fat.

○ **What is the normal Pco$_2$ in pregnancy?**

30 to 34 mm Hg from chronic mild hyperventilation, presumably as a result of progesterone and in later stages abdominal pressure.

○ **What is the predominant change in the lung volumes in pregnancy?**

Decrease in functional residual capacity by as much as 15% to 25%. Tidal volume increases by 40%.

○ **What are the normal changes heard during heart auscultation during pregnancy?**

Exaggerated split S1, systolic ejection murmur heart at the left sternal border (90%), soft/transient diastolic murmurs (20%). All harsh murmurs should be taken seriously and worked up before attributing to pregnancy.

○ **What are the expected changes in volume of the cardiovascular system of a pregnancy patient?**

Cardiac output increased by 30% (first trimester); increased by 50% (second trimester).
Stroke volume increases by 25% while **hematocrit** drops because of hemodilution.
Plasma volume increases by 50%.
Heart rate increased by 12 to 18 bpm.
Systolic and diastolic blood pressure decrease by 10 to 15 mm Hg during the second trimester, but gradually returns to baseline in the third trimester.

○ **What effect does pregnancy have on BUN and creatinine?**

Both are decreased. This is the result of increased renal blood flow and increased glomerular filtration rate.

○ **What white blood cell count is expected during pregnancy?**

15,000 to 20,000 are considered normal during pregnancy

○ **What are the normal physical changes in the cervix during pregnancy?**

Softening and cyanosis. (Chadwick sign—bluish discoloration of the vagina and cervix during pregnancy.)

○ **What is the main ophthalmologic change that occurs during pregnancy?**

Corneal thickening.

○ **What are the main changes to the gastrointestinal system of a pregnant patient?**

Decreased gastric emptying and GI motility leading to GERD and constipation.

○ **Can iodinated radiodiagnostic agents be used in pregnant patients?**

No. They should be avoided because concentration in the fetal thyroid can cause permanent loss of thyroid function.

○ **What are the five parameters included in a biophysical profile (BPP) to access late pregnancy fetal well-being?**

1. Nonstress test (NST)
2. Amniotic fluid level
3. Gross fetal movements
4. Fetal tone
5. Fetal breathing

○ **What is oxytocin and its action?**

It is a powerful uterotonic agent that stimulates uterine contractions during labor and elicits milk ejection by myoepithelial cells of the mammary ducts.

○ **When does labor begin?**

Labor begins with the onset of regular, rhythmic contractions leading to serial dilatation and effacement of the cervix. Thus, contractions alone do not qualify for onset of labor.

○ **What is the term used for sporadic uterine contractions that are most felt in the third trimester but are not accompanied by changes in the cervix?**

Braxton–Hicks contractions.

○ **What are the four stages of labor and delivery?**

Stage I: Onset of labor to complete dilation of the cervix
Stage II: Cervical dilation to birth
Stage III: Birth to delivery of placenta
Stage IV: Placenta delivery to stability of the mother (~6 hours)

○ **What is considered the LATENT phase of labor and how long does it typically last in primiparous and multiparous women?**

Latent phase begins at the point a woman perceives regular uterine contractions and ends with the onset of the active phase (regular uterine contractions and cervical dilation of 3–4 cm).
Primiparous—average 6.4 hours (prolonged at ≥20 hours)
Multiparous—average 4.8 hours (prolonged at ≥14 hours)

○ **What is the typical rate of cervical dilation during active phase of labor in primiparous and multiparous women?**

Primiparous—1 cm/hr
Multiparous—1.5 cm/hr

○ **What is the most common cause for prolongation of the active phase of labor?**

Cephalopelvic disproportion caused by contraction of a narrowed midpelvis.

○ **What is "effacement" of the cervix?**

The foreshortening and thinning of the cervix as it is drawn upward (intra-abdominally).

○ **What agents may be used to ripen the cervix?**

Both chemical and physical agents. Oxytocics, prostaglandins (especially PGE2), progesterone antagonists (RU-486), and dehydroepiandrosterone are such pharmacologic agents. Laminaria and foley catheter balloons are examples of physical dilators.

○ **Does epidural analgesia affect the course of labor?**

Studies show no effect in the first stage. The second stage appears to be prolonged an average of 20 to 25 minutes. No evidence that this prolongation is harmful to fetus.

○ **What is the largest risk for breech presentation?**

Prematurity. At 28 weeks a majority of fetuses are breech but correct by term. 95% of fetuses at term are in vertex presentation.

○ **What are the three types of breech presentation?**

Frank breech—Thighs flexed, legs extended (most common)
Complete breech—At least one leg flexed
Incomplete (footling) breech—At least one foot below the buttocks with both thighs extended

○ **What are the six movements of delivery?**

1. Descent
2. Flexion
3. Internal rotation
4. Extension
5. External rotation
6. Expulsion

○ **What is the modified Ritgen maneuver?**

It describes the elevation of the fetal chin achieved by placement of the delivering hand between the maternal coccyx and perineal body, whereas the other hand guides the crowning vertex. This technique assists in extension of the fetal head and allows the clinician to control delivery.

○ **What is Leopold's maneuver?**

Palpation of the abdomen in the evaluation of a fetus in transverse lie.

○ **What are the degrees of perineal tears associated with vaginal delivery?**

First degree: Perineal skin or vaginal mucosa

Second degree: Submucosa of vagina or perineum

Third degree: Extends into anal sphincter

Fourth degree: Extends into rectal mucosa

○ **Which type of episiotomy is associated with the lowest amount of blood loss, improved healing time and cosmetic result, and less subsequent dyspareunia?**

Midline (median) episiotomy.

○ **Which type of episiotomy is associated with lesser propensity to extend into the external anal sphincter or rectum?**

Mediolateral episiotomy.

○ **What is the normal fetal heart rate?**

120 to 160 bpm.

○ **If fetal bradycardia is detected during labor and delivery, what is the recommended course of action?**

Place mother in left lateral decubitus position, administer oxygen, give IV fluid bolus.

○ **What is the definition of an acceleration, and is it normal?**

An acceleration must be at least 15 bpm above baseline and last at least 15 seconds. Rapid heart rate can indicate fetal distress; 2 accelerations every 20 minutes are normal.

○ **What causes variable decelerations?**

Transient umbilical cord compression. These often change with maternal position.

○ **How can fetal lung maturity be assessed?**

The Lecithin to Sphingomyelin ratio. At more than 2:1 (L:S) the fetal lungs are mature.

○ **What are the benefits of antepartum corticosteroids in premature babies?**

- Increased lung compliance
- Increased surfactant production
- Less respiratory distress syndrome
- Less intraventricular hemorrhage
- Less necrotizing enterocolitis
- Less neonatal mortality

○ **A baby is born with pink body, blue extremities, and heart rate of 70 bpm. The neonate is mildly irritable (grimaces) and has weak respirations and no muscle tone. What is this patient's Apgar?**

1+1+1+1+0 = 4

APGAR POINTS	0	1	2
MUSCLE TONE	Flaccid	Weak	Strong
HEART RATE	None	<100	>100
IRRITABILITY	None	Mild grimace	Strongly irritable
COLOR	Blue	Extremities Blue	All pink
RESPIRATORY EFFORT	None	Weak	Cry

COMPLICATED PREGNANCY

○ **What is the most common cause of ectopic pregnancy?**

Occlusion of fallopian tube secondary to adhesions.

○ **What are the risk factors for ectopic pregnancy using the mnemonic ECTOPIC:**

E—Endometriosis
C—Congenital anomaly of tubes
T—Tubal or abdominal surgery
O—Other ectopic pregnancy
P—Pelvic inflammatory disease
I—IUD
C—Clinician-assisted reproduction

○ **When and how does an ectopic pregnancy most commonly present?**

6 to 8 weeks. Patients usually present with amenorrhea and sharp, generally unilateral abdominal or pelvic pain. Adnexal mass is not common (found in <50%).

○ **What is the most common site of implantation in an ectopic pregnancy?**

The ampulla of the fallopian tube (95%). Less common sites are abdomen, uterine cornua, cervix, and ovary.

○ **How do β-hCG levels differ in women with ectopic pregnancy versus intrauterine pregnancy?**

Lower in ectopic pregnancy.

○ **What is the most common sign of ectopic pregnancy on transvaginal ultrasound?**

Absence of interuterine pregnancy or gestational sac with β-hCG level >2000 mIU/mL. Adnexal mass or gestational sac in adnexa is less reliable finding. Follow-up ultrasound always recommended in high-risk patients to ensure intrauterine pregnancy.

○ **Who is eligible for methotrexate treatment of an ectopic pregnancy?**

Hemodynamically stable patients with unruptured gestations <3.5 cm in diameter on ultrasound and β-hCG <5000 mU.

○ **What criteria are used for assuring the success of methotrexate?**

Following single-dose therapy, the β-hCG levels should fall by 15% between days 4 and 7 and continue to fall weekly until undetectable.

○ **What are the indications for laparotomy for the treatment of ectopic pregnancy?**

- Unstable patient
- Large hemoperitoneum
- Cornual pregnancy
- Large ectopic (>6 cm)
- Fetal heart sounds

○ **What is the definition of spontaneous abortion?**

Loss of fetus before the 20th week of gestation.

○ **Which classification of abortion presents with vaginal bleeding but the cervical os is closed?**

Threatened abortion. It is defined as uterine cramping or bleeding in the first 20 weeks of gestation without the passage of products of conception or cervical dilatation.

○ **What is the definition of missed abortion?**

No uterine growth, no cervical dilation, no passage of fetal tissue, and minimal cramping or bleeding. Diagnosis is made by the absence of fetal heart tones and an empty gestational sac on ultrasound.

○ **What is the recommended clinical intervention in the setting of incomplete abortion?**

Dilation and curettage is necessary to remove the remainder of tissue.

○ **What percentage of pregnancies result in spontaneous abortion? What is the number one etiology for spontaneous abortion?**

15% to 20%. Genetic defects account for 50% of spontaneous abortions.

○ **What are the independent risk factors for spontaneous abortion?**

- Maternal or paternal age
- Smoking
- Infection
- Maternal systemic disease
- Immunologic parameters
- Drug use

○ **Besides hCG and ultrasound, what other laboratory tests are essential prior to treatment for elective or spontaneous abortion?**

Blood type and Rh status. Immunoglobulin should be administered in Rh-negative women in the event of elective or spontaneous abortion.

○ **At what gestation age is suction or vacuum curettage used to terminate a pregnancy?**

7 to 13 weeks.

○ **What is the most common cause of postabortal pain, bleeding, and low-grade fever?**

Retained gestational tissue or clot.

○ **What is the most likely diagnosis in a patient whose uterus is larger than expected from the history of gestation, has vaginal bleeding, and passes grape-like tissue from the vagina?**

Hydatidiform mole.

○ **Of the types of hydatidiform moles, which has a nonviable fetus present?**

Incomplete.

○ **How does age influence the incidence of hydatidiform mole?**

Women aged 50 years or older have 300- to 400-fold increase in risk. Women younger than 15 years have 6-fold increased risk.

○ **What is the classic ultrasound finding in the presence of complete hydatidiform mole?**

"Grape-like vesicles" or "snowstorm" pattern.

○ **What is the most common malignant gestational trophoblastic disease?**

Gestational choriocarcinoma.

○ **What is the single most useful laboratory test in the evaluation of gestational trophoblastic disease?**

β-hCG. Both molar pregnancies and gestational choriocarcinomas produce β-hCG because of their trophoblastic origin. Complete molar pregnancies often have >100,000 mU/mL. β-hCG can also be used as a tumor marker to correlate the volume of disease and response to therapy.

○ **After nonsurgical treatment for gestational trophoblastic disease and establishment of remission, what is the recommended duration of contraception use?**

9 to 12 months.

○ **With what endocrine abnormalities are moles and other gestational trophoblastic neoplasms associated?**

Hyperthyroidism.

○ **What is the most common presentation of twins?**

Vertex–vertex.

○ **What is the average gestational age at delivery of twins, triplets, and quadruplets?**

Twins: 36 to 37 weeks

Triplets: 33 to 34 weeks

Quadruplets: 30 to 31 weeks

○ **In a woman who is Rh negative and a fetus that is Rh positive, what is the risk?**

Development of Rh isoimmunization leading to fetal anemia, hydrops, and/or fetal death.

○ **Which type of blood test is used to determine the occurrence and degree of fetomaternal hemorrhage?**

Apt or Kleinhauer–Betke test.

○ **When should Rho-Gam be administered in Rh-negative mothers for prophylactic protection?**

28 to 29 weeks, and again within 72 hours of delivery of an Rh-positive baby.

○ **What is the standard dose of Rho-Gam?**

300 mg.

○ **If a woman has a positive screening glucose challenge test, what is the next step?**

3-hour glucose tolerance test.

○ **What criteria are necessary for the definitive diagnosis of gestational diabetes?**

If two or more of the 1-hour, 2-hour, or 3-hour glucose values are abnormal on a 3-hour tolerance test, the patient is diagnosed with GDM. Glycosylated hemoglobin (HgbA1c) is not recommended for screening or confirming diagnosis.

○ **What is the treatment for gestational diabetes?**

Diet, exercise, insulin. Do not give patients oral hypoglycemic because they cross the blood–brain barrier.

○ **In pregnant females with underlying asthma, what is the main focus of management?**

Medications should be used sparingly. However, uncontrolled asthma causes more fetal harm than medications therefore use if necessary.

○ **What viral or protozoal infections require extensive work-up during pregnancy? Define ToRCH.**

To—Toxoplasma gondii

R—Rubella

C—Cytomegalovirus

H—Herpes genitalis

○ **A pregnant female at 32 weeks gestation, presents with uterine contractions over the past 5 hours. Upon examination you note cervical dilatation of 2 cm an effacement of >80%, what is the diagnosis?**

Preterm labor.

○ **What is the definition of preterm delivery?**

Delivery of viable infant before 37 weeks gestation.

○ **What are the known risk factors for preterm labor and delivery?**

- Smoking
- Cocaine use
- Uterine malformations
- Cervical incompetence
- Infection (vaginal or UTI)
- Low prepregnancy weight

○ **What agents can be used in an attempt to stop contractions in preterm labor?**

Magnesium sulfate, calcium channel blockers, β-mimetic adrenergic agents (ritodrine or terbutaline).

○ **What diagnostic evaluation is recommended in suspected premature rupture of membranes (PROM)?**

Speculum examination to look for pooling of amniotic fluid in the posterior fornix. And Nitrazine paper test. In the presence of amniotic fluid, the paper will turn blue and exhibit a ferning pattern under the microscope.

○ **What is the recommended management of women with term PROM?**

Prompt induction of labor.

○ **What is the recommended management of women with preterm premature rupture of membranes (PPROM)?**

If no sign of maternal or fetal distress/infection, expectant management with bed rest and prophylactic antibiotics is preferred.

PPROM is defined at rupture between 20 and 36 weeks.

○ **What is the definition of pregnancy-induced hypertension (PIH)?**

An increase in systolic pressure >30 mm Hg and/or an increase in diastolic pressure >15 mm Hg above baseline, measured on two separate occasions at least 6 hours apart presenting after 20 weeks gestation with no other etiologies associated with elevation in blood pressure.

○ **What is the pharmacologic treatment of choice for chronic hypertension or pregnancy-induced hypertension?**

Methyldopa is first line. Labetalol is an alternative.

○ **What are the nonpharmacologic options for treatment of chronic hypertension or pregnancy-induced hypertension?**

- Sodium restriction to 2 to 3 g per day
- Abstaining from alcohol and tobacco
- Weight restriction
- More frequent prenatal visits and ultrasound surveillance

○ **What is the classic triad of preeclampsia?**

Hypertension (systolic >160 mm Hg or diastolic >110 mm Hg)

Edema

Proteinuria

○ **Besides the classic triad, what other clinical features may be present in preeclampsia?**

Sudden weight gain, headaches, visual disturbances, nausea, vomiting, right upper quadrant pain, hyperreflexia, and decreased urine output.

○ **What symptom separates preeclampsia from eclampsia?**

Seizures.

○ **What is HELLP syndrome?**

Severe preeclampsia with the addition of **H**emolysis, **E**levated **L**iver enzymes, and **L**ow **P**latelets.

○ **What is the most common risk factor for preeclampsia?**

Nulliparity

Other factors include extremes of age (<20 or >35), multiple gestation, DM, and chronic HTN

○ **What is the recommended work-up in preeclampsia?**

24-hour urine protein, CBC, fibrinogen, PT, PTT, LFTs, BUN/creatinine, electrolytes, and uric acid levels.

○ **Should blood pressure be lowered acutely in a preeclampsia patient, and how?**

No. Dangerous hypertension should be gradually lowered with hydralazine, 10 mg IV followed by a drip.

○ **What is the definitive treatment of eclampsia?**

Delivery.

○ **How long should the treatment continue after delivery for a woman with preeclampsia?**

24 hours. The cure for preeclampsia is delivery; however, antihypertensives and antiseizure medications (if started) should be continued until there is no longer a risk to the mother.

○ **If a patient had an eclamptic seizure prior to delivery, how long is she at risk for additional seizures?**

10 days postpartum.

○ **What is the most common cause for painful third-trimester bleeding?**

Abruptio placentae, the premature separation of a normally implanted placenta after the 20th week of gestation but before birth.

○ **What are the risk factors of abruption placentae? Using the mnemonic ABRUPTIONS:**

A—Advanced maternal age
B—Blood pressure (HTN)
R—Rupture of membranes (PROM)
U—Uterine abnormalities
P—Previous abruption placentae
T—Trauma
I—Illicit drug use (cocaine)
O—Overuse of alcohol (>14 drinks/week)
N—Number of births (high parity)
S—Smoking

○ **What are the clinical features of abruption placentae?**

Painful vaginal bleeding (85%)
Others include uterine/abdominal/back pain (if bleeding concealed may be the only symptom)

○ **What is the greatest maternal risk in the setting of abruption placentae?**

Disseminated intravascular coagulation (DIC). The abruption leads to liberation of tissue thromboplastin or consumption of fibrinogen, thereby activating the extrinsic clotting mechanism leading to DIC.

○ **What is the preferred management of abruptio placentae?**

Cesarean section delivery
In addition, blood type, cross match, and coagulation studies in an unstable patient.

○ **What is the diagnosis when the placenta is partially or completely covering the cervical os?**

Placenta previa.

○ **What is the hallmark clinical feature of placenta previa?**

Vaginal bleeding (painless).

○ **What are the risk factors for the development of placenta previa?**

Advanced maternal age (>35)
Smoking
Multiparity
Any process that created scarring of the lower uterine segment (i.e., C-section)

○ **What intervention is contraindicated in the setting of suspected placenta previa?**

Digital vaginal examination.

○ **What percentage of placentas "migrate" up the uterine wall during the growth of pregnancy?**

50%.

○   **What is the preferred method of delivery in cases of placenta previa?**

Cesarean section.

○   **What are the etiologies of uterine rupture (both gynecologic and obstetric)?**

- Oxytocin stimulation
- Cephalopelvic disproportion
- Grand multiparity
- Manual removal of the placenta
- Abdominal trauma
- Prior hysterotomy
- Myotomy
- Previous cesarean section (#1 risk factor)
- Curettage

○   **What are the signs and symptoms of uterine rupture?**

- Fetal distress (#1 sign)
- Unrelenting pain
- Hypotension
- Tachycardia
- Vaginal bleeding

○   **What two findings on physical examination are indicative of uterine rupture?**

1. Loss of uterine contour
2. Palpable fetal part

○   **What are the predisposing factors for amniotic fluid embolism?**

- Advanced maternal age (>35)
- Multiparity
- Cesarean section
- Amniotomy
- Insertion of intrauterine fetal monitoring devices

○   **How does amniotic fluid enter maternal circulation?**

Endocervical veins

Uterine tears or injury

○   **What is the major consequence of amniotic fluid embolism?**

Cardiorespiratory collapse and DIC

80% mortality

○   **What are the maternal risk factors for shoulder dystocia?**

Diabetes, maternal obesity, post-term delivery, excessive maternal weight gain.

Intrapartum risk factors include prolonged second stage of labor, oxytocin use (induction of labor), and midforceps deliveries.

○   **What is the known fetal risk factor for shoulder dystocia?**

Fetal weight

○   **What is the best marker of true dystocia in terms of labor progression?**

Inability to deliver vaginally after full cervical dilation and vertex presentation.

○   **What are the most frequent indications for cesarean section?**

- Repeat cesarean section
- Dystocia
- Failure to progress
- Breech presentation
- Fetal distress

○   **What does VBAC stand for?**

Vaginal birth after cesarean delivery.

○   **What are the risks associated with cesarean section?**

- Higher likelihood of thromboembolic events
- Increased bleeding
- Development of infection

○   **Blood loss during and immediately following delivery can be normal. What defines the diagnosis of postpartum hemorrhage?**

Blood loss requiring transfusion or a 10% drop in hematocrit between admission and postpartum period.

○   **What are the causes of immediate postpartum hemorrhage?**

- Uterine atony (most common)
- Vaginal/cervical lacerations
- Retained placenta or placental fragments

○   **What is the recommended initial treatment for uterine atony and postpartum hemorrhage?**

Uterine massage and compression.

○   **What is the recommended first-line pharmacologic intervention in the setting of postpartum hemorrhage?**

IV oxytocin
Others include IV ergonovine, methylergonovine, or prostaglandins

○   **A patient presents 3 days postpartum with fever, malaise, and lower abdominal pain. On examination, a foul lochia and tender boggy uterus are present. What is the most likely diagnosis?**

Endometritis. Typically occurs 1 to 3 days postpartum.

○ **What is lochia?**

Refers to the uterine discharge/bleeding that occurs after the delivery and represents the sloughing off of decidual tissue. It can last for 4 to 5 weeks.

○ **Is endometritis more common after vaginal delivery or cesarean section?**

5 to 10× more likely after cesarean section.

○ **What is the pharmacologic treatment of endometritis initially and based on response to treatment?**

IV clindamycin plus gentamicin is first line

Ampicillin is added if no response in 24 to 48 hours

Metronidazole is added if sepsis present

○ **What is a preventative measure to reduce risk of postpartum endometritis?**

Single dose of broad-spectrum antibiotic at the time of cord clamping.

REFERENCES

Bader, T. *Ob/Gyn Secrets,* Updated 3rd edition. Elsevier Mosby; 2004.

Beckmann C, Ling F, Smith R, Barzansky B, Herbert W, Laube D. *Obstetrics and Gynecology.* 7th ed. Philadelphia, PA: Lippincott, Williams & Wilkins; 2014.

Bickley L. *Bates' Guide to Physical Examination and History Taking.* 11th ed. Philadelphia, PA: Lippincott, Williams & Wilkins; 2013.

Decherney A, Nathan L, Goodwin TM, Laufer N. *Current Diagnosis and Treatment Obstetrics & Gynecology.* 10th ed. Lange Series. New York, NY: McGraw-Hill; 2007.

DeGowin R, LeBlond R, Brown D. *DeGowin's Diagnostic Evaluation. The Complete Guide to Assessment, Examination, and Differential Diagnosis.* 8th ed. New York, NY: McGraw-Hill; 2004.

Lemcke D, Pattison J, Marshall L, Cowley D. *Current Care of Women Diagnosis & Treatment.* Lange Series. New York, NY: McGraw-Hill; 2004.

Gilbert D, Moellering R Jr, Eliopoulous G. *The Sanford Guide to Antimicrobial Therapy.* 43th ed. Antimicrobial Therapy, Inc., Sperryville, VA; 2013.

Committee on Practice Bulletins—Gynecology. ACOG Practice Bulletin Number 131: Screening for cervical cancer. *Obstet Gynecol.* 2012;120(5):1222–1238.

Siegel R, Naishadham, D, Jemal A. Cancer statistics, 2013. *CA Cancer J Clin* 2013; 63(1):11–30.

Thoma M, McLain A, Louis J, et al. Prevalence of infertility in the US as estimated by the current duration approach and a traditional constructed approach. *Fertil Steril.* 2013;99(5):1324–1331.

UpToDate (online 21.8 – C21.112). www.uptodateonline.com. Accessed June 2013, August 2013.

CHAPTER 9 Musculoskeletal

John Oliphant, MHP, MSEd, PA-C, ATC

GENERAL ORTHOPEDIC CONCEPTS

○ **By definition, a <u>sprain</u> involves injury to what types of connective tissue?**

Those tissues that give support to joints—ligaments and joint capsules.

○ **How are sprains classified?**

First degree: Minor stretching or partial tear of ligaments/capsule without instability when the joint is stressed.

Second degree: Significant stretching and partial tear of ligaments/capsule allowing for partial opening of the joint when stressed.

Third degree: Complete tear of ligaments/capsule with complete opening of joint when stressed.

○ **By definition, a <u>strain</u> involves injury to what two types of connective tissue?**

Muscle or tendon.

○ **What is a valgus deformity?**

Valgus deformity is angulation of an extremity at a joint with the more distal part angled away from the midline.

○ **What is a varus deformity?**

Varus deformity is angulation of an extremity at a joint with the more distal part angled toward the midline.

○ **Are dislocations and sprains more common in children or adults?**

Dislocations and ligamentous injuries are uncommon in prepubertal children as the ligaments and joints are quite strong as compared to the adjoining growth plates. Excessive force applied to a child's joint is more likely to cause a fracture through the growth plate than a dislocation or sprain.

REVIEW OF SALTER–HARRIS FRACTURES

○ **Which type of Salter–Harris fracture has the worst prognosis?**

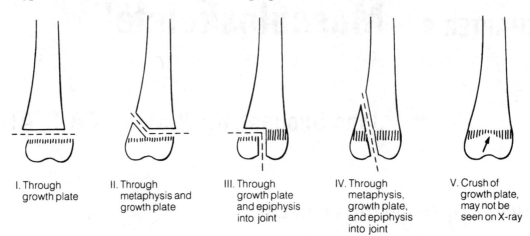

Figure 9-1 (Reproduced, with permission, from Stone CK, Humphries RL. *Current Diagnosis & Treatment Emergency Medicine.* 6th ed. New York, NY: McGraw-Hill; 2008, Fig. 26-2.)

Type V (compression injury of the epiphyseal plate) (see Figure 9-1).

○ **Which type of Salter–Harris fracture is most common?**

Type II (a triangular fracture involving the metaphysis and an epiphyseal separation).

○ **Which type(s) of Salter–Harris fractures can generally be treated with closed reduction and cast immobilization?**

Types I, II, and III.

○ **What is a stress fracture?**

A stress or fatigue fracture is caused by small, repetitive forces that usually involve the metatarsal shafts, the distal tibia, and the femoral neck (though many other bones may be affected). These fractures may not be seen on initial radiographs.

○ **After a fracture, what are the three stages of healing?**

1. Inflammatory
2. Reparative
3. Remodeling

○ **The end of the reparative phase is usually marked by clinical union of the fracture. How is clinical union defined?**

• The fractured bones do not shift on clinical examination
• The fracture site is nontender
• The patient can use the limb without significant pain

○ **What must be present for compartment syndrome to occur?**

Increased pressure within closed tissue spaces compromising blood flow to muscle and nerve tissue. There are three prerequisites to the development of compartment syndrome:

1. Limiting space
2. Increased tissue pressure
3. Decreased tissue perfusion

○ **What are the two basic mechanisms for elevated compartment pressure?**

1. External compression—by circumferential casts, dressings, burn eschar, or pneumatic pressure garments.
2. Volume increase within the compartment—hemorrhage into the compartment, IV infiltration, or edema secondary to injury or because of postischemic swelling.

○ **What intracompartmental pressure indicates a need for emergency surgery?**

Normal pressure within compartments is 0 to 8 mm Hg. It is best to determine the patient's diastolic blood pressure and subtract their intracompartmental pressure to determine what is called their acute compartment syndrome (ACS) delta pressure. Emergency fasciotomy is recommended if the ACS delta pressure is greater than 30 mm Hg.

○ **How do you clinically differentiate between acute compartment syndrome, neurapraxia, and arterial occlusion?**

• The patient will have normal pulses in neurapraxia.
• Decreased pulses in compartment syndrome (though this is a very rare and insensitive finding).
• No pulses in arterial occlusion.
• Stretching the muscles will cause great pain in compartment syndrome but not in neurapraxia.

○ **What fracture is most commonly associated with compartment syndrome?**

The tibia, which often results in anterior compartment syndrome.

○ **What are the early signs and symptoms of compartment syndrome?**

1. Tenderness and pain out of proportion to the injury
2. Pain with active and passive motion
3. Hypesthesia and paresthesia

○ **What are the classic 6 P's of compartment syndrome?**

1. Pain
2. Pallor
3. Pulselessness
4. Paresthesia
5. Pressure
6. Paralysis

Note: Recent evidence indicates that pain and possibly paresthesias may be the most reliable of these.

○ **What 4 C's determine muscle viability?**

1. Color
2. Consistency
3. Contraction
4. Circulation

○ **What are the late signs and symptoms of compartment syndrome?**

1. Tense, indurated, and erythematous compartment
2. Slow capillary refill
3. Pallor and pulselessness

○ **What conditions are in the differential diagnosis of a limp or gait abnormality in a child?**

- Legg–Calvé–Perthes disease (avascular necrosis of the femoral head)
- Osgood–Schlatter disease
- Avulsion of the tibial tubercle
- Infection
- Toxic transient tenosynovitis
- Patellofemoral subluxation
- Chondromalacia patella
- Slipped capital femoral epiphysis
- Septic arthritis
- Metatarsal fracture
- Proximal stress fracture
- Toddler fracture (spiral tibia fracture)

DISORDERS OF THE SHOULDER AND UPPER ARM

○ **What are the four muscles of the rotator cuff?**

1. Supraspinatus
2. Infraspinatus
3. Teres minor
4. Subscapularis

○ **Which bone is most often fractured at birth?**

The clavicle.

○ **What is the most common type of shoulder dislocation?**

Anterior dislocation.

○ **A patient cannot actively abduct her shoulder because of pain and weakness. What injury does this suggest?**

A rotator-cuff tear.

○ **What is the most common joint dislocation?**

Anterior shoulder dislocations account for half of all joint dislocations.

○ **What arm position puts the shoulder joint in the most vulnerable position for an anterior dislocation?**

Abduction and external rotation.

○ **What nerve is usually injured in glenohumeral dislocation?**

Axillary nerve.

○ **What is the most reliable method of diagnosing a posterior shoulder dislocation?**

Performing a physical examination and ordering an axillary view or a transscapular lateral view X-ray along with a standard AP view. A posterior dislocation of the shoulder is often missed with a standard radiographic shoulder series.

○ **In a humeral shaft fracture, what nerve is most commonly injured?**

The radial nerve.

○ **A patient presents with a complaint of pain at the site of the deltoid insertion with radiation into the back of the arm (C5 distribution). On examination, there is increased pain with active abduction from 70 to 120 degrees. X-rays reveal calcification at the tendinous insertion of the greater tuberosity. What is the likely diagnosis?**

Supraspinatus tendonitis (the supraspinatus tendon is the most common tendon affected by calcific tendonitis of the shoulder).

○ **What is the name of the cartilaginous structure of the shoulder that lines the glenoid and provides additional stability to the joint? It has been described as being similar to the meniscus of the knee.**

The glenoid labrum.

○ **What humerus position puts the shoulder in greatest risk of dislocating anteriorly?**

Abduction and external rotation.

○ **Shoulder separations happen at what joint?**

The acromioclavicular joint.

○ **Shoulder dislocations happen at what joint?**

The glenohumeral joint.

○ **What is the best way to position a patient's arm to palpate the subacromial bursa?**

With the humerus held in passive extension.

○ **What muscle forms the anterior wall of the axilla?**

The pectoralis major.

○ **What muscle forms the posterior wall of the axilla?**

The latissimus dorsi.

○ **What muscle is most frequently absent (either totally or partially) because of a congenital anomaly?**

The pectoralis major.

○ **What portion of the biceps is most commonly torn from its bony attachment?**

The long head of the biceps.

○ **Winging of the scapula indicates a weakness of what muscle?**

The serratus anterior muscle.

○ **A positive drop arm test is suggestive of what condition?**

A tear in the rotator cuff (especially the supraspinatus muscle).

○ **What is the likely diagnosis in a patient with significantly restricted range of motion at the shoulder joint 4 weeks after a painful shoulder injury?**

Adhesive capsulitis (frozen shoulder).

○ **What other injuries may occur with an anterior dislocation of the shoulder?**

- Axillary nerve injury
- Axillary artery injury (geriatric patients)
- Compression fracture of the humeral head (Hillsack's deformity)
- Rotator-cuff tear
- Fractures of the anterior glenoid lip
- Fractures of the greater tuberosity of the humerus
- Tear of the glenoid labrum

○ **What type of shoulder dislocation is pictured in the radiograph (see Figure 9-2)?**

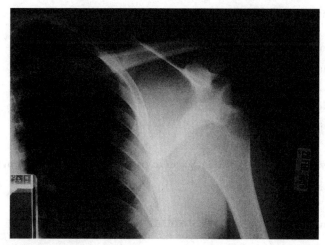

Figure 9-2 (Photo contributed by Kevin J. Knoop, MD MS, reproduced with permission from Knoop KJ, Stack LB, Storrow AB. *Atlas of Emergency Medicine.* 3rd ed. New York, NY: McGraw-Hill; 2010, Fig. 11.5)

This shows an anterior shoulder dislocation. Note the humeral head is anterior and inferior to the glenoid fossa.

DISORDERS OF THE ELBOW AND FOREARM

○ **What is "nursemaid's elbow"?**

A subluxation of the radial head. During forceful retraction, fibers of the annular ligament that encircle the radial neck become trapped between the radial head and the capitellum. On presentation, children hold their arm in slight flexion and pronation.

○ **A patient has a fracture of the proximal third of the ulna. What additional injury should be ruled out?**

A dislocation of the radial head. An anterior dislocation is most common. A proximal ulna fracture with a radial head dislocation is often called a Monteggia fracture.

○ **What is the significance of the fat pad sign seen on a lateral radiograph of the elbow following an injury?**

This indicates the presence of an effusion or hemarthrosis of the elbow joint, suggestive of an occult fracture of the radial head, supracondylar fracture of the humerus, or proximal ulnar fracture.

○ **What is the order of appearance of the ossification centers in the elbow? What approximate age do they appear at?**

Remember the acronym **CRITOE**:
- **C**apitellum (3–5 months)
- **R**adial Head (4–5 years)
- **I**nternal (medial) epicondyle (5–7 years)
- **T**rochlea (8–9 years)
- **O**lecranon (9–10 years)
- **E**xternal (lateral) epicondyle (11–12 years)

○ **Where is the most common site of bursitis?**

The olecranon bursa of the elbow.

○ **What is the usual mechanism of injury in a supracondylar distal humerus fracture?**

A fall on an outstretched arm.

○ **What artery is commonly injured with a supracondylar distal humerus fracture?**

Brachial artery.

○ **What nerves can be injured with a supracondylar humerus fracture?**

- Median nerve
- Radial nerve
- Ulnar nerve

○ **Why is a displaced supracondylar fracture of the distal humerus in a child considered an emergency?**

Because of the high potential for neurovascular compromise that may lead to ischemic injury or nerve palsy.

○ **What nerve injury is associated with a medial epicondyle fracture?**

Ulnar nerve.

○ **What is the most commonly missed fracture in the elbow region?**

A radial head fracture. Like a scaphoid (navicular) fracture in the wrist, radiographic signs of a radial head fracture may not show up for days after the injury. A positive fat pad sign may be the only finding suggestive of this injury.

○ **What upper-extremity joint is most commonly dislocated in children?**

The elbow.

○ **Which epicondyle is involved in tennis elbow?**

The lateral epicondyle.

○ **Which epicondyle is involved in golfer's elbow?**

The medial epicondyle.

○ **What is the most commonly injured bursa of the elbow?**

The olecranon bursa.

○ **Does damage to the olecranon bursa tend to produce diffuse or localized swelling?**

Localized as shown here (Figure 9-3)

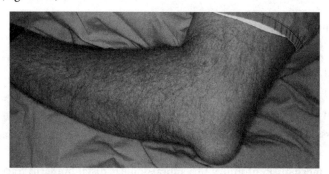

Figure 9-3 (Photo contributed by Selim Suner, MD MS, reproduced with permission from Knoop KJ, Stack LB, Storrow AB. *Atlas of Emergency Medicine.* 3rd ed. New York, NY: McGraw-Hill; 2010, Fig. 12.17.)

○ **Which bone articulates with the humerus in the olecranon fossa?**

The ulna.

○ **What are the three bony articulations of the elbow?**

1. The humeroulnar joint
2. The humeroradial joint
3. The radioulnar joint

○ **Where can the ulnar nerve be best palpated at the elbow joint?**

In the sulcus between the medial epicondyle and the olecranon fossa.

○ **What are the primary muscles that produce active elbow flexion?**

The brachialis and biceps muscles.

○ **What are the primary muscles that produce active elbow extension?**

The triceps muscles.

○ **Besides flexion and extension, what other motions happen at the elbow joint?**

Supination and pronation.

○ **What motor neurons are being evaluated with biceps, brachioradialis, and triceps reflex testing?**

1. Biceps reflex—C5
2. Brachioradialis reflex—C6
3. Triceps reflex—C7

DISORDERS OF THE WRIST AND HAND

○ **What tendons are involved in de Quervain tenosynovitis?**

The abductor pollicis longus and the extensor pollicis brevis tendons.

○ **What is Finkelstein test?**

A test used to determine whether a patient has de Quervain's tenosynovitis. If pain is elicited when the patient grasps his thumb with the fingers of the same hand and deviates his wrist in the ulnar direction then the test is positive.

○ **What is the most common type of peripheral nerve compression?**

Carpal tunnel syndrome which involves compression of the median nerve at the wrist.

○ **Is carpal tunnel syndrome more common in males or females?**

Carpal tunnel syndrome is more often diagnosed in female patients than male.

○ **How is carpal tunnel syndrome treated?**

Splinting the wrist in a neutral position, a course of NSAIDs, or corticosteroid injections may provide relief. If conservative measures do not work, surgical decompression can be performed.

○ **Which fingers are potentially affected by carpal tunnel syndrome?**

The first, second, third, and the radial sides of the fourth finger.

○ **Describe Tinel's tests for carpal tunnel syndrome.**

The examiner percusses the volar aspect of the patient's wrist over the median nerve with the patient's hand hyperextended. A positive test elicits pain and/or paresthesias in the distribution of the median nerve.

○ **Describe Phalenl's tests for carpal tunnel syndrome.**

The patient is asked to hold his/her hands in full flexion at the wrist for approximately 1 minute. A positive test elicits paresthesia along the distribution of the median nerve.

○ **What injury is often referred to as gamekeeper thumb?**

Instability of the ulnar collateral ligament of the MCP joint of the thumb. This may be caused by chronic valgus stresses on the joint, or more commonly an acute injury (such as a fall during skiing) that results in a sudden valgus stress. Often an acute injury of the ulnar collateral ligament of the thumb is referred to as "skier's thumb."

○ **What is a felon and how is it treated?**

A felon is a subcutaneous infection in the pulp space of the fingertip, usually caused by *Staphylococcus aureus*.

○ **How is a felon treated?**

A felon is treated by providing surgical drainage of the pulp space and insertion of a guaze packing strip to promote drainage (this is usually removed in 1 to 2 days). The area should be cultured for both aerobic and anaerobic organisms. The use of an antibiotic is often indicated because of the frequent presence of *Staphylococcus aureus* or other organisms in the wound.

○ **What is the most commonly fractured carpal bone?**

The scaphoid bone (navicular).

○ **How is a scaphoid (navicular) fracture diagnosed?**

Physical examination and radiographs are both useful in making the diagnosis. The initial radiograph frequently appears to be normal. If the patient has tenderness in the anatomical snuff box or pain with axial loading of the thumb, a scaphoid (navicular) fracture should be presumed and the hand splinted. A follow-up radiograph 10 to 14 days after the injury may then reveal the fracture.

○ **What is the most feared complication of a scaphoid (navicular) fracture?**

Avascular necrosis. The more proximal the fracture, the more commonly avascular necrosis occurs.

○ **What is Kienböck disease?**

Avascular necrosis of the lunate with collapse of the lunate secondary to fracture. As with a scaphoid (navicular) fracture, initial wrist X-rays may not demonstrate the fracture. Therefore, tenderness over the lunate warrants immobilization.

○ **What is a boutonnière deformity and how does it usually occur?**

It is a rupture of the extensor apparatus of the PIP joint of a finger. The injury occurs when the PIP joint is forced into flexion and the DIP joint into hyperextension.

○ **How is a boutonnière deformity initially treated?**

By splinting the PIP joint in full extension.

○ **Describe Dupuytren contracture.**

A nodular thickening and contraction of the palmar fascia.

○ **Describe Galeazzi fracture/dislocation.**

A displaced fracture of the distal radius with a dislocation of the distal radioulnar joint.

○ **What are Kanavel's four cardinal signs of infectious digital flexor tenosynovitis?**

1. Tenderness along the tendon sheath

2. Finger held in flexion

3. Pain on passive extension of the finger

4. Finger swelling

○ **What fracture has likely occurred to this individual (Figure 9-4)?**

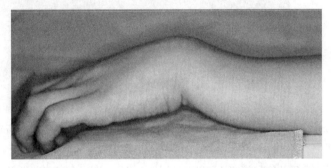

Figure 9-4 (Photo contributed by Cathleen M. Vossler, MD, reproduced with permission from Knoop KJ, Stack LB, Storrow AB. *Atlas of Emergency Medicine.* 3rd ed. New York, NY: McGraw-Hill; 2010, Fig. 11.19.)

A Colles fracture that is a complete fracture of the distal radius in which the fragment is displaced dorsally as shown in the radiograph below (Figure 9-5).

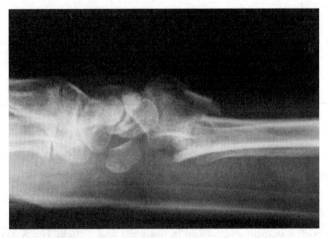

Figure 9-5 (Reproduced, with permission, from Brunicardi FC, Andersen DK, et al. *Schwartz's Priniciples of Surgery.* 8th ed. New York, NY: McGraw-Hill; 2007, Fig. 13.12.)

○ **Active adduction of the thumb tests which nerve?**

Ulnar nerve.

○ **What X-ray views should be obtained when ruling out a lunate fracture in the wrist?**

Anteroposterior, lateral, and two oblique X-rays of the wrist should be obtained if a fracture is suspected.

○ A patient presents with an injury to his second (index) finger after forced flexion. He reports an inability to actively extend the tip of his finger (but he can extend it passively) and presents as below. What is the likely injury (see Figure 9-6)?

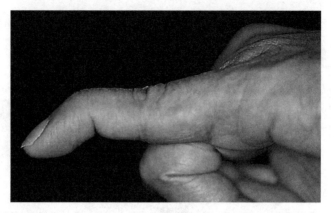

Figure 9-6 (Reproduced, with permission, from Knoop KJ, Stack LB, Storrow AB. *Atlas of Emergency Medicine.* 3rd ed. New York, NY: McGraw-Hill; 2010, Fig. 11.51.)

Mallet finger, which is a result of either a rupture of the distal extensor tendon or an avulsion fraction of the tendon insertion on the distal phalanx with a dorsal plate avulsion.

○ What nerve provides sensations to both the dorsum and volar aspects of the hand?

The ulnar nerve. The radial nerve primarily provides sensation on the dorsum of the hand and the median nerve supplies the volar aspect.

○ A patient presents with a small, soft bump on the dorsum of her wrist. The mass has a jelly-like consistency and is not significantly point tender. What is the likely diagnosis?

A ganglion cyst.

○ In the wrist, what bone is dislocated most often?

Lunate.

○ On an X-ray of the wrist, the AP view shows a triangular shaped lunate. What is the likely diagnosis?

Lunate dislocation.

○ A patient presents with a snapping sensation in the wrist and a click. The X-ray of a patient's hand reveals a 3-mm space between the scaphoid and the lunate. What is your diagnosis?

Scaphoid dislocation.

○ In a boxer's fracture, how much angulation of the fifth metacarpal neck is acceptable.

Opinions vary, but generally less than 30 to 40 degrees is considered acceptable.

○ What ligament in the hand is commonly injured in a fall while skiing?

Thumb MCP joint ulnar collateral ligament rupture (Gamekeeper's thumb).

○ **Why is it important to get radiographic studies after an acute dislocation?**

To rule out other injuries including ligament avulsion, articular fracture, or other signs that might indicate the presence of gross joint instability.

○ **Atrophy of the thenar eminence of the palm may indicate entrapment of what nerve?**

The median nerve.

○ **Atrophy of the hypothenar eminence of the palm may indicate entrapment of what nerve?**

The ulnar nerve.

○ **The median nerve passes through the carpal tunnel at the wrist. Where does the ulnar nerve pass through at the wrist?**

The Tunnel of Guyon.

○ **What important artery passes through the Tunnel of Guyon?**

The ulnar artery.

○ **What do you call an infection that occurs on the posterior distal aspect of a finger, may wrap around the border of the finger nail and often starts with a hangnail?**

A paronychia.

○ **How should one treat a paronychia that has formed an abscess?**

Incision and drainage of the abscess. Antibiotics may be used as well if an associated cellulitis has developed or in the rare situation where systemic signs and symptoms are present.

○ **Do most median nerve injuries occur as a result of acute macro trauma or chronic microtrauma?**

Most median nerve injuries are a result of repetitive movements over time producing chronic microtrauma.

DISORDERS OF THE BACK/SPINE

○ **What is the leading cause of disability for patients under the age of 45 years?**

Chronic lower back pain. Most patients with lower back pain do not need surgery and will recover from their injury within 6 weeks.

○ **What must be checked in a patient with Down syndrome before medical clearance can be given for participation in sports?**

Atlantoaxial instability must be ruled out by means of cervical radiographs and possibly CT scans with the head in various positions. 10% to 20% of children with Down syndrome have unstable atlantoaxial joints.

○ **What vertebrae most commonly sustain compression fractures?**

T11, T12, L1.

○   **A patient in a motor vehicle accident sustains a hyperextension injury to the neck. Plain films reveal a C2 bilateral facet fracture through the pedicles. What is the common name for this type of fracture?**

A hangman's fracture.

○   **What causes Horner syndrome (ptosis, miosis, and anhidrosis)?**

A lesion to the sympathetic pathways that supply the head and neck, including the oculosympathetic fibers.

○   **What spinal level corresponds to the dermatomal innervation of the perianal region? The nipple line? The index finger? The knee? The lateral foot?**

- Perianal region: S2 to S4
- Nipple line: T4
- Index finger: C7
- Knee: L4
- Lateral foot: S1

○   **A patient has difficulty squatting and standing because of quadriceps muscle weakness caused by nerve root compression. At what level is this nerve root compression likely occurring?**

L4.

○   **Where is the most common site of lumbar disk herniations?**

Most clinically important lumbar disk herniations are at the L4 to L5 or L5 to S1 intervertebral levels. Evaluate these patients by checking for weakness of ankle and great toe dorsiflexors (L5). Also check pinprick sensation over the medial aspect of the foot (L5) and the lateral portion of the feet (S1).

○   **A C1 burst fracture from an axial load on the back of the head or hyperextension of the neck is also known as what type of fracture?**

Jefferson fracture.

○   **Where is the most common site of cervical disk herniation?**

Cervical disk herniations are most common at C6 to C7, but also may occur at C5 to C6 and other levels.

○   **Define spondylolysis.**

An acquired unilateral or bilateral defect in the pars interarticularis. This occurs most commonly at the L5 level, but it can occur at other levels as well.

○ **Define spondylolisthesis.**

The forward movement of one vertebral body on the vertebra (see Figure 9-7). Spondylolysis can lead to spondylolisthesis as seen in the diagram below. Spondylolisthesis occurs most commonly when L5 slips forward on S1.

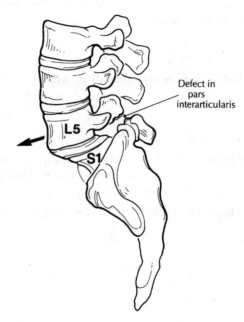

Defect in pars interarticularis

Figure 9-7 (Reproduced, with permission, from Chen MYM, Pope TL Jr, Ott DL. *Basic Radiology*. New York, NY: McGraw-Hill; 2004, Fig. 13.12.)

○ **A patient presents with back pain, leg numbness with weakness, and complaints of incontinence. On examination decreased sphincter tone and perianal numbness is noted. What is your diagnosis?**

Cauda equina syndrome (compression of the L2–S4 nerve roots).

○ **A patient has an avulsion fracture of the spinous process of C7 with a history of a hyperflexion mechanism. Would this likely be a stable or unstable fracture?**

Most isolated spinous process fractures are stable.

○ **A patient suffers a bilateral interfacetal anterior dislocation as a result of excessive cervical flexion. What structures have likely been damaged?**

Cervical vertebrae support ligaments are likely disrupted causing the C-spine to be unstable. Damage to the spinal cord is definitely possible as well.

○ **While providing medical coverage at a soccer game, a player goes down complaining of neck pain after a hard collision with another player and the ground. She does not lose consciousness, has full sensation and motor function in her extremities, but has significant point tenderness directly over her cervical vertebrae. How should you remove this player from the field?**

Apply a stiff extrication collar, strap her to a backboard, and transport her to the hospital via ambulance for imaging studies. She may have a nondisplaced cervical fracture that could shift causing spinal cord damage if she is allowed to move freely.

○ **From what spinal nerve roots does the brachial plexus originate?**

C5 through T1.

○ **Someone with a C5 disk herniation causing right-sided nerve root impingement will likely have pain in what part of his/her body besides the neck?**

The right shoulder.

○ **At what two levels does spinal stenosis most commonly occur?**

L3 to L4 and L4 to L5 interspaces.

○ **What typically causes spinal stenosis?**

It is generally caused by degenerative arthritis (spondylosis) of the spine in older adults with associated osteophyte formation and disk bulging that encroaches on the central canal and the neural foramina.

○ **In patients with significant lumbar spinal stenosis, does walking lead to worsening or improving leg pain?**

Worsening.

○ **Define scoliosis**

A lateral curvature of the spine.

○ **In what gender does scoliosis most commonly occur?**

Female.

○ **Define kyphosis.**

The normal curvature of the thoracic spine where the apex of the curve points posteriorly. Various factors can lead to excessive kyphosis.

○ **When is postural kyphosis (a form of excessive kyphosis that can be voluntarily corrected) most common?**

During adolescences.

○ **In adult females when is excessive kyphosis most common?**

After menopause as a result of osteoporosis and vertebral body fractures.

○ **The C7 neurologic area is responsible for sensation in which part of the body?**

The third finger.

○ **Do cervical, thoracic, or lumbar intervertebral disks have the lowest rate of herniation?**

Thoracic.

○ **Fifty percentage of cervical rotation takes place between what two cervical vertebrae?**

C1 (atlas) and C2 (the axis). The remaining 50% is split up fairly evenly among the remaining five cervical vertebrae.

○ **The 12th ribs articulate with what vertebrae?**

The 12th thoracic vertebrae. Generally the 12 sets of ribs articulate posteriorly with the thoracic vertebrae assigned the same number (i.e., first ribs articulate with T1, second ribs with T2, etc…).

○ **What condition must be ruled out in a middle-aged male with profound limitation in spinal mobility?**

Ankylosing spondylitis.

DISORDERS OF THE HIP AND PELVIS

○ **Describe the leg position of a patient with a femoral neck fracture.**

Shortened, abducted, and slightly externally rotated.

○ **Describe the leg position of a patient with an anterior hip dislocation.**

Mildly flexed, abducted, and externally rotated.

○ **Describe the leg position of a patient with a posterior hip dislocation.**

Shortened, adducted, flexed, and internally rotated.

○ **What is the usual mechanism of injury in a posterior hip dislocation?**

The mechanism of injury is force applied to a flexed knee directed posteriorly.

○ **What nerve and bone injuries are known to be associated with posterior hip dislocation?**

This dislocation is associated with sciatic nerve injury (10%) and avascular necrosis of the femoral head.

○ **Describe the leg position of a patient with an intertrochanteric hip fracture.**

Shortened, externally rotated, and abducted.

○ **Describe a typical patient with a slipped capital femoral epiphysis.**

An obese boy, 10 to 16 years old, with groin or knee discomfort increasing with activity. He may also have a limp.

○ **What is the Young classification system for pelvic fractures?**

The Young system divides pelvic fractures into four categories depending on the type and direction of force.

1. Lateral compression (LC)
2. Anterior–posterior compression (APC)
3. Vertical sheer (VS)
4. Combination mechanical-mixed (CM)

○ **Describe a lateral compression pelvic fracture (LC).**

This fracture is usually caused by a motor vehicle collision in which the car and the patient are broadsided. The lateral force from the collision causes a sacral fracture, iliac wing fracture, or a sacroiliac ligamentous injury and a transverse fracture of the pubic rami. There is no ligamentous injury at the pubic symphysis.

○ **Describe an anterior–posterior compression pelvic fracture (APC).**

APCs are usually caused by a head-on motor vehicle collision. They always include a disruption of the pubis symphysis and usually involve a disruption (of different degrees) of the sacroiliac joint.

○ **Describe a vertical sheer pelvic fracture (VS).**

VSs are usually caused by a fall. They involve an injury of the sacroiliac ligaments and either a disruption of the pubis symphysis or vertical fractures through the pubic rami. The iliac wing is vertically displaced.

○ **What life-threatening injury is associated with vertical sheer pelvic fractures?**

Severe hemorrhage, usually retroperitoneal. Up to 6 L of blood can be accommodated in this space.

○ **Which pelvic fracture is most likely to involve bladder rupture?**

Lateral compression fractures.

○ **Which pelvic fracture is most likely to involve urethral injury?**

Anterior–posterior compression fracture.

○ **Which fracture is associated with avascular necrosis of the femoral head?**

Femoral neck fractures.

○ **What common radiographic views help diagnose a slipped femoral capital epiphysis?**

Evaluation is aided by AP and frog-leg lateral radiographs of both hips.

○ **Which type of hip dislocation is most common: anterior, posterior, lateral, or medial?**

Posterior hip dislocations are the most common, accounting for approximately 90% of all hip dislocations.

○ **A fracture of the acetabulum may be associated with damage to what nerve?**

The sciatic nerve.

○ **Describe the signs and symptoms of pressure on the first sacral root (S1).**

Symptoms of S1 injury include pain radiating to the midgluteal region, posterior thigh, posterior calf, and down to the heel and sole of the foot. Sensory signs are localized to the lateral toes. S1 root compression typically involves the plantar flexor muscles of the foot and toes. The ankle reflex is decreased or absent.

○ **What is the most commonly missed hip fracture?**

Femoral neck fracture.

○ **Where is the most common site of aseptic necrosis?**

The hip.

○ **What must be done to effectively palpate the coccyx and sacrococcygeal joint?**

A rectal examination.

○ **What are the two common tests that can be done on newborn infants to check for instability of the hip joints?**

- Barlow maneuver—The child is positioned on his/her back and the hips are gently adducted and a posteriorly directed pressure applied. If the hip(s) is/are dislocatable, posterior movement and a palpable clunk may be detected as the femoral head exits the acetabulum.
- Ortolani maneuver—The child is positioned on his/her back and the hips are flexed, abducted, and externally rotated. If there is a dislocated hip, the involved hip is unable to be abducted as far as the uninvolved side and there is a palpable click when the hip is reduced.

○ **What is the primary hip flexor muscle?**

The iliopsoas muscle.

○ **What is the primary hip extensor muscle?**

The gluteus maximus muscle.

○ **What is the primary hip abductor muscle?**

The gluteus medius muscle.

○ **What is the primary hip adductor muscle?**

The adductor longus muscle.

○ **Point tenderness and a boggy feeling over the greater trochanter may be indicative of what?**

Trochanteric bursitis.

○ **What are the superior and inferior attachments of the inguinal ligament?**

The superior attachment is at the anterior, superior iliac spines and the inferior attachment is at the pubic tubercles.

○ **What nerve lies midway between the ischial tuberosities and greater trochanters and can best be palpated with the hip in a flexed position?**

The sciatic nerve.

○ **How are the femoral nerve, artery, and vein positioned in relationship to each other?**

Moving from lateral to medial just inferior to the inguinal ligament, first comes the nerve, then the artery, and the most medial structure of the three is the vein.

DISORDERS OF THE KNEE AND LOWER LEG

○ **What long bone is most commonly fractured?**

The tibia.

○ **A 43-year-old female runner complains that she has diffuse, aching <u>anterior</u> knee pain that is worsened when she walks up- or downstairs or when she squats down. There has been no acute trauma, but she has been increasing her running mileage. No effusion is present. What is the probable diagnosis?**

Patellofemoral pain syndrome.

○ **What is the most significant complication of a proximal tibial metaphyseal fracture?**

Arterial involvement, especially when there is a valgus deformity.

○ **Why should one consider aspirating fluid from a knee with an acute hemarthrosis?**

Aspirating fluid from the joint space relieves pressure and pain for the patient and will allow the provider to ascertain whether fat globules are present, indicating a fracture.

○ **What are the four compartments of the leg?**

1. Anterior
2. Lateral
3. Deep posterior
4. Superficial posterior

○ **What is the most common site of compartment syndrome?**

The anterior compartment of the leg.

○ **What are the most common lower-extremity fractures in children?**

Tibial and fibular shaft fractures, usually secondary to twist forces.

○ **What radiograph would one order for a suspected patellar fracture in a child?**

Standard AP and lateral radiographs plus patellar "sunrise" or "skyline" views. Radiographs of the uninvolved knee for comparison should also be done.

○ **What are the differences between an avulsion fracture of the tibial tubercle and Osgood–Schlatter disease (which also involves the tibial tubercle)?**

• Avulsion fractures present with an <u>acute</u> inability to walk. A lateral view of the knee is most diagnostic. Treatment is often surgical.
• Osgood–Schlatter disease is an overuse injury that gradually develops in growing children. It is exacerbated by running, jumping, and kneeling activities. Treatment involves ice, padding, stretching, NSAIDs, rest, and occasionally immobilization.

○ **True/False: Osgood–Schlatter disease often requires surgical intervention?**

False. It is usually a self-limiting condition with symptoms resolving by early adulthood. An enlarged, but painless tibial tuberosity often persists.

○ **What is a toddler fracture?**

A spiral fracture of the tibia without fibular involvement. This type of fracture in toddlers is a common cause of limping or refusal to walk.

○ **With a complete rupture of the medial collateral ligament, what would be felt by the examiner during a valgus stress of the knee?**

Excessive laxity with no firm endpoint.

○ **A female basketball player plants her foot to make a quick change of direction while running down the court. She feels a popping sensation and falls to the ground in pain. Later that day she has a large effusion. Which knee ligament did she likely tear?**

Anterior cruciate ligament.

○ **Which test is more sensitive when used to determine an anterior cruciate ligament tear in the knee: the anterior drawer test or the Lachman test?**

The Lachman test is more sensitive because the stabilizing effect of the hamstrings is eliminated. While the knee is held at approximately 30 degrees of flexion and the distal femur is stabilized, the lower leg is pulled forward. Significant anterior laxity compared to the other knee is evidence of an anterior cruciate ligament tear.

○ **What lower-extremity joint is most commonly affected with pseudogout?**

The knee.

○ **What is the chemical composition of the crystals found in pseudogout?**

Calcium pyrophosphate dehydrate.

○ **What nerve may be injured in a distal femoral fracture?**

Peroneal nerve.

○ **Which is more common, a medial or a lateral tibial plateau fracture?**

The lateral tibial plateau is most commonly fractured. If AP and lateral films are negative, follow up with oblique views if you are suspicious of a tibial plateau fracture.

○ **What nerve may be injured with a knee dislocation?**

The peroneal nerve.

○ **Does a torn meniscus or torn cruciate ligament produce a more dramatic appearing knee effusion?**

A torn cruciate ligament does because of its greater vascular supply.

○ **Are the anterior and posterior cruciate ligaments named based on the location of their attachments to the femur or tibia?**

The tibia.

○ **Is the lateral or medial meniscus injured more frequently and why?**

The medial meniscus is injured far more frequently because of its more firm fixation to the tibia and joint capsule as well as its attachment to the medial collateral ligament. Because the lateral meniscus is smaller, attached more loosely to the tibia and not attached to the lateral collateral ligament, it has more ease of movement and is less prone to injury.

○ **A patient presents with a large area of swelling localized to the front of the knee, between the patella and the skin after a fall directly on her patella. The likely diagnosis is what?**

Prepatellar bursitis.

○ **Do patellar dislocations usually result in the patella going medially or laterally from its normal position?**

Laterally.

○ **Do patellar dislocations occur more commonly in males or females?**

Females.

○ **What four muscles make up the quadriceps?**

1. Vastus lateralis
2. Vastus intermedius
3. Vastus medialis
4. Rectus femoris

○ **What three muscles make up the hamstrings?**

1. Semimembranosus
2. Semitendinosus
3. Biceps femoris

○ **What condition is often a result of avascular necrosis of a segment subchondral bone, typically involving the lateral surface of the medial femoral condyle?**

Osteochondritis dissecans. This condition may also give rise to loose bodies within the joint.

DISORDERS OF THE ANKLE AND FOOT

○ **What is the most common type of ankle injury?**

Sprains, account for the majority of all ankle injuries.

○ **Do most ankle sprains involve ligaments on the lateral or medial side of the joint?**

Most ankle sprains involve the lateral ligaments.

○ **What is the most commonly injured lateral ankle ligament?**

Anterior talofibular ligament.

○ **What is the most common site of <u>stress</u> fractures in the foot?**

Second metatarsal.

○ **A 21-year-old female complains of pain and a clicking sound located at the posterior lateral malleolus. A fullness beneath the lateral malleolus is found. What is the probable diagnosis?**

Peroneal tendon subluxation with associated tenosynovitis.

○ **What is the most helpful physical examination test for determining if an anterior talofibular ligament injury has occurred?**

An anterior drawer test of the ankle will reveal pain and/or laxity if an anterior talofibular ligament injury has occurred.

○ **What are the signs and symptoms for compartment syndrome involving the anterior compartment of the leg?**

Pain on active and passive dorsiflexion and plantarflexion of the foot, and hypesthesia/paresthesia of the first web space of the foot.

○ **What metatarsal fracture is often associated with a disrupted tarsal–metatarsal joint?**

Fracture of the base of the second metatarsal. Treatment may require open reduction and internal fixation.

○ **What fracture is frequently missed when a patient complains of an ankle injury?**

Fracture at the base of the fifth metatarsal, caused by plantar flexion and inversion. Radiographs of the ankle may not include the fifth metatarsal.

○ **Achilles' tendon ruptures occur most commonly in what gender and age group?**

Middle-aged men (especially those that play quick stop and start sports like basketball).

○ **A stress fracture of the second or third metatarsal is suspected but not detected on initial X-rays. How long after the initial examination should a second set of X-rays be ordered?**

3 to 4 weeks.

○ **What tarsal bone is most commonly fractured?**

The calcaneus.

○ **What is the most common injury mechanism that results in a calcaneus fracture?**

A fall from a significant height.

○ **What guidelines are often used to determine if a patient who has suffered an ankle injury needs X-rays?**

The Ottawa ankle rules.

○ **What is the tarsal–metatarsal joint also called?**

Lisfranc joint.

○ **The second metatarsal is the locking mechanism for the mid part of the foot. A fracture at the base of the second metatarsal should raise suspicion of what?**

A disrupted tarsal–metatarsal joint. Treatment may require open reduction and internal fixation.

○ **What is a Jones fracture?**

An avulsion fracture at the base of the fifth metatarsal, usually secondary to plantar flexion and inversion. Also called a ballet fracture, it is the most common metatarsal fracture.

○ **The strong ligaments on the medial side of the ankle are collectively known as what?**

Deltoid ligaments.

○ **What potential complication is of concern in distal tibial (medial malleolus) fractures that are treated without surgery?**

Nonunion at the fracture site.

○ **What is the most common presentation of a Charcot joint?**

A warm, red, swollen ankle with minimal or absent pain and a "bag of bones" appearance on X-ray.

○ **What is the most common cause of a Charcot joint?**

Diabetic peripheral neuropathy.

○ **What nerve is located in the tarsal tunnel?**

The tibial nerve.

○ **What joint is most commonly affected with gout?**

The great (first) toe at the MCP joint.

○ **Describe the signs and symptoms of tarsal tunnel syndrome.**

Insidious onset of paresthesia, as well as burning pain and numbness on the plantar surface of the foot. Pain radiates superiorly along the medial side of the calf. Rest decreases pain.

○ **What ankle motion can lead to injury to the deltoid ligaments?**

Excessive eversion.

○ **Extreme pain on the undersurface of the foot from the calcaneus anteriorly that is often worse with the first few steps of the day or after a prolonged period of standing is likely caused by what condition?**

Plantar fasciitis.

○ **What are the characteristics of a Morton's foot?**

The second toe is longer than the first, which can lead to an increased risk of overuse injuries.

○ **What group of muscles on the lateral part of the lower leg must be strong to prevent excessive ankle inversion?**

The peroneal muscles.

○ **What are the characteristics of a cavus foot (pes cavus)?**

A high medial longitudinal arch, limited tarsal mobility, poor shock absorption qualities, excessive callus build up on the ball and/or heel area caused by increased stresses in these areas.

○ **What two plantar flexing muscles attach into the Achilles tendon?**

The gastrocnemius and soleus muscles.

○ **What is the common name for a laterally deviated first toe or hallucis valgus?**

Bunion.

○   **What are the characteristics of a pes planus foot?**

Flat foot, lowered medial longitudinal arch, often associated with excessive foot pronation.

○   **What type of serious ankle injury is seen in the radiograph below (Figure 9-8)?**

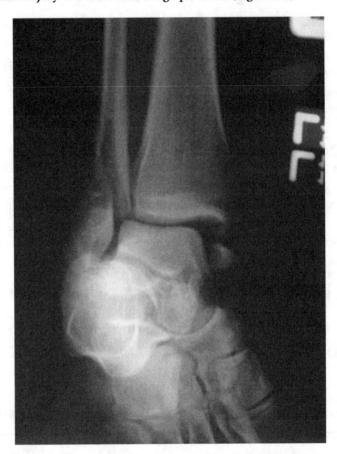

Figure 9-8 (Reproduced, with permission, from Brunicardi FC, Andersen DK, et al. *Schwartz's Principles of Surgery*. 8th ed. New York, NY: McGraw-Hill; 2007, Fig. 42-49.)

A bimalleolar ankle fracture involving the distal tibia and fibula.

INFECTIOUS DISEASE

○   **Where is the most common site of infectious arthritis in adults?**

The knee (although it can occur in other joints such as the hip, shoulder, elbow, and wrist).

○   **What is the most common bacteria implicated in infectious arthritis in adults?**

Staphylococcus aureus.

○   **Where is the most common site of osteomyelitis of the vertebral column?**

The lumbar spine.

O **What bacterial organism is most commonly the cause of osteomyelitis?**

Staphylococcus aureus.

O **What is the most common mechanism that infectious organisms use to reach the bone leading to osteomyelitis?**

By hematogenous spread.

O **What other mechanisms of pathogen transmission can result in osteomyelitis?**

• Spread of organisms from contiguous soft tissue infection
• Direct inoculation of the pathogen into the bone from trauma or surgery

O **What is the best way to determine the organism(s) that may be causing osteomyelitis?**

Bone biopsy of the suspected infection site with sample sent for culture and sensitivity.

O **What are the most common findings of osteomyelitis on X-ray?**

Cortical erosion, periosteal reaction, mixed lucency, and sclerosis. There may also be devitalized bone with radiodense appearance and soft tissue swelling (particularly when osteomyelitis is accompanied by cellulitis or abscess).

O **Where does acute hematogenous osteomyelitis most commonly affect children?**

The long bones.

O **Where does acute hematogenous osteomyelitis most commonly affect adults?**

The vertebrae.

O **What must be done if the patient with osteomyelitis does not respond to antibiotic therapy?**

A surgical decompression of the infected area.

O **What patients are at risk for developing *Salmonella* osteomyelitis?**

Patients with sickle cell anemia.

NEOPLASTIC DISEASE

O **What five primary carcinomas most commonly metastasize to the bone?**

1. Breast
2. Prostate
3. Lung
4. Kidney
5. Thyroid

○   **Where do most metastatic bone tumors occur?**

The spine.

○   **Are cancerous bone lesions generally metastatic or primary tumors when found in older adults?**

Most bone lesions are metastatic in adults.

○   **What is more common: benign or malignant tumors of the bone and soft tissue?**

Benign tumors are more common.

○   **What are lipomas?**

Benign, soft, freely movable, nontender masses composed of adipose (fat) tissue.

○   **What are chondrosarcomas?**

Malignant tumors of the cartilage.

○   **What are osteosarcomas?**

Malignant primary tumors of the bone. They are not metastatic from elsewhere.

○   **With what is nocturnal bone pain often associated?**

Malignancy, but some benign bone lesions can produce nocturnal pain as well.

○   **What part of the skeletal system is affected by Ewing sarcoma, multiple myeloma, and lymphoma of the bone?**

The marrow elements.

○   **What is osteoid osteoma?**

A fairly common benign bone tumor that often occurs in the proximal femur and can present as hip pain that is often worse at night and responds well to NSAIDs.

○   **What population is most likely to develop osteoid osteoma?**

Teenagers. Osteoid osteomas occur two to three times more often in boys than girls.

○   **What has likely occurred if a patient has had dull achy pain for some time associated with a malignant bony lesion and then suddenly has intense pain at the same location after some moderate stress on that bone?**

The patient may have experienced a pathologic fracture.

○   **What bones are most commonly affected by Ewing Sarcoma?**

Ewing Sarcoma is most commonly found in the femur, tibia, fibula, humerus, and pelvis. It occurs less commonly in the hands, feet, and spine.

○   **What is the best way to confirm the diagnosis when a suspicious bony lesion is seen in an imaging study (X-ray, CT, MRI, bone scan, etc…)?**

A bone biopsy must be done (often as an open procedure).

○ **What is the most common primary malignant bone tumor that proliferates through the bone marrow and often results in extensive skeletal destruction, osteopenia, and pathologic fractures?**

Multiple myeloma.

○ **Unicameral or simple bone cysts typically occur before what age?**

20 years of age.

○ **What bones are most commonly found to have unicameral bone cysts?**

Humerus and femur.

○ **How do unicameral bone cysts typically present?**

Pathologic fractures.

OSTEOARTHRITIS

○ **Which is more common: osteoarthritis or rheumatoid arthritis?**

Osteoarthritis is the most common type of arthritis.

○ **What structure is progressively damaged and eroded over time leading to osteoarthritis?**

Articular cartilage.

○ **Which joints of the hands are most commonly affected by osteoarthritis?**

The distal interphalangeal (DIP) joints of the fingers are most commonly affected by osteoarthritis.

○ **What are the bony prominences (caused by osteophytes) at the DIP joints in patients with osteoarthritis called?**

Heberden nodes.

○ **What are some of the common risk factors for developing osteoarthritis?**

- Advancing age
- Obesity
- Repetitive micro joint trauma
- Acute major joint trauma

○ **What are the most common symptoms and signs of osteoarthritis?**

- Joint stiffness
- Joint pain
- Joint deformity

○ **What effect on function can osteophytes have in advanced osteoarthritis?**

The osteophytes can cause a physical obstruction resulting in significantly decreased range of motion in the affected joints.

○ **Does osteoarthritis typically produce a mild or major joint effusion?**

The effusions that occur with osteoarthritis are typically mild.

○ **What findings would commonly be seen on the weight-bearing X-rays of a patient with severe osteoarthritis of the knees?**

- Decreased joint space between the femur and tibia (may be bone-on-bone), especially in the medial compartment
- Osteophytes or spurs at the joint margins
- Sclerosis of the bone

○ **The loss of what motion is often an early sign of the development of osteoarthritis of the hip?**

Internal rotation.

○ **Which of the following joints has the lowest occurrence rate of osteoarthritis (elbows, hands, hips, knees, spine)?**

Elbows because they are non–weight-bearing joints and do not get as much repetitive use as the hands.

○ **What lifestyle changes can help patients with osteoarthritis decrease their symptoms and slow the progression of the condition?**

- Weight loss if the patient is overweight to decrease the stress on the joints
- Avoidance of activities that place heavy impact, torsion, or other stresses on the joints
- Gentle exercise that encourages motion of the joints (gentle yoga, water exercises, exercise bikes, etc…)
- Shock absorbing footwear or shoe inserts to minimize the stress transferred to the weight-bearing joints.

○ **What types of medication may provide some relief for patients suffering with osteoarthritis?**

- Acetaminophen
- Salicylates
- NSAIDs (oral and topical)
- Topical analgesic liquids, creams, balms, and patches
- Glucosamine and Chondroitin (At the time of publication of this book these substances are still being investigated in several studies to determine true efficacy. Most studies to date have shown these substances to be generally safe, but not statistically better than placebo.)
- Intra-articular corticosteroid injections
- Intra-articular hyaluronan injections (for knee joints and possibly hip joints—early studies are under way)
- Colchicine and antimalarial drugs may be useful in particularly challenging cases—additional research is still needed

○ **What surgical treatment options exist for those with severe joint pain and dysfunction that have failed conservative management of their osteoarthritis?**

- Joint replacement surgery (arthroplasty) can provide significant pain reduction and increased function for many patients. There have been especially good outcomes for those undergoing arthroplasty of the hips, knees, and shoulders.
- Joint fusion surgery (arthrodesis) may be a good option to reduce joint pain in some patients, especially those suffering from severe ankle or wrist osteoarthritis. Joint motion will be lost.

OSTEOPOROSIS

○ **What bony abnormalities have occurred in those diagnosed with osteoporosis?**

These patients have a decrease in bone mass with microarchitectural changes that make their skeleton more fragile, resulting in an increased risk of fracture.

○ **What are the most common general types of osteoporosis?**

Primary osteoporosis type 1 generally occurs in postmenopausal women because of the loss of estrogen levels whereas primary osteoporosis type 2 can occur in either gender and is associated with advancing age. Secondary osteoporosis is usually brought on by medications or other diseases that can cause bone loss.

○ **What bones are most commonly fractured in patients with primary osteoporosis type 1?**

The vertebrae and distal radius.

○ **What type of bone is primarily affected by primary osteoporosis type 1?**

Trabecular bone.

○ **What bones are most commonly fractured in patients with primary osteoporosis type 2?**

The hip and pelvis.

○ **What test is generally used to diagnose osteoporosis?**

A DEXA scan (dual-energy X-ray absorptionmetry).

○ **What T-score must someone have before they are diagnosed with osteoporosis?**

−2.5 or less.

○ **What is a T-score measuring?**

A T-score measures the standard deviation difference between a patient's bone mineral density and that of a young-adult reference population.

○ **What percentage of bone loss must occur before decreased bone density is visible with traditional X-rays?**

More than 30%.

○ **What nutritional supplements when combined with resistance exercises and a physically active lifestyle might help prevent the development of osteoporosis?**

Calcium and vitamin D.

○ **What class of medication is commonly used to treat patients with confirmed osteoporosis?**

Bisphosphonates.

○ **When patients have decreased bone mineral density, but not decreased enough to be diagnosed with osteoporosis, what other condition might they be diagnosed with?**

Osteopenia.

○   **What types of exercise are most effective in preventing osteoporosis?**

Weight bearing and resistance exercises.

RHEUMATOLOGIC CONDITIONS

○   **Describe the classic bony changes that occur in the hands of someone suffering from rheumatoid arthritis.**

Ulnar deviation and subluxation at the MCP joints.

○   **Describe the classic bony changes that occur in the feet of someone suffering from rheumatoid arthritis.**

Claw toes and hallux valgus.

○   **Describe the systemic manifestations that can occur with rheumatoid arthritis?**

- Vasculitis
- Pericarditis
- Pulmonary disease

○   **Besides a rheumatoid factor, what other lab values are commonly obtained when working up a patient for possible rheumatoid arthritis?**

- Erythrocyte sedimentation rate (ESR)
- Anti-citrullinated peptide/protein antibodies (ACPA)
- C-reactive protein (CRP)

○   **A patient presents with a painful joint and his provider aspirates some synovial fluid from the affected joint. The fluid is analyzed using a compensated polarized light microscope and needle-shaped negatively birefringent crystals are seen. What condition does this patient likely have?**

Gout.

○   **What is the chemical composition of the crystals found in the joint of a patient suffering from gout?**

Monosodium urate.

○   **What is the treatment for acute gout?**

Indomethacin, naproxen, or other NSAIDs. For those intolerant of NSAIDs, colchicines is effective as well, but many patients experience nausea, vomiting, and/or diarrhea. Glucocorticoids may be used in select patients who are unable to use either NSAIDs or colchicine.

○   **What medications are commonly used to prevent future gout attacks?**

A xanthine oxidase inhibitor such as allopurinol or febuxostat is typically first-line preventative treatment. When not contraindicated (as in chronic kidney disease), a uricosuric therapy such as probenecid could be used. There are other options that may be added to or substituted for those above in specific patients.

○   **What joint is most commonly the site of an initial gout attack?**

The first metatarsal phalangeal joint.

○ **Examination using polarized microscopy of synovial fluid aspirated from a painful, swollen joint showing positively birefringent rhomboid-shaped crystals is associated with what condition?**

Pseudogout.

○ **What is the chemical composition of the crystals found in the joint of someone suffering from pseudogout?**

Calcium pyrophosphate dihydrate.

○ **What joints are most commonly affected by pseudogout?**

- Knee
- Wrist
- Elbow

○ **What is the recommended treatment for pseudogout that is affecting one or two joints?**

Joint aspiration followed by intra-articular glucocorticoid injection. Adjuvant treatment with NSAIDs or colchicine may also be used.

○ **What autoimmune disorder commonly affects women of childbearing years; may affect multiple organs and commonly present with a facial rash, photosensitivity, arthralgias, and the presence of antinuclear antibodies?**

Systemic lupus erythematous (SLE).

○ **The joints of what body parts are most affected by SLE?**

- Knees
- Hands/fingers
- Wrists

○ **What is Felty syndrome?**

Rheumatoid arthritis with splenomegaly and neutropenia.

○ **If a patient presents with multiple joint arthralgias, as well as excessive dryness of the mouth and eyes, what condition must be ruled out?**

Sjögren syndrome.

○ **A middle-aged female patient presents with swelling, stiffness, and pain in her fingers, wrists, and elbow joints as well as taut, shiny skin, and fatigue. What is her likely diagnosis?**

Scleroderma (systemic sclerosis).

○ **A 65-year-old female presents to an urgent care center with complaints of fatigue, low-grade fever, decreased appetite with a 10-lb weight loss, as well as pain and stiffness in her neck, shoulders, and pelvic area. What condition do you suspect?**

Polymyalgia rheumatic.

○   **What condition is characterized by inflammation of striated muscles in the proximal limbs and neck and elevated enzymes including CK, AST, ALT, and LDH?**

Polymyositis.

○   **What condition is far more common in women, is characterized by diffuse muscle tenderness, heightened sensitivity to touch in many different areas of the body, fatigue, and often depression?**

Fibromyalgia.

○   **Describe the three general subcategories of juvenile rheumatoid arthritis (JRA).**

- Pauciarticular-onset JRA is diagnosed in those patients with involvement of less than five joints after 6 months of illness. This is the most common type of JRA and actually has several subgroups.
- Polyarticular-onset JRA is diagnosed in patients with involvement of more than four joints after 6 months of illness. This is the second most common type of JRA and also has several subgroups.
- Systemic-onset JRA (formerly called Still disease) is associated with arthritis in any number of joints, rash, and intermittent fever. This is the least common form of JRA.

○   **What condition is characterized by inflammation of the medium (and sometimes small) sized arteries, occurs most commonly in middle-aged males, presents with fever, fatigue, weakness, weight loss, abdominal pain, arthralgias, arthritis, skin lesions, renal insufficiency, hypertension, and edema?**

Polyarteritis nodosa (PAN).

○   **What condition is a seronegative arthritis that is often seen in combination with urethritis and conjunctivitis? This condition is often precipitated by a sexually transmitted disease (often linked to *Chlamydia trachomatis*) or gastroenteritis and may present with lesions in multiple locations (mouth, penis, extremities), swollen toes and heel pain.**

Reactive arthritis (post-infectious arthritis with urethritis and conjunctivitis was formerly known as Reiter syndrome).

REFERENCES

Beaty JH, Kasser JR. *Rockwood and Wilkins' Fractures in Children*. Philadelphia, PA: Lippincott Williams & Wilkins; 2010.

Becker MA. Clinical manifestations and diagnosis of gout. In: Basow D, ed. *UpToDate*. Waltham, MA: UpToDate; 2013.

Becker MA. Prevention of recurrent gout. In: Basow D, ed. *UpToDate*.Waltham, MA: UpToDate; 2013.

Becker MA. Treatment of acute gout. In: Basow D, ed. *UpToDate*. Waltham, MA: UpToDate; 2013.

Becker MA, Ryan NM. Treatment of calcium pyrophosphate crystal deposition disease. In: Basow D, ed. *UpToDate*. Waltham, MA: UpToDate; 2013.

Beutler A, Stephens MB. General principles of fracture management: Bone healing and fracture description. In: Basow D, ed. *UpToDate*. Waltham, MA: UpToDate; 2013.

Bloom J. Metacarpal neck fractures. In: Basow D, ed. *UpToDate*. Waltham, MA: UpToDate; 2013.

Chorley J. Elbow injuries in the young athlete. In: Basow D, ed. *UpToDate*. Waltham, MA: UpToDate; 2013.

DeLaney TF, Hornicek FJ, Mankin HJ, et al. Clinical presentation, staging, and prognostic factors of the of the Ewing sarcoma family of tumors. In: Basow D, ed. *UpToDate*. Waltham, MA: UpToDate; 2013.

Derby R, Beutler A. General principles of fracture management. In: Basow D ed. *UpToDate*. Waltham, MA: UpToDate; 2013.

deWeber K. Lunate fractures. In: Basow D, ed. *UpToDate*. Waltham, MA: UpToDate; 2013.

Fox R, Creamer P, Moschella SL, et al. Clinical manifestations of Sjögren's syndrome: Extraglandular disease. In: Basow D, ed. *UpToDate*. Waltham, MA: UpToDate; 2013.

George A. Bone and joint complications in sickle cell disease. In: Basow D, ed. *UpToDate*. Waltham, MA: UpToDate; 2013.

Goldenberg DL. Clinical manifestations and diagnosis of fibromyalgia in adults. In: Basow D, ed. *UpToDate*. Waltham, MA: UpToDate; 2013.

Hochman M. Approach to imaging modalities in the setting of suspected osteomyelitis. In: Basow D, ed. *UpToDate*. Waltham, MA: UpToDate; 2013.

Hoppenfeld S. *Physical Examination of the Spine and Extremities*. East Norwalk, CT: Appleton-Century-Croft/Prentice-Hall, Inc., 1976.

Hunder GG. Clinical manifestations and diagnosis of polymyalgia. In: Basow D, ed. *UpToDate*. Waltham, MA: UpToDate; 2013.

Kalunian KC. Pharmacololologic therapy of osteoporosis. In: Basow D, ed. *UpToDate*. Waltham, MA: UpToDate; 2013.

Kay J. Clinical manifestations and diagnosis of Felty's syndrome. In: Basow D, ed. *UpToDate*. Waltham, MA: UpToDate; 2013.

Kedar S, et al. Horner's syndrome. In: Basow D, ed. *UpToDate*. Waltham, MA: UpToDate; 2013.

Lehman TJA. Classification of juvenile rheumatoid arthritis (JRA/JIA). In: Basow D, ed. *UpToDate*. Waltham, MA: UpToDate; 2013.

Lalani T. Overview of osteomyelitis in adults. In: Basow D, ed. *UpToDate*. Waltham, MA: UpToDate; 2013.

Lewiecki EM. Osteoporotic fracture risk assessment. In: Basow D, ed. *UpToDate*. Waltham, MA: UpToDate; 2013

Mathison DJ, Agrawal D. General principles of fracture management: Fracture patterns and description in children. In: Basow D, ed. *UpToDate*. Waltham, MA: UpToDate; 2013.

Merkel PA. Clinical manifestations of and diagnosis of polyarteritis nodosa. In: Basow D, ed. *UpToDate*. Waltham, MA: UpToDate; 2013.

Miller ML, Vleugels RA. Clinical manifestations of dermatomyositis and polymyositis in adults. In: Basow D, ed. *UpToDate*. Waltham, MA: UpToDate; 2013.

Nigrovic PA. Overview of hip pain in childhood. In: Basow D, ed. *UpToDate*. Waltham, MA: UpToDate; 2013.

Robinson J, Kothari MJ. Clinical features and diagnosis of cervical radiculopathy. In: Basow D, ed. *UpToDate*. Waltham, MA: UpToDate; 2013.

Rosenfeld SB. Clinical features and diagnosis of developmental dysplasia of the hip. In: Basow D, ed. *UpToDate*. Waltham, MA: UpToDate; 2013.

Sarwark JF, ed. *Essentials of Musculoskeletal Care,* 4th edition. Rosemont, IL: American Academy of Orthopaedic Surgeons; 2010.

Schiff D. Clinical features and diagnosis of neoplastic epidural spinal cord compression, including cauda equina syndrome. In: Basow D, ed. *UpToDate*. Waltham, MA: UpToDate; 2013.

Schur PH, Gladman DD. Overview of the clinical manifestations of systemic lupus erythematosus in adults. In: Basow D, ed. *UpToDate*. Waltham, MA: UpToDate; 2013.

Sexton DJ. Vertebral osteomyelitis and discitis. In: Basow D, ed. *UpToDate*. Waltham, MA: UpToDate; 2013.

Stracciolini A, Hammerberg EM. Acute compartment syndrome of the extremities. In: Basow D, ed. *UpToDate*. Waltham, MA: UpToDate; 2013.

Taylor PC. Clinically useful biologic markers in the diagnosis and assessment of outcome in rheumatoid arthritis. In: Basow D, ed. *UpToDate*. Waltham, MA: UpToDate; 2013.

Thomas CL, ed. *Tabor's Cyclopedic Medical Dictionary,* 17th edition. Philadelphia, PA: F.A. Davis Company; 1993.

Tis JE. Overview of benign bone tumors in children and adolescents. In: Basow D, ed. *UpToDate*. Waltham, MA: UpToDate; 2013.

Varga J. Overview of the clinical manifestations of systemic sclerosis (scleroderma) in adults. In: Basow D, ed. *UpToDate*. Waltham, MA: UpToDate; 2013.

Yu DT. Reactive arthritis (formerly Reiter syndrome). In: Basow D, ed. *UpToDate*. Waltham, MA: UpToDate; 2013.

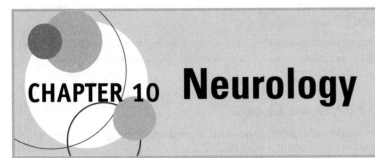

CHAPTER 10 Neurology

Angela Conrad, MPA, PA-C

○ **What are the reversible causes of dementia?**

While normal pressure hydrocephalus, brain tumors, hypothyroidism, neurosyphilis, and vitamin B_{12} deficiency are reversible causes of dementia, they are less commonly seen. Nevertheless, diagnostic studies should be used to rule them in or out as the underlying cause of dementia since early diagnosis can prevent progression or even reverse cognitive impairment.

○ **What is the most common cause of dementia in Western countries?**

Alzheimer disease is the most common cause of dementia, followed by vascular dementia and dementia associated with Parkinson disease. Alzheimer disease is the primary cause of dementia in 60% to 70% of all cases of dementia.

○ **What are the risk factors for Alzheimer disease?**

Increasing age, female gender, Down syndrome (Trisomy 21), and family history are risk factors for Alzheimer disease.

○ **What are the characteristic pathologic features associated with Alzheimer disease?**

Alzheimer disease is characterized by abnormal metabolism and deposition of β-amyloid proteins resulting in the formation of neuritic or senile plaques and neurofibrillary tangles.

○ **What is often the first sign of Alzheimer disease?**

A patient's family members are usually the first to note an impairment in recent memory, initially being disoriented to time and then to place. However, a small percentage (<25%) of patients present with complaints unrelated to memory, such as organizational difficulty, word-finding difficulty, and navigational difficulty.

○ **What are the manifestations of the late stages of Alzheimer disease?**

As the disease progresses, patients develop psychiatric symptoms, such as delusions, hallucinations, and paranoia. Patients may also develop seizures.

○ **What are the clinical features common to subcortical dementia?**

Subcortical dementias are characterized by movement disorders in conjunction with mild memory loss, slowed thoughts, and depressed mood. Language and visuospatial functions are preserved.

○ **What are the causes of subcortical dementia?**

Parkinson disease, Huntington disease, hypothyroidism, normal pressure hydrocephalus, and multiple sclerosis are all common known causes of subcortical dementia. Other causes of subcortical dementia include inflammatory, vascular, and infectious processes.

○ **What types of neurologic deficits are found with cortical dementias?**

Cortical dementias are associated with loss of higher cortical functions, such as language. Patients have varying degrees of aphasia, agnosia, and apraxia. Alzheimer disease is the most common type of cortical dementia.

○ **Which medications are recommended to improve the cognitive dysfunction associated with Alzheimer disease?**

Acetylcholinesterase inhibitors, such as donepezil (Aricept) or rivastigmine (Exelon), address the deficits associated with degeneration of cholinergic neurons.

○ **Which medications are indicated for the management of the behavioral disturbances seen in association with Alzheimer disease?**

Antipsychotic medications, such as haloperidol (Haldol) or risperidone (Risperdal), can be used to address hallucinations, delusions, or aggression. Antidepressants and anxiolytics can also be used to address symptoms of depression and anxiety, respectively.

○ **What are the common symptoms associated with dementia with Lewy bodies?**

Dementia with Lewy bodies is characterized by varying cognitive impairment, visual hallucinations, and signs of Parkinsonism (i.e., bradykinesia, tremor, and rigidity). Lewy bodies are intraneuronal cytoplasmic inclusions that contain similar proteins that are found in Alzheimer disease and Parkinson disease.

○ **What medication is used to treat motor symptoms associated with Lewy body dementia?**

Antiparkinsonian medications (levodopa or anticholinergic medications) are used to treat motor symptoms of Lewy body dementia.

○ **What class of medications should be avoided in patients with Lewy body dementia?**

Antipsychotic medications should be avoided since they will exacerbate the extrapyramidal symptoms.

○ **What are the risk factors associated with vascular (or multi-infarct) dementia?**

Risk factors for multi-infarct dementia include a history of hypertension, diabetes, peripheral vascular disease, or other evidence of advanced atherosclerotic disease.

○ **What is an important historical distinction between vascular dementia and Alzheimer disease?**

The onset of symptoms can be helpful to distinguish between the two disorders. Alzheimer disease has a slowly progressive loss of cognitive function, whereas patients with multi-infarct dementia have acute episodes of neurologic deterioration that progress in an irregular stepwise manner with each ischemic insult.

○ **What is Huntington disease?**

Huntington disease is an autosomal dominant inherited condition characterized by a movement disorder (choreiform movements) in addition to progressive memory loss.

○ **What are the physical examination findings associated with AIDS dementia?**

Behavioral changes (social withdrawal) and motor symptoms can be seen. Ataxia, increased muscle tone, and hyperreflexia can all be seen during the early stage of the disease; however, the motor symptoms become much more pronounced as the disease progresses to later stages.

○ **What are the typical findings on cerebrospinal fluid analysis for a patient with AIDS dementia?**

Mild to moderate elevations in protein levels (≤200 mg/dL), modest mononuclear pleocytosis (≤50 cells/μL), and the presence of oligoclonal IgG bands.

○ **What are the common, underlying characteristics associated with cerebral palsy?**

Cerebral palsy refers to a chronic condition characterized by impaired muscle tone, strength, and coordination of movements. It is associated with a cerebral injury that can occur either before birth, during birth, or in the perinatal period.

○ **What are the most common causes of cerebral palsy?**

Intrauterine hypoxia, intrauterine bleeding, infections, toxins, congenital malformations, neonatal infections, neonatal hypoglycemia, and kernicterus. The underlying etiology is never identified in about 25% of cases.

○ **What is the most common clinical manifestation seen in cerebral palsy?**

The most common manifestation of cerebral palsy is spasticity of the limbs, which can involve one or more limbs. Spasticity can present as a monoplegia, hemiplegia, paraplegia, or quadriplegia.

○ **What type of neurologic deficits can be associated with cerebral palsy?**

Associated neurologic deficits can include seizures, varying levels of mental retardation, ranging from mild to severe. Patients can have various language, vision, speech, sensory, and hearing deficits.

○ **What physical examination findings can be seen with cerebral palsy?**

Spasticity, hyperreflexia, and ataxia.

○ **What are the most common causes of death in patients with cerebral palsy?**

Aspiration pneumonia and multiple infections occurring simultaneously.

○ **What is involved in the management of cerebral palsy?**

The goal is to maximize the patient's functionality. This can improve through occupational, physical, and speech therapies. Managing seizures with medications. Oftentimes spasticity can be managed with botulin injections. It is also important to offer support programs for family as well as educational programs for the patient.

○ **What is the most common form of facial paralysis?**

Bell palsy is an idiopathic lower motor neuron facial weakness.

○ **What are the signs and symptoms commonly associated with Bell palsy?**

Signs and symptoms include unilateral facial paralysis, impaired taste, decreased lacrimation, or hyperacusis.

○ **What is Ramsay Hunt syndrome?**

Ramsay Hunt syndrome is a facial nerve palsy associated with a herpes zoster infection in the facial nerve and the geniculate ganglion. Patients have an eruption of an erythematous vesicular rash involving the ear, external auditory canal, and face.

○ **How can you differentiate between a central facial palsy and a peripheral facial palsy?**

A peripheral facial palsy is a lower motor neuron lesion affecting the entire side of the face ipsilateral to the lesion. A central facial palsy is an upper motor neuron lesion affecting the lower part of the face contralateral to the lesion. Central facial palsies are often associated with motor weakness of the upper extremity on the same side as the facial palsy.

○ **What are the predisposing factors associated with Guillain–Barré syndrome?**

Predisposing factors include minor acute infections (i.e., upper respiratory infection or gastrointestinal infection). It has also been reported in patients with recent herpes, CMV, and Epstein–Barr viral infections as well as recent immunizations.

○ **What are the signs and symptoms associated with Guillain–Barré syndrome?**

Guillain–Barré syndrome is characterized by an ascending symmetrical lower-extremity weakness. Bulbar muscles can also be involved, resulting in facial weakness and dysphagia. If the diaphragm is involved, patients will present with respiratory insufficiency. Deep tendon reflexes will be depressed or absent. Patients may also complain of sensory loss, in a "glove-and-stocking" distribution. Sensory losses are generally less severe than muscle weakness.

○ **What clinical findings would help to rule out Guillain–Barré syndrome as a diagnosis for a patient with the new onset of weakness?**

Pertinent negatives would include a markedly asymmetrical pattern of weakness, bowel or bladder incontinence at the onset of symptoms, and/or a well-defined sensory level.

○ **What is a characteristic finding on cerebrospinal fluid (CSF) analysis for patients with Guillain–Barré syndrome?**

The CSF will show an elevation in protein levels without an elevation in the white cell count.

○ **Does early treatment with intravenous immunoglobulin (IVIg) or plasmapheresis accelerate the recovery for patients diagnosed with Guillain–Barré syndrome?**

Yes, IVIg or plasmapheresis will shorten the recovery time as well as decrease the likelihood of long-term neurologic disability.

○ **What is the prognosis for patients with Guillain–Barré syndrome?**

Approximately 85% of patients have a full recovery. Less than 5% of patients will die. Advanced age, respiratory insufficiency requiring ventilator support, and rapid progression of symptoms are all associated with a poor prognosis.

○ **What role do corticosteroids have in the treatment of Guillain–Barré syndrome?**

Corticosteroids are associated with adverse outcomes and may actually delay recovery and are therefore contraindicated in the treatment of Guillain–Barré syndrome (an acute inflammatory polyneuropathy); chronic inflammatory demyelinating polyneuropathy, however, is responsive to corticosteroids.

○ **What medical conditions can be associated with myasthenia gravis?**

Hyperthyroidism, disseminated lupus erythematous, tumors of the thymus, and rheumatoid arthritis.

○ **What is the hallmark of myasthenia gravis?**

Fluctuating weakness and fatigability of voluntary muscle activity, with involvement of ocular, bulbar, limb, or respiratory muscles. Bulbar involvement presents as dysarthria and dysphagia.

○ **What is the underlying pathophysiology of myasthenia gravis?**

Myasthenia is characterized by autoantibodies to acetylcholine at the neuromuscular junction. Accordingly, there is a block in neuromuscular transmission as well as a decrease in the number of functioning receptors, which accounts for the fatigable weakness.

○ **What conditions or medications are associated with exacerbations of myasthenia gravis?**

Minor infections, pre-menses, pregnancy, stress, and hot weather can all lead to an exacerbation. Medications that are associated with exacerbations include quinine, quinidine, procainamide, propranolol, lithium, tetracycline, and aminoglycoside antibiotics.

○ **What physical examination findings are consistent with myasthenia gravis?**

Fatigability of the affected muscle(s) with persistent activity and slight increase in strength with rest. Sensation and reflexes are not typically affected.

○ **A 32-year-old female patient presents with diplopia and ptosis, which are both worse by the end of the day. She also notes dysarthria if she has been talking a lot. What diagnostic test is indicated for the evaluation of this patient?**

The most commonly used test is the edrophonium or Tensilon test.

○ **What additional diagnostic studies can be used for a patient with suspected myasthenia gravis?**

Acetylcholine receptor antibodies are elevated in up to 90% of patients; repetitive nerve stimulation will show a decrement in response amplitude. A single fiber EMG, which is a specialized EMG that analyzes individual muscle fiber's firing pattern, is the most sensitive test.

○ **What is the treatment of choice for myasthenia gravis?**

The treatment of choice is pyridostigmine (Mestinon).

○ **What are additional treatment options for the management of myasthenia gravis?**

Thymectomy will provide symptomatic relief or remission. Corticosteroids can be used for patients who are nonresponders to anticholinesterase medications.

○ **What is myasthenic crisis?**

Patients in myasthenic crisis have significant impairment in respiratory function, requiring intubation and ventilator support. Plasmapheresis is also indicated.

○ **What is the clinical presentation of mononeuropathy simplex and multiplex?**

Mononeuropathy simplex involves one peripheral nerve (motor and sensation), whereas mononeuropathy multiplex presents with asymmetric involvement of multiple peripheral nerves.

○ **What are the different types of diabetic neuropathy?**

Polyneuropathy (mixed sensory, motor, and autonomic in 70% of cases and primary sensory in 30% of cases) and mononeuropathy (multiplex vs. simplex).

○ **What is the classic presentation of a diabetic sensory neuropathy?**

The classic presentation is a symmetric loss of function in a stocking-glove distribution. Sensation is affected primarily, with a loss of vibratory sense, pain, and temperature. The lower extremities are generally affected first, followed by the upper extremities. Patients complain of numbness, tingling, and other paresthesias.

○ **What is the treatment for diabetic polyneuropathy?**

The key to treatment is maintaining optimal glycemic control; painful paresthesias can be treated with anticonvulsants, antidepressants, and/or topical capsaicin cream.

○ **What complications are associated with a diabetic sensory polyneuropathy?**

Complications include foot ulcerations; because of the sensory neuropathy, patients are unaware of minor trauma to the feet which can progress to ulcerations.

○ **What is sympathetic regional pain syndrome?**

Sympathetic pain after tissue injury such as soft tissue trauma, myocardial infarction, or fracture. There are two types. Type 1 is described as pain to the area of injury that may spread, does not follow a single nerve distribution. Type 2 is described as a burning, persistent pain that is a result of trauma to a nerve.

○ **What are the symptoms associated with sympathetic regional pain syndrome?**

Severe pain, which may be accompanied by swelling, change in blood flow (temperature changes in affected area), and local sweating.

○ **What is the first-line treatment for sympathetic regional pain syndrome?**

Physical therapy, occupational therapy, and exercising the affected limb. Topical lidocaine has shown to be beneficial in some cases as well as glucocorticoid course.

○ **What are the common causes of acute or new onset headaches?**

Causes of acute onset or new headache include subarachnoid hemorrhage, meningitis/encephalitis, hematoma, tumor, and acute-angle closure glaucoma.

○ **What are the common causes of subacute headaches that generally develop over weeks to months?**

Causes of subacute onset headache include temporal (or giant cell) arteritis, intracranial mass lesions (primary or metastatic tumors, abscesses), and neuralgia (trigeminal neuralgia or postherpetic neuralgia).

○ **What are the most common causes of chronic headaches that can occur intermittently over years?**

Migraines, cluster headaches, and tension headaches.

○ **What are the common precipitating factors for migraine headaches?**

Common precipitating factors include certain foods and food additives, fasting, menses, medications (oral contraceptives and nitroglycerin), stress, and bright lights.

○ **A 56-year-old man presents with a mild to moderate dull headache that has steadily progressed over the past month. The headache is worse when he gets up in the morning or with coughing and sneezing. He also notes the recent onset of nausea and vomiting. What is the most likely diagnosis?**

An intracranial tumor. Most often the headache is described as pain worsened by position changes or increases in intracranial pressure (such as coughing or sneezing).

○ **A 67-year-old woman complains of intermittent episodes of pain in her cheek and jaw that feel like a "lightning bolt hit her face." The pain is triggered by eating or touching her face. Her physical examination is unremarkable. What is the most likely diagnosis?**

Trigeminal neuralgia is associated with severe facial pain in the distribution of the trigeminal nerve; most commonly affecting V2 or V3. Episodes of pain may be triggered by any sort of sensory stimulus to the face, that is, touching, chewing, talking, shaving, cold weather, or wind.

○ **What is the first-line treatment for the patient described in the previous question?**

First-line treatment would be carbamazepine with dosing between 400 and 1200 mg/day.

○ **A 26-year-old woman complains of a dull, throbbing right-sided headache that lasts for hours but is relieved by sleep. The headache is associated with nausea, vomiting, and sensitivity to light and sound. She has similar headaches at least once a month and says that prior to the headache, there are "holes in her vision" along with "zigzag lines." What is the most likely diagnosis?**

Migraine headache. Approximately 20% of patients experience a visual aura prior to the onset of pain. Migraines with an aura are classified as classic migraines, whereas migraines without an aura are classified as common migraines.

○ **What is the clinical presentation of a common migraine headache?**

Common migraines, now referred to as migraine without aura, occur more frequently than classic migraines. About 70% of all migraine-type headaches are common migraines. Common migraines are associated with unilateral pulsatile pain, nausea, vomiting, phonophobia, and photophobia. There is usually a strong family history of migraine headaches.

○ **What is the abortive treatment for migraine headaches?**

Mild analgesics, such as nonsteroidal anti-inflammatory medications or acetaminophen, are effective in relieving headache pain. Other first-line options are the 5-HT agonists or triptans, that is, sumatriptan. For analgesics and triptans to be effective, they must be administered at the onset of the headache. Antiemetics are helpful as well.

○ **What are the contraindications for the use of 5-HT agonists or triptans?**

Poorly controlled hypertension, coronary artery disease, or peripheral vascular disease.

○ **What are the indications for the use of prophylactic medications in the management of migraine headaches?**

Frequent headaches (more than one per week), headaches difficult to control, or for patients who cannot tolerate triptans or ergot alkaloids.

○ **What classes of medications are effective for prophylactic management of migraines?**

Beta-blockers, tricyclic antidepressants, anticonvulsants, and calcium channel blockers.

○ **What is the recommended treatment for migraines during pregnancy?**

Migraines during pregnancy should be treated with opiates. Sumatriptan is safe if used within the first trimester. All other migraine treatments have risks of teratogenicity or complications with the pregnancy.

○ **A 39-year-old man presents with intermittent episodes of severe headaches around the left eye and temple. His symptoms typically last less than an hour and resolve on their own. The headaches awaken him nightly for several days in a row then he is headache-free for a couple of months before another "round" begins. What is the most likely diagnosis?**

Cluster headaches present with severe nonthrobbing headaches that typically occur at the same location and the same time each day. Headaches generally last for a few minutes up to a couple of hours. The headaches occur daily for weeks to months before they spontaneously resolve; patients may be pain-free for months to years.

○ **What are the associated signs and symptoms seen with cluster headaches?**

Conjunctival injection, tearing, and nasal congestion ipsilateral to the headache. Horner syndrome (anhidrosis, miosis, and ptosis) can also be seen on the affected side.

○ **What are the abortive therapy options to treat cluster headaches?**

100% oxygen, sumatriptan, or dihydroergotamine.

○ **What is the role of corticosteroids in the treatment of cluster headaches?**

Prednisone can be initiated at the beginning of a cluster cycle to effectively eliminate the patient's symptoms; most patients will be pain-free within 2 days.

○ **What are the presenting signs and symptoms associated with tension headaches?**

Patients describe a nonthrobbing, bilateral headache ("tight band") without the associated visual disturbances, nausea, and vomiting seen in conjunction with migraine headaches.

○ **What types of medications are effective in the treatment of tension headaches?**

Acetaminophen, nonsteroidal anti-inflammatory drugs, and ergotamine can be helpful as abortive therapy for tension headaches; tricyclic antidepressants and beta-blockers can be used for prophylaxis.

○ **What is the differential diagnosis for fever, headache, and nuchal rigidity?**

Bacterial meningitis, aseptic meningitis, encephalitis, and brain abscess.

○ **What are the most common pathogens associated with bacterial meningitis in a neonate?**

Group B *Streptococcus,* **Escherichia coli**, *Listeria.*

○ **What are the most common pathogens associated with bacterial meningitis in adults 20 to 50 years of age?**

Streptococcus pneumoniae and *Neisseria meningitidis.*

○ **What are the most common bacterial pathogens for adults who are older than 50 years or immunocompromised?**

Streptococcus pneumoniae, Neisseria meningitidis, **Haemophilus influenzae***, Listeria,* and gram-negative bacilli.

○ **What is the most common cause of meningitis in patients with AIDS?**

Cryptococcus neoformans.

○ **What risk factors are associated with bacterial meningitis?**

Exposure during delivery (***Escherichia coli***, group B *Streptococcus*); colonization from respiratory tract, sinusitis, otitis (*Streptococcus pneumoniae*); crowded conditions (military, college-*Neisseria meningitidis*); head trauma (*Staphylococcus*), and neurosurgical procedures (*Staphylococcus,* gram-negative organisms).

○ **What are the presenting signs and symptoms associated with bacterial meningitis?**

Fever, nuchal rigidity, headache, altered mental status, photophobia, nausea, and vomiting; cranial nerve palsies and seizures can be seen in 40% of patients.

○ **Which pathogen associated with bacterial meningitis presents with a petechial and purpuric rash?**

Neisseria meningitidis

○ **What are the signs of meningeal irritation?**

Kernig and Brudzinski signs are used to assess for meningeal irritation. Kernig is performed by having the patient supine with the hip and knee flexed; pain and resistance to extension of the knee is considered a positive sign. Brudzinski is performed with the patient supine; forward flexion of the neck results in involuntary flexion of the hips and knees is considered a positive sign. These signs may not be present in very young or very old patients or in patients who have severe impairment in consciousness.

○ **What is the gold standard diagnostic procedure used to establish the diagnosis of bacterial meningitis?**

Lumbar puncture for cerebrospinal fluid analysis; gram stain will identify the organism in 60% to 90% of the time. Perform LP with CSF analysis first unless contraindicated.

○ **What are the contraindications to performing a lumbar puncture for a patient with suspected bacterial meningitis?**

It is contraindicated in some patients who have increased intracranial pressure (papilledema, focal deficits, or altered mental status) such as those with an intracranial mass. However, patients with pseudotumor cerebri benefit from repeated LPs. Other contraindications to lumbar puncture include local skin infection, coagulopathies, and spinal cord mass lesions. Any delay or contraindication to performing a lumbar puncture necessitates obtaining blood cultures followed by empiric antibiotic therapy.

○ **What are the cerebrospinal fluid (CSF) findings in bacterial meningitis?**

Elevated WBC (>1000 cells/mm^3), decreased CSF glucose (<45 mg/dL), and elevated CSF protein levels (>200 mg/dL). Serum glucose levels should be checked at the time of lumbar puncture to correlate the CSF and serum glucose levels. The CSF-to-blood glucose ratio is normally 0.6; in bacterial meningitis, this ratio is less than 0.4.

○ **What is the recommended antibiotic treatment for a newborn (<1 month old) with bacterial meningitis?**

Ampicillin and cefotaxime.

○ **What is the recommended antibiotic treatment for an 18-year-old patient with bacterial meningitis?**

Cefotaxime (or ceftriaxone) and vancomycin.

○ **What is the recommended antibiotic treatment for a 60-year-old adult with bacterial meningitis?**

Ampicillin, cefotaxime (or ceftriaxone), and vancomycin.

○ **What role do corticosteroids play in bacterial meningitis?**

Dexamethasone has been shown to decrease the morbidity and mortality, in particular patients with pneumococcal meningitis.

○ **What complications are associated with bacterial meningitis?**

Impaired mental status/cognition, cerebral edema, seizures, focal neurologic deficits, sensorineural hearing loss, and brain abscess.

○ **What type of prophylaxis is indicated for meningitis secondary to *Neisseria meningitidis* or *Haemophilus influenzae*?**

Prophylaxis with rifampin is indicated for any close contacts of patients with meningococcal meningitis or meningitis caused by *H. influenzae*.

○ **What type of vaccination is required for the prevention of bacterial meningitis?**

Vaccination for *Streptococcus pneumoniae* and *Haemophilus influenzae* are recommended for children aged 2 to 15 months. Vaccination for *Neisseria* meningitidis is recommended for children 1 to 18 years. Vaccination for *S. pneumoniae* is recommended for adults 65 years and older.

○ **What is the most common cause of aseptic meningitis?**

The most common cause of aseptic meningitis is enterovirus (90%); herpes simplex virus (HSV), varicella zoster virus (VZV), mumps, HIV, EBV, and West Nile virus can also cause aseptic meningitis.

○ **What are the cerebrospinal fluid (CSF) findings in aseptic meningitis?**

The WBC is modestly elevated with a predominance of lymphocytes (100–1000 cells/mm^3); CSF protein is usually normal but can be slightly elevated (<80–100 mg/dL); CSF glucose to blood glucose ratio is normal.

○ **What is the most common cause of encephalitis?**

Herpes simplex virus type 1 is the most common; arboviruses (West Nile Virus. St. Louis, eastern equine, western equine) can also cause encephalitis.

○ **What are the presenting signs and symptoms consistent with encephalitis?**

Headache, progressive alterations in mental status, and focal neurological deficits (cranial nerve palsies, hemiparesis); seizures are common.

○ **What will CSF studies show in patients with encephalitis?**

CSF findings will be similar to findings seen with aseptic meningitis. There will be increased WBCs (<250/mm^3) of predominantly lymphocytes; CSF glucose will be normal and CSF protein levels can be normal or slightly elevated.

○ **What is the recommended treatment for encephalitis?**

Based on the causative agent, but most commonly acyclovir.

○ **What is the most common involuntary movement disorder?**

Essential tremor.

○ **What is the etiology of essential tremor?**

The underlying etiology is unknown; about 50% of patients have a positive family history that is consistent with an autosomal dominant pattern of inheritance.

○ **What are the clinical features of essential tremor?**

Bilateral involvement of the upper extremities with sparing of the legs; tremor is usually symmetric although one side can be affected more than the other. The patient can also present with voice tremors and head tremors (yes–yes or no–no).

○ **What are the recommended treatments for essential tremor?**

Propranolol and primidone.

○ **How can essential tremor be differentiated from Parkinson disease?**

Resting tremor, bradykinesia, rigidity, and micrographia are all absent in patients with essential tremor.

○ **What is Tourette syndrome?**

Chronic and often lifelong syndrome consisting of motor and/or verbal tics.

○ **What is the age of onset for Tourette syndrome?**

Typically it presents between 2 and 15 years of age (80% of cases, motor tics; 20% of cases, vocal tics).

○ **How can Tourette syndrome be differentiated from Sydenham chorea?**

Sydenham chorea occurs after a streptococcal infection and is self-limiting, resolving within 6 months.

○ **What is the first-line treatment for severe Tourette syndrome?**

The first-line treatment is clonidine. Mild cases are not treated with medications, but with family and patient education.

○ **What is the most common cause of Parkinson disease?**

Idiopathic degeneration of dopamine-producing neurons in the substantia nigra.

○ **What is the peak age of onset of Parkinson disease?**

The peak age is in the early 60s; onset ranges from 35 to 85 years of age.

○ **What are the risk factors for Parkinson disease?**

Male gender, history of prior head injury, exposure to pesticides, and positive family history.

○ **What factors are associated with a decreased incidence of Parkinson disease?**

Smoking, coffee consumption, use of NSAIDs, and estrogen replacement in women who are postmenopausal.

○ **What medications are associated with Parkinsonism symptoms?**

Conventional antipsychotics; haloperidol and perphenazine have the highest risk.

○ **What signs and symptoms are associated with Parkinson disease?**

Rigidity, bradykinesia, shuffling gait, and resting tremor.

○ **What is cogwheel rigidity?**

Brief interruptions in muscle resistance during the assessment of passive movement.

○ **What type of nonmotor symptoms are seen in association with Parkinson disease?**

Depression, sleep disturbances, cognitive impairments, and autonomic dysfunction.

○ **What are the signs of autonomic dysfunction in Parkinson disease?**

Orthostatic hypotension, urinary urgency, constipation, and excessive sweating.

○ **What is the first-line treatment for Parkinson disease?**

Levodopa-carbidopa or a dopamine agonist.

○ **What complications are associated with levodopa-carbidopa treatment?**

Transient fluctuations in Parkinsonism symptoms occurring at varying times throughout the day ("on–off" phenomena) and dyskinesia. It is also associated with nausea and vomiting.

○ **Which class of drugs is indicated in the management of a patient with Parkinson disease who has a debilitating tremor as the predominant symptom?**

Anticholinergics.

○ **What are the indications for the surgical treatment of Parkinson disease?**

Intractable tremor and drug-induced motor fluctuations or dyskinesias.

○ **What is the preferred surgical procedure for Parkinson disease?**

Deep brain stimulation.

○ **What is the pattern of inheritance for Huntington disease?**

Autosomal dominant.

○ **What type of hyperkinetic movement disorder is characterized by rapid, nonpatterned, dancelike movements?**

Chorea.

○ **What is the usual age of onset for Huntington disease?**

Age 25 to 45.

○ **What is the average lifespan for a patient with Huntington disease once there is the onset of symptoms?**

15 years.

○ **What are the primary symptoms associated with Huntington disease?**

Chorea, dysarthria, and gait disturbances.

○ **How do clinical features change as Huntington disease progresses to an advanced stage?**

Choreiform movements become less prominent; dystonia, rigidity, spasticity, bradykinesia, and myoclonus may begin.

○ **What types of behavioral issues are common with Huntington disease?**

Depression, suicidal ideations, aggressiveness, psychosis, and dementia.

○ **What is the treatment for the choreiform movements associated with Huntington disease?**

Dopamine-blocking agents, such as haloperidol or chlorpromazine, can be used to treat chorea. However, they are not routinely used because they may actually aggravate motor symptoms.

○ **What is the age of onset for multiple sclerosis?**

Usually between 20 and 40 years of age.

○ **What are the diagnostic criteria for multiple sclerosis?**

At least two or more documented episodes of neurologic symptoms and examination findings affecting distinct areas of the central nervous system; symptoms must last at least 24 hours and the interval between episodes needs to be separated by at least 1 month.

○ **What is the underlying etiology for multiple sclerosis?**

The cause is unknown; however, several viral autoimmune and genetic factors have been implicated.

○ **What is the most common clinical type of multiple sclerosis?**

Relapsing remitting.

○ **What are the common presenting symptoms associated with multiple sclerosis?**

Paresthesias, gait disorders (unsteadiness, disequilibrium), focal weakness, sudden loss of vision in one eye, and incoordination.

○ **What common physical examination findings are seen with multiple sclerosis?**

Hyperreflexia, ataxia, extensor response (positive Babinski), impaired rapid alternating movements, impaired vibration, and proprioception.

○ **What is dysdiadochokinesia?**

The inability to perform rapid alternating movements.

○   A 28-year-old female patient presents with a 1-week history of diplopia and vertigo. Three months earlier, she had an episode of blurred vision that resolved spontaneously after 2 days. Physical examination was remarkable for nystagmus and bilateral horizontal gaze palsy on adduction. The remainder of her neurologic examination was normal. An MRI was obtained (see Figure 10-1). What is the most likely diagnosis?

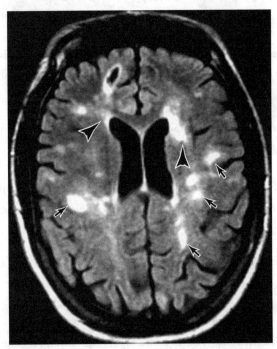

Figure 10-1 (Reproduced, with permission, from Simon RP, Greenberg DA, Aminoff MJ. *Clinical Neurology.* 6th ed. New York, NY: McGraw-Hill; 2009, Fig. 5-2B.)

Multiple sclerosis; the initial presentation was consistent with optic neuritis. Note the signal abnormalities in the white matter, which are consistent with multiple sclerosis.

○   A patient with multiple sclerosis describes an electric shocklike sensation that runs down her back to her legs when she flexes her neck forward. What is this phenomenon called?

Lhermitte sign.

○   What are the findings on examination of the cerebrospinal fluid for a patient with multiple sclerosis?

Mild pleocytosis and the presence of oligoclonal bands.

○   What neurophysiologic tests are indicated in the evaluation of a patient with suspected multiple sclerosis?

Evoked potentials will show slowed conduction because of demyelination. Visual evoked potentials will evaluate the integrity of the optic nerve, brainstem evoked responses evaluate the integrity of the auditory nerve, and somatosensory evoked potentials evaluate the integrity of peripheral sensory pathways.

○   A 34-year-old woman develops blurred vision associated with unilateral retro-orbital pain that is worse with eye movement. On physical examination, her visual acuity is decreased but extraocular eye movements are intact. Funduscopic examination reveals mild papillitis but no exudates or hemorrhages. What is the most likely diagnosis?

Optic neuritis.

○ **What is the treatment of choice for an acute exacerbation of multiple sclerosis?**

Corticosteroids; intravenous methylprednisolone, followed by a prednisone taper.

○ **Which pharmacologic intervention is used as a disease-modifying agent in the treatment of multiple sclerosis?**

Interferon has been shown to decrease the number of lesions seen on MRI as well as the number of exacerbations experienced by the patient.

○ **What is the treatment for the spasticity associated with multiple sclerosis?**

Lioresal (Baclofen).

○ **What is the most common cause of seizures in infants and children?**

Febrile seizures are most common between the ages of 3 months and 5 years.

○ **What is the most common cause of seizures in adults older than 65 years?**

Cerebrovascular disease (ischemic strokes more than hemorrhagic strokes).

○ **What type of seizure disorder is characterized by a sudden loss of postural muscle tone?**

Atonic seizures; may present with a sudden head drop or complete collapse associated with falling.

○ **What type of symptoms can be seen with simple partial seizures?**

Motor, sensory, autonomic, or psychic.

○ **A patient initially experiences clonic movements of the hand, which then spread to involve the forearm and upper arm. What is this phenomenon called?**

Jacksonian march; reflective of seizure involvement spreading to neighboring areas of the motor cortex.

○ **What is Todd paralysis?**

Following a motor seizure of an extremity, there is a focal transient paralysis of the involved muscles that can last from several minutes up to 36 hours.

○ **What happens to the level of consciousness during a simple partial seizure?**

Consciousness is preserved.

○ **What type of autonomic symptoms can be seen with a simple partial seizure?**

Pupillary dilation, pallor, flushing, sweating, vomiting, and urinary incontinence.

○ **What type of psychic symptoms can be seen in association with a simple partial seizure?**

Memory distortions (i.e., déjà vu), fear, detachment, depersonalization, and illusions (objects may appear to grow larger or smaller).

○ **Which type of seizure disorder is characterized by focal seizure activity accompanied by impaired consciousness?**

Complex partial seizures.

○ **What are automatisms?**

Automatisms are involuntary muscle activities seen in association with complex partial seizures; typical automatisms include lip smacking, chewing, picking, or fumbling with clothing.

○ **A 6-year-old child is brought to your office by her mother. The mother states that for the past 6 months she and the girl's teacher have frequently noticed the child staring into space. Each episode lasted about 15 seconds and was associated with eye blinking. What is the most likely diagnosis?**

Absence seizures.

○ **What is the recommended first-line treatment for the patient described in the previous question?**

Ethosuximide or valproic acid is recommended as first-line medications for absence seizures.

○ **A 22-year-old female patient presents with recurrent episodes of altered consciousness during which time she would smack her lips and fumble with her clothing, according to witnesses. She was not responsive during these episodes and afterward she would remain confused for up to an hour. What is the most likely diagnosis?**

Complex partial seizure.

○ **What medications can be used as first-line treatment for the patient described in the previous question?**

Carbamazepine, phenytoin, lamotrigine, and valproic acid are all first-line treatment options for complex partial seizures.

○ **A 25-year-old male patient is brought to the emergency department by his brother. They were watching a football game when he suddenly lost consciousness and fell to the floor. He was initially rigid before beginning to "shaking all over" for about a minute or two. He was sleepy and disoriented afterward. What is the most likely diagnosis?**

Generalized tonic–clonic seizure.

○ **What is the recommended first-line treatment for the patient described in the previous question?**

Valproic acid, lamotrigine, and topiramate.

○ **What type of seizure disorder is characterized by 30 minutes of continuous seizures or frequent seizures that occur without full restoration of consciousness?**

Status epilepticus.

○ **In addition to the "ABCs," what pharmacologic intervention is recommended for the first-line treatment of status epilepticus?**

Lorazepam.

○ **What is the definition of a transient ischemic attack?**

TIAs have been redefined as the acute onset of a neurological deficit that resolves within an hour without a residual deficit.

○ **A patient presents with the loss of vision in the left eye, which he describes as "someone pulling a shade down over his eye." The episode resolved spontaneously within 30 minutes. What is this neurological symptom called?**

Amaurosis fugax.

○ **Amaurosis fugax is consistent with pathology involving which blood vessel?**

Ipsilateral carotid artery; debris from an atherosclerotic plaque in the internal carotid can embolize to the central retinal artery.

○ **What is the risk of stroke following a transient ischemic attack?**

10% to 15% during the first 3 months; however, most strokes occur within the first 2 days following a TIA.

○ **What are the types of stroke?**

Ischemic (more common) and hemorrhagic.

○ **What is the most common cause of ischemic stroke?**

Atherosclerosis.

○ **What is the most important risk factor for stroke secondary to atherosclerosis?**

Hypertension, systolic or diastolic; increased blood pressure can triple the risk of stroke.

○ **What cardiac conditions are associated with increased stroke risk?**

Mural thrombus postinfarction, atrial fibrillation, endocarditis, and paradoxical emboli via a patent foramen ovale.

○ **What hematologic conditions are associated with increased risk for stroke?**

Thrombocytosis, polycythemia, and sickle cell disease; hypercoagulopathy is also associated, but it is uncommon.

○ **What is a lacunar infarct?**

Lacunar infarcts are strokes that are secondary to small vessel disease.

○ **What are common locations for lacunar infarcts?**

Basal ganglia, thalamus, and pons.

○ **What are the signs of an anterior cerebral artery stroke?**

Contralateral sensorimotor deficit affecting the leg and urinary incontinence.

○   **What are the signs of a middle cerebral artery stroke?**

Contralateral sensorimotor deficit affecting the arm, cranial nerve VII palsy, visual field deficit, and language disturbances.

○   **What type of language deficit is seen with a middle cerebral artery stroke affecting Broca area in the dominant hemisphere?**

Expressive (nonfluent) aphasia; presentation may vary from word-finding difficulty to total mutism.

○   **What type of language deficit is seen with a middle cerebral artery stroke affecting Wernicke area in the dominant hemisphere?**

Receptive aphasia. Patients will not be able to follow commands since their ability to understand language will be lost; speech will be fluent but nonsensical.

○   **What type of visual field deficit is seen with a middle cerebral stroke?**

Contralateral homonymous hemianopsia.

○   **What are the signs of a posterior cerebral artery stroke?**

Contralateral visual field deficit (homonymous hemianopsia with or without macular sparing), and visual agnosia; cortical blindness can be seen with bilateral involvement.

○   **What is prosopagnosia?**

The inability to recognize familiar faces; it is seen with a posterior cerebral artery stroke.

○   **What are the signs of vertebrobasilar insufficiency?**

Cranial nerve palsies (diplopia, dysarthria), hemiplegia or quadriplegia, and altered mental status.

○   **A patient presents with the acute onset of quadriplegia. He is able to communicate only by blinking or moving his eyes up and down. What is the most likely diagnosis?**

Locked-in syndrome; consistent with a pontine stroke.

○   **What is the key diagnostic study in the evaluation of an acute stroke?**

Noncontrast CT scan of the head to distinguish an ischemic from hemorrhagic stroke.

○ A 59-year-old male patient with a history of diabetes and chronic atrial fibrillation presented with the acute onset of a left hemiparesis involving the upper arm. There is a right-sided facial nerve palsy involving the lower face. A noncontrast CT scan of the head was obtained (see Figure 10-2). What is the most likely diagnosis?

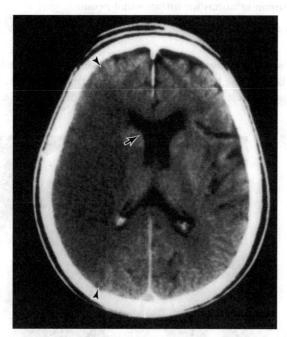

Figure 10-2 (Reproduced, with permission, from Simon RP, Greenberg DA, Aminoff MJ. *Clinical Neurology.* 6th ed. New York, NY: McGraw-Hill, 2009; Fig. 9-14A.)

Acute ischemic stroke.

○ **What vascular territory is involved in the patient described in the previous question?**

Middle cerebral artery (MCA). The wedge-shaped density changes on CT are consistent with the vascular territory for the middle cerebral artery; symptoms are also consistent with an MCA stroke.

○ **What is the recommended treatment of an asymptomatic carotid bruit?**

Aspirin.

○ **What is the recommended long-term treatment for transient ischemic attacks secondary to cardiac emboli?**

Warfarin.

○ **What is the time window to administer recombinant t-PA to treat an acute stroke if contraindications have been ruled out?**

3 hours from the onset of symptoms.

○ **What are contraindications for the use of thrombolytics in the management of an acute stroke?**

Poorly controlled hypertension (systolic BP > 185 mm Hg; diastolic BP > 110 mm Hg), major surgery within past 2 weeks, prior intracranial hemorrhage, other intracranial disease (history of trauma), history of bleeding from either the gastrointestinal or genitourinary tracts within past 3 weeks, and abnormal coagulation profile.

○ **What is the most common cause of intracerebral hemorrhage?**

Hypertension.

○ **What are the most common locations for intracerebral hemorrhages?**

Basal ganglia (most common), thalamus, pons, and cerebellum.

○ **A 62-year-old, hypertensive man presented with the acute onset of a severe headache associated with nausea and vomiting. By the time he arrived in the emergency department, he was lethargic and not able to follow commands. A noncontrast CT scan of the head was done (see Figure 10-3). What is the most likely diagnosis?**

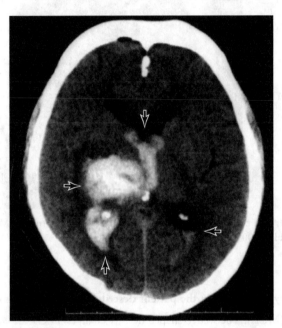

Figure 10-3 (Reproduced, with permission, from Simon RP, Greenberg DA, Aminoff MJ. *Clinical Neurology.* 6th ed. New York, NY: McGraw-Hill; 2009, Fig. 9-18.)

Intracerebral hemorrhage in the area of the thalamus with extension into the ventricles. (Primary extension into right lateral and third ventricle; although there is some extension into the occipital horn of the left lateral ventricle.)

○ **When is surgical decompression indicated in the management of an intracerebral hemorrhage?**

Cerebellar hemorrhages require decompression to avoid brainstem compression; surgery is not indicated for bleeds in the basal ganglia, thalamus, or pons.

○ **In addition to hypertension, what are other causes for intracerebral hemorrhages?**

Trauma, arteriovenous malformations, amyloid angiopathy, recreational drug use (amphetamines or cocaine), anticoagulation therapy, and coagulopathies.

○ **What is the most common cause of a nontraumatic subarachnoid hemorrhage?**

Congenital berry aneurysms.

○   **What additional congenital abnormalities may be seen with berry aneurysms?**

Polycystic kidney disease and coarctation of the aorta.

○   **What are the most frequent locations for intracranial aneurysms?**

Middle cerebral artery (29%), internal carotid artery (16%), anterior communicating artery (15%), basilar artery (14%), and anterior cerebral artery (9%).

○   **A 44-year-old patient presented with the "worst headache of her life." The headache came on suddenly and was associated with neck stiffness and vomiting. There was nuchal rigidity on examination, but no focal motor or sensory deficits. What is the most likely diagnosis?**

Subarachnoid hemorrhage.

○   **What is the first-line diagnostic study indicated in the evaluation of a possible subarachnoid hemorrhage?**

Noncontrast CT scan of the head; will be diagnostic in at least 90% of patients.

○   **For patients who have a suspected subarachnoid hemorrhage but a nondiagnostic CT scan, which diagnostic study is indicated?**

Lumbar puncture with cerebrospinal fluid analysis.

○   **What are the typical findings on analysis of cerebrospinal fluid (CSF) for a patient with a subarachnoid hemorrhage?**

Grossly bloody CSF and an elevated opening pressure; xanthochromia will be seen with centrifuged CSF.

○   **What is the definitive diagnostic study used in the evaluation of a subarachnoid hemorrhage?**

Four-vessel angiography.

○   **What is the recommended treatment of an intracranial aneurysm?**

Surgical clipping or endovascular placement of a coil into the aneurysm.

○   **What complications are associated with a subarachnoid hemorrhage?**

Vasospasm, hydrocephalus, recurrent hemorrhage, and seizures.

○   **What pharmacologic intervention is recommended to minimize the effects of vasospasm?**

Nimodipine, a calcium channel blocker, can help to minimize the ischemic effects associated with vasospasm.

○   **What is a concussion?**

Injury to the body or head that results in a force to the brain, it can be accompanied by transient loss of consciousness; but not always.

○   **What are the symptoms of a concussion?**

Headache, dizziness (feeling off balance), confusion, retrograde/antegrade amnesia, and blurred vision. Symptoms typically resolve within 7 to 10 days postinjury.

○ **What are the indications for CT scan of the head in a patient with a suspected concussion?**

Prolonged loss of consciousness (>1 minute), persistent headache, altered mental status, repeated episodes of vomiting postinjury, history of repeated head injury/severe mechanism, or signs on physical examination of basilar skull fracture .

○ **What is the acute management of patients with concussion?**

Rest, symptomatic treatment (for headaches and nausea), no contact sports, and decreased exposure to technology (television, cellular phones, computers, and electronic games). Athletes should be symptom free while at rest and exercise before returning to sports activities. Many states have laws requiring the patient be reevaluated and cleared before starting sports activities, and at times a stepwise progress for returning to activities is followed.

○ **What is post concussion syndrome?**

Symptoms of headache, dizziness, difficulty concentrating, and fatigue that begins days to weeks after a head injury and can last weeks to several months.

○ **For patients with post concussion syndrome complaining of headache and dizziness, what is the first-line treatment?**

Although narcotics can be used to treat headache, this is not suggested because of the potential of dependence. The best treatment would be acetaminophen as first line. Treatment for the dizziness consists of vestibular exercises as well as promethazine (Phenergan), which acts as a vestibular suppressant.

○ **What is delirium?**

Delirium is an acute state of confusion usually secondary to an underlying neurological or medical illness. Diagnosis is made by the presence of acute fluctuating confusion, inattention, and altered level of consciousness or disorganized thinking.

○ **What are the two subtypes of delirium?**

Hyperactive subtype—an example would be a patient in alcohol withdrawal. These patients have hyperarousal, hallucinations, and agitation. Whereas patients with the hypoactive subtype are quiet, apathetic, and display slow psychomotor skills, such as a patient with opiate intoxication.

○ **What are the risk factors for delirium?**

Age greater than 65 years, baseline cognitive dysfunction, impaired hearing/vision, malnutrition, underlying illness, and immobility. Sixty-six percent of patients with delirium also have dementia.

○ **What are common etiologies of delirium?**

Medications (prescribed or illicit), alcohol/benzodiazepine withdrawal, electrolyte abnormalities, liver/kidney failure, hypercapnia, hypoxia, systemic infections (UTI in elderly, pneumonia, etc.), stroke, seizures, end of life, and unfamiliar setting (inpatient status).

○ **What diagnostic studies are indicated in a patient with delirium?**

After obtaining an appropriate history and physical examination, your diagnostic studies should include laboratory studies to evaluate for the potential etiologies mentioned above. Also, consider a CT scan of the head to rule out the possibility of brain mass versus hemorrhage and lumbar puncture to rule out encephalitis/meningitis.

○ **What is the appropriate treatment for patients with delirium?**

Treatment should focus on the etiology and findings from diagnostic studies. However, focusing on the patients risk factors to minimize delirium is important. This can include hearing and visual aids, family members visiting the patient to decrease anxiety, encouraging open curtains during the day to minimize sundowning, display visible clocks, and mobilizing the patient if able.

○ **What are the common causes of syncope?**

Vasovagal, situational, carotid sinus syncope, orthostatic hypotension, decreased cardiac output, arrhythmias, neurologic, and psychiatric diseases. Vasovagal is the most common cause of syncope.

REFERENCES

Aminoff MJ, Greenberg DA, Simon RP. *Clinical Neurology.* 8th ed. New York, NY: McGraw-Hill; 2012.

Fauci AS, Kasper DL, Hauser ST, et al. *Harrison's Principles of Internal Medicine.* 18th ed. New York, NY: McGraw-Hill; 2012.

Fiebach NH, Kern DE, Thomas PA, Ziegelstein RC. *Barker's, Burton, and Zieve's Principles of Ambulatory Medicine.* 7th ed. Philadelphia, PA: Lippincott Williams & Wilkins; 2007.

Hay WW, Levin MJ, Sondheimer JM, et al. *Current Diagnosis and Treatment in Pediatrics.* 21st ed. New York, NY: McGraw-Hill; 20011.

Mumenthaler M, Mattle H, Taub E. *Fundamentals of Neurology: An Illustrated Guide.* New York, NY: Thieme; 2006.

CHAPTER 11 Psychiatry/ Behavioral Science

Daniel Thibodeau, MHP, PA-C, DFAAPA

ANXIETY DISORDERS

○ **What are the two most common behavior problems seen by general practitioners?**

Anxiety and depression.

○ **What are the recognized DSM-IV Anxiety Disorders?**

- Panic disorder
- Specific phobia
- Social phobia
- Generalized anxiety disorder
- Acute stress disorder
- Post-traumatic stress disorder
- Anxiety disorder caused by medical condition
- Substance-induced anxiety disorder

○ **What is the average age at onset of separation anxiety?**

The average age is 8 to 9 years. They exhibit severe distress when separated from their parent (usually mother). Many times they will complain on abdominal pain, nausea, vomiting, and diarrhea to avoid going to school.

○ **Do patients with mild anxiety attacks require medication?**

In general, no. It can usually be managed with psychotherapy alone. Behavioral or cognitive-behavioral therapy is the treatment of choice.

○ **When should treatment be initiated for panic attacks?**

- When it impairs function.
  - Medical history
  - If agoraphobia is present or developing
  - If major depression or a personality disorder is present
  - If the patient reports significant suicidal ideation
  - If the patient voices a strong preference for medication management
- Tricyclic antidepressant is a first-line treatment

○ **A 24-year-old male presents complaining of pleuritic pain, palpitations, dyspnea, dizziness, and tingling in his arm, legs, and lips. What is the potential diagnosis?**

Hyperventilation syndrome. This is frequently associated with anxiety. Decreased carbonate levels in the blood cause the tingling. This should always be a diagnosis of exclusion.

○ **A 20-year-old female complains of shortness of breath, tachypnea, tachycardia, tremors, and dizziness with symptoms climbing to maximum severity within 10 minutes. What is the diagnosis?**

Panic disorder. Panic disorders are not always linked to an event, although commonly associated with agoraphobia, social phobia, and mitral prolapse.

○ **Are panic attacks more common in the male or female population?**

Females. Women are twice as likely to suffer from panic attacks.

○ **What percentage of patients with primary anxiety disorders will have a history of DSM-IV TR depressive disorder?**

40% to 50%. The comorbidities of anxiety disorders with other psychiatric disorders are high.

○ **Generalized anxiety disorder (GAD) presents with what symptoms?**

- Excessive anxiety and worry
- Difficulty controlling worry
- Restlessness
- Easily fatigued
- Difficulty concentrating
- Irritability
- Muscle tension
- Sleep disturbance

○ **Name a few substances that might mimic generalized anxiety disorder when ingested.**

Nicotine, caffeine, amphetamines, cocaine, and anticholinergic. Alcohol and sedative withdrawal can also mimic GAD.

○ **What are some risk factors for post-traumatic stress disorder (PTSD)?**

Female, prior history of trauma, family history of anxiety.

○ **A 25-year-old male presents with flashbacks and nightmares of an experience while he was overseas. He has been having a hard time sleeping at night and has been avoiding planning another trip. What would be your leading diagnosis?**

PTSD

○ **John has just come back from the war in Iraq and has been diagnosed with PTSD. What would be the first-line treatment medication for John?**

- Selective serotonin reuptake inhibitors (SSRIs)
- Sertraline, Paroxetine, Fluoxetine, Fluvoxamine

○ **Can a person acquire post-traumatic stress disorder (PTSD) if he/she did not actually witness a disturbing event/trauma?**

Yes, according to the DSM-IV, one can experience PTSD if an event, such as a violent personal assault, a serious accident, or the serious injury of a close friend or family member is learned of indirectly. PTSD can also occur after a person hears of a life-threatening disease affecting a friend or family member.

○ **What distinguishes acute stress disorder (ASD) from post-traumatic stress disorder (PTSD)?**

- ASD symptoms must occur within 4 weeks of the traumatic event, whereas PTSD may have a delayed onset.
- ASD symptoms must remit within 4 weeks of their initial presentation, symptoms that last longer than 4 weeks may indicate PTSD.

○ **A 28-year-old woman who was raped 6 months ago has been psychologically sound thus far. She now suddenly develops recurrent flashbacks of the rape, nightmares, intense fear, avoidance of all men, a diminished memory of the rape, and an exaggerated startle response. Is this woman experiencing PTSD?**

Yes. This is a delayed onset of PTSD.

○ **What is an intense, irrational fear or aversion to a particular object or situation, other than a social situation?**

Specific phobia.

○ **What is social phobia?**

Social phobia is characterized by an extreme anxiety response in situations in which the affected person may be observed by others.

○ **What is the most common nonpharmacologic treatment for most phobias?**

Behavioral or cognitive-behavioral psychotherapies.

ATTENTION-DEFICIT DISORDERS

○ **What is the most common emotional, cognitive, and behavioral disorder treated in youth?**

Attention-deficit/hyperactivity disorder (ADHD).

○ **What other disorders does data suggest youth with ADHD are at risk for developing?**

Studies suggest that youth with ADHD are at risk for developing other psychiatric difficulties in childhood, adolescence, and adulthood including delinquency as well as mood, anxiety, and substance-use disorders.

○ **What are the clinical findings of ADHD?**

- Inattentiveness, distractibility, impulsivity, and hyperactivity that is out of the reasonable boundaries for patients within their development stage.
- Other common symptoms include low frustration tolerance, shifting activities frequently, difficulty organizing, and daydreaming.

○ **Is psychological testing necessary for the routine diagnosis of ADHD?**

No, but psychometric testing can be valuable in narrowing the differential diagnosis and identifying comorbid learning difficulties.

○ **What comorbid diseases would you also find in a patient with ADHD?**

Oppositional defiant disorder, conduct disorder (greater severity), mood disorders, and childhood anxiety are some of the more common diseases.

○ **What class of drugs is most commonly prescribed for the treatment of ADHD?**

Stimulants.

○ **What accounts for the most referrals to child psychiatrist?**

Attention-deficit/hyperactivity disorder (ADHD). ADHD accounts for 30% to 50% of child psychiatric outpatient cases.

AUTISTIC DISORDERS

○ **Which gender has a greater prevalence of autism?**

Men are three to four more times more likely than girls to have autism.

○ **What are some of the early signs of autism?**

In early stages of childhood the children are often mute (50%). In later stages, the child has social deficits and difficulty with social interaction, eye contact, and defective imitation.

○ **What percentage of autistic children will be able to function independently?**

20%.

○ **What percentage of autistic adults will be able to function independently?**

Only 1% to 2%.

○ **What are the two strongest associations of autism with medical conditions are with two strongly genetic disorders?**

Fragile X syndrome and tuberous sclerosis.

EATING DISORDERS

○ **What are the two types of anorexia nervosa?**

- Restricting type
- Binge-eating/purging type

○ **The onset of anorexia nervosa is bimodal. What are the two peaks?**

- Early Adolescence (12–15 years)
- Adolescence and early adult hood (17–21 years)

○ **What percentage of patients with anorexia are women?**

90%.

○ **Besides vomiting (purging), what are the other methods for weight loss that patient's with anorexia use?**

Misuse of laxatives, diuretics, or enemas.

○ **What are some signs on examination that may be present in anorexia?**

Emaciated appearance, hypotension (orthostatic at times), bradycardia, lanugo, salivary gland hypertrophy, peripheral edema, and dental enamel erosion.

○ **What are some commonly seen laboratory abnormalities in anorexia?**

- Hematology—Leukopenia
- Chemistry
  - Elevated—liver functions, HCO_3, carotene, cholesterol
  - Lower—chloride, potassium, zinc, estrogen, T_3 and T_4

○ **What is the most common psychiatric comorbidity in anorexia?**

Anxiety disorders.

○ **What are the two types of bulimia nervosa?**

1. Purging type

2. Non-purging type—associated with fasting and/or excessive exercising; without the use of laxatives or diuretics

○ **What percentage of patients with bulimia nervosa are female?**

98% to 100%.

○ **What is the only medication that is approved for the treatment of bulimia nervosa?**

Fluoxetine 60 mg daily.

○ **What are some of the more common physical examination and laboratory abnormalities associated with bulimia?**

- Physical examination—dehydration appearance, dental erosion, oropharyngeal irritation, gastrointestinal bleeding
- Laboratory abnormalities—electrolyte abnormalities, metabolic alkalosis, decreased serum chloride and potassium, metabolic acidosis in patients taking laxatives

○ **What findings in a female patient who presents with parotid gland swelling and eroding tooth enamel might you expect?**

Bulimia, which is associated with elevated serum amylase and hypokalemia. The enlarged parotid is referred to as the "chipmunk appearance."

MOOD DISORDERS

○ **What is an adjustment disorder?**

It is the development of emotional or behavioral symptoms in response to stressors, which occur within 3 months of the onset of stressors.

○ **What are some risk factors for individuals with adjustment disorder?**

Prior stress, childhood experience that was stressful and mod or eating disorders. Any family unity disruption (divorce, death, living with in-laws) and prior exposure to war without PTSD.

○ **What are common comorbidities of adjustment disorder?**

Cluster B personality disorder, substance or alcohol abuse, somatoform and factitious disorders, and psychosexual disorder.

○ **What is the behavioral and pharmacologic therapy for a patient with an adjustment disorder?**

Psychodynamic psychotherapy and antidepressants (SSRIs).

○ **What are the two required symptoms for the diagnosis of depression?**

Depressed mood and loss of interest or pleasure for at least a 2-week period of time.

○ **At what age range are the rates of depression in men and women the highest?**

25 to 44 years old.

○ **What are some of the risk factors for depression?**

A family history of depression or alcoholism, a recent negative life experience, personality disorder, early childhood trauma, and postpartum depressive states.

○ **What are some of the signs and symptoms of a major depressive event?**

Depressed mood, anhedonia, change in appetite and sleep, change in energy, body activity, feelings of worthlessness, decreased concentration, and suicidal ideation.

○ **A patient is being evaluated for depression. Would there be any reason to evaluate the patient's thyroid?**

Yes. Up to 40% of patients with depression will show evidence of subclinical hypothyroidism. Most of these patients will benefit for thyroid supplementation.

○ **What is the correlation with the number of depressive episodes and the incidence of reoccurrence?**

About 50% of patients with one depressive episode will have a recurrence, and about 90% of patients who have had three episodes can be expected to have a fourth, with the average number of lifetime events being five.

○ **What class of drugs is commonly used as a first-line treatment for depression?**

Selective serotonin reuptake inhibitors (SSRIs).

○ **What are some second-line treatment options for depression?**

Monoamine oxidase inhibitors (MAO) and TCAs. Be careful as these medications have several side effects.

○ **When would electroconvulsive therapy (ECT) be considered for the treatment of depression?**

ECT is used as a primary treatment when (1) an urgent need for a rapid response exist, (2) there is less risk with ECT than with other treatment alternatives, (3) there is a patient history of better response to ECT, or (4) there is a strong patient preference for its use.

○ **What are the eight common medical causes of depression?**

1. Stroke
2. Viral syndromes
3. Corticosteroids
4. Cushing disease
5. Antihypertensive medication
6. SLE
7. Multiple sclerosis
8. Subcortical dementias, such as Huntington and Parkinson diseases, and HIV encephalopathy

○ **Major depression and bipolar affective disorders account for what percentage of suicides?**

50%. Another 25% are because of substance abuse and another 10% are attributed to schizophrenia.

○ **What is dysthymic disorder?**

A depressed mood for most of the day, for more days than not, as indicated either by subjective account or observation made by others, for at least 2 years. The severe symptoms of depression, such as delusions and hallucinations are absent.

○ **What are some risk factors for dysthymic disorder?**

More common in first-degree relative or in those with history of major depression; age of onset before 45 years.

○ **What are the symptoms most commonly encountered in dysthymic disorder?**

Low self-esteem, low self-confidence, social withdrawal, loss of pleasure or interest, chronic fatigue or tiredness, feelings of guilt, difficulty thinking, and decreased activity.

○ **What is the common class of drugs that are given for dysthymia?**

SSRIs.

○ **What percentage of inpatients with dysthymia recovers after 2 years?**

40%.

○ **Which has an earlier onset, bipolar disorder or unipolar disorder?**

Bipolar. Onset of bipolar disorder is usually in the patient's twenties or thirties; onset of unipolar disorder is usually between ages 35 and 50 years.

○ **Differentiate between bipolar I, bipolar II, and cyclothymic.**

- Bipolar I: Episodes of mania cycling with depressive episodes
- Bipolar II: Episodes of hypomania cycling with depressive episodes
- Cyclothymic: Hypomania and less severe episodes of depression

○ **Are the majority of affective disorder patients bipolar or unipolar?**

Unipolar (80%).

○ **Which is most commonly the first episode of bipolar disease, mania or depression?**

Mania. Depression is rarely the first symptom. In fact, only 5% to 10% of patients who develop depression first go on to have manic episodes.

○ **First-degree relatives of bipolar patients have a greater risk for which mental illness?**

Bipolar I, bipolar II, and major depressive disorder.

○ **Are bipolar patients at risk for suicide?**

Yes. In fact, they are two to three times more likely to commit suicide compared with general population.

○ **Other than classic mania, what can lithium be used to treat?**

Bulimia, anorexia nervosa, alcoholism in patients with mood disorders, leukocytosis in patients on antineoplastic medication, cluster headaches, and migraine headaches.

○ **Postural tremor is a major side effect of lithium. How is this side effect controlled?**

Minimize the dose during the workday and give small doses of beta-blockers.

○ **Should people who are physically active have their lithium dosage increased or decreased?**

Increased. Lithium, a salt, is excreted more than sodium in sweat.

○ **True/False: A patient starting lithium will be expected to gain weight?**

True. All psychotropic medications cause weight gain, hence, lithium's usefulness in combating anorexia nervosa.

○ **Lithium toxicity begins at what level?**

14 mg/L. Above this level nausea, diarrhea, vomiting, rigidity, tremor, ataxia, seizures, delirium, coma, and death can occur.

○ **What are some renal side effects of lithium?**

Lithium causes polydipsia and polyuria in about 60% of patients; it persist in 20% to 25%.

PERSONALITY DISORDERS

○ **Is there a genetic link to patients with antisocial personality disorder?**

Yes, patients who have a father with an antisocial disorder or alcoholism are more likely to have it even if the father was not around to raise the child.

○   **True/False: Patients with antisocial personality disorders have a higher rate of substance abuse.**

True.

○   **A 24-year-old man who has a history of antisocial personality disorder along with a substance abuse history is concerned about his long-term prognosis. What can you tell him?**

Most patients will have some improvement and 30% to 40% will significantly improve their symptoms as they reach their mid-thirties to forties.

○   **A 30-year-old patient who you are seeing in your clinic had expressed that she does not interact in social situations because of a fear of not being liked. In addition, she is obsessed with thoughts of wondering if people like her. This causes the patient to feel socially inept and inferior. What is her diagnosis?**

Avoidant personality disorder.

○   **Which gender is more likely to have avoidant personality disorder?**

Women.

○   **Are patients with avoidant personality disorder capable of functioning in a normal environment?**

Yes. Many patients with this disorder manage to adapt to their problems and show little impairment, assuming they exist in a favorable interpersonal and occupational environment.

○   **What percentage of the general population is diagnosed with borderline personality disorder?**

1% to 2% of the general population.

○   **What is the most common clinical symptom of a patient with a borderline personality disorder?**

Commonly, impulsivity, inappropriate or intense anger, and chronic feelings of emptiness or boredom.

○   **What is a commonly reported historical fact that most patients with borderline personality disorder admit to in their childhood?**

Sexual, physical, and/or emotional abuse.

○   **Are suicidal gestures common in borderline personality patients?**

Yes. In fact, the more they occur, the more serious they become with 10% of these cases becoming successful.

○   **A 27-year-old woman who is a controlling individual will ask friends to do things that she herself thinks are unpleasant, and tries to draw attention toward herself with superficial sexuality-type behaviors. When rejected, she will display disappointment to the point of throwing a childish temper tantrum. What is the patient's diagnosis?**

Histrionic personality disorder.

○   **True/False: Histrionic patients are often introverts:**

False. They are quite extroverted and at times neurotic.

○ **What are some other psychiatric disorders that accompany patients with histrionic personalities?**

Depression and anxiety can be common diagnoses.

○ **What is a narcissistic personality disorder?**

It is a pattern of behavior that exhibits grandiosity, a feeling of being greater than what is reality, requires excessive admiration, and is critical of others who challenge them. There is also a lack of empathy toward others.

○ **Which gender is more common in a narcissistic personality disorder?**

Men.

○ **Which diagnoses can be confused with narcissistic personality disorder?**

Hypomania can often manic this as well as antisocial personality disorder.

○ **Is psychopharmacologic therapy beneficial in a narcissistic personality?**

No.

○ **What is the prognosis for a narcissistic patient?**

Many of the patients will actually worsen as they get older, typically in their forties. Depression is also common.

○ **Obsessive-compulsive disorders (OCD) generally begin at what age?**

25 years.

○ **What gender do obsessive-compulsive disorders predominate?**

Men.

○ **What are some common obsessions?**

Dirt and contamination, order and symmetry, religion and philosophy, and daily decisions. Unfortunately, compulsion does not relieve the anxiety of the obsession.

○ **Have medications been effective in treating OCD?**

No. SSRI's are felt to have some benefit in reducing the characteristics of perfectionism and ritualizing that can be seen in OCD.

○ **Is there a familial relationship in patients with paranoid personality disorder?**

There seems to be a relationship with family members who have a history of schizophrenia and/or delusional disorders.

○ **A patient who is unable to express his anger, has few close friends, is indifferent to praise from others, is absentminded, and is emotionally cold and aloof probably has which kind of personality disorder?**

Schizoidia.

○ **What is a differentiating characteristic of schizoid when compared to schizophrenia?**

Schizoid patients do not have a need or behavior that dangers or involves others, whereas schizophrenia does.

○ **Are first-degree relatives of schizophrenics more likely to have schizoidia or schizophrenia?**

Schizoidia, at a ratio of 3:1.

○ **Tom is a 14-year-old adolescent who has been exhibiting behavior that is unusual, along with odd beliefs and feels that he possesses magical abilities. What is the most likely diagnosis for Tom?**

Schizotypal personality disorder.

○ **What are some more common disorders in patients with schizotypal disorders?**

Anxiety and substance abuse are common problems.

○ **Which class of medications can be helpful in managing a patient with schizotypal disorder?**

Thus far, effective pharmacotherapy has not been demonstrated, although antipsychotics are used at times.

PSYCHOSES

○ **Can patients with delusional disorder have hallucinations?**

Yes, tactile and olfactory hallucinations can be present in these patients.

○ **What are some types of delusions?**

Erotomanic, grandiose, jealous, persecutory, somatic, and mixed.

○ **What are some differential diagnoses with delusional disorder?**

Schizophrenia, schizoaffective, mood disorders, psychoses, and substance abuse.

○ **Which classes of drugs are used to help control delusions?**

Antipsychotics, particularly the atypical antipsychotics.

○ **What percentage of melancholic episodes are associated with hallucinations and/or delusions?**

20%.

○ **Cite an example for each of the following perceptual disturbances: illusion, auditory hallucination, tactile hallucination, and somatic hallucination.**

- Illusion: A kitten is perceived as a dragon. (false perception)
- Auditory hallucination: The patient claims to hear people talking when no one is around. (They are perceived as being external to the patient; clear voices are often reported)
- Tactile hallucination: The patient feels like insects are crawling on his skin. (characteristic of cocaine and amphetamine intoxication)
- Somatic hallucination: The patient thinks that there is someone behind him every time he walks into his house. (visceral, intracerebral, or kinesthetic sensations are often referred to the influence of persecutors)

○ **What is the difference between schizophrenia and schizophreniform disorder?**

Schizophreniform disorder implies the same signs and symptoms as schizophrenia, yet these symptoms have been present for less than 6 months. The impaired functioning in schizophreniform disorder is not consistent. Schizophreniform disorder is generally a provisional diagnosis with schizophrenia following.

○ **What are some characteristics of schizophrenia?**

Delusional disorder, hallucinations (usually auditory), disorganized thinking, loosening of associations, disheveled appearance, and the inability to realize thought and behaviors are abnormal.

○ **What are the duration criteria for Schizophrenia?**

Continuous signs of the disturbance persist for at least 6 months. The 6-month period must include at least 1 month of symptoms that meet the symptoms.

○ **What are the six criteria for diagnosing schizophrenia?**

- Characteristic symptoms
  ○ delusions, hallucinations, disorganized speech, grossly disorganized or catatonic behavior, negative symptoms
- Social/occupational dysfunction
- Duration
  ○ 6-month period with at least 1 month of symptoms listed above
- Schizoaffective and mood disorder exclusion
- Substance/general medical condition exclusion
- Relationship to a pervasive developmental disorder consideration

○ **What percentage of patients with schizophrenia become chronically ill?**

60% to 80%. Men are at a greater risk for chronic illness.

○ **The onset of schizophrenia generally occurs by what age?**

80% of schizophrenics develop the disease before their early twenties. The disease is very rare after age 40.

○ **What are the five causes of schizophrenia?**

1. Viral infection in the CNS
2. Problem during pregnancy that affects the neuronal development
3. Head injury
4. Seizure disorder
5. Street drugs

○ **What psychiatric problems are associated with violence?**

Acute schizophrenia, paranoid ideation, catatonic excitation, mania, borderline and antisocial personality disorder, delusional depression, post-traumatic stress disorder, and decompensating obsessive–compulsive disorder.

○ **What is the average age of onset for schizophrenia?**

- Men: 18 to 25 years
- Women: 25 to 35 years

○ **What are the ages that are considered late and very late for the onset of schizophrenia?**

- Late: after age 45
- Very late: after age 65

○ **What percentage of schizophrenics is successful at suicide?**

10% to 13%.

○ **What are some secondary reasons for acute psychosis?**

Viral and bacterial infections, CNS infections, parasites, medications, anticholinergics, hallucinogens, over-the-counter stimulants, metabolic disorders, and traumatic brain injury.

○ **What are "hallmark" signs and symptoms of schizophrenia?**

Delusions, hallucinations, disorganized speech and thoughts, and negative symptoms (deficits of normal function but not psychotic).

○ **What class of medications is the first-line treatment of schizophrenia?**

Antipsychotics.

○ **What are the five criteria for brief psychotic disorder? (brief reactive psychosis)**

1. Precipitating stressful event
2. Rapid onset of the psychosis
3. Affective lability and mood intensity
4. Symptoms that match the stressful event
5. Resolution of symptoms once the stressor is removed, generally within 2 weeks

○ **What brain lesion sites are most commonly associated with psychosis?**

The temporolimbic system, caudate nucleus, and frontal lobes.

○ **List some life-threatening causes of acute psychosis:**

WHHHIMP:

Wernicke encephalopathy
Hypoxia
Hypoglycemia
Hypertensive encephalopathy
Intracerebral hemorrhage
Meningitis/encephalitis
Poisoning

○ **What signs and symptoms suggest an organic source for psychosis?**

Acute onset, disorientation, visual or tactile hallucinations, age under 10 or over 60 years, and any evidence suggesting overdose or acute ingestion, such as abnormal vital signs, pupil size and reactivity, or nystagmus.

○ **When are women at the greatest risk for psychiatric illness?**

The first few weeks postpartum. A psychiatric illness most often occurs in patients who are primiparous, have poor social support, or have a history of depression.

○ **When does postpartum psychosis begin?**

Within a week to 10 days following childbirth. A second, smaller peak occurs 5 to 7 months later, correlating with the first menses postpartum. The risk of psychosis is lowest during pregnancy.

SOMATOFORM DISORDER

○ **A 30-year-old woman complains of calf pain, headache, shooting pain when flexing her right wrist, random epigastric pain, bloating, and irregular menses, all of which cannot be explained after medical examination. What is the diagnosis?**

Somatization disorder, many unexplained medical symptoms involving multiple systems. To diagnose a patient with somatization disorder, one must have four or more unexplained pain symptoms. Symptoms generally begin in childhood and are fully developed by age 30. This is more common in women than in men.

○ **What percentage of primary care patients exhibit some form of somatizations in clinic visits?**

25%.

○ **What is a classic type of patient who presents with somatoform disorder?**

Young, unmarried, nonwhite from a rural area who is uneducated.

○ **What is the treatment of somatoform disorder?**

It is extremely difficult. First, you have to detect the disorder and then convince the patient that they have this problem. Second is to have the patient exhibit more than two to three office visits that are legitimate problems. Make sure to examine all symptoms and order test as needed, and lastly prescribe any medications that may help the said illness and monitor for improvement.

OTHER BEHAVIORAL DISORDERS

○ **What are some criteria to meet in an acute stress disorder (ASD)?**

- Primary: Patient has to be witness to a traumatic event or involved. The event has to involve the patient's fear or helplessness.
- Secondary: While during this event, the patient has a sense of detachment, will be in a daze and not able to function normally, and have a detachment from memory about the event. This may also cause the patient to have recall of the event, flashbacks, and reminders of the trauma. This experience will create a significant impairment for the patient.

○ **If a patient has an ASD from an event, what is he/she likely to develop?**

Up to 80% of these patients will later be diagnosed with PTSD.

○ **What are the four categories of child maltreatment?**

Child neglect, physical abuse, emotional abuse, and sexual abuse.

○ **How many children die each year as a result of abuse?**

1500.

○ **What are some parental factors that lend to child abuse?**

Lower parental education, mental illness, alcoholism, and substance abuse.

○ **In what percentage of child sexual abuse cases is the abuser known by the child?**

90%. In 50% of such cases, the mother is also abused.

○ **In addition to the history, physical examination, laboratory tests, and collection of physical evidence, what need to be done in cases of child sexual abuse?**

File a report with child protective services and law enforcement agencies. Provide emotional support to the child and family. Give a return appointment for follow-up of STD cultures and testing for pregnancy, HIV, or syphilis as indicated. Assure follow-up for psychological counseling by connecting the child/family to the appropriate services in your area.

○ **Is violence more likely between family members or nonfamily members?**

Family members: 20% to 50% of the murders in the United States are committed by members of the victims' families. Spouse abuse is as high as 16% in the United States.

○ **What is the epidemiology of domestic violence?**

95% of the victims are women. An estimated 4 million women are battered each year. Domestic abuse is the number one cause of injuries to women. Their intimate partner kills more than half of all women murdered in the United States.

○ **What are the clinical clues for domestic violence?**

Any evidence of injury during pregnancy or late entry into prenatal care. Injuries presenting after significant delay or in various stages of healing; especially to the head, neck, breasts, abdomen, or areas suggesting a defensive posture, such as bruises on the forearms. Vague complaints or unusual injuries, such as bites, scratchers, burns, or rope marks.

○ **What is the standard of care for victims of domestic violence currently recommended by JCAHO, the AMA, and the CDC?**

- Establish a confidential system to identify DV victims
- Document the abuse
- Collect physical evidence
- Evaluate safety issues and potential for lethality or suicide
- Formulate a safety plan with the victim
- Advise the victim of all his/her options and resources
- Refer for counseling and other services, including legal assistance
- Coordinate with law enforcement
- Transport to a shelter if desired or needed
- Follow-up with a domestic violence advocate

○ **What are the prodromes of violent behavior?**

Anxiety, defensiveness, volatility, and physical aggression.

○ **What are the only reliable indicators of a potentially violent patient?**

Male gender, history of violence, and history of substance abuse. Cultural, educational, economic, and language barriers to effective patient/staff communication can increase the patient's frustration and lower his/her threshold for violence as can trivialization of the patient or the family's concerns.

○ **Bereavement generally lasts how long?**

6 months. Full melancholic syndrome, hallucinations, and suicidal ideation are not common in bereavement.

○ **When do you medically treat uncomplicated bereavement?**

When the symptoms mimic depression and last for more than 13 months. This would be the expected time that uncomplicated bereavement should subside.

○ **Who is more successful at suicide, men or women?**

Men (a 3:1 men-to-women ratio). However, women attempt suicide three times as often as men.

○ **True/False: Fantasies frequently precede suicidal acts**

True.

○ **What percentage of patients with melancholia attempt suicide?**

15%.

○ **What is the number one cause of death for African American men between the ages of 10 and 24 years?**

Firearm injury. The overall homicide rate for young men in the United States is more than seven times that of the next developed country.

○ **Do intentional or unintentional causes account for more firearm-related deaths?**

Intentional causes account for 94% of firearm deaths, suicide for 48%, and homicide for 46%. Unintentional firearm injuries account for about 4%. Only 1% of firearm deaths occur as a result of legal intervention. The number of firearm-related fatalities has more than doubled in the last 30 years.

○ **What are risk factors for homicide?**

Someone they know, someone of the same race, and usually during an argument or fight, kills most homicide victims. Drugs or alcohol are important cofactors as is the presence of a handgun.

○ **What are the relative risks for suicide and homicide if a gun is kept in the home?**

Suicide is five times more likely. Homicide is three times more likely. The victim is 43% more likely to be a member of the family than an intruder. In the case of domestic violence, a gun at home increases the risk of homicide 20-fold.

SUBSTANCE ABUSE DISORDERS

○ **What is the prevalence of alcoholism in the United States?**

10% to 15% is the lifetime prevalence, and 10% of men and 3.5% of women are alcoholic.

○ **What age range has the highest prevalence of drinking problems?**

18- to 29-year-olds have the greatest prevalence.

○ **What laboratory changes are suggestive of alcoholism?**

Look for an increase in ALT, AST, alkaline phosphate, amylase, bilirubin, cholesterol, GGT, LDH, MCV, PTT, triglycerides, uric acid, and a decrease in BUN, calcium, coagulopathy, hematocrit, magnesium, phosphorus, platelet count, and protein.

○ **What do higher blood concentrations of alcohol or other CNS depressants cause mild impairment of?**

Mild impairment of motor skills and slowing of reaction time, followed by sedation, decreased motor coordination, impaired judgment, diminished memory, and other cognitive effects.

○ **Describe the signs and symptoms of CNS depressant withdrawal.**

- Anxiety or psychomotor agitation
- Tremor
- Craving
- Autonomic hyperactivity
- Insomnia
- Hallucinations
- Nausea or vomiting
- Seizures
- Delirium

○ **What is the difference in the treatment methods between alcohol withdrawals compared with sedative hypnotic withdrawal?**

Alcohol withdrawal is treated with benzodiazepine, carbamazepine, or paraldehyde. Sedative hypnotic withdrawal is treated with the substitution of a long-acting barbiturate.

○ **What is the most effective long-term treatment program for alcoholism?**

Alcohol anonymous.

○ **What should you do when handling intoxicated, violent, psychotic, or threatening patients?**

Conduct careful histories and physicals with attention to mental status. Look for evidence of trauma, toxic ingestion, or metabolic derangement. Historical sources (e.g., family, paramedics, mental health workers, police, or medical records) may need to be accessed. Patient may need to be physically or chemically restrained to obtain an adequate examination and to ensure the safety of the patient and the provider.

○ **What is the most common mental illness in large cities?**

Substance abuse.

○ **A patient presents with tearing eyes, a runny nose, tachycardia, muscle aches, abdominal pains, nausea, vomiting, diarrhea, insomnia, pupillary dilation, and leukocytosis. What is the diagnosis?**

Opiate and/or opioid withdrawal. Treat with methadone or dolophine. Clonidine may blunt some of the side effects.

○ **Wild and abundant dreams may result from withdrawal of what drugs?**

Antidepressants. Other side effects of withdrawal are anxiety, akathisia, bradykinesia, mania, and malaise.

○ **What percentage of deaths has been associated with tobacco abuse?**

25%.

○ **What are some of the more common diseases associated with tobacco use?**

Coronary heart disease, oral cancers, dental disease, emphysema, lung cancer, and low birth weight in pregnant women.

MISCELLANEOUS

○ **What are the components of the multiaxial diagnostic system?**

- Axis I: Symptoms and syndromes comprising a mental disorder, including substance abuse/addiction
- Axis II: Personality and developmental disorders underlying the axis I diagnosis
- Axis III: Physical medical problems/conditions that may or may not contribute to the axis I diagnosis
- Axis IV: Psychosocial factors
- Axis V: Adaptive ability/disability

○ **What is the most common cause of catatonia?**

Affective disorder.

○ **What is a previously healthy patient most likely suffering from when he becomes suddenly and intensely excited, goes into a delirious mania, develops catatonic features, and a high fever?**

Lethal catatonia. Such patients have a 50% death rate without treatment. Treat these patients with ECT.

○ **How is lethal catatonia differentiated from neuroleptic malignant syndrome?**

By the timing of the hyperthermia. In lethal catatonia, severe hyperthermia occurs during the excitement phase before catatonic features develop. In neuroleptic malignant syndrome, hyperthermia develops later in the course of the disease with the onset of stupor.

○ **In infancy, simple repetitive reactions like nail-biting, thumb-sucking, masturbation, or temper tantrums are manifestations of what psychological reaction?**

Adjustment reactions. These are responses to separation from the caregiver and are often associated with developmental delay.

○ **What is the prevalence of conduct disorder?**

10%. It is more common in boys and is hereditary.

○ **Children with conduct disorders will probably develop what adult disorder?**

Antisocial personality disorder. About 40% will have some pathology as adults.

○ **What is a conversion disorder?**

An internal psychological conflict that manifests itself through somatic symptoms. Voluntary motor or sensory functions are affected. Examples include weakness, imbalance, dysphagia, and changes in vision, hearing, or sensation. These symptoms are not feigned or intentionally produced. They are also not fully explained by medical conditions.

○ **What are the five Kübler-Ross stages of dying?**

1. Denial
2. Anger
3. Bargaining
4. Depression
5. Acceptance

○ **What psychiatric disease is the most hereditary?**

Idiopathic enuresis. If one parent has enuresis, there is a 44% chance that the child will also have the disease. If both parents have it, the likelihood increases to 77%.

○ **What is enuresis?**

- Repeated voiding of urine into bed or clothes.
- The behavior is clinically significant as manifested by either a frequency of twice a week for at least 3 consecutive months or the presence of clinically significant distress or impairment in social, academic, or other important areas of functioning.
- Chronological age is at least 5 years.
- The behavior is not due excessively to the direct physiological effect of a substance.

○ **What is an extreme case of factitious disorder?**

Munchausen syndrome. The patient may actually try to cause harm to themselves (e.g., by injecting feces into their veins) and are very accepting/seeking of invasive procedures. Munchausen by proxy is another example. In this disease, the patient seeks medical care for another, usually a child.

○ **Give examples of the following thought disorders: perseveration, nonsequiturs, derailment, tangential, speech, neologism, private word usage, and verbigeration.**

Perseveration—"I've been wondering if the mechanical mechanisms of this machine are mechanically sound. Mechanically speaking, I must understand the mechanisms." (A repetition of certain words or phrases is found in the natural flow of speech.)

Nonsequiturs—Q: "Are you nervous about the upcoming boards?" A: "Why no, the king of France is an excellent king." (The patient's answers are unrelated to the questions asked.)

Derailment—"I first became interested in the study of medicine after mom bought me a toy ambulance. Toys can be very dangerous, especially if they are very small and can be swallowed. I've been having difficulty swallowing lately." (The patient suddenly switches lines of thought, though the second follows the first.)

Tangential speech—A: "Those are nice clothes you're wearing today." B: "Of course I'm wearing clothes today." A: "I mean, I like the outfit you have on." B: "I think everyone should wear clothes, except on Friday, because Friday is casual day at my office." (Conversations are on the right subject matter; however, the responses are inappropriate to the previous questions or comments.)

Neologism—"I'm going to explaphrase (explain by paraphrasing) the meaning of agnonoctaudiophobia (things that go bump in the night)." (Neologisms are meaningless combinations of two or more words to invent a new word.)

Private word usage—"I can't believe the loquacious way he is formicating those tripods." (Words and/or phrases used in unique ways.)

Verbigeration—"I have been studying, have been studying, have been studying, for hours for hours hours hours." (The patient repeats words, especially at the end of thoughts, thoughts, thoughts, thoughts.)

○   **Matching:**

1. Hypomania	a. One or more hypomanias plus one or more major depressive symptoms
2. Melancholia	b. A mild manic episode
3. Bipolar II	c. Deep depression and vegetative characteristics
4. Unipolar mania	d. Manic episodes only
5. Cyclothymia	e. Many mild episodes of hypomania and depression

Answers: (1) b, (2) c, (3) a, (4) d, (5) e.

○   **A patient is brought in because she believes butterflies are landing all around her. The butterflies talk to her and tell her to love everyone. She denies suicidal ideation and any desire to harm herself or other. She has no record of harming people in the past. Can this person be institutionalized against her will?**

No. Unless the patient is a danger to herself or others, she cannot be confined to an institution despite questionable mental status.

○   **What is the difference between a malingering and a factitious disorder?**

A malingerer's incentive is external, such as workman's compensation. The goal of someone with a factitious disorder is to enter into the sick role. Both involve feigning illness.

○   **According to Holmes and Rahe, what are life's top- 10 most stressful events?**

1. Death of spouse or child
2. Divorce
3. Separation
4. Institutional detention
5. Death of close family member
6. Major personal injury or illness
7. Marriage
8. Job loss
9. Marital reconciliation
10. Retirement

REFERENCES

Ebert ML, Nurcombe B, Leckman JF. *Current Diagnosis and Treatment, Psychiatry.* 2nd ed. New York, NY: McGraw-Hill; 2008.
Fauci Anthony S., Longo Dan L. *Harrison's Principles of Internal Medicine* [Online]. 18th ed. New York, NY: McGraw-Hill; 2012.
McPhee SJ, Papadakis M. *Current Medical Diagnosis and Treatment 2009.* New York, NY: McGraw-Hill; 2009.

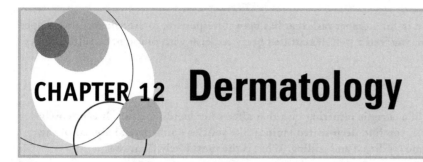

CHAPTER 12 Dermatology

Kimberly K. Dempsey, MPA, PA-C

ECZEMATOUS ERUPTIONS

○ **A 5-year-old female presents with a 3-cm, hyperpigmented, scaling plaque located at the umbilicus. You also note she has smaller similar lesions on bilateral ear lobes at the site of her ear piercings. Her mother states this is extremely pruritic. What is the most likely diagnosis?**

Allergic contact dermatitis secondary to a nickel allergy.

○ **What is the appropriate treatment of contact dermatitis caused by poison ivy?**

Topical treatment with a mid- to high-potency topical steroid depending upon severity is effective for limited or early lesions. Oral steroids are indicated for more severe cases. Oral antihistamines provide relief from pruritus. It is essential that all clothing that may have come in contact with the oils be washed.

○ **A 17-year-old female presents complaining of a rash. On physical examination, you find well-demarcated erythematous plaques covered with a fine, silvery scale. When the scale is lifted, it exhibits pinpoint bleeding. What is the most likely diagnosis?**

Plaque psoriasis.

○ **A 13-year-old male presents with erythema and yellow, scaly plaques located in his eyebrows, eyelids, and nasolabial folds. What is the most likely diagnosis?**

Seborrheic dermatitis.

○ **A mother presents with her 4-year-old child complaining of a pruritic rash that interferes with the child's sleep. On physical examination, the child has red scaling plaques located in bilateral antecubital and popliteal fossae. Overall the skin is dry. What is the most likely diagnosis?**

Atopic dermatitis.

○ **What is the first-line treatment for atopic dermatitis?**

First-line treatment is an appropriate strength topical steroid. Antihistamines should be used to control pruritus. In addition, the use of soap free products for bathing and thick emollients for moisturization is recommended.

○   **A mother brings her 6-month-old in for a diaper rash that has been unresponsive to over-the-counter diaper creams. On physical examination, you find a well-demarcated beefy red rash with pinpoint satellite papules. What is the causative organism?**

Candida albicans.

○   **A 20-year-old female complains of a chronic recurring rash that affects her hands and feet. It is intensely pruritic. On physical examination, you find deep-seated tapioca-like vesicles on the lateral aspects of the fingers and toes. There is also some erythema and scaling. What is the most likely diagnosis?**

Dyshidrotic eczema.

○   **A 24-year-old male presents with a dry, lichenified plaque on his left wrist that is pruritic. He states it started as an insect bite. This has been present for several months. What is the most likely diagnosis?**

Lichen simplex chronicus.

PAPULOSQUAMOUS DISEASES

○   **What are the most common causes of erythema multiforme?**

- **Infection,** especially herpes simplex, Mycoplasma
- **Drugs** such as sulfonamides, NSAIDS, phenytoin, barbiturates, and salicylates
- **Malignancy**
- **Idiopathic**

○   **A 30-year-old female presents with multiple tender, nodular lesion on the anterior surface of her lower legs bilaterally. They range in size from 1 to 5 cm. Newer lesions are red in color, while older lesions appear darker and bruise-like. There is associated leg pain. She has been developing these lesions over the past 5 weeks. What is the most likely diagnosis?**

Erythema nodosum. This is a hypersensitivity reaction to various stimuli such as infectious organisms, drugs, malignancies, and connective tissue diseases. Many times the cause is idiopathic.

○   **A 17-year-old male patient complains of spreading spots. They began several months ago on his upper back and have spread to involve the upper chest and upper arms. There are no associated symptoms; he is just concerned that he is becoming "spotted." On physical examination, you see 2-mm, oval, tan macules with fine scaling. What is the best way to confirm your suspected diagnosis?**

The best way to confirm the diagnosis is to perform a KOH Prep with 10% to 20% KOH. Visualization of hyphae (usually shortened) and spores is confirmatory; this is the classic "spaghetti and meatball" appearance of tinea versicolor.

○   **What are the treatment alternatives for tinea versicolor?**

Treatment options include antifungal shampoo such as selenium sulfide or ketoconazole 2% left on for 10 minutes before washing. This can be done daily for up to 2 weeks. Topical imidazoles such as ketoconazole, econazole, and oxiconazole can be applied twice daily for 2 weeks. For severe, recurrent, or intractable cases PO ketoconazole 400 mg can be used.

○   **A mother presents with her 6-month-old infant complaining that the patient gets frequent welps on her skin. On physical examination, the patient exhibits urticarial lesions with firm stroking of the skin and any pressure that is placed on the skin. What is the most likely diagnosis?**

Pressure urticaria. This is a form of dermatographism.

○ **A 20-year-old female patient complains of a spreading rash. She states it started with a dry scaling patch on the abdomen that was larger than the current lesions. Now she has smaller dry scaling patches located on her chest and back. She denies any associated symptoms. What is the smaller, 2 to 5 mm, most likely diagnosis?**

The characteristic rash of pityriasis rosea begins with a "herald patch," which is usually 2 to 5 cm. Within a week or two, smaller lesions distributed over the torso and proximal extremities develop along the cleavage lines ("Christmas tree" distribution). These are scattered scaling patches that may be asymptomatic or mildly pruritic.

○ **A 14-year-old male presents to the emergency department with 103.1°F fever and dysphagia. He appears ill and has small vesicles on the nasal and oral mucosa. He has a rash on his face and chest with dusky red papule and small vesicles surrounded by macular erythema. Some of the vesicles have coalesced forming bullae. Several bullae have ruptured leaving behind denuded skin. What is the most likely diagnosis?**

Stevens–Johnson syndrome (SJS)/toxic epidermal necrolysis (TEN) are considered to be variants of the same disorder. Patients may initially present with SJS and evolve into TEN depending on the degree of epidermal detachment.

○ **A 25-year-old male patient presents with a well-defined oval violaceous lesion located in the groin. He states that it is pruritic and occurred approximately an hour after taking acetaminophen for a headache. He states this has happened before under similar circumstances. What is the most likely diagnosis?**

Fixed drug eruption.

○ **What is the etiology of Stevens–Johnson syndrome (SJS)/toxic epidermal necrolysis (TEN)?**

Infections, drugs, malignancies, and idiopathic.

○ **A PA is examining a patient who is suspected of having Pemphigus vulgaris. The PA rubs the patient's skin causing the epidermis to separate and exposing a raw base. What is this examination technique called?**

Nikolsky sign.

○ **A 77-year-old man presents to your clinic complaining of multiple fluid-filled blisters to the flexor surfaces of his forearms. He states that he has had itching to these areas for about 1 week. On examination, you see multiple tense bullae to the flexor surfaces of the arms with an irritated erythematous base. What is the most likely diagnosis?**

Bullous pemphigoid.

○ **What is the treatment of choice for bullous pemphigoid?**

Oral steroids are the treatment of choice until blistering ceases. Pruritus can be controlled with oral antihistamines.

ACNEIFORM LESIONS

○ **What are the typical clinical manifestations of hidradenitis suppurativa?**

Typical skin lesions include open comedones, particularly the double comedones, and tender abscesses that may drain purulent or seropurulent material. Patients usually present with a painful boil. Sinus tracts may also form. These lesions are most common in the axillae, anogenital region, and under the breast.

○ **What is the best treatment for the large fluctuant cysts of hidradenitis suppurativa?**

Incision and drainage.

○ **What is the best treatment for the comedonal lesions (white heads and black heads) of acne vulgaris?**

Topical retinoids are the treatment of choice for comedonal acne. Topical benzoyl peroxide and salicylic acid preparations have a mild comedolytic effect.

○ **What are the side effects of tetracycline antibiotics that are commonly used to treat inflammatory acne?**

Side effects include dental staining in children younger than 9 years, GI upset, photosensitivity, pseudotumor cerebri, and vulvovaginal candidiasis. Minocycline has the added side effects of blue-gray skin pigmentation of the skin or mucosa, lupus-like reactions, and vertigo.

○ **A 35-year-old male presents with a complaint of frequent facial flushing in response to spicy foods, alcohol, and sun exposure. In addition, he has experienced a new onset of acne. On physical examination, you find several small red papules and pustules on bilateral cheeks. There are no comedones present. What is the most likely diagnosis?**

Acne rosacea.

○ **A patient presents complaining of an itchy red rash that started after she returned from vacation. She did not use any different soaps or perfumes while on vacation, but she did use a hot tub several times during the week. On physical examination, you find small red papules on the trunk and bilateral lower extremities, worse in areas covered by the bathing suit. What organism is most likely the cause of this rash?**

Pseudomonas aeruginosa.

INSECTS/PARASITES

○ **A 22-year-old female patient complains of intense generalized itching that worsens at night. On physical examination, she has erythematous papules on her hands and feet including the palms and soles. Some have become eczematized. She also has papules and nodules around the umbilicus and in the genital area. Close examination reveals a linear lesion in the webspace on her hands. What is the best test to confirm your diagnosis?**

To confirm your diagnosis of scabies, an intact burrow or papule should be scraped and the scraping should be placed on a glass microscope slide with mineral oil or KOH. Visualization of a mite, eggs, or feces is diagnostic for scabies.

○ **What is the appropriate treatment for a patient diagnosed with scabies?**

Appropriate treatment is application of 5% permethrin cream applied from the neck to toes and left on overnight (8 hours) and then washed off. All people who live in the same residence should be treated at the same time. After the treatment, carpets and upholstered furniture should be vacuumed and sheets and clothing should be washed in hot soapy water. This treatment should be repeated in 1 week to kill any mites that have hatched in the interim. Oral antihistamines can be prescribed to ameliorate pruritus.

○ **What is the treatment of choice for pediculosis capitis (head lice)?**

1% permethrin (which is available OTC).

○ **A patient presents with a large red lesion with an area of central necrosis on her right forearm. She states it started as a small red bump after a bug bite. What is the most likely cause of her current condition?**

Brown recluse spider.

NEOPLASMS

○ **A 62-year-old male tennis player with androgenetic alopecia presents with small scattered areas of skin-colored hyperkeratotic scale. When scraped, they are tender. The texture is that of sandpaper when palpated. What is the most likely diagnosis?**

This presentation is consistent with actinic keratosis.

○ **A 64-year-old male presents with multiple brown plaques on his back. He states they are not painful unless one gets caught on clothing. They have never bled or become irritated. On physical examination they are brown, warty plaques with a greasy, stuck-on appearance. What is the most appropriate treatment?**

Treatment of seborrheic keratoses is considered cosmetic since there is no malignant potential. Cryotherapy eradicates these lesions nicely, but they have a tendency to recur.

○ **A 50-year-old man presents with two pearly papules: one on the nostril and another on the nasolabial fold. These papules are smooth and dome-shaped with some overlying telangiectasias. Your patient states that these have been growing slowly. What is the most likely diagnosis?**

Basal cell carcinoma (BCC) is the most common cutaneous malignancy. These lesions most likely represent the most common variant of BCC, nodular basal cell carcinoma.

○ **Nevi should be examined for what characteristics when evaluating for atypia?**

Asymmetry: One-half is unlike the other half

Border irregularity: Irregular, scalloped, or poorly defined borders

Color variation: Variations in color present (tan, brown, black, white, red) Diameter: >6 mm in acquired after the age of 1 year

Evolving: Mole that looks different from the rest or is changing

○ **What are the risk factors for melanoma?**

- Fair complexion
- History of sunburns
- More than 50 moles
- Atypical moles
- Family history of melanoma

○ **A patient presents with a brown-black linear longitudinal pigmentation under the nail onto the proximal nail fold. What is the most likely diagnosis?**

This is consistent with a Hutchinson sign, which is an indicator of subungual melanoma. However, it is not pathognomonic. Diagnosis is made histologically.

○ **A 45-year-old woman presents with a growing 10-mm, asymmetric, dark-brown papule with black spots on her right shoulder. The borders are irregular. It is asymptomatic. What is the next step in treating this patient?**

The lesion is suspicious for melanoma and should be biopsied.

○ **A 64-year-old male presents with several small, well-defined plaques that are scaly and difficult to visualize. They are located on the dorsum of his hands, scalp, and ears. What is the most appropriate treatment?**

First-line treatment for actinic keratosis is cryotherapy.

○ **A 74-year-old female presents with a complaint of a pink lesion on her face. On physical examination you note a firm, pearly pink papule with telangiectasias. The border of the nodule appears rolled. What is the most likely diagnosis?**

Nodular basal cell carcinoma.

○ **What is the appropriate treatment of basal cell carcinoma?**

The goal of treatment is complete removal of the lesion. If the lesion is well circumscribed, it can be surgically removed in the office. However, complex tumors may required Mohs surgery.

HAIR AND NAILS

○ **A patient presents with the complaint of losing her hair. On physical examination, you note that there is a smooth patch of loss of hair and also note the presence of small "exclamation hairs." What is the likely diagnosis?**

Alopecia areata.

○ **You suspect your patient may have onychomycosis. What is the best way to confirm your diagnosis?**

Clinical diagnosis must be confirmed by laboratory examination. The preferred method of confirmation can be achieved by the isolation of fungus on culture medium. KOH examination of subungual debris or nail plate can be used to confirm the presence of hyphae.

○ **What is the most appropriate treatment for a healthy patient with onychomycosis?**

Terbinafine 250 mg/day for 6 weeks (fingernails) and 12 weeks (toenails).

○ **A patient presents with a red, tender, and indurated lateral nail fold that has purulent drainage on his ring finger. What is the most likely diagnosis?**

Paronychia is inflammation surrounding the nail.

○ **What is the most common causative organism of paronychia?**

Staphylococcus aureus.

○ **A 28-year-old female presents with a complaint of hair loss. Her hair sheds excessively when brushing and with minimal traction. She states that she is otherwise healthy since having her gallbladder removed 6 months ago. On physical examination, there are no areas of alopecia noted but the hair is thinly distributed. What is the most likely diagnosis?**

Telogen effluvium.

○ **A 6-year-old boy presents with diffuse patchy scaling in the scalp with areas of black dot alopecia. What is the most likely diagnosis?**

Tinea capitis is extremely common in school-aged children especially those from the inner city. There is usually posterior cervical lymphadenopathy associated with this infection. Diagnosis is confirmed with a fungal culture.

○ **What is the first-line treatment for tinea capitis?**

Griseofulvin (15 mg/kg/day for 6–8 weeks) and an antifungal shampoo (ketoconazole 2% or selenium sulfide 2.5%) two to three times a week.

VIRAL DISORDERS

○ **A 22-year-old female presents with a complaint of bumps in the genital region. On physical examination, you find cauliflower-like papules in a perivaginal distribution. What are the treatment options for this condition?**

Genital warts can be treated with podophyllin resin in tincture of benzoin cryotherapy, CO_2 laser therapy, podofilox, or imiquimod cream.

○ **A 5-year-old child develops a rash that starts on the face and quickly spreads to the trunk. The lesions begin as small vesicles on a red base. After a couple of days the lesions crust over, but new ones are still forming. What is the most likely diagnosis?**

Chicken pox (varicella zoster virus).

○ **A 4-year-old boy who recently had a few days of bright red cheeks now has a lacy appearing rash on both upper extremities. There are no associated symptoms. What is the most likely causative organism?**

This represents erythema infectiosum or fifth disease.

○ **A mother brings her 14-year-old boy to you a week after you prescribed ampicillin for his pharyngitis. Mom says he developed a rash over his torso, arms, legs, and even the palms of his hands. Upon examination, the patient has an erythematous, macular, and papular rash. What is the most likely diagnosis?**

Infectious mononucleosis.

○ **A 72-year-old woman has a painful red rash with vesicles on erythematous bases in a bandlike distribution on the right side of her lower back, which spreads down and out toward her hip. What is the most likely diagnosis?**

Shingles or herpes zoster disease.

○ **A 65-year-old female presents with vesicles on an erythematous base located on the tip of her nose. She states she had a prior occurrence of shingles. What are possible complications?**

Vesicles at the tip of the nose is Hutchinson sign. This indicates that the varicella zoster virus resides in the nasociliary branch of the ophthalmic nerve. Complications include ocular inflammation and corneal denervation. This is a medical emergency and needs immediate referral.

○ **What is the causative organism of verruca vulgaris?**

Verruca vulgaris is caused by the human papilloma virus (HPV).

○ **An otherwise healthy 8-month-old infant runs a high fever (105°F) and presents to the emergency department (ED). Her physical examination is completely normal and laboratory testing fails to find any signs of infection or dehydration. Two days later the fever subsides and a rash of oval pink macules begins on the trunk. These quickly become confluent. Within 48 hours, the rash subsides. What is the causative organism?**

The causative organism of roseola (exanthem subitum) is HHV-6 and HHV-7.

○ **A patient with AIDS presents with a grayish-white "corduroy-like" plaque on the lateral borders of her tongue that does not scrape off. What is the most likely diagnosis?**

Oral hairy leukoplakia, which is caused by EBV infection of the oropharynx.

○ **What are the appropriate recommendations for the preventions of herpes zoster?**

The CDC recommends that anyone aged 60 and over should have the vaccine to prevent herpes zoster (shingles). This is a one-time vaccine.

○ **A patient with chronic eczema presents with a complaint of a new, painful rash and a fever. On physical examination, you notice a few vesicular lesion and several that are erythematous and crusted with a punched out appearance. These lesions are located on the upper extremities and face. What is the most likely diagnosis?**

Eczema herpeticum.

○ **An unvaccinated 4-year-old boy presents after a week of cold symptoms and malaise. His temperature is 104°F. On physical examination, he has an erythematous maculopapular rash on his face, neck, and shoulders. The rash is mildly pruritic and blanches with pressure. On the buccal mucosa you notice small gray macules on a red base. What is the appropriate treatment?**

This child has rubeola (measles). This is a viral exanthem and appropriate therapy consists of supportive measures including maintaining hydration, antipyretics, and vitamin A supplements.

BACTERIAL INFECTIONS

○ **What are major risk factors for the development of a carbuncle?**

Risk factors for the development include obesity, immunosuppression, hyper-IgE, chronic granulomatous disease, and malnutrition.

○ **What is the most frequent causative organism in cases of impetigo?**

Staphylococcus aureus or group A Streptococcus.

○ **A mother brings her 4-year-old girl to you because she has a terrible rash. The child's face has patches of shallow erosions covered in a thick, honey-colored crust. Just 2 days ago, these lesions were small red papules. What is the appropriate treatment?**

Impetigo is common in children and usually occurs on exposed areas of skin. Most limited cases can be treated with topical mupirocin antibiotic ointment. However, extensive disease should be treated with system antibiotics such as cephalexin or amoxicillin plus clavulanic acid. For penicillin-allergic patients, use erythromycin, clarithromycin, or azithromycin.

○ **A patient has a history of recurrent abscesses. The abscesses have cultured positive for methicillin resistant *Staphylococcus aureus* (MRSA). What is the appropriate recommendation to suppress recurrences?**

Bleach baths two to three times a week can help reduce the bacterial load on the skin and thereby reduce outbreaks. Alternatively, mupirocin ointment in the anterior nares for 1 week each month can suppress outbreaks.

○ **What is the appropriate treatment for a cyst/abscess that occurs just above the gluteal fold in the sacrococcygeal region?**

Appropriate treatment for a pilonidal cyst is incision and drainage (I&D) of the cyst. The incision should extend to the subcutaneous tissue with removal of all hair and debris. The wound should be packed. No antibiotics are necessary unless there is an associated cellulitis. Follow-up with a surgeon shortly after I&D is recommended since the recurrence rate is high.

○ **What is the initial treatment for staphylococcal scalded skin syndrome (SSSS)?**

Oral or IV penicillinase-resistant penicillin, first- or second-generation cephalosporins, or clindamycin are appropriate. Modification may be made after sensitivities are determined. In patients with severe infection, hospitalization is required often times in burn units with special attention given to fluid and electrolyte management, pain management, and infection control.

○ **A 2-year-old girl has significant perianal erythema and small discrete red papules in the gluteal area. She has also been constipated because she is withholding her bowel movements due to pain. What is the most likely diagnosis?**

Perianal staphylococcal/streptococcal infection.

○ **What is the inciting event for the development of decubitus ulcers?**

Decubitus ulcers result from ischemia caused by prolonged exposure to pressure.

○ **You suspect that your 4-year-old patient has staphylococcal scalded skin syndrome (SSSS). What is the appropriate initial therapy?**

First-line therapy is initiation of a first- or second-generation cephalosporin or clindamycin. The antibiotic may be modified on the basis of cultures and sensitivities once they are attained. Neonates, infants, and children with severe disease should be hospitalized with attention to hydration, pain management, infection control, and wound care.

OTHER DERMATOLOGIC DISORDERS

○ **Upon routine examination, a 76-year-old female patient is found to have thickening and brown hyperpigmentation of the skin on the neck and axillae. This finding can be a marker for what disorders?**

Acanthosis nigricans is most commonly associated with obesity and insulin resistance. However, endocrine disorders, drug administration, and malignancy should also be considered.

○ **A 45-year-old female presents with a shiny, red-brown plaque with a yellow atrophic center located on her anterior lower left leg (pretibial). She reports that the lesion began as a small bump and has grown to its current size. What laboratory tests should be ordered?**

Necrobiosis lipoidica can be associated with diabetes. Therefore, laboratory testing should include plasma glucose, Hgb A1c, and insulin levels.

○　**A mother complains that her 2-month-old infant has transient mottling of the skin. On physical examination, you find lacy erythema on the lower extremities that blanches with pressure. When the infant is warmed, the erythemal resolves. What is the most likely diagnosis?**

Cutis marmorata.

○　**On physical examination, a 2-month-old infant has a reticulated vascular pattern on both lower extremities with a decreased circumference of the left lower extremity. The vascular patter on the right resolves with warming; however, it does not resolve on the left. What is the most likely diagnosis?**

Cutis marmorata telagiectasia congenita.

○　**An infant with a port wine stain (PWS) in the distribution of the first branch of the trigeminal nerve (V1). What is the most likely diagnosis?**

Sturge–Weber syndrome (SWS).

○　**A patient presents with a history of a rash that has occurred three times in the last month. He describes the rash as intensely pruritic. The lesions are transient and the rash resolves completely within a few days. On physical examination, he only has few lesions remaining from the most recent episode. They are well-circumscribed erythematous wheals. What is his most likely diagnosis?**

Urticaria.

○　**A 40-year-old male with no regular health care presents with yellow-brown plaques and papules located over the MCP joint tendons and over his elbows. What disorder is associated with the suspected diagnosis?**

Xanthomas in a younger adult is associated with familial hyperlipidemia. Since this patient is 40 years old, he most likely has the heterozygous form.

○　**A 5-year-old African American boy presents with a sharply demarcated 5-mm annular macule with complete loss of pigment on his right knee. He also has a well-defined 2-mm hypopigmented macule located on his right temporal area. There is no scaling or erythema noted. What is the most likely diagnosis?**

This patient most likely has vitiligo.

○　**What examination technique is used to help confirm a diagnosis of suspected vitiligo?**

Wood's lamp examination in a completely darkened room without windows will show accentuation of vitiligo lesions.

○　**A patient presents with a red pedunculated papule that has a collarette of scale. She states that it appeared less than a week ago and has been growing rapidly. She reports that it bleeds profusely in response to minor trauma. What is the first-line treatment?**

Treatment for pyogenic granuloma includes shave excision followed by electrodessication to achieve hemostasis and prevent reoccurrence.

○ **What are the diagnostic criteria for Kawasaki disease?**

Fever for 5 days or more with at least four of the following:
- Bilateral injected conjunctiva
- Red fissured crusted lips, hyperemia of oropharynx, and red strawberry tongue
- Erythema and/or edema of the extremities
- Skin manifestations (diffuse macular and papular, erythematous eruption, diffuse urticarial rash, or scarlet fever-like rash)
- Cervical lymphadenopathy

○ **What is the appropriate treatment strategy for a patient diagnosed with Kawasaki disease?**

Treatment is directed toward reducing inflammation and preventing damage to the arterial wall. Standard treatment regimen includes intravenous immunoglobulin (IVIG) and aspirin.

○ **A 6-year-old boy presents with palpable purpura on bilateral lower extremities. He also complains of pain and mild swelling in his ankles and knees. Today, he is experiencing some abdominal discomfort as well. He is recuperating from streptococcal pharyngitis. What is his most likely diagnosis?**

Henoch-Schönlein purpura (HSP) is a vasculitic disorder that primarily affects children between the ages of 2 and 11 years.

○ **You are examining a 6-month-old infant with a chief complaint of a spreading rash. There is a family history of type 2 diabetes in the mother, neurofibromatosis 1 in the father, and hypertension in the paternal grandfather. On physical examination, you find a total of 12 light tan macules on the torso ranging in size from 5 to 9 mm. The infant also has small tan macules in the inguinal and axillary areas. The remainder of the physical examination is normal. What is the most likely diagnosis?**

Neurofibromatosis 1 (NF1).

○ **What side effects are associated with topical corticosteroids?**

Atrophy, striae, telangiectasia, erythema, and hypopigmentation of the skin are common side effects. Topical corticosteroids used on the eyelid can cause cataracts and glaucoma. Systemic side effects from overuse include hypothalamic–pituitary–adrenal axis suppression.

○ **A 5-year-old boy presents with small discrete erythematous papules in a perioral and nasolabial distribution. What is the appropriate first-line treatment?**

The appropriate first-line treatment for perioraldermatitis is a topical antibiotic such as erythromycin, clindamycin, and metronidazole. In more severe cases, oral erythromycin or tetracyclines (in patients older than 8 years) are required.

○ **What is the most common side effect of treating perioral dermatitis with a topical steroid?**

A granulomatous perioral dermatitis results from treatment with a topical steroid.

○ **An 89-year-old bedridden nursing home patient is found to have a superficial ulceration involving only the epidermis located in the sacral region. What is the most likely diagnosis?**

This most likely represents a stage II decubitus ulcer.

REFERENCES

Paller AS, Mancini AJ. *Hurwitz Clinical Pediatric Dermatology: A Textbook of Skin Disorders of Childhood and Adolescence.* 3rd ed. London: Elsevier Saunders; 2006.

Habif TP, Campbell JL, Chapman MS, Dinulos JG, Zug KA. *Skin Disease: Diagnosis and Treatment.* 2nd ed. Philadelphia, PA: Elsevier Mosby; 2005.

Wolff K, Johnson RA. *Fitzpatrick's Color Atlas and Synopsis of Clinical Dermatology.* 6th ed. New York, NY: McGraw-Hill; 2009.

Pryor JP, Todd B, Dryer M. *Clinician's Guide to Surgical Care.* Lange Series. New York, NY: McGraw-Hill; 2008.

CHAPTER 13 Hematology/Oncology

Anthony E. Brenneman, MPAS, PA-C

ANEMIA

○ **A 23-year-old thin female presents with easy fatigability, exercise intolerance, brittle nails and craving ice chips, and lettuce. Her diet consists primarily of fruits and vegetables because of a concern for weight gain. What would be the best treatment?**

Iron replacement.

○ **A 43-year-old male presents with iron deficiency anemia. What primary history of present illness question do you ask?**

Have you noticed blood in your stools; black or tarry stools.

○ **You are asked to counsel a patient who cares the diagnosis of sickle cell anemia. What health maintenance advice would you provide to minimize the use of emergency room and hospitalizations?**

Continuity of care—use of regular clinician checkups; regular slit-lamp examinations; vigorous oral hydration during periods of extreme exercise, exposure to heat or cold, emotional stress, or infection; vaccination early in life.

○ **A teenage male that is asplenic secondary to sickle cell disease presents with fever and cough. Treatment was started using amoxicillin-clavulanate. Primary concern is for what infectious cause?**

Community acquired pneumonia—likely pneumococcal.

○ **A 74-year-old female with long-standing rheumatoid arthritis that has been difficult to control is seen in the office. She is noting fatigue and exertional intolerance. What laboratory finding do you anticipate and secondary diagnosis?**

Anemia of inflammation.

○ **What treatment is best for a 74-year-old female with chronic and now an acute flare of rheumatoid arthritis? She also complains of fatigue and exertional intolerance and her hemoglobin is 10.8 (12–15.5).**

Treatment of the rheumatoid arthritis. With improvement in the inflammation process, the anemia of chronic disease should self-correct. If the hemoglobin drops below 10, then a transfusion is warranted.

○ **When gathering information about a patient's functional status, a well-founded criteria for measuring performance is called:**

Karnofsky scale.

○ **Physical findings in a patient with pernicious anemia may include:**

Skin that is "lemon yellow" because of jaundice and pallor.

○ **An African American woman presents to your office to establish care. She indicates that she carries the diagnosis of sickle cell anemia. In addition to laboratory work, a full history and medication list, what area(s) of the physical examination would be most important to examine?**

The lower extremities for leg ulcers and/or scarring.

○ **In performing a history in a patient suspected of a hemolytic disorder, what family history questions would be useful to ask?**

Is there a history of family members with jaundice, anemia, and gallstones?

○ **One of the best ways to improve community health and reduce childhood anemia is through the elimination of what environmental source?**

Environmental lead.

○ **A 25-year-old male complains of chronic fatigue, easy bruising and has had increasing nose bleeds. He is unclear exactly when his fatigue started, but noted that he had been traveling in India where he had severe diarrhea and thinks this is when it began. He states he was given an antibiotic to treat it called chloramphenicol. What additional physical finding would you expect to find?**

Pallor.

○ **A 25-year-old male complains of chronic fatigue, easy bruising and has had increasing nose bleeds. He is unclear exactly when his fatigue started, but noted that he had been traveling in India where he had severe diarrhea and thinks this is when it began. He states he was given an antibiotic to treat it called chloramphenicol. What laboratory would you order and what finding would you anticipate?**

CBC, resulting in pancytopenia.

○ **A patient who is vegan and has a megaloblastic anemia found in laboratory studies would best be treated with:**

Cobalamin (Vitamin B_{12}).

○ **A patient is found to have a megaloblastic anemia after presenting with fatigue and pallor. A diagnosis of nontropical sprue is made. What is the best form of treatment?**

Folate plus a gluten-free diet.

COAGULATION DISORDERS

○ **Physical findings in a patient with thrombocytopenia may include:**

Petechiae and ecchymoses in the extremities.

○ **In a patient suspected of having a hemostasis disorder, what useful information would be gathered in the family history?**

Bleeding manifestations or venous thromboembolisms.

○ **Evaluation of a hemostatic disorder should be initiated when:**

1. A patient or physician suspects a bleeding tendency.

2. A bleeding tendency is discovered in one or more family members.

3. An abnormal coagulation assay result is obtained in either a routine examination or preparation for surgery.

4. A patient has unexplained diffuse bleeding following surgery or trauma.

○ **What are the two common clinical manifestations a patient may bring up in their history in a patient with von Willebrand disease?**

Epistaxis and excessive bleeding secondary to razor nicks.

○ **On physical examination with a patient who is suspected of having a hemostatic disorder, where is a clinician most likely to see petechiae or ecchymosis and why?**

The lower extremities because of the hydrostatic pressure being greatest.

○ **A 38-year-old female presents with pale mucous membranes, epistaxis, and scattered petechiae on her arms, legs, and torso that do not blanch to palpation/pressure. What laboratory abnormality would you anticipate?**

Thrombocytopenia.

○ **A 37-year-old female presents with pale mucous membranes, epistaxis, and scattered petechiae on her arms, legs, and torso that do not blanch to palpation/pressure. Laboratory findings note a hemoglobin, hematocrit, and white count in the normal range. Platelet count is <30,000. What is the likely diagnosis?**

Idiopathic thrombocytopenic purpura.

○ **What clinical intervention would be the best option for a patient who is diagnosed with idiopathic thrombocytopenic purpura whose platelet count averages 55,000 over 3 to 4 months?**

Observation in patients with no active or regular signs of bleeding and counts that remain above 50,000, observation is the best approach.

○ **A 20-year-old female presents with a platelet count of 18,000, epistaxis, and oozing gums. She also notes purpura that she states has been present for over 4 weeks to her extremities and abdomen. What is the recommended initial treatment?**

Glucocorticoid therapy.

○ **A 20-year-old college female is admitted to the hospital with high fever, disoriented, and a history of complaining of severe headache and neck pain. She now has signs of nuchal rigidity. She is started on appropriate antibiotic therapy and is moved to the ICU. A physical examination a few hours later reveals petechiae, ecchymoses, and oozing round her IV catheter sites. You are concerned for:**

Disseminated intravascular coagulation (DIC).

○ **In the above case, what laboratory studies would help to support the diagnosis?**

Platelet count, prothrombin time, aPTT, fibrin degradation products, and protease inhibitors.

○ **What treatment regimen would you recommend in this case?**

Aggressive treatment of the underlying cause (meningitis), along with replacing coagulation factors, fibrinolytic proteins, and platelets as these are rapidly consumed in DIC.

MALIGNANCIES

○ **An infiltrative lesion of the skin in a patient with leukemia is called:**

Leukemia cutis.

○ **A 67-year-old male complains of headache not responding to therapy, pruritus, feeling weak, and occasionally dizzy. Routine labs are drawn and are notable for an increased hemoglobin, hematocrit, and erythrocyte count. Platelets are also increased and he has a basophilia on white count. What is the most likely diagnosis?**

Polycythemia vera.

○ **The most common complication of a patient with polycythemia vera is:**

Thrombotic events.

○ **In patients with uncomplicated polycythemia vera, what is the current general approach to treatment?**

1. Hydroxyurea for myelosuppression
2. Aspirin for thromboembolic prevention
3. Allopurinol to control pruritus
4. Phlebotomy for volume reduction

○ **What environmental factors have been established as agents leading to AML?**

Tobacco smoking, high-dose radiation exposure, chronic benzene exposure, and some chemotherapeutic agents.

○ **A 57-year-old male presents with a several month history of increasing fatigue, weakness, dyspnea on exertion, easy bruising, anorexia with weight loss, and intermittent fevers. He has been treated with several rounds of antibiotics with no improvement. What findings would you anticipate when reviewing a CBC?**

Anemia, thrombocytopenia, and a decreased leukocyte count with increased myeloblasts.

○ **While doing a social history on a patient, you learn that he is a farmer. He indicates that he regularly applies organophosphates and herbicides to his crops. While direct evidence has yet to be scientifically established, there is an increased incidence of what type of cancer?**

Lymphoma.

○ **What thorough physical examination should be performed on a farmer who uses organophosphates and herbicides?**

All lymph nodes.

○ **While examining this patient, you note enlarged nodes in the inguinal and supraclavicular regions. The patient was unaware of them. Why is this?**

In the presence of extranodal disease of lymphoma, the nodes are typically nontender and rubbery. Since there is no discomfort, the patient is less likely to note them until they are quite enlarged.

○ **Using the Ann Arbor Staging System for this patient (enlarged nodes in the inguinal and supraclavicular regions), what disease stage would they be given?**

Stage III.

○ **The WHO classification identified three major categories of lymphoid malignancies, these are:**

B-cell neoplasms, T- and natural killer (NK) cell neoplasms, and Hodgkin lymphoma.

○ **A 53-year-old female presents with complaints of back pain and lower leg discomfort, weakness, and fatigue. A radiograph of the lower extremity is obtained and reveals a darkened area that circular and appears "cutout" from the bone. What finding do you believe this is and what disease do you associate this with?**

A lytic lesion of multiple myeloma.

○ **The standard of treatment for patients diagnosed with multiple myeloma is:**

Autologous hematopoietic stem cell transplant.

○ **A volunteer is interested in donating blood. What physical examinations must be completed to determine eligibility?**

Temperature, pulse, blood pressure, and weight. In addition, general appearance for illness or influence of drugs and alcohol should be assessed.

○ **What laboratory value must also be collected on potential donors of blood products?**

Hemoglobin concentration.

○ **A new donor to the blood bank is a 20-year-old female. She is 5′ 6″, weighs 128 lbs, and BP is 110/60. This is her first time donating blood. What common reactions might you anticipate in this woman?**

Weakness, cool skin, and diaphoresis.

○ **After donating a unit of blood for the first time, a 20-year-old female is noted to be dizzy and pale. You take her blood pressure and pulse. She is noted to be hypertensive and bradycardic. This finding is consistent with:**

A vasovagal reaction to the donation.

○ **Treatment for the young woman who is found to be hypertensive, bradycardic, dizzy, and pale following donation would consist of:**

Fluids, rest, rechecking vitals till return to baseline, and no strenuous activity for the rest of the day to prevent relapse.

REFERENCES

Lichtman MA, Kipps TJ, Seligsohn U, et al. *Williams Hematology.* 8th ed. New York, NY: McGraw-Hill Education; 2010.

Longo DL, Fauci AS, Kasper DL, et al. *Harrison's Principles of Internal Medicine.* 18th ed. New York, NY: McGraw-Hill Education; 2012.

Papadakis MA, McPhee SJ, Anemia, Iron Deficiency. Quick Medical Diagnosis & Treatment, McGraw-Hill Education; 2013. http://www.accessmedicine.com/quickam.aspx.

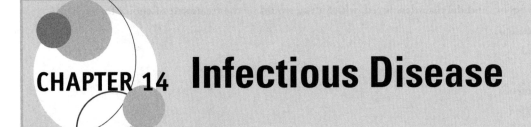

CHAPTER 14 Infectious Disease

Alexis Moore, MPH, PA-C

FUNGAL DISEASE

○ **What are some of the clinical conditions that can present with candidiasis?**

Oral thrush, vulvovaginitis, esophagitis, and mucocutaneous candida, candida funguria, candida endocarditis.

○ **What is the microscopic appearance of *Candida albicans*?**

Either as a singular oval budding yeast or as pseudohyphae (elongated).

○ **What risk factors are associated with the development of invasive or systemic candidiasis?**

Bone marrow transplantation, treatment with broad-spectrum antibiotics, Foley catheters, recent abdominal or other surgery, advanced kidney disease (1).

○ **A male patient with AIDS (CD4 160), presents with substernal odynophagia, gastroesophageal reflux, and nausea. His tongue and buccal mucosa have thickly coated white plaques that are removable when scraped with a tongue blade. His presentation is consistent with which disorder?**

Esophageal candidiasis secondary to immune compromised state.

○ **How is a diagnosis of esophageal candidiasis best confirmed?**

By upper GI endoscopy with biopsy and fungal and viral cultures (2).

○ **Of the five types of candidal disorders listed, which drug would be the treatment of choice for each?**

1. Oral *candidiasis*
2. Esophageal
3. Vaginal
4. Mucocutaneous
5. Disseminated

1. (Clotrimazole troches, nystatin suspension), fluconazole
2. Fluconazole of itraconazole
3. Nystatin, clotrimazole, miconazole (uncomplicated), fluconazole (severe, immune suppressed)
4. Ketoconazole
5. Amphotericin B or fluconazole

Fluconazole, <u>caspofungin</u> (echinocandin class) (3).

○ ***Cryptococcus* is transmitted to humans by what method?**

Inhalation of contaminated soil, usually by bird droppings.

○ **Which species of *Cryptococcus* causes most human infections?**

Cryptococcus neoformans.

Cryptococcus gattii—immunocompetent persons living in the United States' Pacific Northwest Region.

○ **What would a patient's chest X-ray reveal during the early stages of a *Cryptococcus* infection?**

A solitary nodule or diffuse noncalcified infiltrates may be visualized (4).

○ **What is the drug(s) of choice for the treatment of *Cryptococcus*?**

Amphotericin B for 2 weeks followed by fluconazole for 6 weeks or amphotericin B and flucytosine (5).

○ **A 23-year-old male native of Mexico presents to the ED with a complaint of fever and headache. He reports that his main occupation is seasonal migrant work along the west coast primarily in the states of California and Oregon, where he was most recently 4 weeks ago. He is currently visiting his brother who moved to NYC a year ago. Based on his history you suspect that the patient may be at risk for cryptococcal infection. How can you quickly rule out cryptococcal meningitis as a source of his complaint?**

The *Cryptococcal* Antigen Lateral Flow Assay (*CrAg* LFA) is a rapid dipstick *test* for the detection of *cryptococcal* antigen. 70% to 90% of patients with Cryptococcus test positive with this method. Use of the test helps hasten the work-up for meningitis in the clinical setting. CSF sampling is the other modality for diagnosing cryptococcal meningitis (6).

○ **Where is *histoplasmosis* more commonly found in the United States?**

Eastern and central United States, particularly in Mississippi, Ohio, and Missouri Valley areas.

○ **How does the *histoplasmosis* spore spread?**

Any activity that will cause the spores to move from their original site such as dry, windy conditions, demolition of old buildings, and barns where birds and bats have helped the spores proliferate.

○ **What test is used to accurately diagnose *histoplasmosis*?**

Cultures either from blood, marrow, tissue, or sputum via bronchoalveolar lavage.

Urine Antigen assay >90% sensitivity in immunocompromised individuals.

○ **What is the drug of choice for the treatment of a *histoplasmosis* infection?**

Amphotericin B.

Itraconazole (immunocompromised) therapeutic and prophylactic) (7).

○ **What is the newer and more appropriate species for a *pneumocystis* infection in humans?**

Pneumocystis jirovecii. Pneumocystis carinii infects only rats and not humans.

○ **What is the most common opportunistic infection in children and infants with HIV?**

Pneumocystis carinii pneumonia (PCP).

○ **What is the definitive diagnostic test for *pneumocystis* infection?**

Obtaining a respiratory tract specimen, either by tissue sample or by aspiration of secretions.

○ **What is the drug of choice for the treatment of *pneumocystis* infection?**

Oral trimethoprim—sulfamethoxazole, mild to moderate disease; Trimethoprim—sulfamethoxazole IV, poorly tolerated oral therapy.

○ **What if the patient is sulfa allergic or cannot tolerate the medication?**

Alternate drug to use would be pentamidine.

○ **A 32-year-old male has an insidious onset of fever, fatigue, and nonproductive cough over a 4-week period. At presentation he is febrile and breathing deeply. He reports a history of intermittent IV drug abuse over a 10-year period. His chest X-ray is remarkable for bilateral diffuse interstitial infiltrates and lab studies indicate an LDH of 450 U/L. What is the most likely diagnosis in this patient?**

Pneumocystis pneumonia.

○ **What other clinical work-up should be done on this patient?**

HIV-AB testing.

○ **How is the diagnosis of pulmonary *zygomycosis* made?**

By biopsy, zygomycosis fungal infections may manifest in the cutaneous, GI, pulmonary and cerebral systems; rhinocerebral is the most common.

○ **Rhinocerebral zygomycosis is associated with which chronic disease?**

Rhinocerebral zygomycosis is associated with diabetes and acidotic states. More than half of the patients with rhinocerebral zygomycosis present in DKA (8).

○ **The greatest risk factor for the development of aspergillosis infection is?**

Stem cell or organ transplantation (9).

BACTERIAL DISEASE

○ **How is botulism contracted, and what are the principal clinical features?**

It is contracted by:

- consumption of contaminated foods where contents have been canned, smoked, or vacuum packed.
- injury from nonsterile objects (wound botulism).
- in infants, from intestinal colonization by *Clostridium botulinum* via lack of normal intestinal flora permitting this colonization or through the consumption of honey.
- Inhalation (bioterrorism) (10).

The clinical features are that of a descending paralysis with complete ophthalmoplegia, bulbar, and somatic palsy.

○ **What is the best test to use to confirm a diagnosis of botulism?**

Foodborne—toxicity testing of serum samples.

Toxicity testing and culture—for stool, gastric aspirate, or food samples for presence of *C. botulinum* (11).

○ **What is the treatment for adult foodborne illness caused by *Clostridium botulinum*? For infant botulism?**

For adults and infants greater than 1 year old—Heptavalent antitoxin (A-G)-Foodborne and wound
For infants less than 1 year old—Botulism immune globulin (Big-IV or Baby-BIG) (12).

○ **If treating a botulism skin borne infection, what class of antibiotics should you avoid?**

Aminoglycosides because they may potentiate the toxin leading to exacerbation of neurological symptoms.

○ **How do symptoms of botulism exposure unfold?**

Within 12 to 36 hours of ingestion development of dry mouth nausea and vomiting followed by cranial nerve paralysis causing diplopia, blurred vision, fixed, or dilated pupils. Symmetric descending paralysis, motor weakness, and eventual respiratory collapse are the final sequelae if left untreated.

○ **What are the "5 D's" of botulism?**

Dysphagia, dysphonia, visual disturbances, diplopia, and dilated, fixed pupils.

○ **What is the most common cause of sexually transmitted disease in the United States?**

Chlamydia trachomatis infections.

○ **Can *Chlamydia* bacteria grow independently?**

No, they are obligate intracellular pathogens.

○ **What are the two most common forms of transmission of *Chlamydia*?**

Close contact either sexually or via the birth canal.

○ **A newly sexually active 17-year-old female presents with complaint of vague pelvic pain, dysuria, frequency, and urgency. Pelvic examination is remarkable for cervicitis, and presence of cervical motion tenderness. Her urine sample is negative for nitrites, has greater than 5 to 10 WBC/hpf and 3+ leukocyte esterase but no bacteria. What is the most likely pathogen involved with this finding?**

Chlamydia trachomatis, if PID is suspected then the patient should also be treated for gonorrhea and anaerobes most notably those contributing to bacterial vaginosis.

○ **A 19-year-old male has a 3-day history of scrotal pain and swelling associated with dysuria and fever. His physical examination is remarkable for a moderately enlarged scrotum that is erythematous and pain that is relieved by elevation of the testicle. What disorder does this patient have and what agent is the most likely cause?**

Epididymitis, Chlamydia trachomatis, or *Neisseria gonorrhoeae.*

○ **What is the drug of choice for the treatment of sexually transmitted *Chlamydia*?**

Azithromycin.

○ **What is the treatment of neonatal conjunctivitis caused by *Chlamydia trachomatis*?**

Oral erythromycin.

○ **Describe the lesions associated with chlamydia.**

Painless, shallow ulcerations, papular or nodular lesions, and herpetiform vesicles that wax and wane.

○ **Describe the lesions associated with lymphogranuloma venereum (LV).**

LV caused by *Chlamydia* presents as painless skin lesions with lymphadenopathy. Lesions may be papular, nodular, or herpetiform vesicles. Sinus formation, involving the vagina and rectum, are common in women because lack of symptoms in the primary and secondary stages of the disease.

○ **As a medical relief aid assigned to an encampment for victims of the Haitian earthquake, over a 3-day period, you observe several members of the camp develop diarrhea that has the appearance of colorless "rice water" stools. There is no complaint of abdominal pain, but many are dehydrated and have suspected electrolyte abnormalities. What would be the leading diagnosis?**

Vibrio cholera outbreak.

○ **What is the most common mode of contamination of patients infected with *Vibrio cholera*?**

Contaminated water or food (uncooked or raw shellfish, dried fish, and vegetables held in ambient heat).

○ **What is the treatment for a patient with confirmed or suspected cholera?**

Aggressive oral hydration along with electrolyte replenishment. If severe infection, oral doxycycline (one-time dose) or tetracycline can be used.

○ **What are the signs and symptoms of *diphtheria*?**

Gradual onset of symptoms of sore throat, cervical lymphadenopathy, and low-grade fever with progression to exudative pharyngitis, high fever, and malaise. A gray-colored pseudomembrane may form in the oropharynx with possible respiratory compromise. Powerful exotoxins directly affect the heart, kidneys, and nervous system. Diphtheria infection may lead to paralysis of the intrinsic and extrinsic eye muscles, which may be confused with bulbar palsy caused by *Clostridium botulinum*. Botulism does not cause fever.

○ **What confirmatory test is run for the diagnosis of *diphtheria*?**

Culture, usually from the nose, throat, or mucous membrane lesion.

○ **A family recently immigrated from Brazil to the United States and presents with their 4-year-old daughter who has a cough and worsening hoarseness of her voice for the last 5 to 7 days. They are concerned that she is no longer eating because it hurts to swallow. On physical examination she is febrile with a temperature of 101.8°F and has multiple throat exudates that coalesce into a gray membranous growth encompassing most of the tonsils and pharynx. What is the likely cause of this patient's symptoms?**

Diptheria caused by *Corynebacterium diphtheriae* in the unimmunized and is endemic to Brazil, Dominican Republic, Ecuador, Haiti, and Paraguay (13, 14).

○ **What are the three considerations for the treatment of *diphtheria*?**

1. Antitoxin—before cultures are back and have high suspicion
2. Antibiotics—erythromycin or penicillin G
3. Immunization

○ **Do individuals with close contact to a *diphtheria* patient need prophylaxis therapy?**

Close contacts must be observed for up to a week for any signs of infection, and nasal and pharyngeal swabs cultured for diphtheria, and administer prophylaxis treatment with erythromycin for 7 to 10 days, or IM penicillin G.

○ **What percentage of patients with *gonococcal* genital infections have concomitant *Chlamydia trichomatous* infections?**

46%. This is why the treatment for *gonorrhea* includes ceftriaxone and azithromycin or doxycycline to cover both infections.

○ **What is the most common type of *gonorrhea* infection that can be seen in newborns?**

Conjunctivitis (purulent).

○ ***Neisseria gonorrhea* is confirmed by what type of laboratory test?**

Gram stain (higher sensitivity in symptomatic men) and culture. You will see gram-negative diplococci.

○ **A 10-year-old girl presents to your facility with a history and physical examination that is consistent with vaginitis producing thick, purulent yellow discharge. What is the most likely pathogen involved? What other concerns should the parents and clinician have?**

The vaginitis with discharge as described is consistent with <u>Neisseria</u> *gonorrhea* infection. A 10-year-old girl who presents with this profile should create a high degree of suspicion for sexual abuse, as this type of vaginitis is abnormal in a prepubescent child.

○ **What is the recommended initial treatment for cases of gonorrhea?**

Third-generation cephalosporins (specifically ceftriaxone) plus either or azithromycin (1 g PO × 1 dose) or doxycycline (100 mg BID for 7 days) for presumptive coinfection with *Chlamydia*.

○ **What is the most common physical examination finding in an adult patient with disseminated gonorrhea?**
Septic arthritis.

○ **The hallmark triad of disseminated gonococcal infection is?**

Tenosynovitis, dermatitis, and polyarthralgias without purulent arthritis.

○ **Describe the skin lesions found in a patient with disseminated gonococcemia.**

Painless umbilicated pustules with red halos, lasting approximately 3 to 4 days.

○ **What is the course of treatment for disseminated *gonorrhea*?**

7-day course of ceftriaxone or cefotaxime with azithromycin or doxycycline for chlamydia, If suspicion for meningitis, 10 to 14 days of treatment is recommended.

○ **What is the most common cause of bacterial enterocolitis in the United States?**

Salmonella infection.

○ **How is *Salmonella* transmitted?**

It is transmitted by humans and usually comes from contaminated water or food.

○ **Name the three types of infections that occur as a result of *Salmonella*.**

Enterocolitis, typhoid, and septicemia.

○ **What are the features of typhoid fever?**

Remember BIRDS FLEW:

Bradycardia	**F**ever
Insidious onset	**L**eukopenia
Rose spots	**E**pidemic
Dicrotic pulse	**W**idal reaction
Splenomegaly	

○ **Name the signs and symptoms for salmonella enterocolitis.**

Fever, diarrhea, and abdominal pain.

○ **What test do you order to confirm a diagnosis of *Salmonella*?**

Stool cultures most common. You can also obtain blood and urine cultures if examination is consistent.

○ **Which has a longer incubation period, staphylococci or salmonellae?**

Salmonellae; it is generally ingested in small doses and then multiplies in the GI tract. Symptoms occur 6–48 hours after ingestion. *Staphylococcus aureus* has an incubation period of just 3 hours.

○ **What is the first-line treatment for salmonella enterocolitis?**

Fluid and electrolyte replenishment.

○ **What is the pharmacological treatment for persistent salmonellosis?**

Ampicillin, TMP-SMX, ciprofloxacin.

○   **In general, antibiotics should be avoided with what infectious diarrhea?**

Salmonella. However, clear exceptions are severe cases of diarrhea in immunocompromised patients and in children younger than 6 months.

○   **Which part of the GI tract does *Shigella* sp. infect more often?**

The colon.

○   **A patient presents with diarrhea, high fever, headache, lethargy, and confusion. Lumbar puncture is normal. A CBC with differential has a band count of 45% and a blood culture is positive for *Escherichia coli*, what is the most likely cause of the diarrhea?**

Shigella. Blood cultures in shigella diarrhea virtually never isolate the organism. In instances where cultures are positive, *Escherichia coli* is more likely to be the bacterium. Perhaps this is because of the fact that while Shigella is locally quite invasive at the mucosal level, it is very poorly invasive at the systemic level. Resident *E. coli* in the gut, however, take advantage of the disrupted mucosa and invade the blood stream.

○   **What is the microscopic makeup of *Shigella* sp.?**

It is a facultative anaerobe, gram-negative, bacillus.

○   **What is the primary transmission route of *Shigella*?**

Fecal–oral.

○   **In diagnosing *Shigella*, what will a stool culture most likely yield?**

It will show fecal leukocytes, which is consistent with a colitis picture.

○   **Do you treat *Shigella* with antibiotics?**

In general, no, if the disease is self-limiting to less than 72 hours. Should the infection be prolonged, if there is significant diarrhea, dysentery, or an immunocompromised patient, and then antibiotics are used to shorten the duration of the illness and reduce the amount of fecal leukocytes in the stool.

○   **What is the treatment for *Shigella* sp.?**

TMP-SMX or ciprofloxacin (if resistant).

○   **What are the possible complications of Shigella infection?**

Toxic megacolon, intestinal obstruction, seizures (pediatric patients) reactive arthritis (15).

○   **What causes tetanus?**

Clostridium tetani. This organism is a gram-positive anaerobe and rod shaped; characteristically, it is vegetative and a spore former, producing the endotoxin tetanospasmin. The endotoxin induces the disinhibition of the motor and autonomic nervous systems and results in the clinical symptoms exhibited in tetanus.

○   **What is the incubation period of tetanus?**

Hours to months, with most cases occurring in 8 days. The shorter the incubation period, the more severe the disease.

○ **What is the most common presentation of tetanus?**

"Generalized tetanus" with pain and stiffness in the trunk and jaw muscles. Trismus develops and results in risus sardonicus ("The Devil's Smile").

○ **Outline the treatment for tetanus:**

Wound: Debridement

Respiratory: Administer succinylcholine for immediate intubation if required.

Immunotherapy: Human tetanus immune globulin will neutralize circulating tetanospasmin and the toxin in the wound. However, it will not neutralize toxin fixed in the nervous system. Dose TIG 3000 to 5000 units. Prescribe tetanus toxoid, 0.6 mL IM, at 1 week and 6 weeks and 6 months.

Antibiotics: *Clostridium tetani* is sensitive to cephalosporins, tetracycline, erythromycin, and penicillin, but metronidazole is considered the drug of choice with penicillin G as an alternative (16, 17).

Muscle relaxants: Administer diazepam or dantrolene to help with the tetanic spasms.

Neuromuscular block: Prescribe pancuronium bromide, 2 mg plus sedation. Vercorium, short acting and cause less autonomic complications (18).

Autonomic dysfunction: Prescribe magnesium sulfate, 70 mg/kg IV load labetalol, 0.25 to 1.0 mg/min IV; or; then

1 to 4 g/hr continuous infusion is used to treat autonomic dysfunction. Administer MS, 5 to 30 mg IV infusion every 2 to 8 hours; and clonidine, 1.3 mg every 8 hour per NG.

Note: Fatal cardiovascular complications have occurred in patients treated with beta-adrenergic blocking agents alone. Adrenergic blocking agents used to treat autonomic dysfunction may precipitate myocardial depression.

○ **Distinguish the key differences between strychnine and tetanus poisoning.**

Tetanus poisoning produces constant muscle tension, whereas strychnine produces tetany and convulsions with episodes of relaxation between muscle contractions.

○ **What are the signs and symptoms of tularemia?**

Indurated skin ulcers at the site of inoculation, regional lymphadenopathy, fever, shaking chills, cough, hemoptysis, SOB, rales or pleural rub, hepatosplenomegaly, and a maculopapular rash.

○ **What is the treatment for tularemia?**

Streptomycin. Gentamycin, alternative choice and for outpatient therapy. Mortality rate is 5% to 30% without antibiotic treatment.

○ **What is the most common symptom of tularemia?**

Skin sores at the site of inoculation and lymphadenopathy (75%). Other symptoms include pneumonia, lesions in the GI system, infection of the eyes, fever, and headache.

○ **How is tularemia most commonly transmitted?**

Via ticks, deer flies, and rabbits. Tularemia is caused by *Francisella tularensis*.

○ **What is the most frequent complication of tularemia?**

Lymph node suppuration.

○ **What is the most common cause of cellulitis?**

Group A B-hemolytic-*Streptococcus pyogenes*. *Staphylococcus aureus* can also cause cellulitis though it is generally less severe and more often associated with an open wound.

○ **What is the most common cause of cutaneous abscesses?**

Staphylococcus aureus.

○ **What percentage of dog and cat bites become infected?**

About 5% of dog bites and 80% of cat bites become infected, because of the depth of puncture from cats having sharper narrower teeth. *Pasteurella multocida* is the causative agent for 30% of dog bites and 50% of cat bites.

○ **An 8-year-old child received a kitten as a new pet and was bitten a week later. A tender papule develops at the site. She now presents with headache, fever, malaise, and tender regional lymphadenopathy. What is the diagnosis?**

Cat-scratch disease. This condition usually develops 3 days to 6 weeks following a cat bite or scratch. The papule typically blisters and heals with eschar formation. A transient macular or vesicular rash may also develop.

○ **What is thought to be the mode of inoculation in cat-scratch disease?**

Rubbing the eye after contact with a cat.

○ **What is the probable cause of an animal bite infection arising that develops in less than 24 hours? More than 48 hours?**

Less than 24 hours: *Pasteurella multocida* or streptococci. More than 48 hours: *Staphylococcus aureus.*

○ **What is the most common cause of gas gangrene?**

Clostridium perfringens.

○ **What are the neurological features of brucellosis?**

Mainly a chronic meningitis and the vascular complications thereof. However, cranial neuropathies, demyelination, and mycotic aneurysms have all been described.

○ **How is brucellosis spread?**

By ingestion of contaminated milk and milk products. It may also be spread by contact with an infected animal (usually cattle). *Brucella melitensis* is the culprit.

○ **A 43-year-old male attended a food tasting seminar where several varieties of raw and unpasteurized cheeses were sampled. Three to four weeks later he presented to his doctor's office complaining of diffuse muscle aches, low back pain, night sweats, and intermittent fever. Based on his exposure history, what would be on your differential for his presentation?**

Brucellosis, based on his history of exposure to raw milk products.

○ **A 31-year-old man stepped on a nail at his job. The nail pierced through his sneaker and into his foot. His tetanus status is up to date. What is your main concern?**

Infection with *Pseudomonas* that can lead to osteomyelitis. Pseudomonal infection is most commonly associated with hot, moist environments, such as sneakers and moisture in socks.

○ **What is the most common causative bacterium associated with right-sided endocarditis in IV drug abusers?**

Staphylococcus aureus. Left-sided endocarditis in IV drug abusers is usually due to *Escherichia coli, Streptococcus, Klebsiella, Pseudomonas,* or *Candida.*

○ **What are the major Jones criteria used to diagnose rheumatic fever?**

Carditis, chorea (Sydenham), erythema marginatum, migratory polyarthritis, and subcutaneous nodules. The diagnosis requires either two major or one major and two minor with evidence of previous streptococcal infection.

○ **What are the five major manifestations of acute rheumatic fever that must be present to bolster clinical suspicion of the disease?**

- Migratory arthritis (predominantly involving the large joints)
- Carditis and valvulitis (e.g., pancarditis)
- Central nervous system involvement (e.g., Sydenham chorea)
- Erythema marginatum
- Subcutaneous nodules

(18)

○ **After finishing the prescribed dosage of penicillin for pharyngitis, your patient's repeat culture still grows *Streptococcus.* What should you do?**

Nothing. Most people are asymptomatic carriers and in most cases it is inconsequential.

○ **What is the cause of chancroid?**

Haemophilus ducreyi. Patients with this condition present with one or more painful necrotic lesions. Suppurating inguinal lymphadenopathy may also be present.

○ **What is the most common infectious disease complication of both measles and influenza?**

Pneumococcal pneumonia.

○ **Do household pets transmit *Yersinia*?**

Yes, generally via scratches or bites from cats.

○ **A 30-year-old male presents with a 1-week history of lymphadenitis and fever. His fever is currently 105°F. His history is otherwise unremarkable except a report given by his family members that several dead squirrels were removed from his property in the past few weeks. What illness might you suspect this patient has?**

Cases of human plague (*Yersinia pestis*) are sometimes heralded by squirrel die-offs. A squirrelly die-off occurs when the organism is introduced into a highly susceptible mammalian population, causing a high mortality rate among infected animals. This is referred to as epizootic plague.

○ **A 20-year-old woman presents to the emergency department with nausea, vomiting, abdominal pain, and tachycardia. She reports an accidental overdose of oral iron supplements. She is admitted to the hospital and a day later becomes septic. What organism is the most likely cause of her sepsis?**

Yersinia enterocolitica. The growth of *Y. enterocolitica* appears to be enhanced after exposure to excess iron. This combined with intestinal damage to the mucosa by the iron may play a role in pathogenesis.

○ **What is the treatment for *Yersinia* sp.?**

Streptomycin, gentamycin, patients intolerant of aminoglycosides, use doxycycline or tetracycline.

○ **What is Weil disease?**

Weil syndrome is the less common variety of leptospirosis, with icterus, marked hepatic and renal involvement along with a bleeding diathesis being the main features, and hence the name leptospirosis ictero-hemorrhagica.

○ **What is the most common neurological feature of leptospirosis?**

Aseptic meningitis (present in over 50%).

○ **What clinical feature of leptospirosis sets it apart from other infections of the nervous system and hints at the diagnosis?**

Hemorrhagic complications. These are not uncommon, and intraparenchymal and subarachnoid hemorrhages have been reported.

○ **Which organisms produce focal nervous system pathology via an exotoxin?**

Clostridium diphtheria, Clostridium botulinum, Clostridium tetani, Staphylococcus aureus plus wood and dog ticks (*Dermacentor A* and *B*).

○ **How should you treat a patient who has been bitten by a wild raccoon?**

Wound care, tetanus prophylaxis, RIG, 20 IU/kg (1/2 at bite site and 1/2 IM), and HDCV, 1 cc IM.

○ **Do animal bites from birds, reptiles, or rodents (hamster, squirrel, mouse, rat, gerbil, guinea pig, rabbit) require the rabies vaccine?**

No, these types of animal bites do not carry rabies.

○ **Describe the skin lesions associated with a *Pseudomonas aeruginosa* infection.**

Hemorrhagic vesicles or pustules with necrotic ulcerations in the center and erythematous borders.

○ **Why is needle aspiration preferred over incision and drainage for a fluctuant, acute cervical lymphadenitis?**

Development of a fistula tract is possible if the patient has atypical mycobacterium or cat-scratch fever instead of bacterial lymphadenitis.

○ **What is the cause of granuloma inguinale?**

The bacterium *Klebsiella granulomatis* some use an older classification *Calymmatobacterium granulomatis*.

○ **Infections with which enteric or venereal bacterias may result in reactive arthritis?**

Salmonella typhimurium or enteritidis, Streptococcus viridans, group A Streptococcus, Mycoplasma pneumonia, Chlamydia trachomatis, Yersinia enterocolitica or pseudotuberculosis, Campylobacter, and Shigella flexneri.

○ **What triad is associated with Reiter syndrome?**

Nongonococcal urethritis, polyarthritis, and conjunctivitis. Conjunctivitis is the least common and occurs in only 30% of the patients. Acute attacks respond well to NSAIDs.

○ **What is the treatment for persistent *Escherichia coli*?**

Trimethoprim with sulfamethoxazole (TMP-SMX).

○ **What is the treatment for *Giardia lamblia*?**

Tinidazole, metronidazole quinacrine (no longer commercially available in the United States).

○ **What gastrointestinal illness is associated with the ingestion of seafood such as clams or crabs but primarily oysters?**

Acute, explosive diarrhea accompanied by nausea, vomiting, and abdominal cramps because of the infection with Vibrio parahaemolyticus. Severe infections are treated with doxycycline, tetracycline, or ciprofloxacin.

○ **What are the antibiotics of choice in a wound resulting from a skin diving incident?**

Ciprofloxacin or TMP-SMX.

○ **What is the most common gram-negative aerobe found in cutaneous abscesses?**

Proteus mirabilis.

○ **Describe the Gram stain appearance of *Staphylococcus aureus*.**

Gram-positive cocci in grapelike clusters.

○ **Which type of diarrhea-causing disease may be transmitted by pets?**

Yersinia.

○ **Which organism typically is not involved in causing abscesses? Does *Haemophilus influenzae* typically cause abscesses?**

No.

○ **The most common pathogen transmitted in cat bites is?**

Pasteurella multocida.

○ **What percentage of untreated group A-hemolytic streptococcal infections will progress to rheumatic fever?**

3%. Increased incidence of the disease is noted in lower socioeconomic areas.

○ **What prophylaxis treatment is indicated for household or close contacts of individuals infected with meningococcal meningitis to prevent further outbreaks?**

Rifampin ciprofloxacin or ceftriaxone are used as chemoprophylaxis for contacts.

○ **Why does therapy for tuberculosis (TB) take several months, when other infections usually clear in a matter of days?**

Because the mycobacterium divide very slowly and have a long dormant phase, during which time they are not responsive to medications.

○ **What is the typical timeframe for symptoms to appear for patients with TB?**

1 to 6 months.

○ **What are some of the classic symptoms of TB?**

Fevers, chills, cough, night sweats, weight loss, or poor weight gain.

○ **What are some radiographic findings on chest X-ray in a patient with TB?**

- Early infection studies may be normal, exhibit hilar adenopathy or pulmonary infiltrates.
- Pleural effusion progression can include evidence of cavitary lesions and miliary disease.

○ **What type of bacteria is TB?**

It is an acid-fast bacillus.

○ **Name the two types of lesions found in TB.**

1. Exudative lesions—Usually seen at the site of the lung that produces inflammatory reaction of the local tissue.
2. Granulomatous lesions—These are giant cells that have tubercle bacilli around the cells. Over time, these cells will heal but will leave fibrotic or calcified tissue behind.

○ **What percentage of primary infections do not progress to active disease?**

90%.

○ **Which drug remains the cornerstone of TB treatment regimens?**

Rifampin.

○ **What is the most common nonadverse side effect of rifampin?**

Orange discoloration of urine and tears.

○ **What is the triple drug treatment for INH nonresistant pulmonary TB, and how long should a patient remain on each drug?**

Isoniazid, 6 months

Rifampin, 6 months

Pyrazinamide, 2 months.

For patients: Resistant to INH: rifampin or rifabutin, pyrazinamide, and ethambutol for 6 to 9 months
HIV-positive patients, INH rifampin, pyrazinamide, and ethambutol for 2 months then INH and rifamycin for 4 months.

○ **If the result of a patient's initial PPD reading is 3 mm of induration and then 15 mm of induration following the placement of the second PPD 2 weeks later, which reading should be considered the more reliable?**

The second study with an induration of 15 mm. With time, in a person with a past TB infection, the body has diminished skin sensitivity to the tuberculin solution and the individual may test negative with PPD administration.

The placement of a second PPD may stimulate the appropriate positive response in those with prior exposure and avoid a second PPD response being interpreted as a new infection. This is what is referred to as the "booster phenomenon." The boosted result is considered to be the reliable result.

○ List the four groups of atypical mycobacterium, the common bacteria in each group, where it is found, the physical effects, and what drug it used to treat

Group with Name	Name of Bacteria	Environment	Physical Effects	Drug of Choice
Group I Photochromogens	*M. kansasii*	Unknown	Resembles Pulmonary TB infections	Anti-TB drugs
	Mycobacterium marinum	Swimming pools Seafood processors aquariums	Ulcerating skin lesions at abrasions	Doxycycline minocycline
Group II Scotochromogens	*M. scrofulaceum*	Environmental water sources	Cervical adenitis	Surgical excision of affected lymph node
Group III Nonchromogens	*M. avium* *M. intracellulare*	Water and soil Water and soil	Pulmonary infection similar to TB	Clarithromycin or AzithromycinPlus rifabutin
Group IV Rapidly growing bacteria	*M. fortuitum*	Soil and water	Skin and soft tissue punctures	Amikacin
	M. chelonei	Soil and water	Immuno-compromised patients and patients with prosthetics and indwelling catheters	Azithromycin

○ **What regions of the United States have more cases of coccidiomycosis?**

Typically the Southwest states (Arizona, New Mexico, Southern California) and some in the Ohio valley. It is sometimes referred to as Valley fever or the San Joaquin fever.

○ **How is the diagnosis of coccidiomycosis made?**

By culture or staining of sputum, bronchoalveolar lavage or tissue, and by a positive serology.

○ **What is the treatment for a pulmonary infection caused by *coccidiomycosis*?**

Amphotericin B, fluconazole, or itraconazole (less adverse effects), is used for serious infections. Minor infections do not require medications.

○ **What is the cause of granuloma inguinale?**

Klebsiella granulomatis. Onset occurs with small papular, nodular, or vesicular lesions that develop slowly into ulcerative or granulomatous lesions. Lesions are painless and are located on mucous membranes of the genital, inguinal, and anal areas.

○ **A 55-year-old male native of the Philippines presents with two to three well-demarcated, reddish, hypopigmented lesions to his right ear and shoulder. He reports loss of feeling and numbness to the area of the lesions. What is the most likely cause of his problem?**

Leprosy (*Mycobacterium leprae*).

○ **What is the mode of transmission for leprosy?**

It is through human-to-human contact in close quarters and that the mode of transmission is theorized to be via respiratory droplets. The disease may also be acquired through prolonged contact with infected patients.

○ **What are the two forms of leprosy?**

Tuberculin and lepromatous.

○ **What is the treatment for leprosy?**

Dapsone. Rifampin or clofazimine in combination

PARASITIC DISEASE

○ **List three common protozoa that can cause diarrhea.**

1. *Entamoeba histolytica*—Found worldwide. Although half of the infected patients are asymptomatic, the usual symptoms consist of N/V/D/F, anorexia, abdominal pain, and leukocytosis. Determine the presence of this organism by ordering stool tests and performing an ELISA for extraintestinal infections. Treatment is with metronidazole or tinidazole followed by chloroquine phosphate.

2. *Giardia lamblia*—Found worldwide. This organism is one of the most common intestinal parasites in the United States. Symptoms include explosive watery diarrhea, flatus, abdominal distention, fatigue, and fever. The diagnosis is confirmed via a stool examination. Treatment is with metronidazole.

3. *Cryptosporidium parvum*—Found worldwide. Symptoms are profuse watery diarrhea, cramps, N/V/F, and weight loss. Treatment is supportive care. Medications may be needed for immunocompromised patients.

○ **What is the most common intestinal parasite in the United States?**

Giardia. Cysts are obtained from contaminated water or by hand-to-mouth transmission. Symptoms include explosive foul-smelling diarrhea, abdominal distention, fever, fatigue, and weight loss. Cysts reside in the duodenum and upper jejunum.

○ **What are the characteristic features of cerebral amebiasis, and what is the pathogenic organism?**

Cerebral amebiasis is usually a secondary infection, resulting from patients with primary intestinal or hepatic amebiasis. The causative organism is *Entamoeba histolytica*, which produces trophozoites that travel to the brain through the bloodstream. The clinical features are that of intracerebral abscess formation causing focal neurological signs. Frontal lobes and basal nuclei are common sites of abscess formation.

○ **What is the treatment for amebiasis with neurological involvement?**

Entamoeba histolytica is treated with metronidazole, emetine, and chloroquine. *Naegleria* species is treated with amphotericin and rifampicin.

○ **Besides the intestinal and cerebral manifestations related to *Entamoeba histolytica*, what is another potential complication related to this parasite?**

The development of a liver abscess, which may produce a clinical presentation of right upper quadrant pain, fever, weight loss, and an enlarged liver that is tender to palpation.

○ **Which parasite may be found in 25% to 50% of women, causes a watery, foul-smelling vaginal discharge, and has the microscopic appearance of a pear-shaped organism with four flagellates anteriorly?**

Trichomonas vaginalis.

○ **What is the antibiotic of choice for this type of infection?**

Metronidazole.

○ **Where is the hookworm *Necator americanus* infection acquired?**

In areas where soil contains human fecal waste and individuals walk barefoot. Patients commonly present with chronic anemia, cough, low-grade fever, diarrhea, abdominal pain, weakness, weight loss, eosinophilia, and guaiac-positive stools. A diagnosis is confirmed if ova are present in the stool. Treatment includes Albendazole or pyrantel pamoate.

○ **What are the signs and symptoms of *Trichuris trichiura*?**

This hookworm lives in the cecum. Complaints include anorexia, abdominal pain especially RUQ, insomnia, fever, diarrhea, flatulence, weight loss, pruritus, eosinophilia, and microcytic hypochromic anemia. Examining for ova in the stool makes a diagnosis. Mebendazole is the treatment of choice.

○ **A 25-year-old male patient attended a hunting event at which game meats and pork were served. He now reports to clinic and is symptomatic with N/V/D/F. Physical examination is remarkable for urticaria, myalgia, splinter hemorrhages, muscle spasm, headache, and a stiff neck. What additional physical finding would confirm his diagnosis?**

Periorbital edema is pathognomonic for infection with *Trichinella spiralis*. Patients may have acute myocarditis, nonsuppurative meningitis, and catarrhal enteritis bronchopneumonia. Laboratory studies may reveal leukocytosis, eosinophilia, ECG changes, and elevated CPK. Diagnosis is confirmed with a latex agglutination, skin test, complement fixation, or bentonite flocculation test. A stool examination is not helpful after the initial GI phase for confirming the diagnosis.

○ **How are tapeworms transmitted into humans?**

They are usually acquired by ingesting undercooked fish, which has the larvae present. The larvae then proliferate. In the cases of cysticercosis and hydatid disease, the eggs are ingested.

○ **Which is the most common tapeworm in the United States?**

Hymenolepis nana (dwarf tapeworm). Infections are spread via fecal/oral spread and occur in institutionalized patients, typically children.

○ **These three species of hookworms *Ancylostoma duodenale*, *Necator americanus*, and *Ancylostoma ceylanicum*, all affect humans and are responsible for which hematologic clinical presentation?**

Anemia.

○ **Hookworm is associated with what sort of anemia?**

Iron deficiency anemia.

○ **Fish tapeworm (*Diphyllobothrium latum*) is associated with what type of anemia?**

Pernicious anemia (B-12 deficiency).

○ **Roundworm is associated with what GI problem?**

Small bowel obstruction.

○ **In general, what kinds of education can you provide to patients to prevent infections that arise from hookworms?**

Beef and pork products must be cooked thoroughly as well as hands washed properly. Farmers contribute to reducing spread by ensuring that cows and pigs avoid ingesting human waste.

○ **Name the four types of malaria, and which one is the most prevalent?**

1. *Plasmodium falciparum* (most prevalent)
2. *P. vivax*
3. *P. ovale*
4. *P. malariae*
5. ***Plasmodium knowlesi*, a parasite of macaque monkeys, is now recognized to cause occasional illnesses, including some severe disease, in humans in Southeast Asia.**

○ **What is the most deadly form of malaria?**

Plasmodium falciparum.

○ **What is the vector for malaria?**

The female anopheline mosquito.

○ **What is the lifecycle of *Plasmodium falciparum*?**

1. Female anopheline mosquito bite injects sporozoites into the human bloodstream.
2. Sporozoites migrate to the liver and infect hepatocytes.
3. Merozoites are released from the liver and travel to erythrocytes (asexual phase of reproduction).
4. Proliferation and further release of Merozoites causing more larger scale erythrocyte invasion.
5. Differentiation of some erythrocytic parasites into gametocytes that go on to infect mosquitoes thereby completing the lifecycle.

○ **What laboratory findings are expected for a patient with malaria?**

Normochromic normocytic anemia, a normal or depressed leukocyte count, thrombocytopenia, an elevated sedimentation rate, abnormal kidney and LFTs, hyponatremia, hypoglycemia, and a false-positive VDRL.

○ **How is malaria diagnosed?**

Visualization of parasites on Giemsa-stained blood smears. In early infection, especially with *Plasmodium falciparum*, parasitized erythrocytes may be sequestered and undetectable.

○ **How is *Plasmodium falciparum* diagnosed on blood smear?**
   1. Small ring forms with double chromatin knobs within the erythrocyte.
   2. Multiple rings infected within red blood cells.
   3. Rare trophozoites and schizonts on smear.
   4. Pathognomonic crescent-shaped gametocytes.
   5. Parasitemia exceeding 4% didn't find this denoted in this format (what percentage needed to be exceeded), but rather how to determine viremia by RBC, WBC count, and percentage).

○ **What is the fever pattern in malarial infections?**
   1. Quotidian (typically occurs regularly in a 24-hour period), *Plasmodium falciparum*.
   2. Quartnan (72 hours, periodically), *P. malariae*.

○ **What is the drug of choice for treating *Plasmodium vivax, Plasmodium ovale*, and *Plasmodium malariae*?**
   Chloroquine.

○ **What species of *Plasmodium* is resistant to chloroquine?**
   Falciparum.

○ **How is uncomplicated chloroquine-resistant *Plasmodium falciparum* treated?**
   Artemether–lumefantrine (Coartem, Riamet) most countries this is first line.
   Quinine plus pyrimethamine-sulfadoxine considered an older regimen can still be used in Central America west of Panama Canal, Haiti, and the Dominican Republic as resistance has not occurred as yet (20).

○ **What are the adverse effects of chloroquine?**
   Well tolerated, pruritus (Africans), N/V/abdominal pain, headache, hypotension (parenteral), and rash.

○ **Which hemoglobin confers the greatest possibility of survival in the face of *P. falciparum* malarial infection?**
   Erythrocytes of patients who are heterozygous for sickle cell hemoglobin (sickle cell trait), create an inhospitable environment for the organism and thus these carriers have greater survival rates.

○ **A 5-year-old boy presents with his mother complaining of anal itching especially at night for the last 3 days. After performing the "Scotch tape" test, small whitish worms are adherent to the tape when viewed under a microscope. What diagnosis does this child have?**
   Pinworms.

○ **What is the most common helminth in the United States?**
   Enterobius.

○ **What is the most common physical complaint in individuals with an *Enterobius* infection?**
   Perianal pruritus.

○ **What is the treatment for pinworms?**
   Mebendazole as well as proper teaching about hand hygiene to the patient.

○   **Name the most common form of transmission for toxoplasmosis.**

Ingestion of the cysts via uncooked or cured meats or feline feces.

○   **Is there a risk for transmission of toxoplasmosis from a pregnant woman to the fetus?**

Yes, but only if the mother gets infected during the pregnancy.

○   **Which types of pregnant women are at increased risk for developing toxoplasmosis?**

Women who are cat owners. They must be educated to refrain from cleaning out the cat litter as well as to avoid eating uncooked meats.

○   **What disease of the opthalmic system is consistent with toxoplasmosis infection?**

Retinochoroiditis an inflammation of the retina and vasculature of the eye caused by toxoplasmosis exposure. Presentation may be latent or acute depending on whether infection was congenital or in adulthood.

○   **The presence of tachyzoites on stains collected to diagnose toxoplasmosis usually indicates?**

Active infection, cysts may be present in both acute and chronic conditions.

○   **What pathological findings are seen in the brain biopsy of toxoplasma encephalitis?**

Presence of tachyzoites around the necrotic lesion.

○   **What are some important radiological differences between intracranial toxoplasmosis and lymphoma?**

1. Intracranial toxoplasmosis is usually multiple, whereas lymphomas are usually solitary, at least in the beginning.
2. Enhancement—Both may enhance with gadolinium on the MRI scan; however, toxoplasma lesions are usually ring-like or nodular in comparison with the lesion of lymphoma.
3. Thallium 201 SPECT scan—Lymphomas usually show increased uptake activity in the thallium scans compared to toxoplasmosis.
4. Location—Toxoplasmosis is usually in the deeper structures such as basal ganglia, or the gray white junction, whereas the lymphomas usually present themselves in the periventricular areas. However, biopsy is still necessary to make the diagnosis since imaging studies may overlap.

○   **What is the current recommended treatment for intracranial toxoplasmosis in HIV disease?**

This is usually a combination therapy with sulfadiazine, pyrimethamine, and folinic acid (Leucovorin in the United States).

○   **How is Chagas disease transmitted?**

By the blood-sucking Reduviid "kissing" bug, blood transfusion, vertical transmission mother to child, breastfeeding, consumption of contaminated food or drink A nodule or chagoma develops at the site. Acute findings may include the Romana sign (unilateral edema conjunctivitis, and lymphadenopathy), fever or myocarditis. Latent disease may manifest with CHF and ventricular aneurysms or arrhythmias. Mesenteric plexus involvement can result in megacolon. Laboratory findings include anemia, leukocytosis, elevated sedimentation rate, and ECG changes, such as PR interval, heart block, T-wave changes, and arrhythmias.

○ **What causes swimmer itch (Schistosome dermatitis)?**

- An invading cercariae.
- Schistosomatidae a family that includes many types of flatworms.

○ **What is the vector of trypanosomiasis?**

Tsetse fly.

○ **What is the infectious agent of elephantiasis?**

Nematode microfilaria.

○ **Cysticercosis with CNS involvement is associated with:**

New onset seizure.

○ **Onchocerciasis (from *Onchocerca volvulus*) is associated with what visual deficit?**

Blindness. This is referred to as river blindness.

○ **Chagas disease is associated with:**

Acute myocarditis. *Trypanosoma cruzi* invades the myocardium resulting in myocarditis. Conduction defects may occur.

○ **What is the most frequently transmitted tick-borne disease?**

Lyme disease. The causative agent is a spirochete (*Borrelia burgdorferi*), the vectors are *Ixodes dammini*, *Ixodes pacificus*, *Amblyomma americanum*, and *Dermacentor variabilis*.

○ **What areas of the United States report the highest incidence of Lyme disease?**

New England, the middle Atlantic, upper Midwestern states, and West Coast; Northern California

○ **What are the signs and symptoms of Lyme disease?**

Stage I: In the first month after the tick bite, patients can present with fever, fatigue, malaise, myalgia, headache, and a circular macule or papule lesion with a central clearing at the site of the tick bite that gradually enlarges (erythema chronicum migrans) and may have concentric rings or "bullseye" appearance.

Stage II: (Weeks to months later) This stage involves neurological abnormalities such as meningoencephalitis, cranial neuropathies, peripheral neuropathies, myocarditis, and conjunctivitis to blindness.

Stage III: (Months to years) Migratory oligoarthritis of the large joints, neurological symptoms such as subtle encephalopathy (mood, memory, and sleep disturbances) polyneuropathy, cognitive dysfunction, and incapacitating fatigue.

○ **How is Lyme disease diagnosed?**

Immunofluorescent and immunoabsorbent (ELISA) assays identify the antibodies to the spirochete. Western Blot confirms and is more specific for *Borrelia burgdorferi*. Treatment includes doxycycline or tetracycline, amoxicillin, IV penicillin (V in pregnant patients), or erythromycin.

○ **What is the vector and causative organism of Lyme disease?**

The vector is *Ixodes dammini*, and the organism is *Borrelia burgdorferi*. It is the most frequently transmitted tick-borne disease.

○ **Which two diseases are transmitted by the deer tick, *Ixodes dammini*?**

Lyme disease and babesiosis.

○ **At which stage of Lyme disease does neurological involvement occur?**

The second and third stages. Second-stage cranial neuropathies, meningitis, and radiculoneuritis. Third-stage encephalitis, and a variety of CNS manifestations including stroke like syndromes, extrapyramidal, and cerebellar involvement.

○ **Describe the skin lesion seen in Lyme disease.**

A large distinct circular skin lesion called erythema chronicum migrans. It is an annular erythematous lesion with central clearing.

○ **When does ECM show up in Lyme disease?**

Stage I, which is 3 to 32 days after the bite.

○ **Can Lyme disease reoccur?**

Yes, but because of reinfection not relapse.

○ **How do patients present with babesia infection?**

With symptoms similar to malaria: intermittent fever, splenomegaly, jaundice, and hemolysis. The disease may be fatal in patients without spleens. Treatment is with clindamycin and quinine.

○ **What is the pattern of paralysis induced by tick bite or exposure?**

Ascending paralysis. The venom that causes the paralysis is probably a neurotoxin. A conduction block is induced at the peripheral motor nerve branches and thereby prevents the release of acetylcholine at the neuromuscular junction; 43 species of ticks have been implicated as causative agents.

○ **During which months are the incidence of RMSF the highest?**

April through September.

○ **What tick-borne disease is also harbored in wild rabbits?**

Tularemia.

○ **A patient presents with sudden onset of fever, lethargy, a retro-orbital headache, myalgias, anorexia, nausea, and vomiting. She is extremely photophobic. The patient has been on a camping trip in Wyoming. What tick-borne disease might cause these symptoms?**

Colorado tick fever. This is caused by a virus of the genus *Orbivirus* and the family Reoviridae. The vector is the tick *Dermacentor andersoni*. The disease is self-limited; treatment is supportive.

○ *Dermacentor andersoni* (wood tick) is a pesky arthropod associated with four tick-borne illnesses! Name these illnesses and the cause of each:

1. Rocky Mountain spotted fever (RMSF)—caused by *Rickettsia rickettsii; Dermacentor andersoni* is a vector.

2. Tick paralysis—caused by a neurotoxin. The symptoms, consisting of ascending paralysis with decrease or loss of DTRs, are similar to those associated with Guillain–Barré syndrome.

3. Q fever—caused by *Coxiella burnetii* (a Rickettsiae).

4. Colorado tick fever—caused by an arbovirus.

○ **Which condition resembles Guillain–Barré syndrome, the appropriate treatment of which results in miraculous complete improvements often within a day?**

Tick paralysis, which results in an ascending paralysis within a few days of attack by the tick *Dermacentor* (hard tick). This releases a toxin in its saliva, which is responsible for the neuromuscular blockade. Removal of the tick within hours, results in resolution of the weakness.

○ **What is the common name for *Dermacentor andersoni*?**

Wood tick.

○ **What causes Q fever?**

Coxiella burnetii, also known as *Rickettsia burnetii*. It is found in the *Dermacentor andersoni* tick.

○ **What kind of tick transmits Rocky Mountain spotted fever (RMSF)?**

The female andersoni tick which transmits *Rickettsia rickettsii*.

○ **Where do the majority of Rocky Mountain spotted fever cases come from?**

North Carolina, South Carolina, Tennessee, Oklahoma, and Arkansas comprise 56% of all cases.

○ **What are the most common symptoms in RMSF?**

Fever and headache, with headache occurring in 90% of patients.

○ **A patient presents a 40°C fever and a erythematous, macular, and blanching rash which becomes deep red, dusky, papular, and petechial. The patient is vomiting and has a headache, myalgias, and cough. Where did the rash begin?**

Rocky Mountain spotted fever (RMSF) rash typically begins on the flexor surfaces of the ankles and wrists and spreads centrally to the arms, leg, and trunk.

○ **Which test confirms RMSF?**

Immunofluorescent antibody staining of a skin biopsy or serologic fluorescent antibody titer. The Weil–Felix reaction and complement fixation tests are no longer recommended.

○ **Which antibiotics are prescribed for the treatment of RMSF?**

Tetracycline or chloramphenicol. Antibiotic therapy should not be withheld pending serologic confirmation.

○ **What antibiotic is used to treat Rocky Mountain spotted fever in a patient allergic to tetracycline?**

Chloramphenicol.

○ **A 24-year-old male patient presents with a painless ulcer to the glans penis. He reports that his last sexual encounter was approximately 3 weeks ago. What is the most likely diagnosis associated with this lesion?**

Primary chancre from syphilis. These generally erupt within 2 to 10 weeks from exposure.

○ **What is the most common lesion that is seen in secondary syphilis?**

Condyloma lata—flat wart like lesions that are mainly found in the genital or anal regions.

○ **What are some signs and symptoms of secondary syphilis?**

Maculopapular rash usually found on the trunk, and extremities and including the soles and palms of the feet is the most common finding of secondary syphilis. Others include patchy "moth like" alopecia, fevers, chills, myalgias, weight loss, headache, and malaise.

○ **A patient is infected with *Treponema pallidum*. What is the treatment?**

The type of treatment depends upon the stage of the infection. Primary and secondary syphilis are treated with benzathine penicillin G (2.4 million units IM × 1 dose) or doxycycline (100 mg BID PO for 14 days). Tertiary syphilis is treated with benzathine penicillin G, 2.4 million units IM × 3 doses each 1 week apart.

○ **Is the vasculitis that is seen in syphilis, a large or a small vessel disease?**

Both. Large vessel (Heubner arteritis) is caused by adventitial lymphocytic proliferation of large vessels and is commonly seen in the late meningovascular syphilis. The small vessel (Nissl–Alzheimer) vasculitis is the dominant vasculitic pattern in the paretic neurosyphilis.

○ **What is the recommended treatment for neurosyphilis?**

Intravenous penicillin G. Follow-up CSF examinations are mandatory.

○ **What complication may arise from the treatment of syphilis especially early syphilis infection with penicillin?**

Jarisch–Herxheimer reaction usually occurs within 24 hours of treatment with penicillin for syphilis infection. The reaction consists of an acute febrile illness where the patient may also present with malaise, headache, arthralgia, and may produce a temporary worsening of present neurological deficits. The reaction is because of a release of endotoxin when large numbers of spirochete are lysed during the penicillin treatment.

○ **What are the five infectious diseases that give false-positive treponemal tests (FTA, MHA-TP, TPI) for syphilis?**

Yaws, pinta, leptospirosis, rat-bite fever (*Spirillum minus*), and Lyme disease.

○ **What are the five diseases that give false-positive results on <u>screening</u> tests (VDRL, RPR) for syphilis?**

Infectious mononucleosis, connective tissue diseases, tuberculosis, endocarditis, and intravenous drug abuse.

○ **A woman comes to your office frantic because her husband has just received a positive reactive VDRL result. They have been happily married for 35 years and she can't believe he has been unfaithful. Is it at all possible that he has been loyal to his wife?**

Yes. False-positive tests can occur if the patient has had a viral or mycoplasma infection in the near past, if the patient is an IV drug user, or if the patient has SLE. The presence or absence of syphilis can be confirmed with the fluorescent treponemal antibody absorption test (FTA-ABS).

VIRAL DISEASE

○ **In the United States, Cytomegalovirus (CMV) is the most common cause of what type of infections?**

Congenital infections.

○ **Name the forms of transmission of CMV in the different stages of life—fetus/infant, adolescent, and adult:**

Fetus/infant—across placenta, during birth from canal, or through breast milk

Adolescent—saliva, person to person

Adult—sexual contact; both semen and cervical discharge, blood transfusions, and organ transplants

○ **Name the forms of anomalies in infants with CMV, and what percentage of infants with CMV present with these problems?**

Seizures, deafness, jaundice, microcephaly, and purpura. About 20% of the infants with CMV will have one of these conditions. Hearing loss 50% of symptomatic neonates at birth (19).

○ **How is the diagnosis of CMV made?**

By the use of immunofluorescent antibody tests known as "shell vials." An alternative test is the PCR assay.

○ **Name two CMV-related illnesses that can affect AIDS patients.**

CMV colitis and retinitis. In other immunocompromised patients it can cause pneumonitis and hepatitis.

○ **What is the treatment for CMV infections?**

Ganciclovir is the first-line treatment. Valganciclovir can be used as an alternate drug and also in retinitis cases.

○ **What causes infectious mononucleosis?**

Epstein–Barr virus (EBV).

○ **Are there any other illnesses that EBV can cause?**

Yes, Burkitt lymphoma, nasopharyngeal cancer, B-cell lymphomas, and non-Hodgkin lymphoma and hairy leukoplakia seen more commonly in HIV and AIDS patients.

○ **How is EBV transmitted?**

Through the saliva.

○ **What percentage of Americans have the antibody to fight against EBV?**

90% to 95%.

○ **What patients are at risk to get the virus?**

Immunocompromised, first few years in life as a child, and lower socioeconomic classes.

○ **Name the hallmark characteristics seen in patients with EBV (infectious mononucleosis).**

Fever, sore throat, malaise, cervical lymphadenopathy, and anorexia.

○ **A 17-year-old adolescent boy who has recently been diagnosed with infectious mononucleosis. He is in high school and plays for the football team. What are some considerations that need to be addressed for all patients with mono, and what do you need to tell your patient?**

All patients who have infectious mono need to have a careful examination of the spleen, which can enlarge, and in some cases of mono rupture. In rare cases, hepatomegaly can occur. The patient has to be held from playing any contact sport until the virus has subsided and he has been reevaluated to resume contact sports.

○ **What is the average length of illness in infectious mononucleosis?**

56% to 60 days.

○ **How is the diagnosis of EBV made?**

Two methods: one by hematologic and measuring the numbers of abnormal lymphocytes on smear and second by immunologic. There is a heterophile antibody test and an EBV-specific antibody test.

○ **What is the treatment for EBV?**

Mainly supportive care, hydration, pain medications for sore throat, acetaminophen for fever, and prevention of injury of splenic injury.

○ **What causes erythema infectiosum?**

It is parvovirus B19 and is referred to as "fifth disease" or "slapped cheek syndrome."

○ **Is there a test that can determine erythema infectiosum?**

Yes, the detection of IgM antibodies could be run; however, it is mainly a diagnosis on examination.

○ **Is there a specific treatment for fifth disease?**

No, it is only supportive care of any symptoms.

○ **What is the most common site of a herpes simplex I infection?**

The lower lip. These lesions are painful and can frequently recur since the virus remains in the sensory ganglia. Recurrences are generally triggered by stress, sun, and illness.

○ **What is the main transmission of HSV-1 and HSV-2?**

HSV-1: Contact with oral secretions or HSV-1 lesion, oral genital contact
HSV-2: Sexual contact

○ **Where does HSV lie dormant within the body?**

It is held latent in the sensory ganglion cells.

○ **What STD pathogens cause painful ulcers?**

Type II genital herpes and chancroid.

STD	Ulcer	Node
Genital herpes	Painful	Painful
Chancroid	Painful	Painful
Syphilis	Painless	Less painful
Lymphogranuloma venereum	Painless	Moderately painful

○ **Name the different forms of HSV-1 and HSV-2.**

HSV-1	HSV-2
Gingivostomatitis	Genital herpes
Herpes labialis	Neonatal herpes
Keratoconjunctivitis	Aseptic meningitis
Encephalitis	
Herpetic whitlow	
Herpes gladiatorum (from wrestling contact)	
Esophagitis and pneumonia (in immunocompromised patients)	

○ **A 27-year-old woman who is 36 weeks pregnant and has a past history of HSV-2 but has been symptom free for the last several months. What considerations do you have to make in this patient's case?**

She may need a caesarean section if by term she has either active lesions present or positive viral cultures.

○ **What is the treatment for patients with HSV?**

Acyclovir.

○ **Is there any advantage for long-term suppressive therapy for a patient with HSV?**

Yes, long-term therapy can be helpful in reducing the number and severity of outbreaks. Valacyclovir and famciclovir are drugs of choice.

○ **What is the mode of transmission of HIV from mother to child?**

There are three methods by which a mother may transmit HIV to her child: Transplacentally before birth, during the birth process from exchange of blood or body fluids, postpartum through breast-feeding.

○ **To reduce vertical transmission of HIV, what protocol should be followed during the intrapartum, peripartum, and postpartum phases of pregnancy?**

All HIV-positive women should receive at a minimum, AZT in the second and third trimesters, during labor and delivery and the neonate should receive 6 weeks of AZT prophylaxis treatment.

○ **Describe the pathophysiologic features of HIV.**

HIV attacks the T4 helper cells. The genetic material of HIV consists of single-stranded RNA. HIV has been found in semen, vaginal secretions, blood and blood products, saliva, urine, cerebrospinal fluid, tears, alveolar fluid, synovial fluid, breast milk, transplanted tissue, and amniotic fluid. There has been no documentation of infection from casual contact.

○ **How quickly do patients infected with HIV become symptomatic?**

5% to 10% develop symptoms within 3 years of seroconversion. Predictive characteristics include a low CD4 count and a hematocrit less than 40. The mean incubation time is about 8.23 years for adults and 1.97 years for children younger than 5 years.

○ **A 30-year-old man, who has no significant medical history and is taking no medication, presents with multiple painful vesicular lesions on an erythematous base to right side of his thorax. The lesions are arranged in a linear formation and follow a dermatomal distribution. What should you be most concerned about?**

Varicella zoster in an adult may indicate immune suppression HIV should be suspected. Other causes to consider for this presentation include varicella "chicken pox," atypical measles, atopic dermatitis, and syphilis.

○ **An HIV-positive patient presents with a history of weight loss, diarrhea, fever, anorexia, and malaise. She is also dyspneic. Laboratory studies reveal abnormal LFTs and anemia. What is the most likely diagnosis?**

Mycobacterium avium intracellulare. Laboratory confirmation is made by an acid-fast stain of body fluids or by a blood culture.

○ **What are the signs and symptoms of CNS cryptococcal infection in an AIDS patient?**

Headache, depression, lightheadedness, seizures, and cranial nerve palsies. A diagnosis is confirmed by an India ink stain of CSF, a fungal culture, or by a testing for the presence of cryptococcal antigens in the CSF.

○ **What is the most common retinal finding in AIDS patients?**

Cotton wool spots. It has been proposed that the cotton wool spots are associated with PCP. These findings may be hard to differentiate from the fluffy, white, often perivascular retinal lesions that are associated with CMV.

○ **What is the most common cause of retinitis in AIDS patients?**

Cytomegalovirus. Findings include photophobia, redness, scotoma, pain, or a change in visual acuity. On examination, fluffy white retinal lesions may be evident.

○ **What is the most common opportunistic infection in AIDS patients?**

Pneumocystis carinii (PCP). Symptoms may include a nonproductive cough and dyspnea. A chest X-ray may reveal diffuse interstitial infiltrates, or it may be negative. Although Gallium scanning is more sensitive, false positives occur. Initial treatment includes TMP-SMX. Pentamidine is an alternative.

○ **What is HAART?**

HAART is an acronym for **H**ighly **A**ctive **A**nti**r**etroviral **T**herapy. This is a combination of antiretroviral medications that can nearly completely suppress HIV viral replication. Mainstay medications used are nucleoside reverse transcriptase inhibitors non-nucleoside reverse transcriptase inhibitors and protease inhibitors.

○ **What is PEP and when can it be used?**

PEP is an acronym for **P**ost **E**xposure **P**rophylaxis. It is a combination of HIV medications used to try to prevent HIV infection in individuals who have been exposed to the HIV virus. It should be used as soon as possible but definitely within 72 hours.

○ **What is the most common gastrointestinal complaint in AIDS patients?**

Diarrhea. Many of the medications used to treat HIV have GI side effects. Hepatomegaly and hepatitis are also typical. Conversely, jaundice is an uncommon finding. Cryptosporidium and isospora are the common causes of prolonged watery diarrhea.

○ **What is the current recommended treatment for intracranial toxoplasmosis in HIV disease?**

This is usually a combination therapy with sulfadiazine, pyrimethamine, and leucovorin (folinic acid).

○ **What is the nature of CNS lymphoma in AIDS?**

They are almost all tumors of B-cell origin. They may be large cell immunoblastic, or small noncleaved cell lymphoma.

○ **Which virus is considered responsible for AIDS-associated CNS lymphoma?**

Epstein–Barr virus (EBV).

○ **What is the meaning of the term reverse transcriptase in the description of HIV?**

Under normal circumstances, the transcription of a protein in a human cell occurs in a forward direction going from DNA to RNA. In reverse transcriptase, the transcription proceeds from RNA to DNA. HIV is a reverse transcriptase or a "retrovirus" that needs to be incorporated into the human genome by the reverse transcription before replicating.

○ **What life-threatening infection is most commonly associated with AIDS patients?**

Pneumocystis carinii pneumonia (PCP).

○ **What often causes a change in visual acuity in AIDS patients?**

Cytomegalovirus.

○ **Which type of malignancy is most commonly associated with AIDS?**

Kaposi sarcoma, followed by non-Hodgkin lymphoma.

○ **How many years does a patient usually live after being diagnosed with HIV?**

It depends. Life expectancy in a 20-year-old on therapy is about 29 additional years. However, patients who start therapy and are diagnosed with a CD4 count less than 100 cells/mm^3 have an average of 12 extra years, those with a count of 200 cells/mm^3 or higher have an average of 30 extra years, and those with a history of injectable drug use have comparatively lower extra years (12 years).

○ **Describe the AIDS dementia complex, which is also known as HIV-I encephalopathy:**

A progressive disease caused directly by HIV-I. It is present in one-third of AIDS patients and is characterized by recent memory impairment, concentration deficit, elevated DTRs, seizures, and frontal release signs.

○ **What is the most common cause of focal encephalitis in AIDS patients?**

Toxoplasma gondii.

○ **What is the risk of transmission of HIV from an HIV-infected person following a needle stick exposure?**

0.3% to 0.5% on average. (Although this varies depending on needle gauge and depth and site of insertion.)

○ **What are the most common adverse effects of AZT in an AIDS patient?**

Granulocytopenia and anemia.

○ **What signs indicate an HIV-positive patient is at increased risk for opportunistic infections like PCP?**

An absolute CD4 count of less than 200 and a CD4 lymphocytic percentage of less than 20.

○ **What immunizations are recommended for patients with HIV?**

IPV and Td every 10 years
TDAP—one dose
Influenza vaccine yearly, pneumococcal vaccine once
Hepatitis B vaccine for at-risk patients
HAV
Varicella
Meningococcal HPV—women 9–26
Hib and MMR are optional
(CDC)

○ **At what point should AZT treatment begin in an asymptomatic patient with HIV?**

When the CD4+ count reaches 350 cells/mm^3.

○ **What is the prophylactic regime of choice for PCP in patients with AIDS?**

Trimethoprim-sulfamethoxazole DS should be started when the CD4+ count reaches 200 cells/mm^3.

○ **At what point should prophylaxis treatment against *Mycobacterium avium intracellulare* and toxoplasmosis be started in patients with AIDS?**

When the CD4+ count reaches 100 cells/mm^3.

○ **Immunocompromised patients can safely be given which vaccines?**

Killed or inactivated vaccines: Diphtheria

Haemophilus influenzae

Influenza

Pneumococcal

Enhanced inactivated polio

Hepatitis pertussis tetanus

It may be easier to remember the vaccines that should be avoided. The following are live, attenuated vaccines: Oral polio and MMR, smallpox, zoster.

○ **Human papillomavirus (HPV) originates as tumors from what type of cell?**

Squamous cells.

○ **How is HPV transmitted?**

Skin-to-skin contact, usually sexual contact.

○ **What is the cause of condylomata acuminata?**

Papillomavirus.

○ **Which types of HPV cause carcinoma of the cervix and penis?**

Types 16 and 18.

○ **What medium is used to detect occult premalignant lesions caused by HPV?**

Acetic acid preparation.

○ **What is the main treatment for HPV?**

Podophyllin or Imiquimod (Aldara). Genital warts can be either burned off or cryotherapy used.

○ **What is the vaccine for the prevention of HPV, and what types of HPV does it protect against?**

The vaccine Gardisil is available and protects against HPV 6 and 11 (genital warts) and 16 and 18 (cervical cancer). The vaccine is administered to females between the ages of 9 and 26 years.

○ **What strain of influenza is more common in adults? In children?**

Adults: Influenza A

Children: Influenza B

○ **What strain of influenza is most virulent?**

Influenza A.

○ **Influenza epidemics and pandemics are generally associated with which strain of influenza?**

Influenza A.

○ **Which pharmacologic agents are recommended for the prevention of influenza and have a spectrum of coverage for both Influenza A and B?**

Oseltamivir and Zanamivir both provide chemoprophylaxis for Influenza A and B.

○ **Amantadine is 70% to 90% effective in preventing which strain of influenza?**

Influenza A. Amantadine should be prescribed as chemoprophylaxis in immunocompromised patients who are not vaccinated or as a supplement to vaccination. It can also be given to healthy unvaccinated people who want to avoid the flu. Over the last few years, the use of amantadine for the treatment of influenza has fallen out of favor because of the higher resistance (over 90%) to the drug. Not recommended for use by CDC 2013, because of the 92% resistance to Influenza A.

○ **When should the influenza vaccine be given?**

In September or October, about 1 to 2 months before the influenza season begins. The vaccine is protective against influenza A and B.

○ **What is a contraindication to the administration of the influenza vaccine?**

A history of anaphylactic hypersensitivity to eggs or egg products.

○ **How is the influenza virus transmitted?**

By respiratory droplets.

○ **Name the signs and symptoms of a patient with influenza.**

Sudden onset fever, chills, malaise, nonproductive cough, myalgias, headache, and sore throat.

○ **What is a potential respiratory complication to influenza?**

Bacterial pneumonia.

○ **What is the most common pathogen for this type of pneumonia?**

Staphylococcus aureus.

○ **Name two drugs approved for the treatment of influenza.**

Oseltamivir (Tamiflu) and zanamivir (Relenza).

○ **What is the most common clinical finding on examination in a patient with mumps?**

Parotid gland swelling.

○ **What are some prodromal symptoms in patients with mumps?**

Fever, malaise, and anorexia.

○ **What is a key examination that must be done in a male patient with mumps?**

You must examine the scrotum to look for acute orchitis.

○ **Besides orchitis in men, what is another potentially serious complication related to mumps?**

Meningitis.

○ **How is mumps transmitted?**

Respiratory droplets. It has a high-peak incidence in the winter months.

○ **What is the treatment for mumps?**

There is no treatment. If orchitis occurs, immediate consultation with a urologist in indicated. If suspicion for meningitis, appropriate treatment for the infection is warranted.

○ **How can mumps be prevented?**

By giving the live attenuated mumps vaccine as scheduled. This is usually the MMR vaccine.

○ **Explain the pathophysiology of rabies.**

Infection occurs within the myocytes for the first 48 to 96 hours. It then spreads across the motor endplate and ascends and replicates along the peripheral nervous system, axoplasm, and into the dorsal root ganglia, spinal cord, and CNS. From the gray matter, the virus spreads by peripheral nerves to tissues and organ systems.

○ **Rabies viral replication has an affinity for which areas of the body?**

Areas or sites of bountiful nerve innervation such as the salivary glands.

○ **What is the characteristic histologic finding associated with rabies?**

Eosinophilic intracellular lesions within the cerebral neurons called Negri bodies are the sites of CNS viral replication. Although these lesions occur in 75% of rabies cases and are pathognomonic for rabies, their absence does not eliminate the possibility of rabies.

○ **The hallmark lesion of CNS rabies is:**

The Negri body that are eosinophilic inclusions found in the cytoplasm of neuronal brain cells and contain the rabies virus.

○ **What are the signs and symptoms of rabies?**

Incubation period of 12 to 700 days with an average of 20 to 90 days. Initial signs and symptoms are fever, headache, malaise, anorexia, sore throat, nausea, cough, and pain or paresthesias at the bite site.

In the CNS stage, agitation, restlessness, altered mental status, painful bulbar and peripheral muscular spasms, bulbar or focal motor paresis, and opisthotonos are exhibited. As in the Landry—Guillain–Barré syndrome, 20% develop ascending, symmetric flaccid, and areflexic paralysis. In addition, hypersensitivity to water and sensory stimuli to light, touch, and noise may occur.

The progressive stage includes lucid and confused intervals with hyperpyrexia, lacrimation, salivation, and mydriasis along with brainstem dysfunction, hyperreflexia, and extensor planter response.

Final stages include coma, convulsions, and apnea, followed by death between the fourth and seventh day, for the untreated patient.

○ **What are the two major forms in which CNS rabies may evolve?**

The encephalitic or "furious" form is punctuated by delirium states with periods of resolution to lucidity and is common in 80% of rabies sufferers. The "dumb" or paralytic form manifests with ascending paralysis similar to Guillain-Barré, and initially spares cortical function.

○ **What is the diagnostic procedure of choice in rabies?**

Fluorescent antibody testing (FAT) of biopsy sample from the neck area has 60% to 80% sensitivity. Isolation of rabies virus from saliva or CSF.

○ **How is rabies treated?**

Wound care includes debridement and irrigation. The wound must not be sutured; it should remain open. This will decrease the rabies infection by 90%. The immunoglobulin RIG 20 IU/kg, half at wound site and half in the deltoid muscle, should be administered along with the rabies vaccine HDCV, 1 mL doses IM on days 0, 3, 7, 14, also in the deltoid muscle and one at 28 days for immunocompromised individuals. Previously vaccinated individuals who have been reexposed to rabies and require prophylaxis treatment should only receive the vaccine and not a combination of immunoglobulin and vaccine usually given to nonimmunized individuals.

○ **Describe the intracorporeal dissipation of the rabies virus.**

The virus spreads centripetally up the peripheral nerve into the CNS. The incubation period for rabies is usually 30 to 60 days with a range of 10 days to 1 year. Transmission usually occurs via infected secretions, saliva, or infected tissue. Stages of the disease include upper respiratory tract infection symptomatology, followed by encephalitis. The brainstem is affected last.

○ **What animals are the most prevalent vectors of rabies in the world? In the United States?**

Worldwide, dog is the most common carrier of rabies. In the United States, animal species that transmit rabies vary by geographic distribution; however, the skunk has become primary carrier. In descending order, other sources of rabies include bats, raccoons, cows, dogs, foxes, and cats.

○ **What would you expect to find in the hippocampus of a patient with rabies?**

Negri bodies. Incubation for rabies is 30 to 60 days. Treatment includes cleaning of the wound, rabies immune globulin, and human diploid cell vaccine. Remember, half the rabies immune globulin goes around the wound; the other half goes IM.

○ **Since 1980, how many individuals in the United States have survived from rabies without post exposure prophylaxis?**

None, it is 100% fatal.

○ **What is the etiology of roseola infantum?**

It is a virus caused by the herpes virus 6 or 7.

○ **What are the hallmark features of the virus?**

High-spiking fevers up to a week followed by a rose-pink maculopapular rash.

○ **An 8-month-old infant is brought to clinic by her mother who is concerned about a pink maculopapular rash that developed on her daughter's face and has spread to her trunk and body in the last 24 hours. She reports that while responsive to Tylenol, her daughter had a fever for 2 to 3 days prior to the rash with temperatures averaging between 103.5°F to 104°F. How should the clinician advise this mother regarding her child's condition?**

The parent should be told that the condition is self-limiting and is called roseola infantum—a rash that appears after the abrupt cessation of a few days of high fevers and is caused by the herpes 6 or 7 virus.

○ **What are some other physical examination characteristics associated with roseola?**

Pharyngeal and tonsillar injection without exudates, and lymphadenopathy.

○ **Is there a specific treatment for this virus?**

No. Supportive care and treatment of the fever with acetaminophen is appropriate.

○ **What are the two types of rubella?**

Rubella (German measles) and congenital rubella syndrome.

○ **How is the virus spread?**

Through respiratory droplets and through the placenta in congenital rubella syndrome.

○ **Name some potential congenital defects as a result of rubella.**

Patent ductus arteriosus, cataracts, deafness, and mental retardation.

○ **At what stage are these defects more likely to occur in pregnancy?**

In the first trimester.

○ **How would you test for congenital rubella syndrome in a pregnant woman?**

The presence of IgM antibody indicates a recent infection. Amniocentesis analysis can detect if the virus is in the fluid.

○ **What measure can be taken for preventing rubella?**

Vaccination of the rubella live attenuated virus prior to pregnancy. Women are advised to delay becoming pregnant for one month after receiving rubella immunization.

○ **What is the characteristic of a rash caused by measles?**

It is a maculopapular rash.

○ **How is the virus transmitted?**

Respiratory droplets from coughing and sneezing.

○ **Which vitamin deficiency will cause a worsening of the measles virus?**

Vitamin A.

○ **What are some prodromal signs and symptoms that present with measles?**

A course of 10 to 14 days will start a presentation of fevers, conjunctivitis, coryza, and coughing and transitory Koplik spots.

○ **What are Koplik spots?**

They are small, reddish, irregular spots with white centers and a "table salt appearance" that can be seen on the buccal mucosa, near the molars approximately 2 days before the rash of measles.

○ **Name some complications of measles.**

Encephalitis, pneumonia, and otitis media.

○ **Describe the signs and symptoms of varicella (chicken pox).**

Onset of varicella rash 1 to 2 days after prodromal symptoms of slight malaise, anorexia, and fever. The rash begins on the trunk and scalp, appearing as faint macules and later becoming vesicles. They are classically described as having the appearance of "dew drops on a rose petal."

○ **What is zoster?**

Zoster is the recurrent infection of the Herpes virus. This virus will break out commonly in a single dermatome and begin with pain to the dermatome, followed by a vesicular, red-bordered rash that will crust over a 14-day period. Postherpetic neuralgia is a potential long-term complication.

○ **What is the most reliable method for diagnosing varicella-zoster?**

In a majority of cases the diagnosis is made clinically.

○ **What is the treatment in immunocompetent children and in adults?**

In children, no treatment is necessary, only supportive care.
In adults, course of acyclovir for varicella to reduce the course of the virus. In zoster, famciclovir and valacyclovir can be used.

○ **Which patients are recommended to receive the varicella vaccine and the zoster vaccine?**

Varicella—children aged 1 to 12 years.
Zoster—adults older than 60 years.

○ **What is the typical clinical presentation of progressive multifocal leukoencephalopathy (PML)?**

PML commonly presents with focal neurological signs such as hemisensory or motor signs, and visual field deficits.

○ **Which virus is responsible for causing PML?**

JC virus, which is a polyomavirus (formerly papovavirus), that infects oligodendrocytes.

○ **PML is seen in which other immune disorders?**

Cell-mediated immune deficiency. It is thus seen in HIV disease, chronic myeloid leukemia, Hodgkin disease, chemotherapy patients, and rarely sarcoidosis.

○   **What are the common radiological features of PML?**

Hypodensities in the subcortical white matter on the CT scan. T1 images on the brain MRI are hypointense and T2 images are hyperintense. They are nonenhancing and usually start in the parietooccipital region of the subcortical white matter.

○   **Which virus is considered responsible for tropical spastic paraparesis (TSP)?**

Human T cell lymphotrophic virus type 1.

○   **What are the modes of transmission of HTLV 1?**

Vertical: mother to child
Horizontal: through sexual contact and blood transfusion

○   **To which group of viruses does the poliovirus belong?**

Poliovirus is an enterovirus that belongs to the picornavirus group.

○   **What are the four other infectious causes of paraparesis?**

Syphilis, tuberculosis with Pott disease of the spine, leptospirosis, and VZV.

○   **What is epidemic pleurodynia (Bornholm disease)?**

An upper respiratory tract infection followed by pleuritic chest pain and tender muscles. Coxsackie viruses are a group of enteroviruses responsible for the epidemic myalgia (Bornholm disease) where pleurodynia is also a common feature. Specifically, the disease is thought to occur because of a Coxsackie group B virus.

○   **What is the cerebral spinal fluid (CSF) characteristic of polio?**

In the acute stages, it is associated with a lymphocytic pleocytosis, elevated protein, and normal glucose. There may be a neutrophilic response very early in the disease. Chronic residual polio has normal CSF.

○   **What is the cause of epidemic keratoconjunctivitis?**

Adenovirus.

○   **What is the most common cause of foodborne viral gastroenteritis?**

Norwalk virus commonly found in shellfish.

○   **What are the four pathogens contributing to domestically acquired foodborne illnesses resulting in hospitalization?**

1. *Salmonella* (nontyphoidal)
2. *Norovirus*
3. *Campylobacter spp.*
4. <u>*Staphylococcus*</u> *aureus*

(CDC 2013)

○ **What is the Jarisch–Herxheimer reaction?**

Headache, fever, myalgia, hypotension, and an increased severity of syphilis symptoms that occurs after taking benzathine penicillin G for the treatment of syphilis. The reaction may result in neurological, auditory, or visual changes.

○ **How should a patient with a black widow spider bite be treated?**

Consider antivenin, IV calcium gluconate, and IV opiates plus IV benzodiazepines.

○ **How should a jellyfish sting be treated?**

Rinse with saline. Apply 5% acetic acid (vinegar) locally to the wound for approximately 30 minutes. In addition, corticosteroid agents may be applied topically. No antibiotics are necessary. Tetanus prophylaxis.
Chironex fleckeri antivenin only for this coelenterate.

○ **What is the differential diagnosis of a ring lesion on CT scan?**

Toxoplasmosis, lymphoma, fungal infection, TB, CMV, Kaposi sarcoma, and hemorrhage.

○ **Name four enterotoxin-producing organisms that can cause food poisoning.**

1. *Clostridium*
2. *Staphylococcus aureus*
3. *Vibrio cholerae*
4. *Escherichia coli*

○ **What is the most common presentation of cryptococcosis?**

Fungal meningitis with *Cryptococcus neoformans*.

○ **What prophylactic medication would you recommend to a patient traveling to Costa Rica?**

Mefloquine, 250 mg, once a week. Treatment should begin 1 week before travel and continue 6 weeks after returning. Mefloquine, not chloroquine, is now the drug of choice because of the resistance of chloroquine in some regions. Check with the CDC for specific information.

○ **What preventive measures would you recommend to a patient planning a trip to Mexico?**

Avoidance of water, ice, foods prepared in water, and raw or prepeeled fruits and vegetables. Prophylactic antibiotics are not routinely recommended. However, if they are a necessity, ciprofloxacin is the drug of choice. Otherwise, treatment with antibiotics should begin with the onset of symptoms, as should rehydration.

○ **A friend is headed to Benin on the west coast of Africa. What immunizations and prophylactic treatments must she receive before departing?**

Hepatitis A vaccine

Oral polio vaccine

Tetanus-diphtheria vaccine

Live oral typhoid vaccine

Measles vaccine

Yellow fever vaccine

Mefloquine prophylaxis for malaria

○ **At what concentration is ozone damaging to your health?**

10 ppm. Initial effects are tearing, pulmonary edema, and pain in the trachea.

○ **Which immunizations do healthy senior citizens need?**

Tetanus booster every 10 years, influenza vaccination every year, and a pneumococcal vaccination.

○ **Which vaccine should be administered to postsplenectomy patients?**

Pneumococcal vaccine.

○ **What five vaccines should be administered to adults?**

1. Hepatitis B vaccine: Give to high-risk patients (health care workers, homosexuals, and IV drug users) Hepatitis A (MSM)

2. Influenza vaccine: Give annually to elderly patients and patients with chronic illnesses

3. MR: Give to all patients without immunity (most often required by school institutions)

4. Pneumococcal vaccine: Give once to patients older than 65 years and patients with chronic illnesses

5. Tetanus/diphtheria: Give all adults a primary series and a booster every 10 years

○ **Other than immunocompromised patients, who should not receive live vaccines?**

Pregnant women. Oral polio vaccine should be avoided in anyone in close contact with an immunocompromised person because of the virus's ability to spread.

○ **A patient comes in for vaccinations and has a URI and a fever of 37.5°C. Can you administer vaccines to this patient?**

Yes. URI or gastrointestinal illness is not a contraindication to vaccination. Fever may be as high as 38°C and the vaccine still administered. Likewise, the use of antibiotics or recent exposure to illness is not a reason to delay vaccination.

○ **When administering the Mantoux skin test to a person with HIV, what induration indicates a positive reaction?**

Greater than 5 mm. In individuals with risk factors for TB, induration must be >10 mm. For those with no risk factors, induration must be >15 mm to be positive.

REFERENCES

1. Medscape eMedicine Disseminated Candidiasis. 2013 http://emedicine.medscape.com/article/213853-overview.
2. McPhee SJ, Papadakis MA, eds. *Current Medical Diagnosis and Treatment 2013* (Chapter 36). New York, NY: McGraw-Hill; 2013.
3. *Ibid.*
4. UpToDate Cryptococcal pneumonia. http://www.uptodate.com/contents/cryptococcal-infection-outside-the-central-nervoussystem?detectedLanguage=en&source=search_result&search=uptodate+cryptococcal+pneumonia&selectedTitle=1~150&provider=noProvider. Waltham, MA; 2013.
5. *Ibid.*
6. McPhee SJ, Papadakis MA, eds. *Current Medical Diagnosis and Treatment 2013* (Chapter 31). New York, NY: McGraw-Hill; 2013.
7. *Ibid* (Chapter 36).
8. eMedicine-Medscape Zygomycosis. http://emedicine.medscape.com/article/232465-clinical.
9. McPhee SJ, Papadakis MA, eds. *Current Medical Diagnosis and Treatment 2013* (Chapter 36). New York, NY: McGraw-Hill; 2013.
10. McPhee SJ, Papadakis MA, eds. *Current Medical Diagnosis and Treatment 2013* (Chapter 33). New York, NY: McGraw-Hill; 2013.

11. Centers for Disease Control and Prevention: Botulism. www.cdc.gov/ncidod/dbmd/diseaseinfo/files/**botulism**.PDF. Bethseda, MD; 2012.

12. UpToDate Botulism. http://www.uptodate.com/contents/botulism?detectedLanguage=en&source=search_result&search=Botulism+treatment&selectedTitle=1~66&provider=noProvider. Waltham, MA; 2013.

13. UpToDate Diphtheria. http://www.uptodate.com/contents/epidemiology-pathophysiology-and-clinical-manifestations-of-diphtheria.

14. Medscape—eMedicine Diphtheria. http://emedicine.medscape.com/article/963334-overview. 2013.

15. UpToDate Shigella. http://www.uptodate.com/contents/image?imageKey=ID%2F69134&topicKey=ID%2F2718&rank=1~107&source=see_link&search=shigella&utdPopup=true. Waltham, MA; 2013.

16. Medscape E-medicine emedicine.medscape.com/article/229594-medication#2. 2013.

17. UpToDate Tetanus. http://www.uptodate.com/contents/tetanus?detectedLanguage=en&source=search_result&search=Tetanus&selectedTitle=1~150&provider=noProvider#H23. Waltham, MA; 2013.

18. UpToDate Rheumatic fever. http://www.uptodate.com/contents/clinical-manifestations-and-diagnosis-of-acute-rheumatic-fever?detectedLanguage=en&source=search_result&search=Pheumatic+Fever+Jones+criteria&selectedTitle=1~150&provider=noProvider. Waltham, MA; 2013.

19. McPhee SJ, Papadakis MA, eds. Malaria treatment (Chapter 35). *Current Medical Diagnosis and Treatment 2013*. New York, NY: McGraw-Hill; 2013. http://accessmedicine.com/content.aspx?aID=778194&searchStr=malaria. (Current, 2013).

ADDITIONAL READINGS

Fauci AS, Braunwald E, Kasper DL, et al., eds. *Harrison's Principles of Internal Medicine*. 17th ed. New York, NY: McGraw-Hill; 2008. http://www. accessmedicine.com.

Hall JB, Schmidt G, Wood LD. *Principles of Critical Care*. 3rd ed. New York, NY: McGraw-Hill; 2005.

Levinson W. *Review of Medical Microbiology and Immunology*. 10th ed. New York, NY: McGraw-Hill; 2008.

McPhee SJ, Papadakis MA, eds. *Current Medical Diagnosis and Treatment 2009*. New York, NY: McGraw-Hill; 2009.

McPhee SJ, Ganong WF. *Pathophysiology of Disease—An Introduction to Clinical Medicine*. 5th ed. New York, NY: McGraw-Hill; 2006.

McPhee SJ, Papadakis MA, eds. *Current Medical Diagnosis and Treatment 2013*. New York, NY: McGraw-Hill; 2013.

UpToDate TB Treatment. http://www.uptodate.com/contents/treatment-of-pulmonary-tuberculosis-in-hiv-negative-patients?source=see_link.

UpToDate Malaria Treatment http://www.uptodate.com/contents/treatment-of-uncomplicated-falciparum-malaria?detectedLanguage=en&source=search_result&search=Malaria+treatment&selectedTitle=1~150&provider=noProvider.

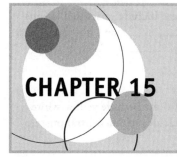

CHAPTER 15 Pediatrics/Geriatrics

Monica Fernandez, MMS, PA-C

PEDIATRICS

THE NEWBORN INFANT

○ **Which days in an infant's life comprise the newborn period?**

The first 28 days. This definition originally set forth by the World Health Organization (WHO) is also known as the neonatal period. Sick or immature infants may require neonatal care for months.

○ **What does the New Ballard Score measure? What six neuromuscular signs does it use?**

Postnatal gestational age. Its six neurological signs are posture, square window, arm recoil, popliteal angle, heel to ear, and scarf sign.

○ **At what times after delivery should the Apgar score be recorded? What is its purpose?**

At 1 and 5 minutes of age, and it may be repeated later if the score remains low. It is used to determine if the infant needs immediate medical attention, and it has no long-term health predictive value.

○ **List the five criteria of the Apgar score.**

Appearance (color)
Pulse
Grimace (response to catheter in nostril)
Activity (muscle tone)
Respiration

○ **What are the normal heart and respiratory rate ranges for a newborn?**

Normal heart rate range is 120 to 160 beats/min and normal respiratory rate is 30 to 60 breaths/min.

○   **There are benign birthmarks that may be observed in a newborn. Some of these include raised red lesions usually over the lower occiput, eyelids or forehead known as _____ and bluish to black pigmented macules over the lower back and buttocks called _____.**

Capillary (strawberry) hemangiomas, Mongolian spots.

○   **There are benign skin eruptions that may be observed in a newborn. Some of these include yellow-white epidermal cysts on the nose known as _____ and erythematous macules with a central pustule or papule called _____.**

Milia, erythema toxicum.

○   **Left untreated, gonococcal ophthalmia neonatorum can lead to severe conjunctivitis and blindness. How is this condition prevented in the newborn?**

By applying erythromycin ophthalmic ointment prophylactically immediately after delivery.

○   **Ear malformations, such as low set or posteriorly rotated ears and preauricular skin tags or pits, should prompt the consideration of which two conditions?**

Genetic disorders (e.g., Down syndrome, Turner syndrome) and hearing loss, respectively.

○   **What is the most common fracture caused by birth trauma?**

Clavicle fracture.

○   **The newborn's hips should be examined for signs of developmental dysplasia of the hip. This is accomplished with the Barlow maneuver and the Ortolani test. Describe these two procedures and the findings that would be considered positive for each one.**

With the infant in supine position, the Barlow maneuver is performed by placing the fingers over the child's greater trochanters holding the hips and knees at a flexion of 90 degree and applying gentle posterior pressure while adducting the hips. The test is positive if the femoral head is felt slipping out of the acetabulum posteriorly. The Ortolani test is performed by abducting the hips while applying gentle upward pressure. The test is positive if the femoral head is felt reentering the acetabulum from a dislocated position.

○   **Jaundice present in the first day of life is always considered pathologic. What two etiologies are most likely when this condition is present?**

Congenital hepatitis or a hemolytic state.

○   **Sixty-five percent of newborns develop neonatal jaundice during the first week of life with bilirubin levels of up to 6 mg/dL, 8% to 10% develop excessive hyperbilirubinemia (bilirubin > 17 mg/dL), and 1% to 2% exhibit levels above 20 mg. What condition may develop if bilirubin levels become extremely high (>25 mg/dL) and what is it characterized by?**

Kernicterus. It is characterized by choreoathetoid cerebral palsy with extrapyramidal movement disorders, auditory disturbances with possible deafness, and variable degrees of cognitive impairment.

○ **How is neonatal jaundice treated? Describe the two most common modalities and when they are used.**

The most common treatment is phototherapy with light in the blue-green spectrum wavelengths (425–275 nm). In extreme hyperbilirubinemia, the infant is admitted to the ICU and exchange transfusion is performed to prevent irreversible neurologic damage.

○ **What is the definition of a preterm birth?**

An infant born before 37 weeks of gestation. Full term is 37 to 42 weeks of gestation and post term is greater than 42 weeks.

○ **What is the most common cause of respiratory distress in a preterm infant?**

Hyaline membrane disease (HMD). It is seen in 5% of infants born between 34 and 35 weeks of gestation and over 50% of those born between 26 and 28 weeks.

○ **Describe the classic CXR findings of HMD.**

Diffuse atelectasis with a "ground glass" appearance.

○ **What is the cause and treatment of HMD?**

HMD is caused by a lack of pulmonary surfactant, which leads to poor lung compliance and atelectasis. It is treated with supplemental oxygen, nasal CPAP, intubation, and administration of artificial surfactant.

○ **Infections known to cause congenital abnormalities are described with the acronym TORCH. What are the components of this acronym?**

Toxoplasmosis
Others (syphilis, coxsackievirus, varicella zoster virus, HIV, parvovirus, HBV and HCV, and other viruses)
Rubella
Cytomegalovirus (CMV)
Herpes simplex virus (HSV)

○ **How do pregnant women acquire toxoplasmosis?**

By ingestion of undercooked meat or contact with cat feces.

○ **If a woman is infected with rubella in the first trimester of pregnancy, what is the probability that the infection will be transmitted to the fetus compared with the second or third trimester? What about infection with syphilis?**

With rubella, there is an 80% chance of transmission in the first trimester, 50% in the second, and 5% in the third.
The rate of transmission to the fetus with syphilis nears 100% and, in the vast majority of cases, it takes place during the first trimester of pregnancy.

○ **Evidence of hearing loss and a "blueberry muffin rash" are seen in newborns who acquired which of the TORCH infections?**

Rubella.

○ **Blood-tinged nasal secretions, saddle nose, diffuse osteochondritis, and Hutchinson teeth (notching of permanent upper two incisors) are seen in newborns that developed which of the TORCH infections?**

Syphilis.

○ **What is the standard of practice during labor and delivery for a woman known to be infected with HSV who has active disease?**

C-section delivery. Vaginal delivery carries a 50% chance of infection for the baby, which leads to significant morbidity and mortality because of pneumonia, meningitis, and/or encephalitis.

GROWTH AND DEVELOPMENT

○ **Describe the <u>gross and fine motor</u> developmental milestones that a child should exhibit by 2, 4, 6, 9, 12, 18, 24, and 36 months of age.**

2 months: Holds head erect and lifts head, turns from side to back. Swipes at objects.

4 months: Rolls from front to back, sits with support. Grasps objects, reaches for and brings objects to mouth.

6 months: Rolls from back to front, sits upright for short periods. Reaches with one hand, transfers objects from hand to hand in midline.

9 months: Crawls, pulls up to stand. Has pincer grasp (thumb and index finger to pick up pellet), eats with fingers.

12 months: Stands, walks. Has mature pincer grasp to pick up pellet, uses cup, tries to build a tower of two cubes.

18 months: Walks upstairs, seats self in chair, throws ball. Uses spoon for solids, dumps pellets from bottle, builds tower of three to four cubes.

24 months: Walks up/down stairs, runs, jumps off floor with both feet, stands on either foot alone, kicks ball on request. Pulls on simple garment, uses spoon for semisolids, builds tower of six to seven cubes.

36 months: Rides tricycle using pedals. Dresses with supervision, eats neatly with utensils, imitates three-cube bridge.

○ **Describe the <u>language and social/cognition</u> developmental milestones that a child should exhibit by 2, 4, 6, 9, 12, 18, 24, and 36 months of age.**

2 months: Coos. Recognizes parents, smiles.

4 months: Orients to voice. Laughs.

6 months: Babbles, is inhibited by the word "no." Exhibits stranger anxiety.

9 months: Says "mama" and "dada" (nonspecific). Waves bye-bye, responds to name, follows one-step command.

12 months: Says "mama" and "dada" with meaning (specific). Points to desired object, uses picture book.

18 months: Speaks 4 to 20 words, names common objects. Understands two-step command. Carries and hugs doll.

24 months: Speaks two-word sentences (two words at 2 years), uses pronouns, verbalizes toilet needs. Points to named objects or pictures.

36 months: Speaks three-word sentences (three words at 3 years), uses prepositions. Refers to self as I, gives first and last name, carries on a conversation.

RECOMMENDED IMMUNIZATION SCHEDULE FOR PERSONS AGED 0 THROUGH 18 YEARS—2013:
(Centers for Disease Control and Prevention, 2013. http://www.cdc.gov/vaccines/schedules/downloads/child/0-18yrs-schedule.pdf)

Vaccines	Birth	1 mo	2 mos	4 mos	6 mos	9 mos	12 mos	15 mos	18 mos	19–23 mos	2–3 yrs	4–6 yrs	7–10 yrs	11–12 yrs	13–15 yrs	16–18 yrs
Hepatitis B (HepB)	◄1ˢᵗ dose►	◄------2ⁿᵈ dose------►			◄--------------------3ʳᵈ dose--------------------►											
Rotavirus (RV) RV-1 (2-dose series); RV-5 (3-dose series)			◄1ˢᵗ dose►	◄2ⁿᵈ dose►												
Diphtheria, tetanus, & acellular pertussis (DTaP: <7 yrs)			◄1ˢᵗ dose►	◄2ⁿᵈ dose►	◄3ʳᵈ dose►		◄------4ᵗʰ dose------►				◄5ᵗʰ dose►				
Tetanus, diphtheria, & acellular pertussis (Tdap: ≥7 yrs)														(Tdap)		
Haemophilus influenzae type b (Hib)			◄1ˢᵗ dose►	◄2ⁿᵈ dose►			◄----3ʳᵈ or 4ᵗʰ dose,----►									
Pneumococcal conjugate (PCV13)			◄1ˢᵗ dose►	◄2ⁿᵈ dose►	◄3ʳᵈ dose►		◄------4ᵗʰ dose------►									
Pneumococcal polysaccharide (PPSV23)																
Inactivated Poliovirus (IPV) (<18 yrs)			◄1ˢᵗ dose►	◄2ⁿᵈ dose►	◄--------------------3ʳᵈ dose--------------------►							◄4ᵗʰ dose►				
Influenza (IIV; LAIV) 2 doses for some					Annual vaccination (IIV only)						Annual vaccination (IIV or LAIV)					
Measles, mumps, rubella (MMR)							◄------1ˢᵗ dose------►					◄2ⁿᵈ dose►				
Varicella (VAR)							◄------1ˢᵗ dose------►					◄2ⁿᵈ dose►				
Hepatitis A (HepA)							◄--------------------2 dose series--------------------►									
Human papillomavirus (HPV2: females only; HPV4: males and females)														(3-dose series)		
Meningococcal (Hib-MenCY ≥ 6 wks; MCV4-D ≥9 mos; MCV4-CRM ≥ 2 yrs.)														◄1ˢᵗ dose►		booster

| | Range of recommended ages for all children | | Range of recommended ages for catch-up immunization | | Range of recommended ages for certain high-risk groups | | Range of recommended ages during which catch-up is encouraged and for certain high-risk groups | | Not routinely recommended |

○ **Which vaccine is routinely administered at birth?**

Hepatitis B. It should be administered to all newborns before hospital discharge.

○ **A child is born to a hepatitis B surface antigen (HBsAg)-positive mother. What is the most appropriate management for this patient?**

Administer HepB vaccine and hepatitis B immune globulin (HBIG) within 12 hours of birth. The child should also be tested for HBsAg and HBsAg antibody 1 to 2 months after completion of the HepB series at age 9 to 10 months.

○ **An unvaccinated 13-year-old adolescent presents to your office to establish care. Should he receive a hepatitis B vaccine if there are no known carriers in his family?**

Yes. A two-dose series of adult formulation Recombivax HB is licensed for use in children 11 through 15 years.

○ **Recommended immunization schedules for vaccines, including minimum age for administration of first dose and intervals between doses, are determined during their clinical trial period before they are licensed for use. List the vaccines that have a minimum age for routine administration of first dose of 6 weeks, 12 months, and 9 years.**

6 weeks: Rotavirus, diphtheria and tetanus toxoid, and acellular pertussis (DTaP), *Haemophilus influenzae* type b (Hib), pneumococcal conjugate vaccine (PCV), and inactivated poliovirus vaccine (IPV).

12 months: Measles, mumps, and rubella (MMR) vaccine, varicella (VAR) vaccine, and hepatitis A (HepA) vaccine.

9 years: Human papillomavirus (HPV) vaccines.

○ **What are the minimum ages for administration of the different meningococcal conjugate vaccines? When is routine administration of this vaccine carried out?**

Six weeks for Hib-MenCY, 9 months for Menactra [MCV4-D], and 2 years for Menveo [MCV4-CRM]. Routine vaccination for healthy individuals is usually carried out at 11 to 12 years of age, with a booster at 16 years.

○ **Which polio vaccine can induce secondary transmission of the vaccine virus?**

Oral polio vaccine (OPV). The use of OPV was discontinued in the United States in 2000, but it is still used in other countries.

○ **How common is vaccine-associated paralytic poliomyelitis?**

About 1 case per 750,000 vaccine recipients.

○ **What is the immunization schedule for the MMR vaccine?**

First dose at age 12 to 15 months and second dose at age 4 to 6 years. The second dose may be administered before the age of 4 if at least 4 weeks have elapsed since the first dose.

CDC CATCH UP IMMUNIZATION SCHEDULE
(Centers for Disease Control and Prevention http://www.cdc.gov/vaccines/schedules/hcp/imz/catchup.html, 2013.)

Vaccine	Minimum Age for Dose 1	Minimum Interval Between Doses			
		Dose 1 to dose 2	Dose 2 to dose 3	Dose 3 to dose 4	Dose 4 to dose 5
Persons aged 4 months through 6 years					
Hepatitis B	Birth	4 weeks	8 weeks and at least 16 weeks after first dose; minimum age for the final dose is 24 weeks		
Rotavirus	6 weeks	4 weeks	4 weeks		
Diphtheria, tetanus, pertussis	6 weeks	4 weeks	4 weeks	6 months	6 months
Haemophilus influenzae type b	6 weeks	4 weeks if first dose administered at younger than age 12 months 8 weeks (as final dose) if first dose administered at age 12–14 months No further doses needed if first dose administered at age 15 months or older	4 weeks if current age is younger than 12 months 8 weeks (as final dose) if current age is 12 months or older and first dose administered at younger than age 12 months and second dose administered at younger than age 15 months No further doses needed if previous dose administered at age 15 months or older	8 weeks (as final dose) This dose only necessary for children aged 12 through 59 months who received 3 doses before age 12 months	
Pneumococcal	6 weeks	4 weeks if first dose administered at younger than age 12 months 8 weeks (as final dose for healthy children) if first dose administered at age 12 months or older or current age 24 through 59 months No further doses needed for healthy children if first dose adminsistered at age 24 months or older	4 weeks if current age is younger than 12 months 8 weeks (as final dose for healthy children) if current age is 12 months or older No further doses needed for healthy children if previous dose administered at age 24 months or older	8 weeks (as final dose) This dose only necessary for children aged 12 through 59 months who received 3 doses before age 12 months or for children at high risk who received 3 doses at any age	
Inactivated poliovirus	6 weeks	4 weeks	4 weeks	6 months minimum age 4 years for final dose	
Meningococcal	6 weeks	8 weeks			
Measles, mumps, rubella	12 months	4 weeks			
Varicella	12 months	3 months			
Hepatitis A	12 months	6 months			
Persons aged 7 through 18 years					
Tetanus, diphtheria; tetanus, diphtheria, pertussis	7 years	4 weeks	4 weeks if first dose administered at younger than age 12 months 6 months if first dose administered at 12 months or older	6 months if first dose administered at younger than age 12 months	
Human papillomavirus	9 years	Routine dosing intervals are recommended			
Hepatitis A	12 months	6 months			
Hepatitis B	Birth	4 weeks	8 weeks (and at least 16 weeks after first dose)		
Inactivated poliovirus	6 weeks	4 weeks	4 weeks	6 months	
Meningococcal	6 weeks	8 weeks			
Measles, mumps, rubella	12 months	4 weeks			
Varicella	12 months	3 months if person is younger than age 13 years 4 weeks if person is aged 13 years or older			

CARDIOPULMONARY SYSTEM

○ **What is the most common form of congenital heart disease in infants?**

Tetralogy of Fallot. It is also the most common cyanotic heart defect.

○ **What is the most common cardiac malformation?**

Ventricular septal defect (VSD). It is more common in males than in females.

○ **Persistence of the normal fetal vessel that joins the pulmonary artery to the aorta after birth is common in children whose mothers contracted rubella in the first trimester of pregnancy. What is this defect called?**

Patent ductus arteriosus (PDA). It is also common in preterm infants weighing less than 1500 g, and it may be seen with VSD in coarctation of the aorta.

○ **Describe the pathognomonic heart murmur heard with VSD.**

Holosystolic, high-pitched murmur heard best along the left sternal border between the third and fifth intercostal spaces.

○ **Describe the classic heart murmur of PDA.**

Machine-like, continuous murmur heard best at the second left intercostal space. It is unaltered by postural changes.

○ **How is VSD treated?**

Most VSDs are small and close spontaneously (30%–70%) in the first 2 years of life or do not need repair. Large shunts are repaired surgically using a prosthetic patch before 2 years of age to prevent pulmonary hypertension.

○ **Spontaneous closure of PDA is common. However, if there is significant respiratory distress or impaired oxygenation, medical or surgical management is usually indicated. If used in the first 10 to 14 days of life, IV _____ or newer preparations of IV _____ is usually effective. Surgical treatment includes transcatheter closure and surgical ligation via thoracotomy.**

Indomethacin, ibuprofen.

○ **List the four classic clinical features of Tetralogy of Fallot.**

1. Large, unrestricted ventricular septal defect (VSD).
2. Aorta overriding the VSD.
3. Right ventricular hypertrophy (RVH).
4. Right outflow obstruction-infundibular pulmonary stenosis.

○ **Describe the classic ECG, CXR, and echocardiogram findings for Tetralogy of Fallot.**

ECG: RVH and right axis deviation.

CXR: Boot-shaped heart caused by RVH and concavity of the upper left heart border caused by the absence of the main pulmonary artery segment.

Echocardiogram: Right ventricular wall thickening, overriding aorta, and VSD.

○   **Children with Tetralogy of Fallot may exhibit episodes of cyanosis called "tet spells." Older children often squat during these episodes, particularly after exercise. Why?**

Squatting increases systemic vascular resistance and temporarily reverses the right-to-left shunt.

○   **What is the most common etiology of bronchiolitis?**

Respiratory syncytial virus (RSV).

○   **Describe the classic CXR findings of bronchiolitis.**

Hyperinflation of the lungs, peribronchial cuffing, subsegmental atelectasis, and mild interstitial infiltrates.

○   **How is bronchiolitis treated?**

Inpatient versus outpatient supportive care depending on severity. If hypoxemia, inadequate feeding, or dehydration is present, the patient should be admitted and given warm, humidified O_2 and nutritional support. If the condition is severe, admission to the ICU and mechanical ventilation with CPAP or endotracheal intubation may be necessary.

○   **When should the antiviral ribavirin be used in patients with bronchiolitis?**

In documented RSV bronchiolitis and severe disease or severe disease risk factors.

○   **Infants who have bronchopulmonary dysplasia or who were premature at birth are considered to be at high risk for RSV disease. Immunoprophylaxis with _____ is available for these infants to prevent serious lower respiratory tract disease and can lower admissions by 45% to 55%.**

Palivizumab (Synagis).

○   **A 4-year-old female is brought to the emergency department by her parents with a 1-day history of rapidly worsening painful difficulty swallowing, fever of 104°F, drooling, and muffled voice. Physical examination reveals an anxious patient with inspiratory stridor and tachypnea. She is sitting in a tripod position (sitting leaning forward with her elbows on her legs). What is the most likely diagnosis?**

Epiglottitis.

○   **What is the most common etiology of epiglottitis?**

Haemophilus influenzae type B (Hib).

○   **Describe the classic radiologic findings of epiglottitis and croup?**

Epiglottitis: Thumb print sign on lateral soft-tissue X-ray of the neck. It is because of swelling of the epiglottis.

Croup: Steeple sign on AP X-ray of the neck. It is because of the subglottic swelling and narrowing.

○   **How is epiglottitis treated?**

Hospital admission with probable intubation. IV antibiotics should also be started with cefotaxime (Claforan), ceftriaxone (Rocephin), or ampicillin/sulbactam (Unasyn) as the usual primary options.

○ **What procedures should be avoided in epiglottitis?**

Anything that would agitate the child, particularly examination of the mouth and neck, which may cause spasms and lead to airway obstruction.

○ **What is the most common etiology of laryngotracheitis (croup)?**

Parainfluenza virus, usually types 1 or 3.

○ **Describe the classic clinical features of croup.**

Slow onset of URI symptoms, hoarseness, seal-like "barking" cough, inspiratory stridor, and low-grade fever.

○ **How is croup treated?**

Single dose of oral or IM dexamethasone, which improves symptoms and the duration of hospitalization in more severe cases. Cool air mist or having the patient sit in a steamed-up bathroom is also part of mainstay of therapy.

GASTROINTESTINAL SYSTEM AND NUTRITION

○ **At how many days after birth should newborns stop losing weight and then return to their birth weight?**

Newborns should stop losing weight by 5 to 7 days of age and return to their birth weight by 10 to 14 days.

○ **Projectile vomiting that occurs within 2 hours of feeding in an infant is often associated with pyloric stenosis. What is the most common age range for this condition to present?**

Between the first 2 and 12 weeks of life.

○ **Give four examples of conditions that should be included in the differential diagnosis for a neonate who has never passed stool.**

Meconium ileus or plug, Hirschsprung disease, intestinal stenosis, and intestinal atresia.

○ **Infectious gastroenteritis in the pediatric patient is most often caused by a viral etiology. What are the two most common pathogens involved?**

Rotavirus and Norwalk virus.

○ **Is regurgitation dangerous in an otherwise thriving neonate? What if the vomitus contains bile?**

No, postprandial spitting and vomiting that resolves spontaneously in healthy newborns is considered benign uncomplicated gastroesophageal reflux. Bile-stained emesis, on the other hand, may indicate an intestinal obstruction and requires immediate evaluation.

○ **A 2-week-old infant is brought to the pediatric office by her parents for irritability, vomiting, and decreased stooling. Mom indicates that the vomitus usually "looks like it has bile in it." Physical examination reveals a rigid, distended abdomen. What is the most likely diagnosis?**

Volvulus (malrotation).

○　**What is the classic abdominal plain film finding for volvulus (malrotation)?**

"Double bubble" sign.

○　**True/False: A neonate's stool color is considered an important clinical sign.**

False. Unless blood is evident, stool color is generally considered insignificant.

○　**A late finding in this condition, the passage of currant jelly stool typically indicates _____.**

Intussusception.

○　**What is the most common cause of abdominal pain in children?**

Constipation.

○　**What is the most common cause of painless lower GI bleeding in an infant or a child?**

Meckel's diverticulum.

○　**What is the most common cause of intestinal obstruction in the first 2 years of life? What part of the intestine is most often involved?**

Intussusception. In 95% of patients, the condition involves telescoping of the ileum into the colon (ileocolic).

○　**Although not always present upon physical examination, the palpation of a sausage-shaped mass in the area of the hepatic flexure usually indicates _____ while the palpation of an olive-shaped mass in the right upper quadrant typically indicates _____.**

Intussusception, pyloric stenosis.

○　**What is the diagnostic test of choice and treatment of choice for intussusception? List the contraindications to this procedure.**

Barium enema. Barium enema reduction under fluoroscopy will successfully treat about 75% of cases. Contraindications are findings of intraperitoneal free air and/or signs of compromised intestine.

OTHER PEDIATRIC DISORDERS

○　**What are the most common etiologies for acute otitis media (AOM)?**

Streptococcus pneumoniae (40%–50%), *Haemophilus influenzae* (20%–30%), and *Moraxella catarrhalis* (10%–15%).

○　**What is first-line antibiotic therapy for confirmed uncomplicated AOM? What are the options for treatment failure?**

Amoxicillin (Amoxil) is considered first-line therapy. Amoxicillin/clavulanate (Augmentin), cefuroxime (Ceftin), and cefdinir (Omnicef) are options for treatment failure.

○　**When is AOM considered recurrent?**

If the child has >3 episodes in 6 months or >4 episodes in 1 year.

○   _____ is considered the antibiotic treatment of choice for confirmed group A beta-hemolytic streptococcus (GABHS) pharyngitis.

Oral penicillin V. A macrolide antibiotic can be used in case of penicillin allergy.

○   **Describe the nonsuppurative and suppurative complications of GABHS pharyngitis.**

Nonsuppurative: Acute rheumatic fever and poststreptococcal glomerulonephritis.
Suppurative: Tonsillar and peritonsillar abscess, sinusitis, and otitis media.

○   **What is the antibiotic treatment of choice for confirmed rheumatic fever?**

Oral penicillin V. A macrolide antibiotic can be used in case of penicillin allergy.

○   **Antibiotic treatment of confirmed GABHS pharyngitis reduces the severity and duration of symptoms and prevents transmission. However, the main goal of therapy is the prevention of _____, which, unlike _____, can be avoided with antibiotic treatment.**

Acute rheumatic fever, poststreptococcal glomerulonephritis.

○   **Describe the pathophysiology of slipped capital femoral epiphysis (SCFE).**

The proximal femoral epiphysis becomes displaced because of a disruption of the growth plate. The epiphysis moves posteriorly and medially.

○   **In terms of epidemiology, what gender and age group has the highest incidence of SCFE? What condition is it correlated with?**

It is most common in adolescent males 11 to 15 years of age. A close correlation has been found between childhood obesity and SCFE.

○   **What are the most common etiologies of bacterial meningitis in neonates, children of ages 1 to 3 months, 3 months to 6 years, and 7 years and older?**

Neonates: _Group B Streptococcus, Escherichia coli, Listeria, Staphylococcus aureus,_ and _Staphylococcus epidermidis._
1 to 3 months: _Group B Streptococcus, E. coli, Listeria, Haemophilus influenzae, Streptococcus pneumoniae,_ and _Neisseria meningitidis._
3 months to 6 years: _S. pneumoniae, H. influenzae, N. meningitidis, Salmonella,_ and _group A Streptococcus._
7 years old and older: _S. pneumoniae, N. meningitides, Listeria,_ and gram-negative bacilli.

○   **In terms of epidemiology, what age group has the highest incidence of meningitis? Are there peaks?**

Incidence is highest between birth and 2 years of age. Peaks occur in neonates and between 3 and 8 months of age.

○   **What is the primary empiric antibiotic treatment option for bacterial meningitis in infants younger than 1 month? And those older than 1 month?**

≤1 month: Cefotaxime or ceftriaxone + ampicillin.
≥1 month: Cefotaxime or ceftriaxone + vancomycin.

○ The administration of _____ to patients with bacterial meningitis before the first dose of antibiotics and its continuation for 4 days leads to improved morbidity and mortality.

Dexamethasone. It should not be given to patients who are less than 3 months of age.

○ What is the most common seizure disorder in children? What is the cause?

Febrile seizure. It is associated with a rapid rise in temperature.

○ What is the primary treatment option for uncomplicated cystitis in children 6 weeks to 13 years of age? How about those 6 weeks and younger?

6 weeks to 13 years old: Oral third-generation cephalosporin such as cefixime (Suprax). Amoxicillin/clavulanate (Augmentin) and TMP-SMX (Bactrim) are alternatives.

≤6 weeks: Hospital admission with full sepsis workup and IV antibiotics (usually with ampicillin and gentamicin).

○ What is the most common etiology of diaper dermatitis ("diaper rash")? How is it treated?

Candida albicans. It is treated with topical nystatin or miconazole. Caregivers should also be educated on good diaper practices including frequent changes and diaper-free time whenever practical.

GERIATRICS

AGING

○ What is the average life expectancy in the United States? Which gender and race have the highest life expectancy?

78 years, with an average of 81 years for women and 76 for men. White women have the highest life expectancy.

○ Overall, life expectancy in the United States has steadily increased in the past century and this trend is expected to continue. What is the percentage of the population that is ≥65 years old? What will it be by the year 2030?

13% currently. It is expected to be 25% by 2030.

○ What percentage of the elderly in the United States are older than 80 years?

13%.

○ What percentage of the elderly live in nursing homes?

5%.

○ **Name the seven basic activities of daily living (ADLs).**

1. Personal hygiene
2. Dressing
3. Eating
4. Transferring

5. Continence
6. Toileting
7. Ambulating

○ **Name the seven basic instrumental activities of daily living (IADLs).**

1. Housekeeping
2. Preparing meals
3. Taking medications
4. Shopping

5. Using the telephone
6. Managing money
7. Transportation

○ **What are the six most prevalent diseases among the elderly?**

Arthritis, diabetes type 2, Alzheimer disease, heart failure, cancer, and Parkinson disease.

○ **The three leading causes of death in the elderly are _____, _____, _____.**

Heart disease is the leading cause, followed by cancer and stroke.

○ **List the physiologic changes of aging by body system and describe their clinical implications.**

Homeostasis: Decreased physiologic reserves. Leads to higher risk for volume depletion and overload and makes the individual more likely to develop complications from injuries and common illnesses.

Temperature: Minimal decrease in body temperature, but increased susceptibility to hypo- and hyperthermia.

Blood Pressure: Rise in systolic blood pressure because of arterial stiffening and widened pulse pressure. Leads to higher risk of orthostatic hypotension, particularly in patients being treated for hypertension.

Integumentary System: Skin thinning and decreased elasticity. Leads to increased risk of infection and bacteremia.

Cardiopulmonary System: Decreased cardiac and pulmonary functional reserves and impairments in swallowing and cough reflexes. Leads to higher risk of aspiration pneumonia.

Genitourinary System: Decreased number and size of nephrons and renal mass, incomplete bladder emptying, and decreased prostatic fluid. Leads to higher incidence of urinary tract infections.

Immune System: Decreased immune response. Leads to atypical disease presentations (e.g., 25% of elderly patients with sepsis are afebrile).

Recommended Adult Immunization Schedule—United States - 2013

(Centers for Disease Control and Prevention, 2013. http://www.cdc.gov/vaccines/schedules/downloads/adult/adult-schedule.pdf)

Note: These recommendations must be read with the footnotes that follow containing number of doses, intervals between doses, and other important information.

VACCINE ▼ AGE GROUP ▶	19–21 years	22–26 years	27–49 years	50–59 years	60–64 years	≥65 years
Influenza*	1 dose annually					
Tetanus, diphtheria, pertussis (Td/Tdap)*	Substitute 1-time dose of Tdap for Td booster; then boost with Td every 10 yrs					
Varicella*	2 doses					
Human papillomavirus (HPV) Female*	3 doses	3 doses				
Human papillomavirus (HPV) Male*	3 doses	3 doses				
Zoster					1 dose	1 dose
Measles, mumps, rubella (MMR)*	1 or 2 doses					
Pneumococcal polysaccharide (PPSV23)	1 or 2 doses					1 dose
Pneumococcal 13-valent conjugate (PCV13)*	1 dose					
Meningococcal*	1 or more doses					
Hepatitis A*	2 doses					
Hepatitis B*	3 doses					

*Covered by the Vaccine Injury Compensation Program.

For all persons in this category who meet the age requirements and who lack documentation of vaccination or have no evidence of previous infection; zoster vaccine recommended regardless of prior episode of zoster

Recommended if some other risk factor is present (e.g., on the basis of medical, occupational, lifestyle, or other indication)

No recommendation

Report all clinically significant postvaccination reactions to the Vaccine Adverse Event Reporting System (VAERS). Reporting forms and instructions on filing a VAERS report are available at www.vaers.hhs.gov or by telephone, 800-822-7967.

Information on how to file a Vaccine Injury Compensation Program claim is available at www.hrsa.gov/vaccinecompensation or by telephone, 800-338-2382. To file a claim for vaccine injury, contact the U.S. Court of Federal Claims, 717 Madison Place, N.W., Washington, D.C. 20005; telephone, 202-357-6400.

Additional information about the vaccines in this schedule, extent of available data, and contraindications for vaccination is also available at www.cdc.gov/vaccines or from the CDC-INFO Contact Center at 800-CDC-INFO (800-232-4636) in English and Spanish, 8:00 a.m. - 8:00 p.m. Eastern Time, Monday - Friday, excluding holidays.

Use of trade names and commercial sources is for identification only and does not imply endorsement by the U.S. Department of Health and Human Services.

The recommendations in this schedule were approved by the Centers for Disease Control and Prevention's (CDC) Advisory Committee on Immunization Practices (ACIP), the American Academy of Family Physicians (AAFP), the American College of Physicians (ACP), American College of Obstetricians and Gynecologists (ACOG) and American College of Nurse-Midwives (ACNM).

VACCINE ▼ INDICATION ▶	Pregnancy	Immuno-compromising conditions (excluding human immunodeficiency virus [HIV])	HIV infection CD4+ T lymphocyte count <200 cells/µL	≥200 cells/µL	Men who have sex with men (MSM)	Heart disease, chronic lung disease, chronic alcoholism	Asplenia (including elective splenectomy and persistent complement component deficiencies)	Chronic liver disease	Kidney failure, end-stage renal disease, receipt of hemodialysis	Diabetes	Healthcare personnel
Influenza*	1 dose IIV annually				1 dose IIV or LAIV annually	1 dose IIV annually					1 dose IIV or LAIV annually
Tetanus, diphtheria, pertussis (Td/Tdap)*	1 dose Tdap each pregnancy	Substitute 1-time dose of Tdap for Td booster; then boost with Td every 10 yrs									
Varicella*	Contraindicated			2 doses							
Human papillomavirus (HPV) Female*		3 doses through age 26 yrs			3 doses through age 26 yrs						
Human papillomavirus (HPV) Male*		3 doses through age 26 yrs			3 doses through age 21 yrs						
Zoster	Contraindicated			1 dose							
Measles, mumps, rubella (MMR)*	Contraindicated			1 or 2 doses							
Pneumococcal polysaccharide (PPSV23)	1 or 2 doses										
Pneumococcal 13-valent conjugate (PCV13)*	1 dose										
Meningococcal*	1 or more doses										
Hepatitis A*	2 doses										
Hepatitis B*	3 doses										

*Covered by the Vaccine Injury Compensation Program.

For all persons in this category who meet the age requirements and who lack documentation of vaccination or have no evidence of previous infection; zoster vaccine recommended regardless of prior episode of zoster

Recommended if some other risk factor is present (e.g., on the basis of medical, occupational, lifestyle, or other indications)

No recommendation

These schedules indicate the recommended age groups and medical indications for which administration of currently licensed vaccines is commonly indicated for adults ages 19 years and older, as of January 1, 2013. For all vaccines being recommended on the Adult Immunization Schedule: a vaccine series does not need to be restarted, regardless of the time that has elapsed between doses. Licensed combination vaccines may be used whenever any components of the combination are indicated and when the vaccine's other components are not contraindicated. For detailed recommendations on all vaccines, including those used primarily for travelers or that are issued during the year, consult the manufacturers' package inserts and the complete statements from the Advisory Committee on Immunization Practices (www.cdc.gov/vaccines/pubs/acip-list.htm). Use of trade names and commercial sources is for identification only and does not imply endorsement by the U.S. Department of Health and Human Services.

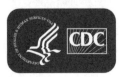

U.S. Department of Health and Human Services
Centers for Disease
Control and Prevention

COMMON GERIATRIC DISORDERS

○ **What is the most common cause of hearing loss in the elderly? What are other causes?**

Presbycusis. Other causes include neoplasm, noise exposure, ototoxic drugs, and otosclerosis.

○ **Define presbycusis. What is its prevalence?**

Age-related hearing loss. It is a progressive, bilaterally symmetrical, sensorineural hearing loss that occurs with aging. 28% to 40% of elderly individuals have hearing loss and its prevalence increases with age.

○ **Describe the consequences of presbycusis in a patient's life. How can they be remedied clinically?**

Bilateral high-frequency hearing loss and decreased ability to understand speech leads to social and emotional problems. Patients should be referred to ENT and/or audiology and hearing aids should be considered.

○ **What are the five most common causes of visual impairment in the elderly?**

Presbyopia, cataracts, age-related macular degeneration (AMD), diabetic retinopathy, and glaucoma.

○ **What are the leading causes of blindness in elderly Caucasians? How about elderly African Americans? And the overall leading cause of blindness worldwide?**

Age-related macular degeneration is the leading cause of blindness in elderly Caucasians. Glaucoma is the leading cause of blindness in elderly African Americans. The overall leading cause of blindness worldwide is cataracts.

○ **Name and describe the treatment of choice for functional vision impairment caused by cataracts.**

Phacoemulsification where the cloudy lens is emulsified with an ultrasonic handpiece and aspirated from the eye. An artificial intraocular lens is then implanted into the space that used to contain the natural lens.

○ **Diabetic retinopathy is a common complication of diabetes and it is the leading cause of blindness in working-aged adults between 20 and 74 years old. What is the most appropriate three-pronged management?**

1. Long-term glycemic control.
2. Annual ophthalmic examinations.
3. Prompt laser therapy treatment of neovascularization.

○ **An elderly patient is diagnosed with stage 1 hypertension. There are no other comorbid conditions. What is the most appropriate management for this patient?**

Diuretic monotherapy + lifestyle modifications. Hydrochlorothiazide is the first-line agent.

○ **An elderly patient who has a history of diabetes type 2 is diagnosed with stage 1 hypertension. What is the most appropriate management for this patient?**

ACE inhibitor/angiotensin-II receptor blocker + lifestyle modifications. ACE inhibitors and angiotensin-II receptor blockers have renoprotective effects.

○ **An elderly patient who has a history of CAD without CHF is diagnosed with stage 1 hypertension. What is the most appropriate management for this patient?**

Beta-blocker monotherapy + lifestyle modifications. Beta-blockers are cardioprotective in patients with CAD.

○ **An elderly patient who has a history of CHF with an ejection fraction <55% is diagnosed with stage 1 hypertension. What is the most appropriate management for this patient?**

ACE inhibitor/angiotensin-II receptor blocker + beta-blocker + lifestyle modifications. If the patient falls under NYHA class III or IV an aldosterone antagonist (usually spironolactone) is also recommended.

○ **What percentage of elderly are ambulatory?**

90%.

○ **What is the percentage of individuals ≥65 years old who sustain falls? And of those ≥80 years old?**

Approximately 30% and 50%, respectively.

○ **Which five pharmacologic agent classes are most commonly implicated in falls?**

Psychotropic agents are the medications most commonly associated with falls. Class Ia antiarrhythmic agents, digoxin, diuretics, and analgesics (particularly opioids) are also commonly associated with this condition.

○ **The vast majority of hip fractures occur in the elderly and most are associated with compromised bone strength because of _____ and _____.**

Osteopenia, osteoporosis.

○ **Hip fractures are associated with high morbidity and mortality. There is a rapid decline in quality of life and _____ of these geriatric patients will die in the first year following the fracture.**

14% to 36%.

○ **What is the most common systemic skeletal disease? What population group is most affected?**

Osteoporosis. It predominantly affects white postmenopausal women.

○ **Why is osteoporosis considered such a significant public health problem?**

It is associated with around 1.5 million fractures annually, usually of the hip and vertebrae. It causes loss of independence, emotional distress, and increased morbidity and mortality.

○ **How does osteoporosis present clinically?**

The disease is usually asymptomatic and up to two-thirds of patients may go undiagnosed. Patients do not experience any pain until a fracture occurs. For this reason, evaluation of risk factors and screening is important.

○ **Dual-energy X-ray (DXA) absorptiometry is considering the standard for measuring bone density and screening for osteoporosis. Results, which are reported as a T-score, define osteoporosis and its severity. List the T-score ranges for normal bone, osteopenia, osteoporosis, and severe osteoporosis.**

Normal bone: T-score > –1
Osteopenia: T-score between –1 and –2.5
Osteoporosis: T-score ≤ –2.5
Severe osteoporosis: T-score ≤ –2.5 with fracture.

○ **What is the first-line pharmacologic treatment option for patients with a DXA T-score of ≤–2.5 or a previous vertebral (frailty) fracture?**

Bisphosphonate + calcium and vitamin D supplementation.

○ **List four examples of bisphosphonates along with their mode of administration.**

Alendronate (Fosamax) and risedronate (Actonel) available as once daily and once weekly PO formulations, ibandronate (Boniva) available as once daily and once monthly PO formulations, and once every 3 months IV formulation; and zoledronic acid (Reclast) given IV once annually.

○ **What is the most common cause of abdominal pain in the elderly?**

Constipation.

○ **What is the most common cause of large bowel obstruction in the elderly? What are other causes?**

Neoplasm. Diverticular disease, colonic volvulus, and fecal impaction are other causes.

○ **Which gender is most likely to suffer from urinary incontinence? What is its prevalence in elderly individuals living in the community versus those living in nursing homes?**

Women. The prevalence is 15% to 30% in the community and 40% to 70% in nursing homes.

○ **_____ is the most common form of incontinence in the elderly.**

Urge incontinence ("overactive bladder").

○ **In addition to behavioral techniques and lifestyle changes, what are the pharmacologic treatments of choice for stress and urge incontinence?**

Stress incontinence: Pseudoephedrine is first line, imipramine (Tofranil) is a secondary option.
Urge incontinence: Anticholinergic agents, with oxybutynin (Ditropan) and tolterodine (Detrol) as preferred agents.

○ **List the acute incontinence etiologies summarized by the pneumonic DIAPPERS. These causes of incontinence are usually reversible.**

Delirium
Infection
Atrophic vaginitis (urethritis)
Psychiatric
Pharmacologic (e.g., diuretics, opioids)
Excess output or endocrine (i.e., diabetes mellitus and insipidus, CHF, and hypercalcemia)
Restricted mobility
Stool impaction

○ **What is the definition of pressure ulcer?**

Localized injury to the skin and/or underlying tissue usually over a bony prominence as a result of pressure or of pressure in combination with shear.

○ **Describe the six stages of pressure ulcers.**

Stage I: Nonblanchable hyperemia.
Stage II: Extension through the epidermis.
Stage III: Full-thickness skin loss.
Stage IV: Full-thickness skin loss with extension into muscle, bone, or supporting structures.
Unstageable: Full-thickness skin loss with base of ulcer covered by eschar or slough.
Suspected deep tissue injury: Area of intact skin that is discolored or blistered.

○ **What are the three most common complications of pressure ulcers?**

Sepsis, cellulitis, and osteomyelitis.

○ **How often should a patient at high risk for pressure ulcers be repositioned?**

At least every 15 minutes sitting and every 2 hours supine.

○ **What are the most common sources of sepsis in the elderly?**

Respiratory > urinary > intra-abdominal.

○ **Among geriatric patients, _____ of those who present with sepsis are afebrile.**

25%.

○ **Compare and contrast delirium and dementia in terms of reversibility, main clinical features, and changes in consciousness.**

Delirium: Potentially reversible. Characterized by acute changes in mental status with a fluctuating course, inattention, disorganized thinking, and the presence of a medical condition as the direct cause. Patients exhibit alterations in the level of consciousness.

Dementia: Irreversible. Characterized by a subacute to chronic progressive decline in memory and at least one other cognitive area (i.e. attention, orientation, judgment, abstract thinking, and personality) in an alert patient. No changes in the level of consciousness.

○ **Management of delirium begins with _____.**

Treatment of the underlying inciting condition.

○ **List three supportive care measures that are highly effective in treating delirium.**

1. Sleep–wake cycle vigilance with a well-lit room during the day and a quiet, dark environment at night.
2. Reorientation by the family and medical staff combined with clocks, calendars, and outside-facing rooms.
3. Prevention of sensory isolation by providing personal eyeglasses and hearing aids.

○ **Chemical restrains should be avoided in delirium, but when necessary, which class of medications is most effective?**

Atypical or typical antipsychotic agents.

○ **What is the most common type of dementia? What percentage of dementias falls under this category?**

Alzheimer disease. It makes up 60% to 70% of dementias.

○ **List the second and third most common types of dementia? Do any other types exist?**

Vascular dementia is the second most common type and cortical Lewy body disease is the third. Other causes of dementia include Parkinson disease, Pick disease, Huntington chorea, and Creutzfeldt–Jakob disease.

○ **The major risk factor in the incidence of Alzheimer disease (AD) is _____.**

Increasing age. Prevalence is 5% to 10% in those ≥65 years old and 30% in those ≥80 years old.

○ **The most common gene associated with late-onset (after age 65) AD is _____, while its less common _____ isoform is protective.**

Apolipoprotein (APO), and APO e2

○ **What is the clinical hallmark and most common presenting symptom of AD?**

Cognitive deficits. Loss of recent memory is the most common presenting symptom, and difficulty with executive function and/or nominal dysphagia usually follows.

○ **Describe the pathological features seen in postmortem studies of patients with AD.**

There is cortical atrophy of the temporal, frontal, and parietal areas seen upon gross examination. Microscopic examination reveals extracellular beta-amyloid senile plaques and intracellular neurofibrillary tangles.

○ **What medication class is considered first-line therapy for mild to moderate AD? And for moderate to advanced disease?**

Cholinesterase inhibitors such as donepezil, galantamine, and rivastigmine are first line for mild to moderate disease. Memantine is first line for moderate to advanced disease as monotherapy or in combination with a cholinesterase inhibitor.

○ **What percentage of dementia patients have comorbid depression?**

Approximately 30%.

○ **Along with psychotherapy, what class of drugs is considered preferred treatment for depression in the elderly? Which agents within this class are considered first line and which should be avoided?**

SSRIs. Sertraline, citalopram, and escitalopram are first-line agents and drugs with long half-lives and those that are activating should be avoided.

REFERENCES

Centers for Disease Control and Prevention (2013). www.cdc.gov.
Epocrates online (2013). www.epocrates.com.
Hay W, Levin M, Deterding R, et al. *CURRENT Diagnosis and Treatment Pediatrics.* 21st edition. New York, NY; McGraw-Hill; 2012.
Longo D, Fauci A, Kasper D, et al. *Harrison's Principles of Internal Medicine.* 18th edition. New York, NY; McGraw-Hill; 2011.
Papadakis M, McPhee S, Rabow M. *CURRENT Medical Diagnosis & Treatment 2014.* New York, NY; McGraw-Hill; 2013.
United States Census Bureau (2013). www.uscensus.gov.

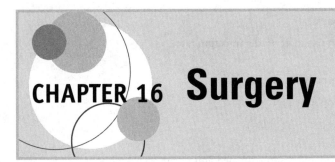

CHAPTER 16 Surgery

Jeffrey Yates, MPAS, PA-C

○ **How many days should sutures remain in the following areas: face, scalp, trunk, hands, back, and extremities?**

Face: 3 to 5 days

Scalp: 5 to 7 days

Trunk: 7 to 10 days

Hands, back, and extremities: 10 days, and 14 days if sutures are placed over a joint.

○ **What is the onset of effect, duration, and maximum dose of the two most commonly used local anesthetics (LAs)?**

Lidocaine: 2- to 5-minute onset of effects with a 1- to 2-hour duration. The maximum dose of 4.5 and 7 mg/kg if epinephrine is added.

Bupivacaine: 3- to 7-minute onset of effects with a duration of 90 minutes to 6 hours. The maximum dose is 2 and 3 mg/kg if epinephrine is added.

○ **What are the lines of Langerhans?**

Lines of tension in the skin that incisions should follow when possible for the best cosmetic results. In the forehead, these lines run horizontally, whereas in the lower face they run vertically.

○ **Why is epinephrine added to local anesthesia?**

To increase the duration of the anesthesia and provide hemostasis. Epinephrine causes vasoconstriction and therefore decreases bleeding and slows the systemic absorption of lidocaine.

○ **Which is more painful to the patient, plain lidocaine or lidocaine with epinephrine?**

Lidocaine with epinephrine, because it has a very low pH. To avoid this pain, buffer the solution with sodium bicarbonate by adding 1 mL of sodium bicarbonate to 9 mL of lidocaine +/− epinephrine. The injection should be administered very slowly and subdermally.

○ **In what areas should you avoid the infiltrative administration of lidocaine with epinephrine?**

Lidocaine with epinephrine should not be used on fingers, toes, ears, nose, or the penis because the limited vascularity in these regions might be compromised.

○ **How should hair be removed prior to wound repair?**

Clip the hair around the wound. A razor preparation can increase the infection rate.

○ **What three elements are common to a surgical infection?**

An infectious agent, a susceptible host, and a closed, poorly perfused space.

○ **Define the term closure by primary intention.**

Primary intention occurs when tissue is cleanly incised and reapproximated and repair occurs without complication. Primary healing is simpler and requires less time and material than secondary healing.

○ **What is meant when a wound is closed by secondary intention?**

Secondary intention occurs in open wounds through formation of granulation tissue and eventual coverage of the defect by spontaneous migration of epithelial cells. Most infected wounds and burns heal in this manner.

○ **What is delayed primary closure?**

When a wound is allowed to heal open under a carefully maintained, occlusive dressing for about 5 days and is then closed as if primarily. Such wounds are less likely to become infected than if closed immediately because their oxygen needs are better met.

○ **What components create the perfect host for a surgical wound infection?**

Areas with or surrounded by poorly vascularized tissue and that have a natural space. The common denominators are poor perfusion, local hypoxia, hypercapnia, and acidosis. Some natural spaces with narrow outlets, such as those of the appendix, gallbladder, ureters, and intestines, are especially prone to becoming obstructed and then infected. The peritoneal and pleural cavities are potential spaces, and their surfaces slide over one another, thereby dispersing contaminating bacteria.

○ **How long can a "clean" wound closure be delayed before proliferation of infection-causing bacteria develops?**

Six (6) hours, though the high vascularity of the face and scalp can allow for longer delays in these areas, typically up to 12 hours.

○ **What factors increase the likelihood of wound infection?**

Dirty, contaminated wounds or wounds with retained foreign bodies. Stellate or crushing wounds, wounds longer than 5 cm, wounds older than 6 hours, and wounds in infection prone anatomic sites are at increased risk.

○ **Which has greater resistance to infection, sutures or staples?**

There are no significant differences in the healing of wounds closed by suture or staples; however, staples do not provide a conduit for infective organisms thereby making them more resistant to infections.

○ **Which factors determine the ultimate appearance of a scar?**

The wounds alignment, either parallel or perpendicular, to the skins tension lines. Static and dynamic tension on surrounding skin. Static tension refers to the width of the wound at rest. Dynamic tension is determined by determining the width of the wound during range of motion of the involved body part. In addition, exposure to UV light will also cause scar hyperpigmentation.

○ **Can tetanus develop after surgical procedures?**

Yes. Although most cases of tetanus in the United States develop after minor trauma, there have also been reports of tetanus following general surgical procedures, especially those involving the abdomen and pelvis.

○ **What are the indications and contraindications to tetanus prophylaxis?**

Consideration for prophylaxis should be made on every patient presenting with a wound, however slight. Patients with clean, minor, wounds should be considered for prophylaxis if their previous dose was taken more than 10 years ago. Prophylaxis should be considered for all other wounds if their previous dose was taken more than 5 years ago. The only contraindication to tetanus prophylaxis is a history of severe systemic reaction after a previous dose.

○ **How long should a repaired laceration need be kept out of the sun?**

Patients should be instructed to keep the repaired area out of the sun during the time of healing, about 2 to 3 months, and also to cover the area with sunblock for the following 6 to 12 months. Sun exposure may cause hyperpigmentation to the wound area.

○ **What organisms are most common in wound infections?**

Staphylococcus, primarily *S. aureus.*

○ **What is the most likely cause of a postoperative fever which occurs (1) the day after the operation (POD 1), (2) 3 days postoperative (POD 3), (3) 5 days postoperative (POD 5), (4) 7 days postoperative (POD 7), and (5) 2 to 3 weeks postoperative?**

1. **W**IND: Atelectasis

2. **W**ATER: Urinary tract infection (UTI)

3. **W**ALK: Deep vein thrombosis (DVT)

4. **W**OUND: Postoperative infection

5. **W**ONDER DRUGS: Hypersensitivity reaction most common caused by antibiotics

Mnemonic: Wind, Water, Walk, Wound, and Wonder drugs

○ **What gas is used to create a pneumoperitoneum during a laparoscopy? Why is this gas used? What are the associated risks?**

Carbon dioxide (CO_2). CO_2 is noncombustible and has a high rate of diffusion, which results in a low risk of gas embolism. The use of CO_2 can also result in tachycardia, increased central venous pressure, hypertension, decreased cardiac output, and occasionally, transient arrhythmias because of its rapid rate of absorption into the systemic circulation, which increases P_{CO_2} and decreases pH. Alternative, and significantly less popular, gases include helium and argon.

○ **A 32-year-old female patient is under general anesthesia for a cholecystectomy. Part way into the operation her body tenses up, she develops tachycardia and a fever of 101.8°F. What anesthetic-related complication is she experiencing and what is the recommended treatment?**

This patient is suffering from malignant hyperthermia, a muscular response to general anesthetics that causes the release of calcium. A patient's susceptibility to malignant hyperthermia may be established with the caffeine–halothane contracture test. Dantrolene may be used prophylactically or in the acute treatment of patient's experiencing this complication. Its effects will inhibit the release of calcium while aiding in the prevention of acute renal failure.

○ **What is the maintenance IV fluid rate for a child weighing 30 kg?**

The 100/50/20 rule would apply in this patient:

100 mL/kg/day for the first 10 kg + 50 mL/kg/day for the next 10 kg + 20 mL/kg/day for the next 10 kg.
    This child should receive 1700 mL/day at an IV flow rate of 71 mL/h.

○ **What is the appropriate bolus for a dehydrated child weighing 15 kg?**

The recommended IVFB for a child is calculated at 20 mL/kg.

20 mL × 15 kg = 300 mL.

○ **What is the composition of sodium in normal saline and lactated ringers IV solutions?**

Normal saline (0.9% sodium chloride) 154 mEq/L.
Lactated ringers 130 mEq/L.

○ **What solutes determine serum osmolality?**

Sodium, chloride, bicarbonate, proteins, and glucose. To a much lesser extent magnesium, calcium, and potassium are also present.

○ **What is the Whipple procedure?**

Pancreaticoduodenectomy. The procedure involves resection of the distal stomach, pylorus, duodenum, proximal pancreas, and the gallbladder, plus a truncal vagotomy. The jejunum is then anastomosed to the stomach, biliary, and pancreatic ducts. This procedure is used for treating pancreatic, duodenal, ampulla of Vater, and common bile duct cancers.

○ **What are the Billroth I and II procedures?**

Billroth I anastomosis is a gastroduodenostomy, and Billroth II is a gastrojejunostomy.

○ **What is the Roux-en-Y operative procedure?**

An end-to-side anastomosis between the distal segment of small bowel and the stomach or esophagus. This forms a Y shape. This procedure is used in gastric bypass surgery for obesity and to treat reflux of bile and pancreatic secretions into the stomach secondary to ductal tumors, injury, obstruction, or infection.

○ **Match the type of transplant to the most appropriate definition.**

1. Autograft
2. Heterotrophic
3. Isograft
4. Orthotopic
5. Allograft
6. Xenograft

a. Donor and recipient are genetically the same
b. Donor and recipient are the same person
c. Donor and recipient are of the same species
d. Donor and recipient belong to different species
e. Transplantation to a normal anatomical position
f. Transplantation to a different anatomical position

Answers: (1) b, (2) f, (3) a, (4) e, (5) c, and (6) d.

○ **What fungal infection is most common in transplant patients?**

Candida albicans.

○ **Differentiate between visceral pain and parietal pain.**

Visceral pain: Diffuse and poorly localized pain caused by the stretching of a hollow viscus. It is frequently associated with autonomic nervous system responses.

Parietal pain: Sharp and localized pain caused by irritation or inflammation of a parietal surface and associated with guarding, rebound, and a rigid abdomen.

○ **What is the most common cause of bleeding in postoperative patients?**

Failure to achieve operative local hemostasis.

○ **What does an increase in pulmonary arterial wedge pressure indicate?**

Fluid overload. Normal pulmonary wedge pressure is 4 to 12 mm Hg. Higher levels can indicate left ventricular failure, constrictive pericarditis, or mitral regurgitation with stenosis.

○ **What are the two most commonly injured genitourinary organs?**

Kidneys and bladder.

○ **A patient presents with fever and shoulder pain 4 days following a splenectomy. What is the most probable postoperative complication?**

Subphrenic abscess. This condition can cause fever as well as irritation to the diaphragm and to the branch of the phrenic nerve that innervates it.

○ **What organisms are most commonly responsible for overwhelming postsplenectomy sepsis?**

Encapsulated organisms: pneumococcal (50%), meningococcal (12%), *Escherichia coli* (11%), *Haemophilus influenzae* (8%), staphylococcal (8%), and streptococcal (7%).

○ **What is a sentinel loop?**

A distended or dilated loop of bowel detected by X-ray that lies near a localized inflammatory process.

○ **What is a delphian node?**

A palpable node on the trachea, which is just above the thyroid isthmus. This is indicative of thyroid disease (malignancy or thyroiditis).

○ **Which types of nodules are more likely to be malignant on a thyroid scan, hot or cold?**

Cold. These cells most commonly do not produce thyroid hormones and do not absorb iodine. This procedure should not be considered confirmatory and fine-needle aspiration (biopsy) is strongly suggested to obtain a diagnosis.

○ **What test should be performed to distinguish a benign cystic nodule from a malignant nodule?**

Fine-needle aspiration with biopsy and cytological evaluation.

○ **What is the sensory innervation to the nipple, umbilicus, and perianal region?**

Nipple: T4
Umbilicus: T10
Perianal: S2 to S4

○ **What is the most common etiology of a solitary thyroid nodule?**

A nodular goiter (50%). Other possibilities to consider include cancer (20%), adenoma (20%), cyst (5%), or thyroiditis (5%).

○ **Which nerve must be located and then avoided when performing a thyroidectomy?**

The recurrent laryngeal nerves, which are located immediately posterior to the gland.

○ **What is the most common type of thyroid carcinoma?**

Papillary carcinoma accounts for about 75% of thyroid carcinomas and statistically present with an excellent prognosis.

○ **A 15-year-old female adolescent comes to your office complaining of a mass in the midline of her neck near the hyoid bone. It is tender and raises when she swallows or if she sticks her tongue out. What is your diagnosis?**

An infected thyroglossal duct cyst. This is a remnant from the embryological descent of the thyroid in the neck. Treatment includes antibiotics, drainage, and then excision once the inflammation subsides if necessary.

○ **What is the most common benign salivary gland tumor?**

Pleomorphic adenomas make up about 85% of these tumors.

○ **What is the most common type of malignant parotid gland tumor?**

Mucoepidermoid carcinoma is the most common malignant tumor of the parotid gland, accounting for 30% of parotid malignancies.

○ **What type of contrast medium should be used to evaluate the esophagus if a perforation is suspected?**

Gastrografin (diatrizoate meglumine). This is an iodinated, water-soluble media that is not harmful in the presence of a mucosal tear.

○ **What are the most significant risk factors for esophageal cancer?**

Age 65 or older, being male, smoking, heavy drinking of alcohol, diets low in the intake of fruits and vegetables, obesity, and acid reflux disease.

○ **Cancer occurs more frequently in which third of the esophagus?**

Adenocarcinoma of the distal esophagus is the most common form of esophageal cancer in the United States.

○ **Which other forms of cancer cell types may occur in esophagus?**

Squamous cell carcinoma most frequently occurs in the proximal region of the esophagus and is less common in the United States but is the most common worldwide.

○ **Which types of cancer metastasize to bone?**

Prostate, thyroid, breast, lung, and kidney. (Remember the mnemonic: "P.T. Barnum Loves Kids.")

○ **What is Hamman sign?**

This sign is associated with a tracheobronchial injury resulting in a pneumomediastinum or pneumopericardium. The sound is heard best over the left lateral position and has been described as a series of precordial crackles that correlate with the cardiac contraction and not respiration.

○ **What is the most common site of rupture in Boerhaave syndrome?**

The left posterolateral wall of the lower third of the esophagus, 2 to 3 cm proximal to the gastroesophageal junction.

○ **What is the most common acute surgical condition of the abdomen?**

Acute appendicitis.

○ **What is the most common cause of appendicitis?**

Fecaliths. Fecaliths are found in 40% of uncomplicated appendicitis cases, 65% of cases involving gangrenous appendices that have not ruptured, and 90% of cases involving ruptured appendices.

○ **How does retrocecal appendicitis most commonly present?**

Dysuria, hematuria, and urinary frequency (caused by the proximity of the appendix to the right ureter). Poorly localized abdominal pain, anorexia, nausea, vomiting, diarrhea, mild fever, and peritonitis are also common signs.

○ **Differentiate between McBurney point, Rovsing sign, the obturator sign, and the psoas sign.**

McBurney point: Point of maximal tenderness in a patient with appendicitis. The location is two-thirds the way between the umbilicus and the iliac crest on the right side of the abdomen.

Rovsing sign: Palpation of LLQ causes pain in the RLQ.

Obturator sign: Internal rotation of a flexed hip causes pain.

Psoas sign: These signs are all indicative of an inflamed appendix. Extension of the right thigh causes pain.

○ **What kind of wound closure should be used in a patient with a perforated appendix?**

Delayed primary closure with direct drainage of the infection. Wound infection occurs in 20% of patients with perforated appendices.

○ **A 27-year-old man who smokes heavily complains of tingling in his fingers. On examination he has cyanotic digits with ulcers forming. What is the diagnosis?**

Thromboangiitis obliterans or Buerger disease. This is a disease that affects young smokers (males 20–40 years of age). Inflammatory changes (vasculitis) in the small- to medium-sized vessels cause constriction or occlusions.

○ **Where is the most common site of intracranial aneurysms?**

The circle of Willis (most common in the anterior communicating artery).

○ **What is the most common type of brain tumor in adults?**

Glioblastoma multiforme (40%). This is additionally the most aggressive (malignant) type of primary brain tumor in adults.

○ **What is the most common primary central nervous system tumor that arises in childhood.**

Medulloblastoma.

○ **What are the most common microorganisms found in brain abscesses?**

Direct extension—Sinus, odontogenic, and otogenic sources: *Streptococcus* species (aerobic and anaerobic), *Bacteroides, Enterobacteriaceae,* and *Pseudomonas.*

Hematogenous spread (Pathogens depend on predisposing source)

Endocarditis—*Streptococcus viridans* and *Staphylococcus aureus*

Pulmonary infections—*Streptococcus, Fusobacterium, Corynebacterium,* and *Peptococcus* species

Cardiac defects with right-to-left shunt—*Streptococcus* species

Intra-abdominal infections—*Klebsiella* species, *E. coli,* other Enterobacteriaceae, *Streptococcus* species, and anaerobes

Urinary tract infections—Enterobacteriaceae and *Pseudomonas* species wound infection—*S. aureus*

Penetrating head trauma

S. aureus is most commonly isolated.

Enterobacteriaceae, other gram-negative bacilli, *S. epidermidis, Clostridium* species, anaerobes, and *Pseudomonas* species may also be found.

Opportunistic infection (organ transplant, HIV, and immunodeficiencies). Common organisms include *Toxoplasma gondii* and *Nocardia, Aspergillus,* and *Candida* species.

○ **Match the following terms with their definitions.**

1. Neurapraxia
2. Axonotmesis
3. Neurotmesis

   a. **Damage to the axon, no damage to the sheath**
   b. **Temporary loss of function, no damage to axon**
   c. **Damage to axon and sheath**

Answers: (1) b, (2) a, and (3) c.

○ **You detect hard mass in the upper outer quadrant of the right breast of a 45-year-old woman. What are the next steps?**

Mammogram followed by a biopsy. The options for biopsy are as follows:

Fine-needle aspiration with cytology—Easily performed, inexpensive, false-negative rate 10%

Large-needle (core) biopsy—Cost-effective, office-based procedure with false-negative rates secondary to sampling errors

Open biopsy—Reliable means of diagnosis when previous attempts are nondiagnostic; performed with local anesthetic through an open incision

○ **What is the most common histologic type of breast cancer?**

Infiltrating ductal carcinoma (80%–90%) with subtypes: medullary, colloid, papillary, and tubular.

○ **A 30-year-old woman comes to you worried that she has breast cancer in both breasts. She is concerned because she experiences soreness in the upper outer quadrants of her breasts and what she describes as "lumpy" feeling upon self-examination with a mild swelling that seems to come and go. Further questioning reveals that her pain begins 1 week before she menstruates and then disappears when her menses is over. What do you tell her?**

She most likely has fibrocystic breast changes but these are frequently clinically indistinguishable from carcinoma. First, provide her reassurance and let her know that fibrocystic changes are not a premalignant syndrome. Secondly, schedule her for a mammogram with plans to perform fine-needle aspiration of suspicious lesions.

○ **Which is the most common type of noncystic breast tumor?**

Fibroadenomas. These are most common in women younger than 25 years and presents as round, rubbery, mobile, nontender masses of 1 to 5 cm in diameter.

○ **What does a high cathepsin D level indicate in a woman with breast cancer?**

These levels serve as an independent prognostic indicator and have been shown to be related to an increased risk of metastasis.

○ **What is the most aggressive form of lung cancer and most likely to be involved in metastasis?**

Small-cell lung cancer comprises about 15% to 20% of lung cancers and is the most aggressive form of the disease. It frequently metastasizes to the liver, bone, and brain.

○ **What is Westermark sign?**

Decreased vascular markings on chest X-ray, indicative of pulmonary embolism.

○ **What is the most common kidney tumor in a child's first year of life?**

Wilms tumor (nephroblastoma).

○ **What is the average age for pediatric patients to develop Wilms tumor?**

Peak occurrence is at 3 years and it is rare after 8 years of age. Children with a localized tumor have a 90% cure rate when treated with surgery and chemotherapy; or with surgery, radiation, and chemotherapy combined.

○ **One to two percent of patients with Wilms tumor will develop secondary malignancies. Which types are most common?**

Hepatocellular carcinoma, leukemia, lymphoma, and soft tissue sarcoma.

○ **What are Grey–Turner and Cullen signs?**

Cullen sign: Periumbilical ecchymosis indicative of intraperitoneal hemorrhage, first recognized in patients experiencing a ruptured ectopic hemorrhage.

Grey Turner sign: Flank ecchymosis that develops in 24 to 48 hours, and is indicative retroperitoneal or intra-abdominal hemorrhage. This is most commonly associated with severe acute pancreatitis, abdominal aortic aneurysm, abdominal trauma, and ruptured ectopic pregnancies.

○ **Serum amylase is frequently elevated in acute pancreatitis. What other conditions can cause a similar rise in amylase?**

Bowel infarction, cholecystitis, mumps, perforated ulcer, and renal failure. Lipase is more specific to pancreatic etiologies.

○ **What are the most common causes of pancreatitis?**

Alcoholism (40%) and gallstone disease (40%). Additional causes of pancreatitis are because of hypercalcemia, hyperlipidemia, iatrogenic pancreatitis, and protein deficiency.

○ **Name some abdominal X-ray findings associated with acute pancreatitis.**

Approximately two-thirds of patients will have an abnormal abdominal radiograph. The most common finding is the presence of a sentinel loop (either of the jejunum, transverse colon, or duodenum). In addition, a colon cutoff sign, an abrupt cessation of gas in the mid or left transverse colon caused by colonic spasm secondary to inflammation of the adjacent pancreas.

○ **What are Ranson criteria?**

A means of estimating the severity and prognosis for patients with acute pancreatitis.

Criteria at initial presentation:

Age > 55 years

LDH > 350 IU/L

WBC > 16,000/mm^3

AST > 250 UI/L

Serum glucose > 200 mg/dL

Criteria developing during first 24 hours:

Hematocrit falling > 10%

Increase in BUN > 8 mg/dL

Serum Ca$^+$ < 8 mg/dL

Arterial PO$_2$ < 60 mm Hg

Base deficit > 4 mEq/L

Fluid sequestration > 6 L

Mortality:

0 to 2 criteria = 2% mortality

3 to 4 criteria = 15% mortality

5 to 6 criteria = 40% mortality

7 to 8 criteria = 100% mortality

○ **What is the most common cause of pancreatic pseudocysts in children and adults?**

Children: The etiology for pancreatitis in children is widely varied with abdominal trauma being the most common case at 23% of the cases. In addition, anomalies of the pancreaticobiliary system (15%), multisystem disease (14%), drugs and toxins (12%), viral infections (10%), hereditary disorders (2%), and metabolic disorders (2%) are also involved in this etiology.

Adults: Acute pancreatitis secondary to alcoholism or gallstone disease is the most common etiology. Pseudocysts are generally filled with fluid and pancreatic enzymes that arise from the pancreas and should be suspected in patients who fail to improve within 1 week of appropriate treatment.

○ **What is the treatment for pancreatic pseudocysts?**

In the absence of symptoms and radiographic evidence of enlargement expectant management for the first 6 to 12 weeks is recommended. The spontaneous resolution is expected in 40% of these cases. For pseudocysts greater than 5 cm or those that persist greater than 12 weeks, treatment with percutaneous catheter drainage or surgical drainage into the stomach or intestine is recommended.

○ **A 44-year-old gentleman presents with a deep, dull pain in the center of his abdomen that radiates to his back and will not go away. He states he has not "felt like himself" for a few weeks and that he has been kind of depressed. He also notes that he has lost a lot of weight, about 30 pounds in 3 weeks. On physical examination you notice that he has mild jaundice, a palpable hepatomegaly, and an abdominal mass in the epigastrium. What is your diagnosis?**

This presentation is classic for carcinoma of the head of the pancreas. The ability to palpate a mass suggests surgical incurability secondary to advanced disease progression.

○ **Where is the most common anatomic and histologic location of pancreatic cancer?**

Head of the pancreas (66%–75%). Pancreatic cancer is generally adenocarcinoma and located in the ducts.

○ **What gender and age group most commonly presents with pancreatic cancer?**

Middle-aged men, 35 to 55 years of age.

○ **What is the overall 5-year survival rate for pancreatic carcinoma?**

10%: However only 60% of these patients have had a complete tumor resection. Tumor location is an important prognostic indicator with tumors of the head and tail having a higher mortality than those involving the head. Patients with metastatic pancreatic cancer who have symptoms of weight loss or pain, the chance of surviving 1 year is less than 20% for those undergoing chemotherapy and less than 5% for those who choose not to receive chemotherapy.

○ **What is Courvoisier law?**

This states that in the presence of (obstructive) jaundice if the gallbladder is palpable, then the jaundice is unlikely to be caused by gallstones.

○ **What is the most common endocrine tumor of the pancreas?**

An insulinoma, only 10% are malignant. The classic diagnostic criteria is "Whipple triad":

1. Hypoglycemic symptoms produced by fasting.
2. Blood glucose < 50 mg/dL during symptomatic episodes.
3. Relief of symptoms with administration of IV glucose.

○ **Where do Glucagonomas arise?**

A glucagonoma is a rare neuroendocrine tumor with nearly exclusive pancreatic localization. Malignant glucagonomas are islet cell pancreatic tumors that originate from the alpha-2 cells of the pancreas.

○ **Which type of operation is associated with a higher incidence of common bile duct injury, laparoscopic cholecystectomy or conventional cholecystectomy?**

Laparoscopic.

○ **What is the typical size of an adrenal carcinoma when diagnosed?**

The mean diameter is 12 cm with an average range of 3 to 30 cm.

○ **What compounds are produced by a pheochromocytomas?**

Catecholamines. This group of chemicals trigger an increase in blood pressure, perspiration, heart palpitations, anxiety, and weight loss.

○ **If vanillylmandelic acid, normetanephrine, and metanephrine are detected in the urine, what is the likely cause?**

Pheochromocytoma.

○ **Where are the majority of pheochromocytomas located?**

90% are found in the adrenal medulla.

○ **What is the pheochromocytoma rule of 10s?**

10% are malignant; 10% are multiple or bilateral; 10% are extra-adrenal; 10% occur in children; 10% recur after surgical removal; 10% are familial.

○ **What is the most common benign liver tumor?**

Hemangioma is the most common benign tumor affecting the liver and are composed of masses of blood vessels that are atypical or irregular in arrangement and size.

○ **All types of hepatomas are associated with underlying liver disease except:**

Fibrolamellar hepatocellular carcinoma, or fibrolamellar carcinoma, is an uncommon malignant neoplasm of the liver.

○ **Hepatic cancer most commonly metastasizes to where?**

The lungs (bronchiogenic carcinoma).

○ **What is the 5-year survival rate for patients with liver cancer who present with a single tumor less than 5 cm in diameter and undergo transplant surgery?**

70%.

○ **Alpha-fetoprotein (AFP) will be elevated in which types of tumors?**

Primary hepatic neoplasms and testicular tumors.

○ **Where will colorectal cancer most commonly metastasize?**

The liver and the lungs.

○ **What is the most common cause of portal hypertension?**

Cirrhosis (85%) secondary to heavy alcohol use. The second most common cause is extrahepatic portal venous thrombosis or occlusion.

○ **What are the most commonly isolated organisms in pyogenic hepatic abscesses?**

Escherichia coli, Klebsiella pneumoniae, Proteus vulgaris, and *Enterobacter aerogenes* most commonly as a result of ascending cholangitis secondary to biliary obstruction.

○ **What clinical sign can assist in the diagnosis of cholecystitis?**

Murphy sign: pain on inspiration with palpation of the RUQ. As the patient breathes in, the gallbladder is lowered in the abdomen and comes in contact with the peritoneum just below the examiner's hand. This will aggravate an inflamed gallbladder, causing the patient to discontinue breathing deeply.

○ **What is the difference between cholelithiasis, cholangitis, cholecystitis, and choledocholithiasis?**

Cholelithiasis: Gallstones in the gallbladder.

Cholangitis: Inflammation of the common bile duct often secondary to bacterial infection or choledocholithiasis.

Cholecystitis: Inflammation of the gallbladder most commonly as a result of gallstones.

Choledocholithiasis: Gallstones that have migrated from the gallbladder to the common bile duct.

○ **What percentage of people with gallstones will eventually require surgery?**

Approximately 30%.

○ **Which ethnic group has the largest proportion of people with symptomatic gallstones?**

Native Americans and Mexican American populations.

○ **What percentage of patients with cholangitis are also bacteremic?**

25% to 40% of patients may present with or develop fever, chills, or rigors.

○ **What is the diagnostic test of choice for a patient suspected of having gallstones?**

Ultrasound is the diagnostic procedure of choice and is very sensitive at seeing abnormalities in the biliary system, including stones or signs of inflammation or infection.

○ **What is the most common etiology of cholecystitis?**

Obstruction of the cystic duct secondary to cholelithiasis.

○ **What are the components of Charcot triad?**

1. Fever
2. Jaundice
3. Abdominal pain

These three components are hallmarks of acute cholangitis.

○ **What is Reynolds pentad?**

Charcot triad plus hypotension and mental status changes.

*Hallmark of acute ascending cholangitis.

○ **What are the majority of gallstones composed of?**

Cholesterol stones are more common in the United States, making up about 80% of all gallstones. They form when there is too much cholesterol in the bile. The remaining are pigmented stones that form when there is excess bilirubin in the bile.

○ **What are the majority of kidney stones made of?**

Calcium oxalate (60%). The remainder consists of uric acid, struvite, cystine, and calcium phosphate.

○ **What percentage of patients with cancer of the gallbladder will also have cholelithiasis?**

75% to 90% of patients diagnosed with gallbladder cancer will have cholelithiasis.

○ **What is the diagnostic test of choice for acute cholecystitis?**

Biliary scintigraphy (hydroxy iminodiacetic acid [HIDA] scan) is the gold standard and provides the highest levels of sensitivity (95%). The HIDA scan uses a gamma-ray–emitting isotope that is selectively extracted by the liver into bile. The labeled bile can then be used to determine if there is cystic duct obstruction or extrahepatic bile duct obstruction, which is based on whether the bile fills the gall bladder or enters the intestine. Clinically the diagnosis is most commonly made using clinical impressions, CBC, and RUQ ultrasound.

○ **How effective is oral dissolution therapy with bile acids for patients with symptomatic gallstones?**

Oral therapy with bile acids can be administered in monotherapy or in combination therapy with bile acids having different mechanisms of action. Monotherapy has shown results of complete dissolution in 19% to 37% of patients whereas combination therapy provided complete dissolution in 63% of patients. The expected dissolution rate is approximately a 1-mm decrease in stone diameter per month of treatment and is assessed by ultrasound every 3 to 6 months. Common side effects with this treatment are diarrhea, increased serum cholesterol levels, and possible hepatotoxicity.

○ **What are the contraindications to extracorporeal shockwave lithotripsy (ESWL) lithotripsy?**

Absolute contraindications include:

acute urinary tract infection or urosepsis
uncorrected bleeding disorders or coagulopathies pregnancy
uncorrected obstruction distal to the stone

○ **What is the most common major complication associated with laparoscopic cholecystectomy?**

Bile duct injury.

○ **Is it possible for gallstones to form in patients' S/P cholecystectomy?**

Yes. Stones may form as a result of bile backing up in the duct and a narrowing of the duct after surgery.

○ **Where is the most common site for fibromuscular dysplasia?**

The renal arteries. Fibromuscular dysplasia is a rare arterial disease that presents in 4/1000 people and is more common in women than in men.

○ **Where is the most common site of a hernia?**

Inguinal (groin) hernia: Making up 75% of all abdominal wall hernias and occurring up to 25 times more often in men than women, these hernias are divided into two different types, direct and indirect.

○ **Do infants and children most commonly present with direct or indirect inguinal hernias?**

Indirect inguinal hernia: An indirect hernia follows the pathway that the testicles made during fetal development, descending from the abdomen into the scrotum. If this pathway does not close, it may remain a possible site for a hernia to develop in later life. Sometimes the hernia sac may protrude into the scrotum. An indirect inguinal hernia may occur at any age.

○ **Differentiate between reducible, incarcerated, strangulated, Richter, and complete hernias:**

Reducible: An uncomplicated hernia that returns, either spontaneously or after manipulation, to its original site.

Incarcerated: Contents of the hernia sac cannot be returned to the abdomen by manipulation.

Strangulated: An incarcerated hernia so tightly constricted as to compromise the blood supply of the hernial sac, leading to gangrene of the sac and its contents.

Richter: An incarcerated or strangulated hernia in which only part of the circumference of the bowel wall is involved.

Complete: A hernia in which the sac and its contents have passed through the hernial orifice.

○ **What are the boundaries of Hesselbach triangle?**

Medial to the inferior epigastric artery, superior to the inguinal ligament, and lateral to the rectus sheath. Hesselbach triangle is the site through which direct hernias pass.

○ **What weakened tissue does a direct hernia pass through?**

The transversalis fascia that makes up the floor of Hesselbach triangle.

○ **Indirect inguinal hernias occur secondary to what defect?**

A failure of embryonic closure of the internal inguinal ring after the testicle has passed through it. This forms a temporary connection called the process vaginalis, which the resulting hernia can then pass through.

○ **Which type of hernia is most common in females?**

Males are 25 times more likely to develop a hernia but in females the direct inguinal hernia is the most common. Although femoral hernias are more common in females than in males, they are still less common than direct hernias.

○ **Of all hernias involving the abdominal wall, which is most likely to strangulate?**

Usually occurring in women, femoral hernias are particularly at risk of becoming irreducible and strangulated.

○ **What type of hiatal hernia is most common, sliding or paraesophageal?**

A sliding hiatal hernia where the stomach and the section of the esophagus that joins the stomach slide up into the chest through the hiatus.

○ **Where is the most common site of duodenal ulcers?**

The first portion of the duodenum (duodenal bulb) accounts for 95% of duodenal ulcers.

○ **What is the most common site for benign gastric ulcers?**

The most common site is the lesser curvature of the stomach; however, they can occur anywhere. Malignant ulcers usually have irregular heaped-up margins that protrude into the lumen of the stomach.

○ **What are the signs and symptoms of intestinal obstruction in the newborn?**

Signs and symptoms of newborn proximal bowel obstruction can be subtle and nonspecific; however, the most common presentation in distal obstruction involves abdominal distention, delayed passage of meconium, and absence of transitional stools (meconium mixed with normal stool content).

○ **What amount of residual volume suctioned from the stomach of a newborn is diagnostic of obstruction?**

Greater than 25 to 40 mL.

○ **A newborn's vomit will be stained with bile if the obstruction is distal to what anatomical structure?**

The ampulla of Vater.

○ **What is the differential diagnosis for neonatal intestinal obstruction?**

Disorders of the small intestine:

Duodenal atresia

Jejunoileal atresia

Malrotation and volvulus

Meconium ileus

Disorders of the large intestine:

Meconium plug syndrome

Anorectal malformation

Hirschsprung disease

Small left colon syndrome

Other causes:

Narcotics

Electrolyte abnormalities

Hypermagnesemia

Hypokalemia

Hypercalcemia

Hypothyroidism

Sepsis

Acute (congestive) heart failure

○ **Where is the most prevalent location for atresia of the bowel?**

The duodenum (40%) is twice as common as in the jejunum (20%) and ileum (20%). In nearly half of all cases multiple congenital anomalies are present (Down syndrome, being the most common).

○ **What is the "double bubble" sign?**

The appearance of a distended stomach and duodenum on the X-ray of a patient with duodenal obstruction. This is classically seen in duodenal atresia of the newborn.

○ **What is the most common cause of bowel obstruction in children?**

Intussusception is the most common cause of intestinal obstruction in infants and children aged 3 months to 6 years.

○ **What are the most common causes of small bowel obstruction in adults?**

The most common causes of mechanical obstruction are adhesions, hernias, and tumors.

○ **Volvulus of the colon most frequently involves which segment?**

The sigmoid colon is the most common site for colonic volvulus (65%) occurring often in patients older than 60 years, with a history of chronic constipation.

○   **Where is the most common site of intestinal obstruction secondary to gallstones?**

Gallstone ileus occurs in the terminal ileum in 55% to 60% of patients. A clinical presentation involves Rigler triad of pneumobilia, small bowel obstruction, and impacted gallstones at the ileocecal valve.

○   **What is the differential diagnosis for a 65-year-old man who has abdominal pain and bloody diarrhea a few days after the repair of an abdominal aortic aneurysm?**

Ischemic colitis is the most likely condition. The most common etiology resulting in this condition is diminished bowel perfusion resulting from low cardiac output and is often seen in patients with cardiac disease or in patients with prolonged shock of any etiology.

○   **Is colovesicular fistula more common among men or women?**

Men (3:1) more than women because a woman's uterus lies between her colon and bladder. This condition is occasionally seen in women S/P hysterectomy.

○   **What is Osler–Weber–Rendu syndrome?**

Also known as hereditary hemorrhagic telangiectasia (HHT) is an autosomal dominant disorder typically identified by the triad of telangiectasia, recurrent epistaxis, and a positive family history for the disorder. The major cause of morbidity and mortality due to this disorder lies in the presence of multiorgan arteriovenous malformations (AVMs) and the associated hemorrhage that may accompany them.

○   **How much blood must be lost in the GI tract to cause melena?**

Between 50 and 100 mL. Normal healthy patients lose 2.5 mL of blood per day in their stools.

○   **What are the most common causes of upper GI bleeding?**

Peptic ulcer disease (PUD), esophageal varices, gastritis, and Mallory–Weiss syndrome account for 90% of all etiologies.

○   **What percentage of patients with upper GI bleeds will stop bleeding within hours of hospitalization?**

About 85% of UGIB will spontaneously stop bleeding within a few hours.

○   **What are the most common causes of rebleeding in patients with upper GI bleeds?**

PUD, esophageal varices, amenia, or shock. Most cases of rebleeding occur within 2 days from the time of the first episode.

○   **What percentage of patients with PUD bleed from their ulcers?**

About 20%, which result in 40% of the deaths related to this condition.

○   **Bleeding ulcers are more predominant in patients with which blood type?**

Type O. The reason is not known.

○   **Where are bleeding duodenal ulcers most commonly located?**

On the posterior surface of the duodenal bulb.

○   **How soon after an episode of duodenal bleeding has occurred can an ulcer patient be fed?**

12 to 24 hours after the bleeding has stopped in a patient who feels hungry.

○ **Which type of ulcer is more likely to rebleed?**

Gastric ulcers are three times more likely to rebleed compared to duodenal ulcers.

○ **What is the surgical treatment of choice for a bleeding peptic ulcer?**

Oversewing the ulcer combined with a bilateral truncal vagotomy and pyloroplasty. Other treatments are proximal gastric vagotomy and Billroth II gastrojejunostomy. The decision to perform surgery is based on the rate of bleed, not on the location of the bleed.

○ **What percentage of patients with large intestinal bleeding will spontaneously stop before transfusion requirements exceed two units?**

90%.

○ **If blood is recovered from the stomach after an NG tube is inserted, where is the most likely location of the bleed?**

A site above the ligament of Treitz (upper GI bleed).

○ **Where do the majority of Mallory–Weiss tears occur?**

In the stomach (gastric cardia), the esophagogastric junction, and the distal esophagus (5%).

○ **What is angiodysplasia and where is it most frequently found?**

It is an acquired condition of focal submucosal vascular ectasia that has a propensity to bleed spontaneously. Most frequently it is located in the cecum and proximal ascending colon. Lesions are generally singular; bleeding is intermittent and seldom massive.

○ **What is the major cause of death in patients with Hirschsprung disease?**

Nonbacterial/nonviral enterocolitis.

○ **Is Hirschsprung disease more common in men or women?**

Men (4:1, men-to-women-ratio).

○ **Are tumors located in the jejunum and ileum more likely malignant or benign?**

Benign. Tumors of the jejunum and ileum comprise only 1% to 5% of all GI tumors. The majority (90%) are asymptomatic.

○ **What is the most common remnant of the omphalomesenteric (vitelline) duct?**

Meckel diverticulum.

○ **What is the Meckel diverticulum rule of 2's?**

2% of the population has it; it is 2 inches long; 2 feet from the ileocecal valve; occurs most commonly in children under 2; and is symptomatic in 2% of patients.

○ **What is the most likely cause of rectal bleeding in a patient with Meckel diverticulum?**

Peptic ulceration of the adjacent ileum caused by ectopic gastric mucosa.

○ **What is the most likely cause of cellulitis of the umbilicus in a pediatric patient with an acute abdomen?**

A perforated Meckel diverticulum.

○ **What is the difference in the prognosis between familial polyposis and Gardner disease?**

Although both are inheritable conditions of colonic polyps, Gardner disease rarely results in malignancy, whereas familial polyposis virtually always results in malignancy.

○ **Clinically, how is right-sided colon cancer differentiated from left-sided?**

Right-sided lesions present with occult blood in the feces, unexplained weakness or anemia, dyspepsia, palpable abdominal mass, and dull abdominal pain.

Left-sided lesions present with gross rectal bleeding, obstructive symptoms, and noticeable changes in bowel habits with the common presentation of "Pencil thin" stools.

○ **Adenocarcinoma develops from adenomatous polyps. What percent of asymptomatic patients have adenomatous polyps when a routine colonoscopy is performed?**

25% with the prevalence increasing with age: At age 50: 30%, age 60: 40%; age 70: 50%; and age 80: 55%.

○ **The advancement to adenocarcinoma of the colon from adenoma is significantly related to the size of the adenoma. What is the risk of developing cancer if a 1.5-cm polyp is found upon colonoscopic examination?**

10%. The risk for developing adenocarcinoma is 1% if the polyp is less than 1 cm, 10% if it is 1 to 2 cm, and 45% if the polyp is greater than 2 cm.

○ **Is a villous, tubulovillous, or tubular adenoma more likely to become malignant?**

40% of villous adenomas will become malignant, compared with 22% of tubulovillous adenomas and 5% of tubular adenomas.

○ **Which are more likely to turn malignant, pedunculated or sessile lesions?**

Sessile lesions are more likely to become malignant.

○ **Where are the majority of colorectal cancers found?**

In the rectum (30%), ascending colon (25%), sigmoid colon (20%), descending colon (15%), and transverse colon (10%).

○ **What is the surgical treatment of choice for cecal cancer?**

Colonic resection from the vermiform appendix to the junction of the ascending and transverse colon.

○ **What is the treatment of choice for a plantar wart?**

Cryosurgery with liquid nitrogen. Additional options include electrodesiccation and curettage, surgical excision, and laser therapy.

○ **Where are soft tissue sarcomas most often found?**

About 60% occur in the arms, legs, hands, or feet.

○ **A 41-year-old patient complains of severe but short rectal spasms but has not noticed any bleeding. He is known to be stressed and overtaxed at work. What is your diagnosis?**

Proctalgia fugax. Proctalgia fugax is transient, severe rectal pain related to spasm of levator ani and coccygeal muscles that may last seconds or up to 20 minutes.

○ **A patient complains of severe pain when defecating. He is constipated, has blood-streaked stools, and a bloody discharge following bowel movements. What is the diagnosis?**

Anal fissure.

○ **Differentiate between mucosal rectal prolapse, complete rectal prolapse, and occult rectal prolapse:**

Mucosal rectal prolapse: Involves only a small portion of the rectum protruding through the anus and have the appearance of radial folds.

Complete rectal prolapse: Involves all the layers of the rectum protruding through the anus. Clinically, this condition appears as concentric folds.

Occult rectal prolapse: Does not involve protrusion through the anus but rather intussusception.

○ **Which are more painful, internal or external hemorrhoids?**

External. The nerves above the pectinate or dentate line are supplied by the autonomic nervous system and have no sensory fibers. The nerves below the pectinate line are supplied by the inferior rectal nerve and have sensory fibers.

○ **Differentiate between first-, second-, third-, and fourth-degree internal hemorrhoids.**

Classification is based upon the following history:

First degree: Presence of only bleeding

Second degree: Bleed and prolapse but reduce spontaneously

Third degree: Bleed, prolapse, and require manual reduction

Fourth degree: Bleed, cannot be reduced, and may strangulate

○ **What portion of the colon most common presents with diverticular disease?**

The sigmoid colon is involved in 95% of patients.

○ **What percentage of patients with diverticula are symptomatic?**

20% and most commonly diagnosed by barium enema radiography or endoscopic procedures.

○ **What percentage of 40-year-olds will have diverticula?**

10% and 65% will have diverticular by the age of 80.

○ **What are the signs and symptoms of diverticulitis?**

Abdominal pain, generally in the left lower quadrant with significant tenderness to palpation, a low-grade temperature, change in bowel habits, nausea, and vomiting. If perforated, patients may have peritoneal signs and appear toxic.

○ **What is the treatment for diverticulitis?**

Specific details of the treatment depend upon the severity of the patient's condition. Generally patients are hospitalized, made NPO, NG tube placed to suction, IV fluids are initiated with broad-spectrum IV antibiotics.

Surgical treatment should be considered for patients who do not improve with medical therapies or develop signs of peritonitis.

○ **Ulcerative colitis has two peaks of incidence. When do they occur?**

The most significant peak is in the second (15–30 years old) decade. A second lower peak occurs during the sixth to eighth decades of life.

○ **What are some extraintestinal manifestations of ulcerative colitis?**

Lesions of the skin and mucous membranes: Erythema nodosum, erythema multiforme, pyoderma gangrenosum, pustular dermatitis, and aphthous stomatitis.
Ocular: Uveitis.
Bone and joint lesions: Arthralgia, arthritis, and ankylosing spondylitis.
Hepatobiliary and pancreatic lesions: Fatty infiltration, pericholangitis, cirrhosis, sclerosis cholangitis, bile duct carcinoma, gallstones, and pancreatic insufficiency.
Hematologic: Anemia (Most commonly iron deficiency anemia).

○ **Kulchitsky cells are the precursors to what tumor?**

Carcinoid tumors arise from *Kulchitsky cells*, granular *cells* within the intestinal and bronchial.

○ **What is the most probable cause of colovesicular fistulas?**

Diverticulitis.

○ **A 47-year-old man complains of impotence as well as pain and coldness in both legs after exercise. What would you expect to find on examination?**

This patient probably has Leriche syndrome, which is a vascular disorder marked by gradual occlusion of the terminal aorta, bilateral iliac arteries, or both; intermittent claudication in the buttocks, thighs, or calves; absence of pulsation in femoral arteries; pallor and coldness of the legs; gangrene of the toes; and, in men, impotence. Symptoms are the result of chronic tissue hypoxia caused by inadequate arterial perfusion of the affected areas.

○ **What is the most commonly obstructed artery in the lower extremity?**

The superficial femoral, which is a branch of the common femoral.

○ **A 64-year-old man presents with jaundice, upper GI bleeding, anemia, a palpable nontender gallbladder, a palpable liver, and rapid weight loss. What is your initial diagnosis and what confirmatory test would you order?**

This is the clinical picture of a tumor of the ampulla of Vater and the results of an ERCP would demonstrate the tumor as an exophytic papillary lesion, an ulcerating tumor, or an infiltrating mass. You would also expect to identify dilation of the biliary and pancreatic ducts.

○ **Testicular torsion occurs most commonly in what age group?**

Teens with the left testicle most commonly involved.

○ **What is the maximum amount of time a testicle can remain torsed without being irreversibly damaged?**

4 to 6 hours.

○ **What are the recommended treatments for the reduction of a testicular torsion?**

Medical: The "Open Book Maneuver."
Surgical: Emergent surgical scrotal exploration.

○ **What percentage of palpable prostate nodules are malignant?**

Nearly 50%. Surgical cure of patients who present with asymptomatic nodules and no metastasis is attempted with radical prostatectomy or radiation therapy.

○ **What are mycotic aneurysms?**

A mycotic aneurysm is a localized, irreversible arterial dilatation caused by destruction of the vessel wall by infection. A mycotic aneurysm can develop either when a new aneurysm is produced by infection of the arterial wall or when a preexisting aneurysm becomes secondarily infected.

○ **Where is mesenteric ischemia more serious, in the small or the large bowel?**

The small bowel. Embolization in the superior mesenteric artery affects the entire small bowel with mortality from small bowel ischemia being nearly 60%. Embolization to the large bowel is not as serious because of the collateral circulation and ischemia of the large bowel rarely result in a full-thickness injury or perforation.

○ **Where do glomus tumors develop?**

Glomus jugulare tumors are rare, slow growing, hypervascular tumors that arise within the jugular foramen of the temporal bone.

○ **What is an ABI, and why is it significant?**

The ankle-brachial index (ABI) is a quick screening test used to evaluate peripheral vascular disease or traumatic arterial injury. It consists of measuring the resting systolic BP in the brachial artery and comparing it to the resting systolic BP in the posterior tibial or dorsalis pedis arteries of the lower extremity. The ABI is calculated by dividing the LE systolic BP by the brachial artery BP. A normal ABI is 1 or greater whereas a value of less than 1 indicates occlusive disease or arterial injury.

○ **What technical factors can affect the accuracy of the ABI?**

Doppler probe pressure, rapid deflation of the BP cuff, and arterial wall calcifications.

○ **What pain medications are not recommended for the treatment of pain arising from acute diverticulitis?**

Opioid pain medications should be avoided, if possible. Their use may increase intraluminal colonic pressure and precipitate constipation and decreased bowel motility.

○ **What are the most common causes of large bowel obstruction?**

Carcinoma, followed by volvulus, diverticulitis inflammatory disorders, and fecal impaction, all of which most commonly occur in the sigmoid.

○ **What is the most common cause of massive upper GI tract hemorrhage?**

Duodenal ulcers.

○ **What layers of the bowel wall and mesentery are affected by regional enteritis?**

All layers.

○ **Which hernia is the most common in women?**

Inguinal hernia. It is also the most common in men.

○ **What is the most common cause of paralytic ileus?**

Abdominal surgery. This is a routine complication following abdominal surgery.

○ **An elderly woman presents with pain in the knee and medial aspect of the thigh. What GI diagnosis should be considered?**

Obturator hernia. This presentation is most common in elderly women and is difficult to diagnose and is frequently missed, which makes these the most lethal of all abdominal hernias (mortality 13%–40%).

○ **Where is the most common site of volvulus?**

The sigmoid colon in nearly 65% of patients.

○ **Describe the location of an indirect inguinal hernia.**

Lateral to the epigastric vessels, protruding through the inguinal canal and commonly into the scrotum.

○ **Describe the location of a femoral hernia.**

Descends through the femoral canal and beneath the inguinal ligament.

○ **Describe the location of a spigelian hernia.**

This is an acquired ventral hernia through the linea semilunaris, the line where the sheaths of the lateral abdominal muscles fuse to form the lateral rectus.

○ **What is a pantaloon hernia?**

A hernia with both direct and indirect inguinal hernia components that occur on the same side.

○ **What is a sliding hernia?**

A hernia in which one wall of the hernia sac includes viscus.

○ **Describe a Richter hernia.**

A hernia involving only one sidewall of the bowel, which can more easily result in bowel strangulation.

○ **Which is the most common type of hernia in children?**

Indirect. Direct inguinal hernias are more common in the elderly.

○ **In the pediatric esophagus, where is a foreign body most commonly lodged?**

The most common site of esophageal impaction is at the thoracic inlet, defined as the area between the clavicles on chest radiograph, this is the site of anatomical change from the skeletal muscle to the smooth muscle of the esophagus. More specifically most foreign bodies (70%) lodge at the cricopharyngeus sling.

○ **Of the following, which is not a common cause of large bowel obstruction: diverticulitis, adhesions, sigmoid volvulus, or neoplasms?**

Adhesions. Adhesions are the most common cause of small bowel obstructions, uncommon in the colon.

○ **Describe the clinical presentation of a patient with sigmoid volvulus.**

Most common in geriatric patients presenting with colicky abdominal pain with a dull discomfort between spasms. Patients commonly have abdominal distention and occasionally vomiting. Characteristic abdominal X-ray findings are a significantly dilated cecum with a distended loop that assumes a "coffee bean" shape.

○ **Describe a typical patient with intussusception.**

It usually occurs in children aged 3 months to 6 years, although the majority are 7 to 8 months old. It is more common in boys (3:1). The typical presentation is a previously healthy infant boy aged 6 to 12 months with sudden onset of colicky abdominal pain 10 to 20 minutes apart with vomiting.

○ **What is the most common anatomical abnormality in the arterial blood supply to the liver?**

The right hepatic artery branches from the superior mesenteric instead of the common hepatic, which arises from the proper hepatic in 15% to 20% of the population.

○ **What is Kehr sign?**

Pain in the shoulder made worse in Trendelenburg. Pain in the left shoulder is a classic presentation indicating splenic injury.

○ **What spinal level provides motor innervation to the diaphragm?**

C3, C4, C5 (Phrenic nerve.) Remember: "3, 4, and 5 keep the diaphragm alive!"

○ **Where are the most common sites of the hematologic spread of breast cancer?**

Bones, liver, and brain.

○ **What characteristics are associated with the best prognosis in breast cancer?**

The (TNM) staging of breast cancer is the most reliable indicator of prognosis.

T1 Tumor < 2 cm

N0 No regional lymph node metastasis

M0 No distant metastasis

○ **What is the most commonly injured nerve during parotidectomies?**

Most serious complications result from damage to the facial nerve (either temporary or permanent paralysis). Injury to the greater auricular nerve results in hypesthesia of the ear.

○ **If medical management fails to relieve symptoms of gastroesophageal reflux after a 1-year trial period, what surgical methods might be attempted?**

Previously antireflux surgery is considered only for patients that did not respond to medical treatment. Currently the following indications are considered:

Young patients who require chronic therapy with proton pump inhibitors for control of symptoms.

Patients in whom regurgitation persists during therapy.

Patients with respiratory symptoms (cough).

Patients with vocal cord damage.

Patients with Barrett esophagus.

The goal of surgical therapy is to restore the competence of the lower esophageal sphincter and the surgical procedure of choice is a laparoscopic Nissen fundoplication.

○ **Other than laparotomy, what invasive examination will confirm suspected mesenteric ischemia?**

For many years, angiography has been considered to be the criterion standard for the diagnosis of acute arterial occlusion with reported sensitivities 74% to 100% and specificity 100%. Currently the noninvasive multidetector row CTA has emerged as a valuable tool for the evaluation of mesenteric ischemia.

○ **What is the most common cause of postsplenectomy (postsplenic) sepsis?**

Streptococcus pneumoniae and *Haemophilus influenzae* to a lesser extent. All postsplenectomy patients should receive the pneumococcal conjugate vaccine (Prevnar), Hib vaccine, and the meningococcal vaccine.

○ **What are the X-ray findings in ischemic bowel disease?**

"Thumb printing" (mucosal dilation) on plain film with dilation of the colon and thickening of the valvulae conniventes.

○ **Which local anesthetic, ester or amide, is responsible for most allergic reactions?**

Ester (Procaine). However, allergic reactions that occur are usually not in response to Procaine, but rather to para-aminobenzoic acid (PABA), which is a major metabolic product of all ester-type local anesthetics.

○ **What are the most common signs and symptoms of mild, moderate, and severe dehydration?**

Symptom/Sign	Mild	Moderate	Severe
Level of consciousness	Alert	Lethargic	Obtunded
Capillary refill	2 seconds	2–4 seconds	>4 seconds
Mucous membranes	Normal	Dry	Cracked
Tears	Normal	Decreased	Absent
Heart rate	Slightly increase	Increased	Very increased
Respiratory rate/pattern	Normal	Increased	Tachypnea
Blood pressure	Normal	Orthostatic	Decreased
Pulse	Normal	Thready	Faint
Skin turgor	Normal	Slow	Tenting
Fontanel	Normal	Depressed	Sunken
Eyes	Normal	Sunken	Very sunken
Urine output	Decreased	Oliguria	Anuria

○ **What are the classic signs and symptoms of a localized infection process becoming more systemic?**

Tachycardia, tachypnea, CO_2 retention, body temperature above 38°C or below 36°C, leukocytosis of 12,000 WBC/mm^3 or higher or below 4000, or a bandemia.

○ **What is the best method to establish a proper differential diagnosis and achieve an accurate diagnosis in a patient with acute abdominal pain?**

Complete a comprehensive history of present illness (HPI), a complete review of systems (ROS), and a past medical history (PMHx) followed by a thorough and detailed physical examination (PE).

○ **What anatomical landmark is used as the division between "upper" and "lower" gastrointestinal bleeding?**

Ligament of Treitz.

○ **What is the target hemoglobin concentration used to establish when a patient experiencing an acute GI Bleed should receive blood and blood product?**

Blood and blood products should be administered early to these patients based upon their clinical status and not laboratory data. Criteria include the presence of impaired end-organ perfusion such as hypotension, oliguria, confusion, and cardiac ischemia.

○ **What is the location of the typically duodenal ulcer that requires emergent surgery?**

They are generally located on the posterior-medial aspect of the first portion of the duodenum and have eroded into the gastroduodenal artery.

○ **What modality is critical in the evaluation and management of gastroesophageal varices and other upper GI bleeding?**

Early endoscopy.

○ **What are the critical evaluation and treatment criteria of a patient presenting with acute chest pain, shortness of breath, fever, dysphagia, and a productive cough s/p 2 days esophagogastroduodenoscopy (EGD)?**

This patient has likely experienced an esophageal perforation and rapid diagnosis, institution of broad-spectrum antibiotics, and aggressive surgical intervention is crucial.

○ **What is the most common cause of an enterocutaneous fistula in a patient with Crohn disease?**

This most common occurs as a complication of abdominal surgery as a result of an anastomotic leak or unrecognized enterotomy.

○ **Are plain radiographic studies always diagnostic in patient's suspected of having an acute bowel obstruction?**

Plain films may only be diagnostic in half of all cases of acute bowel obstruction. They are more sensitive in identifying high-grade (complete) obstructions and much less in detecting low-grade (partial) obstructions.

○ **What is the etiology of a partial bowel obstruction in a patient who has never had a prior abdominal surgery?**

External or internal hernia, tumor, malrotation, volvulus, or intussusception. Malignant tumors are responsible for 20% of SBO.

○ **Explain the "classic" initial appendicitis presentation.**

Initial dull periumbilical discomfort that localizes to sharp right lower quadrant pain. Low-grade fever is common with accompanying malaise and lethargy. After the pain begins the development of nausea is common along with anorexia.

○ **What is the most common cause of acute pancreatitis?**

The passage of biliary precipitates in the form of crystalline sludge or gallstones from the gallbladder into the common bile duct (CBD). This in turn causes obstruction of the pancreatic duct.

○ **Describe the most common symptoms of acute pancreatitis.**

Severe epigastric pain with radiation to the back occur generally 2 hours after eating a fatty meal or 1 to 3 days after an alcoholic drinking binge. In addition, patients commonly report nausea, vomiting, and anorexia. Systemically, fever and tachycardia are common and in the most severe cases hypotension is present.

○ **What two serum biochemical markers are most helpful in obtaining the diagnosis of acute pancreatitis?**

Serum amylase level elevates in 6 to 12 hours from the onset of pain and remain elevated for approximately 10 hours. The levels of serum lipase elevate more slowly and peak in 24 hours, remaining elevated for 2 to 3 weeks.

○ **What are the sonographic findings suggestive of acute cholecystitis?**

a. The presence of gallstones or sludge

b. Gallbladder wall thickening greater than 4 mm

c. Pericholecystic fluid

d. Sonographic Murphy sign

○ **During the evaluation of a patient with suspected cholecystitis, what two findings would strongly suggest the correct diagnosis is cholangitis?**

Elevate bilirubin levels (jaundice) and common bile duct (CBD) dilation.

○ **Describe the basic etiology of a Gallstone ileus.**

A gallstone erodes through the gallbladder wall, through the wall of the duodenum, and migrates to the ileocecal valve, which is the narrowest area of the gastrointestinal tract. As the stone lodges in the ileocecal valve, it causes a small bowel obstruction of the terminal ileum.

○ **What is the appropriate treatment for a patient diagnosed with Fournier gangrene?**

Systemic resuscitation including administration of IV fluids, glucose control, and vasopressor agents in cases of septic shock. In addition, broad-spectrum antibiotics are indicated postsurgically. Definitively, wide surgical excision and debridement with delayed wound closure should be performed.

○ **What are the potential complications of surgical site infections (SSIs)?**

Tissue destruction, failure or prolonged wound healing, incisional hernias, and blood stream infections.

○ **What are the four (4) most common factors that are present in patients diagnosed with abdominal aortic aneurysm (AAA)?**

Atherosclerosis, hypertension, smoking, and being male.

○ **What is the primary indication for conducting CT angiogram in a patient presenting with classic signs and symptoms of an abdominal aortic aneurysm (AAA)?**

Stable hemodynamic status. CTA provides important anatomical information that determines if endovascular repair is indicated.

○   **What are the four (4) clinical patterns associated with acute mesenteric ischemia?**

Arterial embolism, arterial thrombosis, mesenteric vein thrombosis, and nonocclusive mesenteric ischemia.

○   **What are the classic nonspecific symptoms of a lower-extremity deep vein thrombosis (DVT)?**

Stasis is the most significant factor involved in the formation of DVTs with the presentation of leg swelling, pain, fever, erythema, or cyanosis.

○   **What is the most common cause of upper-extremity deep vein thrombosis (DVT)?**

Central venous catheters.

○   **What are the classic venous duplex ultrasound findings present in the diagnosis of a lower-extremity deep vein thrombosis (DVT)?**

Vein incompressibility and lack of phasic flow.

REFERENCES

Britt LD, Peitzman A, Barie P, Jurkovich G. *Acute Care Surgery*. 1st ed. Philadelphia, PA: Lippincott Williams & Wilkins; 2012.
Britt L, Trunkey DD, Feliciano DV. *Acute Care Surgery—Principles and Practice*. New York, NY: Springer-Verlag; 2007.
Doherty GM, Way L. *Current Surgical Diagnosis and Treatment*. 12th ed. New York, NY: McGraw-Hill; 2006.
Silen W. *Cope's Early Diagnosis of the Acute Abdomen*. 22nd ed. Oxford: Oxford University Press Inc; 2010.
Tintinalli MJ, Kelen MG, Stapczynski MJ, Ma MO, Cline MD. *Tintinalli's Emergency Medicine—A Comprehensive Study Guide*. 6th ed. New York, NY: McGraw-Hill; 2004.

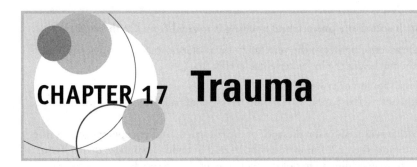

CHAPTER 17 Trauma

Jeffrey Yates, MPAS, PA-C

○ **What percentage of cervical fractures are identified on multislice computed tomography (MCT) that are not seen on plain films?**

Several prospective studies have been completed on this topic and generally it is thought that approximately 50% to 55% of clinically significant fractures where not visualized on plain films but where recognized on MCT. Plain films may be a reasonable imaging screening modality in patients with a low probability of injury; however, numerous studies have found that 75% of the plain radiographic studies will be inadequate and require an MCT for complete visualization. It should be noted that no clinically significant injuries were missed by MCT.

○ **Describe the three types of fractures involving the odontoid process.**

Type I odontoid fracture is an avulsion of the tip of the dens at the insertion site of the alar ligament. Although a type I fracture is mechanically stable, it is often seen in association with atlanto-occipital dislocation and must be ruled out because of this potentially life-threatening complication.

Type II fractures occur at the base of the dens and are the most common type of odontoid fracture. This type is associated with a high prevalence of nonunion because of the limited vascular supply and small area of cancellous bone.

Type III odontoid fracture occurs when the fracture line extends into the body of the axis.

○ **What are the two clinical decision-making criteria used to assess the need for radiographic imaging of the C-spine?**

1. To be clinically cleared using the Canadian C-Spine Rules (CCR), a patient must be alert (GCS 15), not intoxicated, and not have a distracting injury (e.g., long-bone fracture, large laceration). The patient can be clinically cleared providing the following:

   • The patient is not high-risk (age >65 years or dangerous mechanism or paresthesias in extremities).
   • A low-risk factor that allows safe assessment of range of motion exists. This includes simple rear end motor vehicle collision, seated position in the emergency department, ambulation at any time post-trauma, delayed onset of neck pain, and the absence of midline cervical spine tenderness.
   • The patient is able to actively rotate their neck 45 degree left and right.

2. The NEXUS criteria states that a patient with suspected C-spine injury can be cleared provided the following are met:

   • No posterior midline cervical spine tenderness is present.
   • No evidence of intoxication is present.
   • The patient has a normal level of alertness.
   • No focal neurologic deficit is present.
   • The patient does not have a painful distracting injury.

○ **On a lateral C-spine X-ray, how much soft tissue prevertebral swelling is normal from C2 through C4?**

Prevertebral space extends between the anterior border of the vertebra to the posterior wall of the pharynx in the upper vertebral level (C2–C4) or to the trachea in the lower vertebral level (C6).

- At the level of C2, prevertebral space should not exceed 7 mm.
- At the level of C3 and C4, it should not exceed 5 mm, or it should be less than half the width of the involved vertebrae.
- At the level of C6, prevertebral space is widened by the presence of the esophagus and cricopharyngeal muscle. At this level, the space should be no more than 22 mm in adults or 14 mm in children younger than 15 years.
  - Children younger than 24 months may exhibit a physiologic widening of the prevertebral space during expiration; therefore, obtain images in small children during inspiration to assess prevertebral space adequately.

If the prevertebral space is widened at any level, a hematoma secondary to a fracture is the most likely diagnosis.

○ **On a lateral C-spine X-ray, how much soft tissue predental soft tissue swelling is normal?**

The predental space, also known as the atlantodental interval, is the distance between the anterior aspect of the odontoid and the posterior aspect of the anterior arch of C1. This space should be no more than 3 mm in an adult and 5 mm in a child. Suspect transverse ligament disruption if these limits are exceeded.

○ **How much anterior subluxation is allowable on an adult lateral C-spine and still within the normal limits?**

3.5 mm.

○ **On a lateral C-spine plain film, what does "fanning" of the spinous processes suggest?**

This is evident as an exaggerated widening of the space between two spinous process tips and suggests posterior ligamentous disruption.

○ **What are the three most unstable C-spine injuries?**

1. Rupture of the transverse ligament of the atlas.
2. Fracture of the dens (odontoid fracture).
3. Burst fracture with posterior ligamentous disruption (flexion teardrop fracture).

○ **Describe a Jefferson fracture.**

This fracture is caused by a compressive downward force that is transmitted evenly through the occipital condyles to the superior articular surfaces of the lateral masses of C1. The process displaces the masses laterally and causes fractures of the anterior and posterior arches, along with possible disruption of the transverse ligament.

Radiographically, the fracture is characterized by bilateral lateral displacement of the articular masses of C1. The odontoid view shows unilateral or bilateral displacement of the lateral masses of C1 with respect to the articular pillars of C2.

○ **Describe a hangman fracture.**

The name of this injury is derived from the typical fracture that occurs after hangings. Presently, it is commonly caused by motor vehicle collisions and entails bilateral fractures through the pedicles of C2 because of hyperextension.

Radiographically, a fracture line should be evident extending through the pedicles of C2 along with obvious disruption of the spinolaminar contour line.

○ **What is a clay-shoveler fracture?**

Abrupt flexion of the neck, combined with a heavy upper body and lower neck muscular contraction, results in an oblique fracture of the base of the spinous process, which is avulsed by the intact supraspinous ligament. Fracture also occurs with direct blows to the spinous process or with trauma to the occiput that causes forced flexion of the neck.

Radiographically, this injury is commonly observed in a lateral view, since the avulsed fragment is readily evident.

○ **Describe the key features of spinal (neurogenic) shock:**

An acute onset of flaccidity and areflexia with the loss of anal sphincter tone and fecal incontinence. A priapism or loss of bulbocavernosus reflex may also occur. Hypotension with SBPs in the 80 to 100 mm Hg range is common with paradoxical bradycardia at 40 to 60 beats/minute. The classic skin findings are the presence of flushed, dry, and warm peripheral skin.

○ **A trauma patient presents with a decreasing level of consciousness and an enlarging right pupil. What is your diagnosis?**

Probable uncal herniation with oculomotor nerve compression.

○ **The corneal reflex tests what nerves?**

The ophthalmic branch (V1) of the trigeminal (fifth) nerve (afferent), and the facial (seventh) nerve (efferent).

○ **Name five clinical signs of basilar skull fracture.**

1. Periorbital ecchymosis (raccoon eyes)
2. Retroauricular ecchymosis (Battle sign)
3. Otorrhea or rhinorrhea
4. Hemotympanum or bloody ear discharge
5. First, second, seventh, and eighth CN deficits

○ **A trauma patient presents with anisocoria, neurological deterioration, and/or lateralizing motor findings. What should be the immediate treatment?**

1. Immediate intubation (maintain continued C-spine immobilization) with a controlled ventilatory rate. The use of routine hyperventilation should be avoided.
   • Consider pharmacologic paralysis and sedation
2. Obtain venous access and restore intravascular volume.
3. Monitor blood pressure (ICP), oxygen saturation, and neurologic status constantly while obtaining non–contrast-enhanced CT scan.
   • GOALS: MAP between 90 and 100 mm Hg, oxygen saturation 100%, ICP < 20 mm Hg, $PaCO_2$ = 33–37, Hct = 30–34, CVP = 8–14.
4. Control rising intracranial pressures (ICPs)
   • Elevate head-of-bed (HOB) 30 degrees
   • Consider mannitol 25 to 50 g IV q4h
   • Consider phenytoin during the first 7 days only for patients with significant risk factors for post-traumatic seizures (cortical contusion, SDH, penetrating head wound).
   • Determine if the placement of a ventriculostomy catheter is warranted.
5. Determine the need for any acute neurosurgical procedures.
6. Repeat head CT in 24 hours.

○ **How is posterior column function tested? Why is it significant?**

Position and vibration sensation are carried in the posterior columns and are usually spared in anterior cord syndrome. Light touch sensation may also be spared. Pain and temperature sensation cross near the level of entry and are carried in the more posterior spinothalamic tract.

○ **Define increased intracranial pressure.**

Intracranial pressure (ICP) >20 mm Hg.

○ **Where is the most common site of a basilar skull fracture?**

Through the floor of the anterior cranial fossa.

○ **What cardiovascular injury is commonly associated with a sternal fracture?**

Myocardial contusions (blunt myocardial injury).

○ **Which valve is most commonly injured during blunt trauma?**

Aortic valve.

○ **What plain film radiographic finding most accurately indicates traumatic rupture of the aorta?**

Widening of the mediastinum >8 cm.

○ **What is the differential diagnosis of distended neck veins in a trauma patient?**

Tension pneumothorax and pericardial tamponade are the primary conditions with additional possibilities being pulmonary embolism right heart failure. It should be fully understood that JVD may **not** be present in a hypovolemic patient.

○ **What is the most sensitive indicator of compensated shock in children?**

Because cardiac output (CO) depends on both stroke volume (SV) and heart rate (HR), the body typically tries to maintain CO when SV decreases by increasing the HR. A patient in the early stages of shock is typically tachycardic.

○ **What initial IV crystalloid fluid bolus should be administered to children in shock?**

20 mL/kg.

○ **A radial pulse on examination indicates a systolic BP of at least:**

80 mm Hg.

○ **A femoral pulse on examination indicates a systolic BP of at least:**

70 mm Hg.

○ **A carotid pulse indicates a systolic BP of at least:**

60 mm Hg.

○ **What is the most common symptom of patients with a traumatic aortic injury?**

For those patient who are still alive, they frequently complain of retrosternal or intrascapular pain. The most common signs and symptoms are those of acute exsanguinating hemorrhage and shock.

○ **When should amputation be considered in a lower-extremity injury?**

Severe open fractures with popliteal artery and posterior tibial nerve injuries can be treated but multiple surgeries are required. The result is often a leg that is painful, nonfunctional, and less efficient than a prosthesis. Sound clinical judgment from trauma, orthopedic, and vascular surgeons is required to determine the proper course of treatment.

○ **How long does it take to prepare fully cross-matched blood?**

30 to 60 minutes at a minimum.

○ **Should a chest tube be placed into an entrance or exit wound in the appropriate anatomical location rather than making a surgical incision in the chest?**

No. The tube might follow the bullet track into the diaphragm or lung.

○ **Why do simple through-and-through wounds of the extremities far better regardless of the velocity of the bullet?**

The bullet's short path in the tissue results in (1) little or no deformation of slower bullets and (2) less time for higher-velocity bullet to yaw, which results in less tissue damage.

○ **Is the heat from firing a bullet significant enough to sterilize a bullet and its wound?**

No, contaminants from the body surface and viscera can be carried along the bullet's path.

○ **Should intra-articular bullets be removed?**

In most cases they should be removed because of the potential for synovitis to develop, leading to severe damage of articular cartilage.

○ **What artery is usually involved in an epidural hematoma?**

The middle meningeal artery.

○ **Where are epidural hematomas located?**

Between the dura and inner table of the skull.

○ **Where are subdural hematomas located?**

Beneath the dura, over the brain, and in the arachnoid.

○ **What risk is associated with not treating a septal hematoma of the nose?**

Aseptic necrosis followed by absorption of the septal cartilage, resulting in septal perforation referred to as a "saddle-nose deformity."

○ **What are the most commonly injured organs as a result of blunt trauma?**

The spleen, liver, and retroperitoneum.

○ **A patient who was recently hit in the eye during a bar room brawl complains of diplopia when looking up. The injured eye does not appear to be able to look up. What is the diagnosis?**

Orbital blowout fracture with entrapment of inferior rectus or inferior oblique.

○ **What is the LD50 for falling in adults?**

25 to 30 feet.

○ **What clinical history and physical examination findings are most suggestive of a laryngeal fracture?**

Obtaining a mechanism of injury (MOI) of the patient sustaining a direct blow to the anterior or anterolateral neck is highly suggestive of a possible laryngeal injury. The physical examination findings of subcutaneous emphysema, the loss of the normal contour of the thyroid cartilage, and a palpable tracheal defect are most concerning for this condition.

○ **What formula should be used to calculate the estimated fluid requirements for resuscitation of an adult burn victim during the first 24 hours of care?**

Thermal and chemical burns: 2 mL × kg × % BSA involved. One-half of this is given in the first 8 hours, and the second half is given over the next 16 hours.

Electrical burns: 4 mL × kg × % BSA involved. One-half of this is given in the first 8 hours, and the second half is given over the next 16 hours.

*Maintaining urinary outputs of 0.5 to 1 mL/kg/h are good indicators for resuscitation.

○ **What is the adult dose of epinephrine for acute anaphylactic shock?**

0.3 mg of 1:10,000 IV or 0.3 mg of 1:1000 SQ.

○ **How should neurogenic shock be managed?**

The treatment of all patients with a suspected etiology of shock should start with the ABCs of **A**irway, **B**reathing, and **C**irculation. In addition, appropriate fluid resuscitation should be instituted to restore the intravascular volume, blood pressure, and perfusion to vital organs. The use of vasopressors may prove beneficial, and typically vasopressors are required only for a brief 24 to 72 hours. Invasive hemodynamic monitoring may also be indicated but should be based upon the patient's age, associated injuries, and chronic medical conditions.

○ **What is the most common cause of airway obstruction in trauma?**

Unconscious patients: Tongue

Conscious patients: Dentures, avulsed teeth or other foreign bodies, oral secretions, and blood are the most common.

○ **How much lactated Ringer solution should be infused while performing a Diagnostic Peritoneal Lavage (DPL)?**

Adults: 1 L of warmed normal saline

Children: 10 cc/kg of warmed normal saline

○ **What criteria is used to indicate a positive diagnostic peritoneal lavage (DPL)?**

1. 10 mL of gross blood on initial aspiration

2. Greater than 100,000 RBCs

3. Greater than 500 WBCs

4. The presence of bacteria, bile, or food particles

○ **Identify the zones of the neck and the appropriate method of evaluation for penetrating injuries to each zone.**

Zone I: Extends from the clavicles to the cricoid cartilage

Zone II: Extends from the cricoid cartilage to the angle of the mandible

Zone III: Extends from the angle of the mandible to the base of the skull

Treatment: For zone II injuries in patients who present with hemodynamic instability or with "hard signs" (rapidly expanding hematoma), immediate surgical exploration is strongly indicated. Stable patients may be evaluated in the same manner as stable zone I or III injured patients.

For stable patients presenting with injuries in zone I or III, an initial nonoperative evaluation is indicated, most frequently with the use of angiography. Other considerations are the use of computed tomographic (CT) or magnetic resonance (MR) angiography. There is also an emerging role for the use of bedside duplex ultrasound depending upon the experience of the clinician. Any unstable patient with a zone I or III related injury should undergo immediate surgical exploration.

○ **What is the etiology for the cause of death in an untreated tension pneumothorax?**

Decreased cardiac output. As a result of the mediastinal shift, the superior and inferior vena cava are compressed creating an impaired venus return and decreased cardiac output.

○ **What is the best method to open an airway while maintaining C-spine precautions?**

The jaw thrust maneuver with manual C-spine immobilization.

○ **What is the formula for determining the appropriate ET tube size for children older than 1 year?**

The internal diameter of the appropriate endotracheal tube for a child will roughly equal the size of that child's little finger.

Uncuffed ET tube size = (age in years/4) + 4

Cuffed ET tube size = (age in years/4) + 3

○ **What is the correct ET tube size for a 1-year-old child?**

4 to 4.5 mm.

○ **What is the correct ET tube size for a 6-month-old child?**

4 mm.

○ **What is the average distance from the mouth to 2 cm above the carina in men and in women?**

Men: 23 cm; women: 21 cm.

○   **When should blood products be supplemented with fresh-frozen plasma for a trauma patient receiving multiple units of transfused blood?**

A significant amount of ongoing research is being conducted on this topic and the common conclusion is a ratio of 1:1 is optimal, especially in the setting of massive transfusion. For every unit of PRBC a unit of FFP should be infused. Because the time to thaw a unit of FFP is roughly 30 to 60 minutes, most facilities are unable to initially meet this goal and the 1:3 ratio is also acceptable and most commonly recognized.

○   **What is the Cushing reflex?**

The Cushing reflex is a hypothalamic response to ischemia in the brain. It consists of an increase in sympathetic outflow to the heart as an attempt to increase arterial blood pressure and total peripheral resistance, accompanied by bradycardia. The primary features of this reflex are increased systolic blood pressure and bradycardia.

○   **A core temperature of less than 33°C (mild hypothermia) is commonly associated with what complications?**

Metabolic acidosis, tachypnea, tachycardia, mental status changes, impaired coagulation, and decreased urine output. Hypothermia significantly increases a trauma patient's mortality and roughly 66% of patients arrive with below normal body temperature.

○   **What are the six most lethal conditions involved with blunt force thoracic trauma?**

1. Airway obstruction
2. Tension pneumothorax
3. Cardia tamponade
4. Open pneumothorax
5. Massive hemothorax
6. Flail chest

○   **What, potentially life-threatening, conditions are most difficult to diagnose in patients experiencing blunt chest trauma?**

- Traumatic rupture of the aorta
- Major tracheobronchial disruption
- Blunt cardia injury
- Diaphragmatic tear
- Esophageal perforation
- Pulmonary contusion

○   **What are the three components to the Glasgow Coma Scale, and what is the maximum point value for each?**

1. Eye opening: 4 points
2. Verbal response: 5 points
3. Motor response: 6 points

○ **What responses are measured while determining the Glasgow Coma Scale in a patient and what are their numerical values?**

Eyes

1. Does not open eyes
2. Opens eyes in response to painful stimuli
3. Opens eyes in response to voice
4. Opens eyes spontaneously

Verbal

1. Makes no sounds
2. Incomprehensible sounds
3. Utters inappropriate words
4. Confused, disorientated
5. Oriented, N/A converses normally

Motor makes

1. No movements
2. Extension to painful stimuli
3. Abnormal flexion to painful stimuli
4. Flexion/withdrawal to painful stimuli
5. Localizes painful stimuli
6. Follows commands

○ **What results are normal in the oculocephalic reflex?**

Conjugate eye movement is opposite to the direction of head rotation.

○ **When testing a patient's oculovestibular reflex, which direction of nystagmus is anticipated in response to cold water irrigation: toward or away from the irrigated ear?**

Away from the irrigated ear. Recall that nystagmus is defined as the direction of the fast component of saccadic eye movement. (*Remember*: COWS = **C**old **O**pposite, **W**arm **S**ame.)

○ **What does tonic eye movement toward an irrigated ear in response to warm caloric testing in a comatose patient signify?**

Life.

○ **What common finding on a sinus X-ray suggests a basilar skull fracture?**

Blood in the sphenoid sinus with a transsphenoid fracture pattern.

○ **The best view of the zygomatic arch on a face X-ray is:**

Standard facial series are the norm and are obtained with varying angulation of the X-ray beam vector. The Caldwell projection allows for visualization of the orbital floor and zygomatic process above the dense petrous pyramids. A submental vertex view affords excellent detail of the zygomatic arches. However, computed tomography (CT) scans have replaced radiographs in the evaluation of midfacial trauma and are the current modality of choice.

○ **Describe central cord syndrome.**

Traumatically, most commonly caused by severe neck hyperextension and injury to the ligamentum flavum with the following patient presentation:

Arm > leg weakness

Distil > proximal arm weakness

Variable sensory deficits

Bladder dysfunction

Frequently presents with a gradual improvement with traumatic mechanism of injury.

○ **Under what conditions does trench (immersion) foot develop?**

Trench foot occurs when the extremity is exposed for several days to wet or cold conditions at temperatures that are above freezing. The extremity develops superficial damage resembling partial-thickness burns.

○ **Describe pernio (chilblain).**

Exposure of an extremity for a prolonged period of time to dry, cold but above freezing temperatures. Patients develop superficial, small, edematous, painful ulcerations over the chronically exposed areas, most commonly the feet. Sensitivity of the surrounding skin, erythema, and pruritus may also develop.

○ **Describe frostnip.**

The skin becomes numb and blanched and then cessation of discomfort occurs. A sudden loss of the "cold" sensation at the location of injury is a reliable sign of precipitant frostbite. Frostnip will proceed to frostbite if treatment is not initiated.

○ **How is frostnip treated?**

It is treated by warming the affected area(s) by using the hands, breathing on the skin, or by placing the exposed extremities under the armpit. The affected part should not be rubbed because this treatment does not thaw the tissues completely.

○ **What are the proper classifications of frostbite?**

Superficial (first-degree injury): Erythema, edema, waxy appearance, hard white plaques, and sensory deficit.

Partial full-thickness (second-degree injury): Erythema, edema, and formation of blisters filled with clear or milky fluid and which are high in thromboxane. (These blisters form within 24 hours of injury.)

Complete full-thickness (third-degree injury): Damage affecting muscles, tendons, and bone, with resultant tissue loss.

○ **What is the appropriate treatment for frostbite?**

Do not use dry heat! The exposed extremity should be rewarmed rapidly by immersing the affected area in 38° to 41°C circulating water for 20 minutes or until flushing is observed. Elevation of the extremity will minimize the possibility of developing edema. Refreezing thawed tissue greatly increases damage. Remember to provide tetanus prophylaxis.

○ **What are the signs/symptoms of anterior cord syndrome?**

The common etiology is related to an anterior spinal artery infarction or injury. Patients present with paralysis with loss of pain and temperature sensation below the level of the lesion that spares touch, vibration, and proprioception because that blood supply received from the posterior spinal arteries.

○ **What are some common complications of frostbite?**

Wound infection primary with *Staphylococcus aureus*, beta-hemolytic streptococci, gram-negative rods, or anaerobes. Tetanus (frostbite is considered a high-risk wound), hyperglycemia, metabolic acidosis, and tissue loss. In rare cases, rhabdomyolysis and compartment syndrome.

○ **What is the half-life of carboxyhemoglobin?**

4 to 6 hours on room air but can be reduced to approximately 40 minutes with the administration of 100% oxygen.

○ **What is the best method for transporting an amputated extremity?**

Wrap the extremity in sterile gauze, place it in waterproof plastic bag, and then immerse in ice. Do not allow it to freeze.

○ **What organ is most severely affected in a blast injury?**

The lungs.

○ **What organ is most commonly affected in a blast injury?**

The middle and inner ear.

○ **What is the most effective method for decontaminating the skin following particulate radiation exposure?**

Wash with soap and water after removing all clothes.

○ **What is the best emergency treatment of an Ellis III dental fracture in an adult?**

Cover the exposed surface with a calcium hydroxide composition (e.g., Dycal) or a glass ionomer.

Provide immediate dental follow-up and analgesics as needed.

Initiate antibiotics with coverage of intraoral flora (e.g., penicillin, clindamycin).

○ **What are the classic findings of shaken baby syndrome?**

- Failure to thrive
- Lethargy
- Seizures
- Retinal hemorrhages
- CT may show subarachnoid hemorrhage or subdural hematoma from torn bridging veins

○ **How do you treat a patient with a severe, high concentration hydrofluoric acid burn?**

Ensure that the caregivers are adequately protected. Decontaminate the patient with copious amounts of clean water while removing all of their clothing. If calcium gluconate gel is available, apply liberally to the affected area. For digital burns, if calcium gluconate gel is not available, the fingers may be soaked in magnesium hydroxide (Mylanta). Treat inhalation injuries with oxygen and 2.5% calcium gluconate nebulizer.

○ **How should an ocular burn secondary to hydrofluoric acid be treated?**

Generously irrigate with sterile water or saline for at least 15 minutes. Local anesthetic may be required. If pain persists, irrigate with a 1% solution of calcium gluconate.

○ **What electrolyte disorder may occur in a victim of a significant hydrofluoric acid burn?**

Hypocalcemia.

○ **An unconscious 60-year-old patient presents to the emergency department with a head injury. An ECG shows significant ST-segment elevation. What is your main concern?**

Although MI should be considered and is quite probable, do not forget the possibility of an intracerebral hemorrhage. This may also cause significant ST-segment elevation.

○ **A near-drowning victim is comatose and intubated. A diagnosis of severe pulmonary edema is made. What specific pulmonary treatment should be provided in the emergency department?**

It is important to give these patients PEEP early to increase alveolar pressure and alveolar volume. The increased lung volume increases the surface area by reopening and stabilizing collapsed or unstable alveoli.

○ **What laboratory abnormalities may be found with heat stroke?**

ABG analysis may reveal respiratory alkalosis because of direct CNS stimulation and metabolic acidosis because of lactic acidosis, hypoglycemia, hypernatremia, hypokalemia, and hypophosphatemia. CK levels exceeding 100,000 IU/mL are common. Elevated white blood cell counts are common as well as serum uric acid levels, blood urea nitrogen, and serum creatinine in patients whose course is complicated by renal failure myoglobinuria and proteinuria are frequently found on urinalysis.

○ **What distinguishes heat stroke from heat exhaustion?**

Heat stroke is the most severe form of the heat-related illnesses and is defined as a body temperature higher than 41.1°C (106°F) associated with neurologic dysfunction. Heat exhaustion is a milder form of heat-related illness that develops after several hours or days of exposure to high temperatures and inadequate or unbalanced replacement of fluids.

○ **How should a patient with heat stroke be treated?**

Heat stroke is a medical emergency and the rapid reduction of the core body temperature is the cornerstone of treatment because the duration of hyperthermia is the primary determinant of outcome. Appropriate considerations include removal of restrictive clothing and spraying water on the body, covering the patient with ice water–soaked sheets, or placing ice packs in the axillae and groin may reduce the patient's temperature significantly. Patients who are unable to protect their airway should be intubated. Patients who are awake and responsive should receive supplemental oxygen. Intravenous lines may be placed in anticipation of fluid resuscitation and for the infusion of dextrose and thiamine if indicated.

○ **What complications can result from heat stroke?**

Renal failure, rhabdomyolysis, DIC, and seizures. *Remember*: Antipyretics are not recommended to reduce the core body temperature.

○ **A young boy presents for evaluation after suffering a coral snake bite. He has no complaints and appears to be in no distress. What is appropriate management?**

The onset of symptoms may be delayed up to 10 to 12 hours but may then be rapidly progressive. Admit this patient to the intensive care unit and monitor for impending respiratory failure. Coral snake venom has significant neurotoxicity and neuromuscular dysfunction is common. Coral snake antivenom may be very difficult to obtain in some areas and there has been a recent shortage.

○ **Describe the appearance of a coral snake.**

This is a round snake with red, yellow, and black stripes and a black spot on the head, which can easily be mistaken for the nonvenomous milk snake. The mnemonic "Red on yellow, kill a fellow; red on black, venom lack."

○ **Which type of rattlesnake bite leads to most deaths?**

The Western diamondback rattlesnake accounts for nearly all lethal snakebites in the United States. However, it accounts for only 3% of the snakebites seen. Treat with 10 to 20 vials of antivenin.

○ **What are the physical attributes of a pit viper?**

The deep pits on each side of the triangular-shaped head between the eye and the nostril tend to be a commonly recognizable feature. Research indicates that the pits are very sensitive detectors of radiant heat, thereby enabling the snake to find warm-blooded prey in the dark. In addition, a pair of elongated fangs that are folded back against the palate of their triangular-shaped head are a key feature.

○ **What is the recommended dose for steroids for treating patients with acute spinal cord injuries?**

Highly controversial topic and recent studies no longer recommend the use of high-dose steroids for any spinal injury. Previously, high-dose methylprednisolone (Solu-Medrol) 30 mg/kg bolus over 15 minutes followed by 45 minutes normal saline drip. Over the subsequent 23 hours, the patient should receive an infusion of 5.4 mg/kg/h of methylprednisolone.

○ **A cold water drowning patient with a temperature of 29°C develops ventricular fibrillation. Is defibrillation likely to be successful?**

Defibrillation is not indicated for patients experiencing severe hypothermia until they have been appropriately warmed.

○ **A straight (Miller) blade is preferred for intubating children of less than what age?**

Approximately 4 years of age.

○ **What is the Parkland formula for treating a pediatric burn victim weighing less than 25 kg?**

Ringer lactate at 3 mL/% TBSA burned/kg. One-half of this should be infused over the first 8 hours with the remaining infused over the next 16 hours.

○ **How much fluid is required for the maintenance of pediatric patients?**

100 mL/kg/day for each kg up to 10 kg, 50 mL/kg/day for each kg from 10 to 20 kg, and 20 mL/kg/day for each kg thereafter.

○ **A trauma patient, from a high-speed MVC, presents with a complaint of a severe burning pain in the upper extremities and associated neck pain. On physical examination, the patient has good strength in his upper extremities and a significant decrease in sensation at his fingertips. There are no obvious neurologic deficits in the lower extremities with normal rectal tone. Radiographically, the patient's C-spine series is negative. What condition do you suspect and what diagnostic test should you order?**

Central cord syndrome. This injury is common with a hyperextension injury of the spinal cord. Impairment in the upper extremities is usually greater than in the lower extremities and is especially prevalent in the muscles of the hand. Pain and temperature sensations, as well as the sensation of light touch and of position sense, may be impaired below the level of injury. Neck pain and urinary retention are common complaints. MRIs demonstrate direct evidence of spinal cord impingement from bone, a disk, or a hematoma and are the diagnostic modality of choice. CT scanning of the cervical spine shows spinal canal compromise and allows the indirect approximation of the degree of spinal cord impingement.

○ **What is the common patient presentation of a laryngeal fracture and how are they diagnosed?**

Common signs of laryngeal injury include stridor, subcutaneous emphysema, hemoptysis, hematoma, ecchymosis, laryngeal tenderness, vocal cord immobility, loss of anatomical landmarks, and bony crepitus. CT scanning is the imaging modality of choice to assess laryngeal anatomy. The Schaefer classification of laryngeal injuries is based on a combination of the CT and endoscopic findings, which dictate treatment modalities.

○ **When does dysbaric air embolism (DAE) typically occur?**

DAE develops within minutes of surfacing after SCUBA diving. Symptoms are sudden and dramatic; they include loss of consciousness, focal neurologic symptoms (such as monoplegia, convulsions, blindness, and confusion), and sensory disturbances. Sudden loss of consciousness or other acute neurologic deficits immediately after surfacing are because of DAE unless proven otherwise. Treatment includes high flow oxygen and rapid transport for hyperbaric oxygen treatment.

○ **A 2-year-old has jammed a pencil into her lateral soft palate. What complication might develop?**

Penetrating injury to the internal carotid artery (ICA) with resultant neurologic deficit is a well-documented complication in children. In addition to the potential of thrombotic injury, the development of a collection of air in the retropharyngeal space can result in mediastinitis.

○ **In a trauma patient, what is the physical examination finding of dimpling of the unilateral cheek associated with?**

Zygomatic arch fracture.

○ **A patient sustains blunt force trauma to his face and mouth and you observe that a tooth has been fractured. Upon closer examination you note that blood is originating from the tooth and there is no additional intraoral injury. What is the Ellis classification?**

Ellis III fractures involve enamel, dentin, and pulp; patients complain of pain with manipulation, air, and temperature. Pinkish or reddish markings around surrounding dentin or blood in the center of the tooth from the exposed pulp may present.

○ **What is the most common location involved in the malposition of an orotracheal endotracheal tube?**

The right mainstem bronchus is the common location for a tube placed in the trachea; however, the most common location for an improperly placed endotracheal tube is the esophagus.

○ **A scuba diver descends to 33 feet. How many atmospheres of pressure is he experiencing?**

2 atmospheres. Sea level is considered 1 atm and atmospheric pressure doubles every 33 feet. 2 atm = 33 feet; 3 atm = 66 feet.

○ **What are the most common complaints in patients with carbon monoxide poisoning?**

A headache is most common, followed by dizziness, weakness, and nausea.

○ **A patient presents after experiencing trauma to the head. He has an elevated systolic blood pressure and bradycardia. What is this reflex?**

Cushing reflex.

○ **What is the name for a flexion mechanism fracture through the anterior aspect of a vertebral body that is associated with ligamentous damage and an anterior cord syndrome?**

A flexion teardrop fracture occurs when flexion of the spine, along with vertical axial compression, causes a fracture of the anteroinferior aspect of the vertebral body. This fragment is displaced anteriorly and resembles a teardrop. For this fragment to be produced, significant posterior ligamentous disruption must occur. Since the fragment displaces anteriorly, a significant degree of anterior ligamentous disruption exists. This injury involves disruption of all the three columns, making this an extremely unstable fracture that frequently is associated with spinal cord injury.

○ **What nerves control the corneal reflex?**

The afferent limb is V1 (ophthalmic) of the trigeminal nerve; the efferent limb is the facial or seventh cranial nerve.

○ **A patient presents with a hypertension-type neck injury after receiving a blow to the forehead. She complains of weakness in her arms and no weakness in her lower extremities. What is the most likely diagnosis?**

Central cord syndrome.

○ **You are evaluating a patient with an obvious traumatic spinal cord injury. On physical examination, he has motor paralysis, loss of gross proprioception, loss of vibratory sensation on one side, and loss of pain and temperature sensation on the opposite side. What is the likely diagnosis?**

Brown-Séquard syndrome.

○ **A patient presents after sustaining a high-speed traumatic injury to the chest. A systolic murmur over the precordium is auscultated and the patient has a slightly hoarse voice, and her pulse is stronger in the upper extremities. What is the most likely diagnosis?**

Traumatic rupture of the aorta.

○ **What is the most common X-ray finding in traumatic rupture of the aorta?**

Widening of the superior mediastinum.

○ **A patient presents with a history of blunt chest trauma, a 5/6 systolic murmur that radiates to the axillae, and an infarct pattern on ECG. What is the likely diagnosis?**

Traumatic ventricular septal defect.

○ **A patient who has been involved in a motor vehicle accident has X-ray findings of retroperitoneal air with obliteration of the right psoas margin on a flat plate of the abdomen. What is a likely diagnosis?**

Duodenal injury. Patients who are hemodynamically normal should undergo an upper gastrointestinal (UGI) study with a water-soluble contrast (gastrografin).

○ **About how many liters of blood can a patient lose in the retroperitoneal space after sustaining a pelvic fracture?**

4 L before venous tamponade occurs.

○ **What is the most common cause of superior vena cava obstruction?**

Bronchogenic carcinoma.

○ **What laboratory abnormalities are found in times of stress?**

Increased cortisol, glucose intolerance, cholesterol, and platelet adhesion plus impaired lipoprotein ratios.

○ **A patient opens his eyes to voice, makes incomprehensible sounds, and withdraws from painful stimulus. What is his GCS?**

Eyes 3, Voice 2, Motor 4 = 9.

○ **What acronym is commonly used during the evaluation of a patient with suspected rhabdomyolysis?**

MUSCLE = Rhabdomyolysis (evaluation)

Myoglobinuria
Urinalysis
Serum potassium
Creatinine
Lysis sign on CBC (hemolysis)
Enzyme (CPK) increase

○ **A trauma patient has blood at the urinary meatus. What test should be ordered?**

Retrograde urethrogram; 10 mL of radiocontrast solution should be injected into the urinary meatus immediately followed by radiologic evaluation for extravasation.

○ **In blunt trauma, what is the most common renal pedicle injury?**

Renal artery thrombosis.

○ **A trauma patient presents with a "rocking horse" type of ventilation. What is the diagnosis?**

Probable high spinal cord injury with intercostal muscle paralysis.

○ **What is the differential diagnosis for a trauma patient presenting with subcutaneous emphysema?**

Pneumothorax, tension pneumothorax, tracheal/bronchial injury, or pneumomediastinum.

○ **What rib fracture has the worst prognosis?**

The first rib. First and second rib fractures are associated with bronchial tears, vascular injury, and myocardial contusions.

○ **A patient presents to the emergency department after a motor vehicle accident with hematuria and fractures of the left 10th and 11th ribs. What internal organ might be damaged?**

The spleen is the most commonly injured organ in blunt trauma and be especially suspicious of splenic trauma if the 10th or 11th ribs are fractured and the patient has hematuria.

○ **For a trauma victim, what test is most helpful for evaluating retroperitoneal organs?**

CT.

○ **Where should the incision be made to perform a DPL on a trauma patient with a suspected pelvic fracture?**

A supraumbilical incision should be made to avoid insertion of the DPL catheter into a contained pelvic hematoma. Performing a FAST examination may be more clinically appropriate especially if the patient does not have hemodynamically normal vital signs.

○ **What is an absolute contraindication to DPL?**

The only absolute contraindication is the obvious need for laparotomy. Relative contraindications are previous abdominal surgery, morbid obesity, and pregnancy.

○ **What type of intracranial hemorrhage is more common in the geriatric patient?**

Subdural hematomas are most common.

○ **The inability to pass a nasogastric tube in a trauma victim suggests damage to what organ?**

A rupture of the left hemidiaphragm secondary to a diaphragmatic hernia.

○ **What are the primary advantages of performing a digital nerve block?**

Less anesthetic agent is required, better anesthetic effects are obtained, and the tissues do not become distorted.

○ **What nerve block is used to anesthetize of the sole of the foot?**

Tibial nerve block. (Note: Tibial nerve block does not provide anesthesia to the lateral aspect of the heel and foot.)

○ **What is the preferred route for anesthesia for deep lacerations of the anterior tongue?**

Lingual nerve block.

○ **Where is a local anesthetic injected for an ulnar nerve block?**

On the anterior wrist, in the proximal volar skin crease, between the ulnar artery and the flexor carpi ulnaris.

○ **Where is a local anesthetic injected for a median nerve block?**

On the anterior wrist in the proximal volar skin crease, between the tendon of the palmaris longus and the flexor carpi radialis.

○ **A patient presents to your office after stepping on a nail that went right through the shoe and punctured the plantar aspect of the foot. What gram-negative organism would be most commonly involved in this type of injury?**

Pseudomonas aeruginosa.

○ **What are the laboratory criteria for intubating patients and placing them on mechanical ventilation?**

Room air $PaO_2 < 60$ mm Hg or $PaCO_2 > 45$ mm Hg.

Basing your decision to intubate on laboratory criteria alone is a critical error. The clinical indications of a respiratory rate >36 breaths/min, labored respiratory efforts, the use of accessory muscles, and tachycardia are much more significant. The patient's clinical status provides the primary indication for intubation.

○ **What negative pressure must be generated by an intubated patient for weaning to be successful?**

At least 20 to 30 cm of H_2O. Other important factors include PaO_2, arterial saturation, pH, spontaneous respiratory rate, minute volume, tidal volume, and PEEP.

○ **A fire victim suffers from partial- and full-thickness burns over the complete surface of both legs, his entire back, and his entire right arm. What percentage of his body is burned?**

Follow the "rule of 9's". Anterior/posterior legs = 18% × 2 36%
Entire back = 18% Entire right arm = 9% **TBSA 63%**

○ **A patient who has been burned over the entire top of his body (arms and torso, front and back) develops severe difficulty breathing and appears to be going into respiratory arrest. What should be done?**

An emergent escharotomy. The patient is most likely suffering ventilatory restriction because of the circumferential eschar about his chest resulting in constriction of the chest cavity. Anesthesia is rarely required when performing an escharotomy and frequently is performed at the bedside because of its emergent nature.

○ **What is the caloric requirement of a 100-kg firefighter who was burned over 20% of his body?**

3300 kcal. (25 kcal/kg of body weight + 40 kcal/1% burned surface)

○ **What is the 24-hour estimated fluid resuscitation requirement for the above patient?**

2 L in the first 8 hours (250 mL/h) and 2 L in the next 16 hours (125 mL/h). The burn formula gives the requirement as 2 mL/kg body weight X% burned (2 mL X of 100 kg X 20 = 4 L). Give half the volume in the first 8 hours and the other half in the next 16 hours, while maintaining a urine output (UO) of 0.5 to 1 mL/kg/h. If there is a drop in the UO, then the fluids should be increased to maintain the desirable output.

○ **Name the function and spinal innervation level of the biceps, triceps, flexor digitorum, interossei, quadriceps, extensor hallucis, biceps femoris, soleus and gastrocnemius, and rectal sphincter.**

Muscle	Action	Spinal Level
Biceps	Forearm flexion	C5–C6
Triceps	Forearm extensors	C7
Flexor digitorum	Finger flexion	C8
Interossei	Finger adduction/abduction	T1
Quadriceps	Knee extension	L3–L4
Extensor hallucis	Great toe dorsiflexion	L5
Biceps femoris	Knee flexion	S1
Soleus and gastrocnemius	Foot plantar flexion	S1–S2
Rectal sphincter	Sphincter tone	S2–S4

○ **What are the clinical signs of CSF leakage?**

A headache that improves when supine and worsens when sitting up, otorrhea, and rhinorrhea.

○ **How many minutes of cerebral anoxia will result in irreversible brain injury?**

Greater than 4 to 6 minutes.

○ **What do muffled heart tones, hypotension, and distended neck veins indicate?**

This is Beck triad and is classic for pericardial tamponade.

○ **Cricothyroidotomy is not recommended in children under what age?**

Children younger than 10 to 12 years pose a relative contraindication to this procedure.

○ **Is succinylcholine a depolarizing or a nondepolarizing neuromuscular blocking agent?**

Depolarizing. Succinylcholine is the only commonly used depolarizing agent. It binds to postsynaptic acetylcholine receptors, thereby causing depolarization. The material is enzymatically degraded by pseudocholinesterase (serum cholinesterase). Onset is within 1 minute; paralysis lasts 7 to 10 minutes. The recommended adult dose is 1 to 2 mg/kg.

○ **What is the rationale for pretreating a patient with a subpolarizing (defasciculating) dose of a nondepolarizing agent prior to treatment with succinylcholine?**

This primarily reduces the fasciculations secondary to succinylcholine-induced depolarization. In addition, it may also be helpful in decreasing intracranial and intraocular pressure is associated with the administration of succinylcholine.

○ **What dosage of midazolam (versed) causes a loss of consciousness and amnesia during rapid sequence induction?**

0.1 mg/kg; 5 mg is effective for most people.

○ **Etomidate is the recommended agent to obtain sedation and induction while performing rapid sequence intubation. What is the appropriate adult dose?**

0.2 to 0.3 mg/kg.

○ **What is the "defasciculating" or the "priming" dose of vecuronium?**

0.01 mg/kg or commonly 1 mg or 1/10th of the total dose.

○ **What dose of vecuronium should be administered for paralysis (no "priming")?**

0.08 to 0.1 mg/kg providing an NMR effects for 15 to 30 minutes.

○ **What are the primary concepts involved in the initial assessment of the trauma patient?**

1. Rapid primary survey
2. Resuscitation
3. Detailed secondary survey
4. Reevaluation

○ **What is involved in the primary survey of the trauma patient?**

  1. Airway maintenance with C-spine immobilization
  2. Breathing and ventilation
  3. Circulation and hemorrhage control
  4. Disability (neurological status)
  5. Exposure/environmental control

○ **When should the secondary survey be completed?**

  After the primary survey has been established and resuscitation has begun.

○ **What are the absolute indications for performing exploratory laparotomy in a patient with penetrating trauma?**

  Peritonitis, evisceration, impaled object, hemodynamic instability, associated hemorrhage from a natural orifice, pneumoperitoneum.

○ **What regions of the body are evaluated during Focused Abdominal Sonography for Trauma (FAST) examination?**

  1. Subxiphoid area: Pericardium
  2. Left subcostal: Splenorenal recess
  3. Right subcostal: Hepatorenal recess (Morrison pouch)
  4. Suprapubic: Pelvic cul-de-sac

○ **How much intra-abdominal "fluid" is generally required to identify a positive FAST examination?**

  200 mL, however ultrasound examination is highly operator dependent

○ **What is the next diagnostic modality of choice for a hemodynamically stable trauma patient with a positive FAST examination showing intra-abdominal fluid?**

  Computed tomography.

○ **What is the most appropriate management for patients sustaining blunt trauma spleen and liver injuries that are identified by CT with no active extravasation of IV contrast?**

  The vast majority of these patients can be managed nonoperatively at level I or II trauma centers. If the facility does not have the availability of conducting emergent surgery in the event of nonoperative failure the patient should be transferred to a facility that does.

○ **What are the primary goals of damage control surgery?**

  Control of hemorrhage and contamination.

○ **What classification is generally accepted to assist in the determination of difficulty before performing endotracheal intubation?**

  Mallampati.

○ **What is the clinical definition of a massive transfusion protocol in a trauma patient?**

Anticipated needs to potentially transfuse greater than 10 units of packed red blood cells (PRBCs), fresh-frozen plasma (FFP), and platelets at a 1:1:1 ratio.

○ **What are the classifications of hemorrhagic shock?**

Class	I	II	III	IV
EBL	500–750 mL	750–1000 mL	1000–1500 mL	>1500 mL
HR	Normal	100–120	120–140	>140
BP	Normal	↓ Pulse pressure	↓ SBP	Severe hypotension
MS	Anxious	Confused	Very confused	Obtunded
UOP	Normal	Normal	Decreased	Anuric

○ **What is the indication of a positive FAST examination at the Splenorenal recess?**

A dark fluid stripe between the spleen and the kidney.

○ **What two pre-hospital factors dramatically increase the mortality of patients suffering a mild or moderate traumatic brain injury (TBI)?**

Hyperventilation and poorly performed intubation.

○ **What are the clinical indicators for performing pre-hospital or emergency department hyperventilation, before invasive ICP monitoring, in a patient experiencing a traumatic brain injury (TBI)?**

Development of signs or symptoms of herniation; unilateral dilated pupil, asymmetric motor examination, or a declining GCS.

○ **During the acute resuscitation of a patient presenting with a moderate traumatic brain injury (TBI) what intravenous fluid has shown efficacy in decreasing intracranial pressure?**

IVFB of hypertonic saline solution.

○ **What are the contraindications for performing an emergent resuscitative thoracotomy?**

1. CPR > 10 minutes in blunt trauma
2. CPR > 15 minutes in penetrating trauma
3. When the patient's initial EKG rhythm is asystole

○ **What are the risk factors for abdominal compartment syndrome (ACS)?**

Abdominal surgery/trauma, fluid resuscitation >5 L in 24 hours, ileus, pulmonary/renal/hepatic dysfunction, hypothermia, acidosis, and anemia.

○ **What is the most common cause of a patient experiencing a bladder rupture and how do most patients initially present?**

90% of bladder ruptures are caused by motor vehicle accidents and patients most commonly present with hematuria and/or abdominal pain.

○ **What is the most important study to perform in a patient with a suspected bladder rupture?**

If there is blood at the urethral meatus a retrograde urethrogram should be performed to rule out urethral injury. If there is no urethral injury a static CT cystogram may be performed. But in all likelihood a contrast-enhanced CT of the abdomen and pelvis will be performed, to include a CT cystogram, for the evaluation of additional injuries.

REFERENCES

Britt LD, Peitzman A, Barie P, Jurkovich G. *Acute Care Surgery.* 1st ed. Philadelphia, PA: Lippincott Williams; 2012.

Britt L, Trunkey DD, Feliciano DV. *Acute Care Surgery—Principles and Practice.* New York, NY: Springer-Verlag; 2007.

Doherty GM, Way L. *Current Surgical Diagnosis and Treatment.* 12th ed. New York, NY: McGraw-Hill; 2006.

Peitzman AB, Rhodes M, Schwab CW, Yealy DM, Fabian TC. *The Trauma Manual.* 2nd ed. Philadelphia, PA: Lippincott, Williams & Wilkins; 2002.

Tintinalli MJ, Kelen MG, Stapczynski MJ, Ma MO, Cline MD. *Tintinalli's Emergency Medicine—A Comprehensive Study Guide.* 6th ed. New York, NY: McGraw-Hill; 2004.

CHAPTER 18

Pharmacology/ Toxicology

Daniel Thibodeau, MHP, PA-C, DFAAPA

GENERAL PRINCIPLES

○ **What are the two mechanisms of drug metabolism and breakdown?**

Hepatic and renal.

○ **Which enzyme is mostly responsible for drug breakdown in the liver?**

Cytochrome P-450.

○ **What are the three methods of drug excretion from the kidneys?**

Glomerular filtration, proximal renal secretion, and distal tubule reabsorption.

AUTONOMIC NERVOUS SYSTEM

○ **Which transmitter is released at all pre- and postganglionic receptors?**

Acetylcholine. This interaction of acetylcholine with pre- and postganglionic receptors gives the "flight or fight" responses.

○ **What are the two receptors of acetylcholine?**

Muscarinic and nicotinic.

○ **What effect does the sympathetic nervous system have on the cardiovascular system?**

Increases heart rate and contractility. Parasympathetic system would then reverse this and decrease heart rate.

○ **Which organs have both sympathetic and parasympathetic innervations?**

Heart, eyes, bronchial smooth muscle, and GI and GU smooth muscle.

○ **What are some of the main activities of β_1-, β_2-, and α-receptors?**

β_1-Heart regulation

β_2-Smooth muscle relaxation

α-Contraction and constriction, mostly vasoconstriction

○ **What effect does the activation of presynaptic α_2-receptors cause?**

It facilitates the release of norepinephrine.

○ **What are some common anticholinergics side effects?**

Dry eyes, dry mouth, blurred vision, constipation, and urinary retention.

○ **What are some uses of muscarinic antagonists?**

They can be used for problems with urinary frequency, urgency, as well as incontinence.

○ **Name the mechanism of action for neuromuscular blockers**

They act as competitive blockers at the nicotinic receptors to cause muscle relaxation.

○ **What is the mechanism of action for succinylcholine?**

It is a depolarizing neuromuscular blocker. It is commonly used in general anesthesia and rapid sequence intubations.

○ **What is the one potentially fatal side effect of succinylcholine?**

It can cause malignant hyperthermia.

○ **What are the two substances that can activate both α- and β-receptors?**

Epinephrine and norepinephrine. However, norepinephrine has less of an effect on β_2-receptors, making it less effective on actions of bronchospasm like that of epinephrine.

○ **What is the main effect of dopamine?**

It causes renal and coronary vasodilation as well as activates the β_1-receptors of the heart at low doses.

○ **Name the two major actions that norepinephrine play on the cardiovascular system.**

It causes an increase in total peripheral resistance and increases mean arterial pressure.

○ **α-agonists have what type of effect on the cardiovascular system?**

They act by reducing the sympathetic nerve activity, thus lowering blood pressure.

○ **What are the major side effects of α-agonists?**

Postural hypotension and reflex tachycardia are most common.

○ **Why should you worry about giving a β-blocker to a diabetic patient?**

They can stimulate the sympathetic activity of glycogenolysis, gluconeogenesis, as well as lipolysis.

○ **What are some other side effects of β-blockers?**

Bronchoconstriction and decreased heart rate.

○ **What is the clinical presentation of anticholinergic poisoning?**

Mydriasis, tachycardia, hypoactive bowel sounds, urinary retention, dry axilla, hyperthermia, and mental status changes. *Remember*:

Dry as a bone
Red as a beet
Mad as a hatter
Hot as Hades
Blind as a bat

○ **Name a few substances that have anticholinergic properties.**

Antihistamines, cyclic antidepressants, phenothiazine, atropine, tiotropium, and jimson weed.

○ **What ECG abnormality is most common in patients who suffer from anticholinergic toxicity?**

Sinus tachycardia. Other dangerous arrhythmias include conduction problems and V-Tach.

○ **What are the common anticholinergic compounds?**

Atropine, tricyclic antidepressants, antihistamines, phenothiazine, antiparkinsonian drugs, belladonna alkaloids, and some Solanaceae plants (i.e., deadly nightshade and jimson weed).

CARDIOVASCULAR SYSTEM

○ **What are the three groups of diuretics?**

Thiazide, loop, and potassium-sparing diuretics.

○ **How do the thiazide diuretics function?**

They limit the sodium and chloride reabsorption in the ascending loop. This in turn increases the urine production.

○ **What drug is the treatment of choice in hypertension?**

Thiazide diuretics, specifically chlorthalidone and hydrochlorothiazide (HCTZ).

○ **What is a main side effect of thiazide diuretics?**

Hypokalemia and possibly hypotension.

○ **How does the potassium sparing diuretics function?**

They act as an antagonist of aldosterone, which will lead to sodium retention.

○ **The use of ACE inhibitors functions to lower blood pressure by what mechanism?**

They convert angiotensin I to angiotensin II, which acts as an aldosterone antagonist, which in turn lowers pressure by retaining sodium.

○ **Unlike β-blockers, what advantage does ACE inhibitors have for the treatment of hypertension?**

They are ideal for diabetics because they do not affect gluconeogenesis.

○ **Name some major side effects of ACE inhibitors.**

Headache, dizziness, abdominal pain, confusion, renal failure or elevation of creatinine, and erectile dysfunction.

○ **What is one of the most common side effects of ACE inhibitors?**

Cough.

○ **Do angiotensin II receptor antagonists cause cough?**

No.

○ **What is the main physiological effect by calcium channel blockers?**

They reduce cardiac afterload by blocking calcium entrance into cells.

○ **Name some of the most common side effects of calcium channel blockers.**

Headaches, dizziness, hypotension. Anything that you can imagine with the action of vasodilation can occur in calcium channel blockers.

○ **What action do nitrates have on blood vessels and the cardiac cycle?**

They vasodilate, which in turn causes a reduction in cardiac preload. At higher concentrations, nitrates will decrease afterload also.

○ **What drug is the treatment of choice for relieving coronary vasospasm?**

Nitroglycerine.

○ **What forms of nitrates can be given?**

Oral, intravenous, sublingual, and transdermal.

○ **Which nitrate when metabolized turns into cyanide?**

Sodium nitroprusside.

○ **What are the two main side effects of nitrates?**

Headache and hypotension. Another possible side effect is postural hypotension.

○ **What is the main goal in the treatment of coronary artery disease?**

Reduction of myocardial oxygen demand.

○ **What are the three pharmacologic principles in the treatment of heart failure?**

Decreasing the cardiac workload, controlling excess fluid, and enhancement of myocardial contractility.

○ **What are the main effects of ACE inhibitors with regard to heart failure?**

They reduce cardiac workload. This will slow the progression of heart failure, which in turn prolongs survival.

○ **What class of drugs is used as a mainstay in controlling the excess fluid accumulation in heart failure?**

Diuretics.

○ **How do the cardiac glycosides (digoxin and digitoxin) function to improve myocardial contractility?**

They inhibit the Na^+-K^+-ATPase pump, which improves contractility.

○ **A 77-year-old male patient with a history of heart failure has been taking both furosemide and digoxin for several months. Over the past 3 weeks, he has noticed having nausea, fatigue, drowsiness, and blurred vision. What could be the possible problem in this patient?**

Digoxin toxicity.

○ **What effect, if any, do diuretics play on the role of digoxin?**

If a patient on diuretics is not closely monitored for hypokalemia, lower serum potassium levels can have higher than normal therapeutic levels of digoxin, thus leading to possible toxicity.

○ **What are some of the common side effects resulting from digoxin toxicity?**

Arrhythmias, anorexia, nauseam diarrhea, drowsiness, fatigue, and visual disturbances (including a yellow visual appearance).

○ **What is the mechanism of dobutamine in the use of heart failure?**

It increases cardiac output and can be used in cardiac shock.

○ **Name three nonpharmacologic treatments for arrhythmias.**

Pacemakers, implantable defibrillators, and ablation therapy.

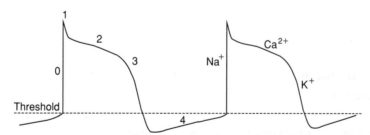

Figure 18-1 (Cardiac action potential. Note the first action potential shows the class of antiarrhythmics and where they have action. Note the second action potential and what electrolyte plays a major role in that part of the action potential. (Reproduced with permission from Stringer JL. *Basic Concepts in Pharmacology.* 3rd ed. New York, NY: McGraw-Hill; 2006: Fig 13-1.))

○ **What is the role of class I antiarrhythmic drugs?**

They are sodium channel blockers.

○ **Class IA drugs such as procainamide and quinidine are useful in what type of arrhythmias?**

Both atrial and ventricular arrhythmias.

○ **Lidocaine is a IB antiarrhythmic. What type of arrhythmias does this drug work best?**

Treatment of ventricular arrhythmias such as ventricular tachycardia, ventricular fibrillation, and ventricular ectopy.

○ **Are drugs like lidocaine effective in the treatment of supraventricular tachycardia?**

No, they have almost no effect on this type of arrhythmia.

○ **What is the mechanism by the class IC medications?**

They are used to suppress ventricular arrhythmias.

○ **What effects do β-blockers have on the sinoatrial (SA) and atrioventricular (AV) nodes?**

They slow the conduction at these sites, thus slowing the refractory period.

○ **β-Blockers are useful in the treatment of which arrhythmias?**

They are useful in tachyarrhythmias as they can slow transmission.

○ **Amiodarone is a potassium channel blocker. Describe how this drug functions as an antiarrhythmic.**

It acts by slowing the repolarization of the action potential without impairing the resting potential prior to depolarization. It is used commonly in atrial fibrillation for rate control as well as some ventricular arrhythmias like ventricular tachycardia (both sustained and nonsustained).

○ **Are calcium channel blockers more effective toward atrial or ventricular arrhythmias?**

Atrial. They slow the conduction at the AV node, which increases the refractory period.

○ **What drug is the treatment of choice for paroxysmal supraventricular tachycardia?**

Adenosine

○ **Does adenosine have a long half-life?**

No, in fact, it is only seconds long, which is why it is favorable in converting SVT.

○ **What are the three drugs that will increase heart rate?**

Atropine, epinephrine, and isoproterenol.

○ **What is the first-line pharmacologic treatment of hypercholesterolemia?**

HMG-CoA reductase inhibitors. These are referred to as the "statins."

○ **What is the effect of statins with respect to cholesterol?**

It lowers serum LDL and plasma cholesterol.

○ **What does niacin do for overall cholesterol levels?**

It lowers both overall cholesterol as well as triglycerides.

○ **What are the two side effects of niacin?**

Flushing of the skin and liver toxicity.

○ **If you have a patient who gets the typical flushing of the skin with the taking of niacin, what can you instruct the patient to do to help reduce this side effect?**

Usually, taking the medication with an 81-mg aspirin will help as well as instructing the patient to take the medication at night.

○ **Gemfibrozil, fenofibrate, and clofibrate, the so-called "fibrates," act to lower what to lipid values?**

They can lower triglycerides and HDL.

○ **Hemostasis consists of what three phases?**

Vascular (from tissue injury), platelet, and coagulation phases.

○ **What is the main synthesis component, which causes the formation of coagulation?**

Thromboxane A_2.

○ **What is the action of nonsteroidal anti-inflammatory drugs?**

They inhibit prostaglandins, which inhibit platelet aggregation and prolong bleeding time.

○ **How do drugs like ticlopidine and clopidogrel work as "blood thinners"?**

They inactivate the platelet adenosine diphosphate receptors, which in turn inhibit platelet aggregation.

○ **Which receptors are critical for the formation of platelet aggregation?**

Glycoprotein IIb/IIIa receptors. They prevent platelet aggregation by blocking fibrinogen and von Willebrand factors.

○ **What is the main side effect of all platelet inhibitors?**

They all can cause bleeding. That is also the main side effect of anticoagulants. Most of the agents are no reversible and need to have a washout period before surgery.

○ **Does heparin interact with the intrinsic or extrinsic coagulation pathway?**

Actually, both. It binds to antithrombin III and inactivates IIa, IXa, Xa, XIa, XIIa, XIII, and III.

○ **What anticoagulant has a longer half-life: heparin or low-molecular-weight heparin (LMWH)?**

Low-molecular-weight heparin.

○ **Which types of patients should avoid the use of LMWH?**

Those with renal impairment or those with bleeding abnormalities.

○ **What is the antidote to heparin?**

Protamine sulfate.

○ **What is the mechanism of action of warfarin?**

It is an antagonist of vitamin K.

○ **If administration of vitamin K is the antidote for warfarin overdose, how long does it take for the anticoagulant properties to take effect?**

At a minimum, 24 hours. Additional measures such as fresh-frozen plasma and platelet transfusions can be given if emergency measures are required.

○ **What is the mechanism of action on thrombolytic agents?**

They act as plasminogen activators to lyse clots that have already formed. The plasminogen will convert to plasmin, which then causes the degradation of fibrin.

○ **What is the main side effect of thrombolytic agents?**

Bleeding, naturally.

○ **What can be a serious life-threatening side effect from streptokinase?**

An allergic-anaphylactic reaction. This is usually because streptokinase is created from a bacterial origin.

○ **Which drugs cause methemoglobinemia?**

Oxidant drugs, such as antimalarials, dapsone, nitrites/nitrates (nitroprusside), and local anesthetics (lidocaine). Methemoglobinemia occurs when the iron moiety of hemoglobin is oxidized from the ferrous to the ferric state.

○ **Which common enzyme deficiency predisposes to the development of methemoglobinemia in the presence of the above drugs?**

G6PD deficiency.

○ **What drugs can induce a chronic cough?**

ACE inhibitors cause chronic cough as a result of the accumulation of prostaglandins, kinins, or substances that excite the cough receptors. (Remember that ACE sitting next to you at the boards!!). β-Blockers evoke bronchoconstriction, and thus coughing, by blocking β_2 receptors. Never give β-blockers to asthmatic patients or other patients with an airway disease.

○ **What is the incidence of cough induced by captopril?**

1% to 2%.

○ **What is the incidence of enalapril-induced cough?**

24.7%.

○ **True/False: Generally, the cough related to ACE inhibitors resolves within a few days of withdrawal of the drug.**

False. The resolution of cough may be slow, taking several weeks.

○ **How does treatment for a cocaine-induced MI differ from a typical MI?**

Both are treated the same except that β-blockers are <u>not</u> used for a cocaine-induced MI secondary to potential unopposed α-adrenergic activity. The tachycardia of a cocaine-associated MI is first treated with benzodiazepine sedation.

○ **A patient has an arterial pH of 7.5 through alkalization, but her urine pH is still low. What electrolyte is probably responsible?**

Potassium. When reabsorbing sodium, the renal tubules will preferentially excrete hydrogen ions into the tubular lumen rather than potassium ions. Thus, potassium should be maintained at 4.0 mmol/L.

○ **What are the absolute indications for Digibind administration in digoxin poisoning?**

Ventricular arrhythmias, hemodynamically significant bradyarrhythmias that are unresponsive to standard therapy, and a potassium level greater than 5.0 mEq/L.

○ **A patient on Digoxin is bradycardic and hypotensive with significantly peaked T waves. What is the initial line of treatment?**

Administer 10 vials of Digibind intravenously while simultaneously treating the presumed hyperkalemia with insulin and glucose, sodium bicarbonate, and Kayexalate. After the Digibind is administered, hyperkalemic-induced arrhythmias may safely be treated with calcium chloride.

○ **What is the antidote for β-blocker poisoning?**

Glucagon. Glucagon receptors, located on myocardial cells, are G-protein–coupled receptors that activate adenylate cyclase, leading to increased levels of intracellular cAMP. Thus, glucagon administration causes the same intracellular effect as β-agonist.

○ **What are potential treatment modalities for a calcium channel blocker poisoning?**

Therapeutic interventions include IV calcium, isoproterenol, glucagon, transvenous pacer, atropine, and vasopressors, such as norepinephrine, epinephrine, or dopamine.

○ **What are the mechanism and treatment for clonidine-induced hypotension?**

Treatment: Includes IV fluid administration and dopamine.
Mechanism: Decreased cardiac output secondary to a decreased sympathetic outflow from the CNS.

○ **What typical eye response is related to clonidine poisoning?**

Pinpoint pupils.

○ **Clonidine is a centrally acting presynaptic α-2 adrenergic agonist that decreases the central sympathetic outflow. Although its primary use is to treat hypertension, clonidine has additional emergency value in blunting withdrawal symptoms from opiates and ethanol. A clonidine overdose closely resembles an overdose with which other class of drugs?**

Opiates.

○ **Toxicity from clonidine (Catapres) usually occurs within what time period?**

Within 4 hours.

○ **Which agent is a useful "antidote" for clonidine overdose?**

Naloxone (Narcan).

○ **True/False: A patient with acute digitalis OD presents with frequent multifocal PVCs, peaked T waves, and a K+ of 6.2 mEq/L. The correct treatment is to first administer CaCl₂, as this is the fastest-acting agent for reducing hyperkalemia.**

False! Although $CaCl_2$ is the fastest-acting agent for decreasing hyperkalemia, don't give any more Ca+ to a patient with digitalis-induced cardiac toxicity.

○ **β-Adrenergic antagonists have three main effects on the heart. Name these effects.**

1. Negative chronotropy
2. Negative inotropy
3. Decrease AV nodal conduction velocity (negative dromotropy)

○ **True/False: β-adrenergic antagonists can cause mental status changes and seizures.**

True.

○ **A cocaine addict presents with chest pain but his ECG is normal. What are the odds that he will have abnormal CPK and CPK-MB isoenzymes?**

6% to 19%.

○ **What is the most common arrhythmia induced by chronic, heavy ethanol bingeing?**

Atrial fibrillation.

○ **What is the antidote for nitrites?**

Methylene blue 1%, 0.2 mL/kg IV over 5 minutes. Severe methemoglobinemia requires an exchange transfusion.

○ **What are the effects of dopamine at various doses?**

1 to 10 mg/kg: Renal, mesenteric, coronary, and cerebral vasodilation
10 to 20 mg/kg: Both α- and β-adrenergic
20 mg/kg: Primarily α-adrenergic

○ **Methylene blue is used to treat:**

Methemoglobinemia.

○ **What are the signs and symptoms of isopropanol poisoning?**

Sweet breath odor (acetone), hypotension, hemorrhagic gastritis, and CNS depression from isopropanol and from its metabolite, acetone.

CENTRAL NERVOUS SYSTEM

○ **What is the main pharmacologic goal in the treatment of Alzheimer disease?**

It is to maintain or elevate the level of acetylcholine by preventing the breakdown of acetylcholine.

○ **Define the following terms: Tolerance, cross-tolerance, and dependence.**

Tolerance is the state by which there is a reduced drug effect with repeated use of the medication. This will necessitate the requirement for more of a medication to produce the same desired result.

Cross-tolerance refers to a patient who is tolerant to one drug will also be tolerant to drugs that are in the same class.

Dependence is signs and symptoms of withdrawal when drug levels fall.

○ **Name the type of medication to use for the following specific seizures: generalized convulsive, partial (simple, complex, secondary), and generalized nonconvulsive.**

Seizure Type	Medication of Choice
Generalized convulsive	Valproate
	Carbamazepine
Partial (includes simple, complex, and secondarily generalized)	Carbamazepine
	Phenytoin
Generalized nonconvulsive	Ethosuximide
	Valproate

○ **How are all these antiepileptic medications metabolized?**

Hepatic.

○ **What are two major conditions that can be seen with the use of carbamazepine?**

Granulocyte suppression and apastic anemia.

○ **Name some common side effects of phenytoin.**

Hirsutism, coarse facial features, and gingival hyperplasia. With higher doses, it can cause ataxia and nystagmus.

○ **Are antipsychotic and neuroleptic drugs considered to be medications that can cure these diseases?**

No. They are not curative; they only allow the patient to function in a more normal state.

○ **What is the mechanism of neuroleptics?**

They are α-blockers, muscarinic, and histamine antagonists.

○ **What is a common side effect with most antipsychotic drugs?**

Extrapyramidal side effects (EPS).

○ **Name the more common EPSs and give some examples of each:**

Dystonia—spasms of the face, neck, tongue, and back
Parkinsonism—rigidity, shuffling gait, and tremor
Akathisia—motor restlessness
Tardive dyskinesia—lip smacking, jaw movements, darting of the tongue, and quick involuntary movements

○ **What is neuroleptic malignant syndrome?**

It is a rare syndrome that is potentially fatal as a result of the use of neuroleptic medications. It becomes more common as the doses of medications increase.

○ **What are some of the signs of neuroleptic malignant syndrome?**

These will present with severe forms of parkinsonism, catatonia, autonomic instability, and in some cases stupor.

○ **What is the mortality rate for a patient with neuroleptic malignant syndrome?**

About 10% to 20%.

○ **What are the three targets for the pharmacologic treatment of Parkinson disease?**

Dopamine replacement therapy, dopamine agonist therapy, and anticholinergic therapy.

○ **Which dopamine crosses the blood–brain barrier (BBB)?**

Levodopa.

○ **Carbidopa does not cross the BBB. How does this drug function?**

It reduces the peripheral metabolism of l-dopa in the bloodstream, which in turn will increase the amount of dopamine going to the brain.

○ **Anticholinergics therapy reduces the effectiveness of uninhibited cholinergic neurons. Describe some of the side effects that these drugs commonly have:**

They are all the muscarinic side effects that you should be familiar with: dry mouth, confusion, constipation, and urinary retention.

○ **The two main anxiolytic and hypnotic drug classes are barbiturates and benzodiazepines. What are the main side effects of these two classes of drugs?**

Sedation and most induce sleep or hypnosis. At higher doses, they can induce medullary depression and death.

○ **What is the mechanism of action of barbiturates?**

They enhance the function of γ-aminobutyric acid (GABA) in the CNS.

○ **What are some potential side effects of barbiturates if not taken appropriately?**

Sedation, hypnosis, coma, suppression of respiration, and death.

○ **A 42-year-old male patient who has been on phenobarbital for the last several years arrives to the emergency department with nausea, vomiting, hypotension, and acute psychosis. By history, you have been told that he has not been taking his phenobarbital that he is normally prescribed. What is the probable diagnosis?**

Withdrawal symptoms secondary to barbiturate use. Other signs and symptoms include seizures and cardiovascular collapse, which can lead to death.

○ **What is the mechanism of action of benzodiazepines?**

They block a specific site associated with $GABA_A$ receptors which increases inhibition.

○ **A 23-year-old female patient presents to the emergency department with a suspected benzodiazepine overdose. She has shallow respirations, is hypoxic, and also has confusion, agitation, and restlessness. What is the antidote that could be given in this scenario?**

Flumazenil.

○ **Name one benzodiazepine does not produce dependence.**

Buspirone.

○ **What is the common mechanism of action of antidepressants and lithium?**

They all act by increasing the concentration of norepinephrine and serotonin.

○ **What are some indications for prescribing serotonin-selective reuptake inhibitors (SSRI)?**

Depression, eating disorders, panic disorders, obsessive–compulsive, and borderline personality disorders.

○ **What is the usual onset of improvement of symptoms after starting tricyclic antidepressants?**

It usually takes 2 to 3 weeks for patients to have a noticeable difference.

○ **How do heterocyclics work as antidepressants?**

They are potent muscarinic cholinergic antagonists, and have weak α_1 and H_1 antagonist properties.

○ **What is the mechanism of action of monoamine oxidase inhibitors?**

They increase levels of norepinephrine, serotonin, and dopamine by preventing the degradation of these products.

○ **What is the one major complication in taking an MAO inhibitor?**

They can cause a fatal hypertensive crisis.

○ **What are some foods that patients on MAO inhibitors should avoid?**

Cheeses, beer, and red wines. Any foods that have higher levels of tyramine or other active amines should be avoided.

○ **What are the three most common drugs that are used in the treatment of bipolar disease?**

Lithium, carbamazepine, and valproate.

○ **What is the major receptor for the mediation of pain?**

μ(mu)-Receptors. The other receptors that have less activity are kappa (κ) and delta (δ).

○ **What are the three main types of narcotics? Give some examples of each:**

1. Agonists—codeine, fentanyl, heroin, morphine, methadone, meperidine

2. Mixed agonist–antagonist—pentazocine, buprenorphine, nalbuphine

3. Antagonists—naloxone, naltrexone, and nalmefene

○ **Name some signs and symptoms from narcotic withdraw.**

Hyperactivity, nausea, vomiting, chills, fever, tearing, runny nose, tremor, abdominal pain, and cramps.

○ **What are the main effects of morphine?**

Analgesia, respiratory depression, spasm of the smooth muscle of the GI and GU tracts, and pinpoint pupils.

○ **What is the potency of fentanyl when compared to morphine?**

It is 80 times more potent but has a much shorter half-life.

○ **What is the indication for the use of methadone?**

It is used for narcotic withdraw and dependence. It acts by reducing the craving for narcotics.

○ **What is the drug of choice to reverse a narcotic overdose?**

Naloxone.

○ **What factors influence the elimination of inhaled anesthetics?**

The rate of ventilation, blood flow, and the solubility of the gas itself.

○ **What is the mechanism of action for local anesthetics?**

They block nerve conduction by the local application of the drug. They do this by blocking the sodium channel of the nerve membrane.

○ **Why should not the 600 mg/day of thioridazine (Mellaril) be exceeded?**

Exceeding this dosage causes retinitis pigmentosa. Thioridazine is a piperidine phenothiazine with low-frequency extrapyramidal effects.

○ **Why is haloperidol one of the preferred neuroleptics?**

It can be used IM in emergencies, plus it has few side effects. It does, however, have a high frequency of extrapyramidal effects.

○ **What is the only neuroleptic with tardive dyskinesia as a side effect?**

Clozapine. Unfortunately, patients taking clozapine can develop agranulocytosis and are at a higher risk for seizures than patients on other neuroleptics. Other side effects include hypotension, anticholinergic symptoms, and oversedation.

○ **What happens when ethanol is combined with an anxiolytic (benzodiazepine)?**

Death can occur because of the combined respiratory depressive effects.

○ **Name another contraindication to benzodiazepine use.**

Known hypersensitivity, acute narrow angle glaucoma, and pregnancy, especially in the first trimester.

○ **What should be used to treat a hypertensive crisis caused by the combination of MAO inhibitors with a known toxin?**

An α- and β-adrenergic antagonist, such as labetalol. Also consider nifedipine or nitroglycerin. If unsuccessful, consider IV phentolamine or sodium nitroprusside.

○ **Name some drugs contraindicated in a patient on MAO inhibitors.**

Meperidine (Demerol) and dextromethorphan can cause toxic reactions, such as excitation and hyperpyrexia. The effects of indirect-acting adrenergic drugs are potentiated, including ephedrine, sympathomimetic amines in cold remedies, amphetamines, cocaine, and methylphenidate (Ritalin).

○ **Name the three common MAO inhibitors (chemical and brand name).**

1. Phenelzine (Nardil)
2. Isocarboxazid (Marplan)
3. Tranylcypromine (Parnate)

○ **Name eight drugs that decrease sexual desire.**

1. Antidepressants
2. Antihypertensives
3. Anticonvulsants
4. Neuroleptics
5. Cimetidine
6. Digitalis
7. Clofibrate
8. High doses or chronic ingestion of alcohol or street drugs

○ **What is the first cardiac finding in a cyclic antidepressant overdose?**

Sinus tachycardia.

○ **How long should a tricyclic antidepressant overdose patient, demonstrating tachycardia and conduction disturbances, be monitored?**

24 hours.

○ **What major tranquilizer displays the most hypotensive tendency?**

Thorazine.

○ **What is the most significant pathophysiologic mechanism of death from cyclic antidepressants?**

Myocardial depression, including hypotension and conduction blocks.

○ **What antibiotic may either increase or decrease lithium secretion?**

Tetracycline.

○ **How is lithium overdose treated?**

Lavage, saline diuresis, furosemide, and hemodialysis. Alkalinization may be appropriate.

○ **Name seven primary actions of cyclic antidepressant overdose.**

1. Inhibition of amine reuptake
2. Sodium channel blockade, which causes negative inotropy
3. Anticholinergic effects, primarily antimuscarinic
4. CNS depression
5. α-Adrenergic antagonism, which contributes further to hypotension
6. GABA antagonism
7. Q-T prolongation

○ **What is the appropriate treatment for QRS widening in tricyclic antidepressant (TCA) poisoning?**

$NaHCO_3$ is administered intravenously for patients with a QRS > 100 ms; 0.5 to 2 mEq/kg are initially administered and repeated until the blood pH is between 7.45 and 7.55. A continuous infusion of $NaHCO_3$, 3 amps in 1 L of D5W, may then be initiated and titrated in over 4 to 6 hours to maintain an appropriate pH. Potassium levels must be closely monitored as supplementation may be required to prevent hypokalemia. To arrhythmias not responsive to the above, consider lidocaine (1 mg/kg IV).

○ **What is the appropriate treatment for TCA-induced seizures?**

Benzodiazepines (clorazepam or diazepam) and barbiturates (phenobarbital) are the agents of choice. Phenytoin is not generally effective but may be tried for recurrent seizures or those unresponsive to treatment. Bicarbonate and alkalosis are the main stays of treatment.

○ **What is the treatment for TCA-induced hypotension?**

Isotonic saline and peptid alkalinization. If the patient is resistant to fluid resuscitation, a direct-acting α-adrenergic agonist, such as norepinephrine, should be started. Dopamine acts in part by releasing norepinephrine. This agent may already be depleted by the reuptake inhibition of the cyclic antidepressant and by stress.

○ **What period of observation is required before medically clearing a TCA overdose?**

6 hours.

○ **What level of lithium is generally considered toxic?**

2 mEq/L.

○ **Will charcoal bind lithium?**

No.

○ **What are the signs and symptoms of lithium toxicity?**

Neurological signs and symptoms include tremor, hyperreflexia, clonus, fasciculations, seizures, and coma. GI signs and symptoms consist of nausea, vomiting, and diarrhea. Cardiovascular effects include ST-T wave changes, bradycardia, conduction defects, and arrhythmias.

○ **What is the treatment for lithium toxicity?**

Supportive care, normal saline diuresis, hemodialysis for patients with clinical signs of severe poisoning, that is, seizures and arrhythmias, renal failure, or decreasing urine output.

○ **What are the typical CNS findings in mild lithium toxicity?**

Rigidity, tremor, and hyperreflexia.

○ **What are the typical CNS findings in severe lithium toxicity?**

Seizures, coma, and myoclonic jerking.

○ **What are the indications for hemodialysis in lithium toxicity?**

Serum lithium level above 4 mEq/L, renal failure, and severe clinical symptoms (stupor, seizures, etc.).

○ **True/False: Permanent neurologic sequelae (encephalopathy) can develop from lithium toxicity.**

True.

○ **A 30-year-old man presents to the emergency department 20 minutes after ingesting 30 tablets of amitriptyline. What is the preferred method of gastric emptying?**

Immediate gastric lavage using a large (34–36 French) orogastric tube. Ipecac should not be used because of the potential for a rapid deterioration in mental status and seizures.

○ **What is the initial treatment for hypotension in antidepressant overdose?**

Intravenous fluids—normal saline or Ringer lactate.

○ **What vasopressor should be used to treat hypotension not responsive to IV fluids in antidepressant overdose?**

Norepinephrine should be used because it is a direct-acting α-adrenergic agonist.

○ **The onset of toxicity of monoamine oxidase inhibitors (MAOI) can occur up to what period of time after ingestion?**

12 to 24 hours.

○ **What over-the-counter cold medications should not be used by people taking MAOIs?**

Decongestants, antihistamines, and products containing dextromethorphan.

○   **A 45-year-old patient presents with a diagnosis of depression, anxiety, and insomnia and is currently taking tramadol, flecainide, and tamoxifen. Can you prescribe an SSRI for her?**

No. SSRIs are cyp 450 2D6 inhibitors. The drugs she is on utilize the cyp 450 2D6 for their metabolism.

○   **Describe the signs, symptoms, and ECG findings associated with lithium toxicity.**

Tremor, weakness, and flattening of the T waves, respectively.

○   **What is the treatment of lithium overdose?**

Saline diuresis and hemodialysis.

○   **What is the difference between low-potency and high-potency neuroleptics and give examples of drugs in each category.**

Low-potency neuroleptics have greater sedative, postural hypotensive, and anticholinergic effects. High-potency neuroleptics have greater extrapyramidal effects.

Low potency: Chlorpromazine (Thorazine)

Medium potency: Perphenazine (Trilafon)

High potency: Haloperidol, droperidol (Inapsine), thiothixene (Navane), fluphenazine (Prolixin), trifluoperazine (Stelazine)

○   **You are considering chemical restraint. List your options:**

Benzodiazepines:

1. Lorazepam (Ativan), 1 to 2 mg IV, or 2–6 mg orally every 30 minutes
2. Midazolam (Versed), 2 to 4 mg IV every 30 minutes
3. Diazepam (Valium), 5 mg IV or orally every 30 minutes

Sedative hypnotics:

Haloperidol (Haldol), 1 to 5 mg IM/IV, titrate to clinical response

Droperidol (Inapsine), 1 to 2 mg IV every 30 minutes

Benzodiazepines may be given in combination with the sedative hypnotics above to both hasten and potentiate their effect. Titrate to effect and monitor appropriately.

○   **Is phenobarbital more quickly metabolized by children or by adults?**

Adults. Neonates are especially slow at metabolizing phenobarbital.

○   **A 32-year-old female patient is prescribed meperidine (Demerol) for an open fracture. The patient is chronically on fluoxetine (Prozac). What is a potential complication?**

The serotonin syndrome.

○   **What signs and symptoms are typical of the serotonin syndrome?**

Agitation, anxiety, altered mental status, ataxia, diaphoresis, incoordination, sinus tachycardia, hyperthermia, shivering, tremor, hyperreflexia, myoclonus, muscular rigidity, and diarrhea.

○ **What are potential pharmacological treatments for the serotonin syndrome?**

Serotonin antagonists, such as methysergide and cyproheptadine. Benzodiazepines and propranolol have also been successfully employed.

○ **A patient ingests a toxic quantity of an MAOI inhibitor and is in a hyperadrenergic state with a blood pressure of 240/160. What is the appropriate treatment?**

Short-acting antihypertensives, such as phentolamine and nitroprusside, should be employed because the patient may soon develop refractory hypotension.

○ **What are the major pharmacological effects of neuroleptics?**

Blockade of dopamine, α-adrenergic, muscarinic, and histamine receptors.

○ **What findings occur with neuroleptic malignant syndrome?**

Altered mental status, muscular rigidity, autonomic instability, hyperthermia, and rhabdomyolysis.

○ **What are the pharmacological effects of barbiturates and benzodiazepines?**

Both enhance chloride influx through the GABA receptor associated chloride channel. Benzodiazepines increase the frequency of channel opening, whereas barbiturates increase the duration of channel opening.

○ **Alkalization of the urine is beneficial in the management of what barbiturates?**

Long-acting barbiturates such as phenobarbital.

○ **What is the pharmacological basis of the anticonvulsant effect of phenytoin?**

Sodium channel blockade. Phenytoin causes an increasing efflux or a decreasing influx of sodium ions across cell membranes in the motor cortex during generation of a nerve impulse.

○ **What are the signs and symptoms of phenytoin toxicity?**

Seizure, heart blocks, bradyarrhythmias, tachyarrhythmias, hypotension, and coma. All dangerous cardiovascular complications of phenytoin OD result from parenteral administration. High levels after PO doses do not cause such signs in a stable patient.

○ **What is the treatment for a phenytoin overdose?**

Systemic support, charcoal, atropine for bradyarrhythmias, and phenobarbital, 20 mg/kg IV, for seizures.

○ **What is the treatment for an opiate overdose?**

Naloxone, 0.4 to 2.0 mg in an adult and 0.01 mg/kg in a child. Naloxone duration of action is about 1 hour. Higher doses and continuous infusion may be required.

○ **What herbal remedies are associated with CNS stimulation?**

Guarance, ma huang, St. John wart, yohimbe, and ginseng.

○ **What four mechanisms induce tricyclic toxicity?**

1. Anticholinergic atropine-like effects secondary to competitive antagonism of acetylcholine
2. Reuptake blockage of norepinephrine
3. A quinidine-like action on the myocardium
4. An α-blocking action

○ **What is the most common neurologic complication of IV drug abuse?**

Nontraumatic mononeuritis (i.e., painless weakness 2–3 hours after injection).

ANTIBIOTICS

○ **Name the four potential adverse effects that can happen with antibiotics.**

Allergic, toxic, idiosyncratic, and changes to the normal body flora.

○ **What is the most common overgrowth of bacteria as a result of antibiotic use?**

The superinfection of *Clostridium difficile*, which is the causative agent of pseudomembranous colitis.

○ **Which laboratory test is the most helpful in determining the proper use of an antibiotic?**

The culture and sensitivity test. This will give you the mean inhibitory concentration for the bacteria, thus narrowing down your choices of antibiotics.

○ **What is the action of antibiotics such as penicillin, cephalosporin, and vancomycin?**

They all work by inhibiting cell wall synthesis of the bacteria.

○ **What is a potentially fatal reaction from penicillin?**

Hypersensitivity reaction.

○ **Name some other common adverse reactions with penicillin use.**

Urticaria, GI intolerance, and skin rashes (usually 72 hours or later).

○ **What are the four syndromes of penicillamine-induced lung toxicity?**

Chronic pneumonitis, hypersensitivity lung disease, bronchiolitis obliterans, and pulmonary renal syndrome.

○ **Which generation cephalosporin can be used to penetrate the CNS?**

Third generation. These are typically used for treatment of infections such as meningitis.

○ **What is the cross reactivity of cephalosporin's in relation to penicillin?**

7% to 18%, depending on the study.

○ **A 73-year-old female with a history of atrial fibrillation and on chronic warfarin therapy is diagnosed with a mild cellulitis of her forearm. You would like to prescribe her a first-generation cephalosporin as the first-line treatment. Is this a good choice for this patient?**

No. Cephalosporins can have an antivitamin K effect. Given that this patient is on chronic warfarin therapy, this may adversely affect her INR and bleeding rate. Your best bet is to choose another antibiotic.

○ **Name some adverse effects of using vancomycin.**

Ototoxicity—tinnitus, hightone deafness, hearing loss, and deafness.

○ **Which class of antibiotics acts by gaining entry into the cells and binds to intracellular proteins?**

Protein synthesis inhibitors, which include aminoglycosides, tetracyclines, macrolides, clindamycin, streptogramins, and chloramphenicol.

○ **Name three potential side effects of aminoglycosides.**

Ototoxicity, nephrotoxicity, and neuromuscular toxicity.

○ **When administering tetracycline, how is the medication to be taken to ensure proper absorption?**

They must be taken on an empty stomach to maximize absorption.

○ **A 15-year-old male adolescent has been diagnosed with acne. One of the possible treatment options is the use of tetracycline. Would this be a good choice for this type of patient?**

No. Tetracycline can cause staining of the teeth, retardation of bone growth, and photosensitivity and should be avoided in children as well as pregnant patients.

○ **Mnemonic for erythromycin for the drug of choice in these bacteria: Legionnaires Camp on My Border**
(*Legionella, Campylobacter, Mycoplasma, Bordetella*).

○ **What is the one bacteria that chloramphenicol is not sensitive in eradicating?**

Pseudomonas aeruginosa.

○ **What is gray baby syndrome?**

It is a fatal syndrome by which infants cannot conjugate chloramphenicol. The antibiotic absorbs into the cerebrospinal fluid. The infants will get abdominal distention, vomiting, cyanosis, hypothermia, decreased respiration, and vasomotor collapse.

○ **Which antibiotic has been listed as the most susceptible in contracting *Clostridium difficile* superinfections?**

Clindamycin.

○ **What is the effect of macrolide antibiotics (erythromycin, clarithromycin) on mucous hypersecretion?**

Some macrolide antibiotics have the ability to down/regulate mucous secretion by an unknown mechanism. This is thought to be because of an anti-inflammatory activity.

○   **Why are quinolones contraindicated in young adults and children?**

Quinolones are contraindicated because they can suppress the epiphyseal plate and cartilage formation in young adults. In all patients, quinolones can cause tendon rupture, most notably Achilles tendon ruptures.

○   **What are the possible side effects?**

Quinolones are contraindicated because they can suppress the epiphyseal plate and cartilage formation in young adults. In all patients, quinolones can cause tendon rupture, most notably Achilles tendon ruptures.

○   **How do quinolones work?**

They inhibit DNA gyrase synthesis, which is responsible for DNA replication of bacteria.

○   **Which bacteria do quinolones effectively kill?**

They are broad-spectrum killers (gram-negative mostly) and most effective in treating respiratory, bone and joint, urinary tract, and prostatitis. Some are effective in treating *Pseudomonas aeruginosa.*

○   **What is the mechanism of action of isoniazid?**

It is a simple inhibitor of mycolic acids, which are responsible for the formation of bacterial cell wall envelopes.

○   **What two side effects are causes of isoniazid?**

Hepatotoxicity and peripheral neuropathy. Both can be reversed by stopping the drug.

○   **What is the antidote for isoniazid-induced seizures?**

Pyridoxine.

○   **What is a serious side effect of rifampin?**

Hepatotoxicity. LFTs need to be monitored while patient is on either rifampin or isoniazid. Rifampin will also turn the urine and secretions orange while on the medication.

○   **What is the drug of choice for the treatment of leprosy?**

Dapsone.

○   **Fungal infections in general are more difficult to eradicate than bacterial infections. How do drugs like amphotericin B and nystatin function?**

They act by binding to ergosterol, which is the principal sterol in fungus.

○   **How can nystatin be taken?**

It is limited to topical applications and oral liquids. Systemic nystatin is too toxic and therefore not used.

○   **What is the most serious and most common toxicity of amphotericin B?**

Nephrotoxicity.

○ **Why do patients with tinea infections that require griseofulvin need to take such a prolonged course of the medication?**

These infections must have new skin, hair, and nails that are new—keratin-containing griseofulvin. This usually takes several weeks to accomplish.

○ **What is the drug of choice for the treatment of trematodes (flukes)?**

Praziquantel.

○ **Name three drugs that can be used for the treatment of nematodes (roundworms).**

Albendazole, mebendazole, and pyrantel. Filarial infections must be treated with Ivermectin or diethylcarbamazine.

○ **What is the mechanism of action of albendazole and mebendazole?**

They inhibit tubulin polymerization in worms, which prevents replication.

○ **What is the treatment for lymphatic filariasis?**

Diethylcarbamazine.

○ **What are the three mechanisms of controlling viral illnesses?**

Vaccination, chemotherapy, and stimulation of the hosts natural resistance mechanisms.

○ **What is the function of reverse transcriptase inhibitors?**

All three types (nucleoside, nonnucleoside, and nucleotide) inhibit the formation of viral DNA from RNA by reverse transcriptase.

○ **Protease inhibitors are commonly used in the treatment and suppression of HIV. How do these medications work?**

They interfere with the production of viral proteins, thus preventing replication of new viral particles.

○ **What is the most effective treatment for HIV?**

The triple drug therapy (or cocktail) is the use of two reverse transcriptase inhibitors, and a protease inhibitor.

○ **What is the most effective prevention method for influenza?**

Vaccination.

○ **Which type of influenza does amantadine work effectively against?**

Influenza A.

○ **Which class of drugs is effective in reducing the length of both influenza A and B?**

Neuraminidase inhibitors. They are effective if the medication can be started within 30 hours of onset of symptoms of flu.

○ **Which antiviral is effective in the treatment of respiratory syncytial virus (RSV)?**

Ribavirin.

○ **How is ribavirin administered?**

By aerosol form.

○ **What is the treatment of choice for *trichomoniasis* and *giardiasis*?**

Metronidazole.

○ **Name some common side effects of metronidazole.**

Nausea, vomiting, and diarrhea. It will also cause your secretions to turn dark or red-brown in color. Some patients will get a metallic taste.

○ **Metronidazole, when mixed with alcohol, will cause a disulfiram-like reaction to occur. What are some symptoms that you should look for in this scenario?**

Abdominal cramping, flushing, vomiting, and headache.

○ **What is the one drug that has shown resistance in treating plasmodium falciparum?**

Chloroquine.

○ **Which antiprotozoal drug must be avoided in patients with G6PD deficiency?**

Primaquine, which can cause hemolytic anemia.

○ **Chloroquine is a commonly prescribed drug for the treatment of malaria. What are two ophthalmologic side effects of the drug that need to be monitored?**

Corneal deposits containing melanin can develop. This can lead to blindness.

○ **What is the main goal of most anticancer drugs?**

They are either cytotoxic drugs, which will block cell replication, or they are drugs, which act on hormonal-sensitive tumors.

○ **Patients undergoing chemotherapy are at risk for bleeding and infections. Why?**

The chemotherapeutic agents' most serious side effect is bone-marrow toxicity. This will cause a drop in the production of all blood products including white cells and platelets.

○ **What are the main gastrointestinal side effects of chemotherapy?**

Nausea and vomiting, which is thought to be a centrally acting effect.

○ **Some chemotherapeutic agents can have cardiotoxicity. Name some possible cardiac effects from these drugs.**

Patients can develop arrhythmias, decreased ventricular function (cardiomyopathy), and focal necrosis of tissue.

○ **Why does hair loss occur so frequently in chemotherapy?**

Most chemotherapeutic agents block the telophase stage of hair production, thus causing a stoppage of hair growth. This will cause hair death. Stopping the chemo will reverse this side effect.

Common chemotherapeutic agents and their serious side effects:

Drug	Side Effect
Cisplatin	Renal tubular damage
Cyclophosphamide	Hemorrhagic cystitis
Doxorubicin/daunorubicin	Cardiotoxicity
Bleomycin	Pulmonary fibrosis
Vincristine	Central nervous system toxicity
Methotrexate	Renal tubular damage

○ **A 66-year-old female patient is currently under treatment for malignant myeloma. Her calcium is measured at 19 mg/dL and she is showing signs of hypercalcemia on examination. What treatment can be given to help lower the calcium level?**

Bisphosphonates, creating the volume status of the patient to be euvolemic are the two initial goals. An additional therapy for life-threatening hypercalcemia is plicamycin.

○ **How do drugs such as Tamoxifen and toremifene act on breast cancer cells?**

They are competitive antagonists of estrogen receptors.

○ **An acute chest pain syndrome can occur with which chemotherapeutic agents?**

Methotrexate and bleomycin.

○ **What are four distinct presentations of bleomycin lung toxicity?**

Chronic pulmonary fibrosis, hypersensitivity lung reaction, acute pneumonitis, and acute chest pain syndrome.

○ **What are the risk factors for methotrexate (MTX) pulmonary toxicity?**

Primary biliary cirrhosis, frequency of administration, adrenalectomy, tapering of corticosteroid therapy, and use in multidrug regimens.

○ **What drug will produce hilar and mediastinal adenopathy as a toxic reaction?**

Methotrexate.

ENDOCRINE SYSTEM

○ **What is the main glucocorticoid and mineralocorticoid produced by the adrenal gland?**

Glucocorticoid—hydrocortisone (cortisol)
Mineralocorticoid—aldosterone

○ **What is the function of glucocorticoids?**

They promote the catabolism of proteins and gluconeogenesis.

○ **Why is there an increased risk of infection for those patients on steroids?**

Glucocorticoids inhibit inflammatory and immunologic responses, which make them more susceptible to infection.

○ **What is a potential long-term complication for chronic glucocorticoid use?**

Osteoporosis.

○ **Where does the primary source of estradiol originate?**

From the ovary.

○ **What are the most common side effects of estrogen use?**

Nausea and vomiting.

○ **Which antiestrogen is used to stimulate ovarian function for the purpose of treating infertility?**

Clomiphene.

○ **What are the most common side effects when using progestins?**

Weight gain, edema, and depression. More serious problems are with the hematologic system. Increased clotting can occur; thrombophlebitis and pulmonary embolus are serious adverse effects of progestins.

○ **Progestin alone used in contraceptives can cause what main side effect?**

Irregular uterine bleeding.

○ **The main androgen in the body is testosterone. What are some of the effects that androgens cause in the body?**

Virilization of women, including deepening of voice, acne, growth of facial hair, and excessive muscle development.

○ **What is the treatment of choice for hypothyroidism?**

Levothyroxine.

○ **Name two medications that inhibit thyroid synthesis.**

Propylthiouracil and methimazole.

○ **What is the most common side effect of insulin?**

Hypoglycemia.

○ **What is the treatment for the crystallization of tissue from repetitive use of insulin at the same site of skin?**

Injections of glucagon to the site will reverse the problem.

○ **What is the mechanism of sulfonylureas in the treatment of diabetes?**

They act to stimulate the cells of the pancreas.

○ **A 65-year-old male patient has a history of diabetes for which he takes metformin. He is having an MI and will be in need of a cardiac catheterization. Is there anything special that this patient needs before the cath?**

Yes. The metformin needs to be stopped prior to the cath as the dye in combination with the metformin can impair renal function.

○ **Describe which histamine receptors act on different systems of the body.**

H_1 receptors act on intestinal and smooth muscle whereas the H_2 receptors control gastric secretions.

○ **What are H_1 antagonists used to treat?**

They are commonly used to treat allergic rhinitis, motion sickness, and in some cases to help induce sleep.

RESPIRATORY SYSTEM

○ **What is the main delivery system for β-agonists for respiratory diseases?**

Inhalation by either aerosol nebulizer or metered dose inhaler.

○ **What is the inhaled drug of choice for the treatment of COPD?**

Ipratropium.

○ **Is cromolyn useful in the treatment of acute asthma attacks?**

No.

○ **True/False: β-adrenergic antagonists in massive overdose may cause severe bronchospasm in normal individuals.**

False.

○ **What conditions or commonly used medications result in an increase in serum theophylline concentration?**

Cimetidine, macrolides, quinolones, verapamil, fever, congestive heart failure, and liver failure.

○ **What drugs, activities, and cooking habits are associated with an increased clearance of theophylline (decreasing the theophylline level)?**

Phenytoin, phenobarbital, cigarette smoking, and charcoal barbecuing.

○ **What is the appropriate initial treatment of theophylline-induced seizures?**

Benzodiazepines and barbiturates. Theophylline-induced seizures warrant hemodialysis or charcoal hemoperfusion.

○ **What is the treatment of theophylline-induced hypotension?**

Fluid administration and β-blockers. Theophylline-induced cardiovascular instability is secondary to β-agonist effects. Therefore, β-blockers can be beneficial in the treatment of arrhythmias and hypotension.

GASTROINTESTINAL SYSTEM

○ **Of all the H2-blockers used for gastrointestinal complaints, which one has the most potential side effects and why?**

Cimetidine because it binds to cytochrome P-450.

○ **What instructions do you need to give patients that you prescribe sucralfate and why?**

They must take on an empty stomach because the drug binds to protein.

○ **What are the two major types of drugs used to treat constipation?**

There are bulk-forming agents, which absorb water and soften the stool, and the second is the cathartics and stimulants, which increase water and electrolytes in the stool to increase bowel motility.

Two other types are saline salts to draw water into the colon, and docusate, which absorbs into stool to soften.

○ **Which drugs are utilized in the treatment of Crohn disease?**

Sulfasalazine, which is metabolized into 5-ASA and sulfapyridine.

MUSCULOSKELETAL SYSTEM

○ **What is the main mechanism of nonsteroidal anti-inflammatory (NSAIDs)?**

They act by inhibiting prostaglandin synthesis.

○ **What are the most common side effects associated with NSAIDs?**

GI upset, bleeding, oliguria, fluid retention, renal insufficiency, decreased sodium excretion, and renal failure. They can also prolong bleeding times.

○ **What is the only nonreversible COX inhibitor?**

Aspirin.

○ **Why are children not to be given aspirin?**

Aspirin can cause Reyes syndrome to occur.

○ **What are some of the characteristics associated with Reyes syndrome?**

CNS damage, liver injury, and hypoglycemia.

○ **What is the incidence of aspirin-induced bronchospasm in patients with nasal polyps?**

Up to 75%.

○ **True/False: In aspirin-induced bronchospasm, there can be cross-reactivity with nonsteroidal anti-inflammatory drugs.**

True.

○ **What is the major side effect associated with the inhalation of N-acetylcysteine?**

Cough and bronchospasm, most likely caused by irritation from the low pH (2.2) of the aerosol solution.

○ **Which acid–base disturbance is typical for salicylate poisoning?**

Mixed respiratory alkalosis, secondary to central respiratory center stimulation, and metabolic acidosis, secondary to uncoupling of oxidative phosphorylation.

○ **What order are the kinetics of elimination for an ASA overdose?**

Zero-order elimination with hepatic enzymatic clearance saturated and renal clearance becoming important.

○ **What is the "magic number" for the dose of a nonenteric-coated ASA that must be exceeded to cause toxicity (mg/kg)?**

150 mg/kg.

○ **What dose of ASA will cause mild to moderate toxicity?**

200 to 300 mg/kg. Greater than 500 mg/kg is potentially lethal.

○ **Is hemodialysis used to treat salicylate toxicity?**

Yes. For severely poisoned patients, that is, coma, ARDS, cardiac toxicity, serum levels > 100 mg/dL, and for patients who are unresponsive to maximal therapy.

○ **What is the treatment for a prolonged prothrombin time in salicylate poisoning?**

Parenteral vitamin K administration. Salicylates inhibit vitamin K epoxide reductase in poisoning, resulting in an ability for the inactive vitamin K epoxide to be regenerated into the active vitamin K.

○ **Can a patient present with salicylate poisoning and a therapeutic level?**

Yes. Patients with chronic salicylate poisoning have a large Vd (volume of distribution) and thus may present with mental status changes and a therapeutic level.

○ **What is the X-ray finding in a patient with salicylate toxicity?**

Noncardiogenic pulmonary edema.

○ **Describe the effects of salicylate poisoning on the central nervous system.**

Lethargy, confusion, seizures, and respiratory arrest.

○ **Salicylate levels should ideally be checked how long after an ingestion?**

6 hours.

○ **What is the minimum toxic dose of salicylates?**

150 mg/kg.

○ **What salicylate level, measured 6 hours after ingestion, is associated with toxicity?**

45 mg/dL.

○ **What acetaminophen level, measured 4 hours after ingestion, is associated with toxicity?**

150 /g/mL.

○ **What are the signs of salicylate poisoning?**

Hyperventilation, hyperthermia, mental status change, nausea, vomiting, abdominal pain, dehydration, diaphoresis, ketonuria, metabolic acidosis, and respiratory alkalosis.

○ **A child presents with lethargy, seizures, and hypoglycemia. He has had viral syndrome symptoms for several days. Mom states she has only been giving him aspirin. What two disorders should be considered?**

Reye syndrome and salicylate intoxication.

○ **When does acetaminophen become toxic?**

When there is no glutathione to detoxify its toxic intermediate.

○ **Would you like to have four Aces?**

Of course! So check ACEtaminophen levels 4 hours after ingestion.

○ **Which type of acid–base disturbance initially occurs with a salicylate overdose?**

Respiratory alkalosis. Approximately 12 hours later, an anion gap metabolic acidosis or mixed acid–base picture may occur.

○ **Is hyperglycemia or is hypoglycemia expected with a salicylate overdose?**

Expect either hyperglycemia or hypoglycemia.

○ **What are the common signs and symptoms of chronic salicylism?**

Fever, tachypnea, CNS alterations, acid–base abnormalities, electrolyte abnormalities, chronic pain, ketonuria, and noncardiogenic pulmonary edema.

○ **A patient presents with an acute salicylate ingestion. What symptoms are expected with a mild, moderate, and severe overdose?**

Mild: Lethargy, vomiting, hyperventilation, and hyperthermia

Moderate: Severe hyperventilation and compensated metabolic acidosis

Severe: Coma, seizures, and uncompensated metabolic acidosis

○ **What is the treatment for a salicylate overdose?**

Decontaminate, lavage and charcoal, replace fluids, supplement with potassium, alkalize the urine with bicarbonate, cool for hyperthermia, administer glucose for hypoglycemia, place on oxygen and PEEP for pulmonary edema, prescribe multiple dose–activated charcoal, and initiate dialysis.

○ **What are the four stages of acetaminophen (APAP) poisoning?**

Stage I: 30 minutes to 24 hours, nausea and vomiting

Stage II: 24 to 48 hours, abdominal pain and elevated LFTs

Stage III: 72 to 96 hours, LFTs peak, nausea, and vomiting

Stage IV: 4 days to 2 weeks, resolution or fulminant hepatic failure

○ **Which measure of hepatic function is a better prognostic indicator in APAP overdose: liver enzyme levels or bilirubin level and prothrombin time?**

Bilirubin level and prothrombin time.

○ **An acutely intoxicated, nonalcoholic, otherwise healthy patient ingests APAP. Is this patient more or less likely to develop hepatotoxicity?**

Less likely. An acute ingestion of alcohol will tie up the P-450 system thereby inhibiting the formation of NAPQI. A chronic alcoholic has an induced P-450 system and will suffer greater APAP hepatic toxicity through increased NAPQI formation.

○ **What is the minimum dose of APAP that can cause hepatotoxicity in the child? In the adult?**

Child: 140 mg/kg. Adult: 140 mg/kg (or about 7.5 g).

○ **What is the antidote for APAP poisoning?**

Mucomist (NAC) 140 mg/kg followed by 17 doses of 70 mg/kg every 4 hours.

○ **According to the Rumack–Matthew nomogram, at what 4-hour APAP level should treatment be initiated?**

150 mg/mL.

○ **What is the treatment goal in the management of osteoporosis?**

First is the prevention of further bone loss, and second is the treatment of the osteoporosis already present.

○ **What is the mechanism of bisphosphonates?**

They inhibit osteoclast activity to prevent further bone destruction.

TOXICOLOGY AND OVERDOSE

○ **What is the most important treatment of all poisoned and toxic patients?**

Supportive care.

○ **What is the difference between methadone and heroin?**

Methadone causes analgesia, but does not cause euphoria. Habituation occurs with both drugs. The withdrawal symptoms of methadone are less severe, but they last longer.

○ **What is the treatment for cocaine toxicity?**

Acidify the urine and administer neuroleptics and phentolamine

Sedate with benzodiazepine

Treat unresponsive hypertension with nitroprusside or phentolamine

○ **Name some over-the-counter and "street" drugs that may produce delirium or acute psychosis.**

Salicylates, antihistamines, anticholinergics, alcohols, phencyclidine, LSD, mescaline, cocaine, and amphetamines.

○ **Hallucinogens affect what neurotransmitter?**

Serotonin.

○ **What is the treatment for a "bad trip" on LSD?**

Constantly remind patients that their perceptions are only distortions because of the drug. This is called "talking down." Chlorpromazine can be used IM for severe or uncontrollable anxiety.

○ **PCP most commonly affects what brain system?**

The vestibulocerebellar system. This has a positive analgesic effect. However, the side effects, including dizziness, muscular incoordination, nystagmus, delirium, anxiety, irritability, and catalepsy, weigh heavily against any positive effect.

○ **How is a patient with PCP overdose treated?**

Acidify the urine with cranberry juice or NH_4Cl, give a benzodiazepine, and restrain the patient.

○ **Which types of nystagmus are expected with a PCP overdose?**

Vertical, horizontal, and rotary. Vertical nystagmus is not common with other conditions/ingestions. The most common findings of a PCP overdose are hypertension, tachycardia, and nystagmus.

○ **How can the pesticide PCP enter the body?**

Through inhalation, skin, and ingestion.

○ **What is the clinical presentation of PCP intoxication?**

Irritation of skin, eyes, and upper respiratory tract, headache, vomiting, weakness, sweating, hyperthermia, tachycardia, tachypnea, convulsions, coma, pulmonary edema, cardiovascular collapse, and death.

○ **Describe the features of the three stages of PCP intoxication:**

Stage I: agitation or violence, normal vital signs

Stage II: tachycardia, hypertension, no response to pain

Stage III: unresponsive, depressed respirations, seizures, death

○ **Should the urine be acidified in the treatment of PCP intoxication?**

Although acidification of the urine is theoretically advantageous, clinical experience has not shown this to be efficacious. Let's call that a "no."

○ **What is a dystonic reaction?**

A very common side effect of neuroleptics seen in the emergency department. It involves muscle spasms of the tongue, face, neck, and back. Severe laryngospasm and extraocular muscle spasms may also occur. Patients may bite their tongues, leading to an inability to open the mouth, to tongue edema, or to hemorrhage.

○ **How do you treat dystonic reactions?**

Diphenhydramine (Benadryl), 25 to 50 mg IM or IV, or benztropine (Cogentin), 1 to 2 mg IV or PO. Remember that dystonias can recur acutely.

○ **A patient has ingested a phenothiazine and arrives hypotensive. What intervention(s) may be considered?**

IV crystalloid boluses usually suffice. Severe cases best managed with norepinephrine (Levophed) or metaraminol (Aramine). These pressors stimulate α-adrenergic receptors preferentially. β-Agonists, such as isoproterenol (Isuprel), are contraindicated because of risks of β-receptor–stimulated vasodilation.

○ **What are some common side effects of phenothiazine use?**

Malaise, hyperthermia, tachycardia, anticholinergic effects, and quinidine-like membrane stabilization. The most dangerous side effect is neuroleptic malignant syndrome.

○ **How should stable ventricular tachyarrhythmias associated with phenothiazine overdose be treated?**

Lidocaine and phenytoin.

○ **What factors and substances decrease theophylline metabolism and increase theophylline levels?**

Factors: Age greater than 50 years, prematurity, liver and renal disease, pulmonary edema, CHF, pneumonia, obesity, and viral illness in children.

Substances: Drugs that increase theophylline levels include cimetidine, erythromycin, allopurinol, troleandomycin, BCPs, and quinolone antibiotics.

In smokers, the theophylline half-life is decreased, which causes the levels of serum theophylline to decrease.

Phenobarbital, phenytoin, rifampin, carbamazepine, marijuana smoking, exposure to environmental pollutants, and the consumption of charcoal-broiled foods can also decrease serum theophylline levels.

○ **Can theophylline be dialyzed?**

Yes.

○ **Why should the use of atropine be considered in a pediatric patient prior to intubation?**

Many pediatric patients develop bradycardia associated with intubation, which can be prevented by pretreatment with atropine (0.01 mg/kg).

○ **What is a "Mickey Finn"?**

A mixture of alcohol and chloral hydrate.

○ **At what rate is alcohol metabolized in an acutely intoxicated person?**

About 20 mg/dL/h.

○ **What is the pharmacological treatment for alcohol withdrawal?**

Benzodiazepines or barbiturates.

○ **What is a normal osmolar gap?**

<10 mOsm.

○ **What is the toxic metabolic end product in methanol poisoning?**

Formic acid.

○ **What cofactor is required to convert formic acid to carbon dioxide and water?**

Folate. Leucovorin, folinic acid, the active form of folate, is preferentially administered at 1 mg/kg. Folate may be substituted at the same dose if leucovorin is not available.

○ **Is sodium bicarbonate (NaHCO$_3$) beneficial in the management of methanol poisoning?**

Yes. In animal models, maintenance of a normal pH through bicarbonate administration decreased toxicity, including visual impairment.

○ **What methanol level mandates dialysis?**

50 mg/dL. Other indications include visual impairment, severe metabolic acidosis, and ingestion of greater than 30 cc.

○ **What cofactors are administered to a patient with ethylene glycol poisoning?**

Thiamine and pyridoxine. These cofactors will aid in transforming glyoxylic acid to nontoxic metabolites. Both are administered intravenously in 100-mg increments.

○ **Name the three clinical phases of ethylene glycol poisoning:**

Stage I: Neurological symptomatology (i.e., inebriation)
Stage II: Metabolic acidosis and cardiovascular instability
Stage III: Renal failure

○ **When should dialysis be initiated for an ethylene glycol poisoning case?**

When the serum level is >25 mg/dL, or when renal insufficiency or severe metabolic acidosis occurs.

○ **What is the toxic dose of naloxone?**

None. Narcan is a safe drug and may be given in large quantities. The usual adult dosage is 2 mg IV; the usual pediatric dose is 0.01 mg/kg. Narcan may precipitate acute withdrawal and may therefore be titrated to effect.

○ **What syndrome is associated with Jimson Weed?**

Anticholinergic poisoning.

○ **What are absolute indications for hemodialysis or hemoperfusion in theophylline toxicity?**

Seizures or arrhythmias that are unresponsive to conventional therapy—a theophylline level >100 µg/mg in an acute overdose or 50 µg/mg in a chronic overdose.

○ **What are the four stages of iron poisoning?**

Stage I (0–6 hours): Abdominal pain, nausea, vomiting, and diarrhea secondary to the corrosive effects of iron. In more severe cases, hematemesis, hypotension and altered mental status.

Stage II (6–24 hours): Quiescent period during which iron is absorbed (in severe poisoning, a latent period may be absent).

Stage III: (12–24 hours): GI hemorrhage, shock, metabolic acidosis, heart failure, CV collapse, coma, seizures, coagulopathy, hepatic, and renal failure.

Stage IV: (4–6 weeks postingestion): Gastric outlet or small bowel obstruction secondary to scarring.

○ **What dose of iron is expected to produce clinical toxicity?**

20 mg/kg of <u>elemental</u> iron. For example, a toddler ingests 10 tablets of 324 mg ferrous sulfate, that is, 20% <u>elemental</u> iron; this equals 648 mg of elemental iron. The dose would be toxic to a 20-kg child at 32.4 mg/kg.

○ **What 4-hour iron level is generally considered toxic?**

300 to 350 µg/dL.

○ **What are the indications for deferoxamine therapy?**

All symptomatic patients exhibiting more than merely transient symptomatology.

Patients with lethargy, significant abdominal pain, hypotension, mental status changes, hypovolemia, or metabolic acidosis.

Patients with a positive KUB.

Any symptomatic patient with a level greater than 300 mg/dL.

○ **What oral chelator reduces iron absorption in animal model studies?**

Magnesium hydroxide or milk of magnesia.

○ **What historical disclosure warrants an evaluation after a hydrocarbon ingestion?**

Coughing. Any patient who coughs after ingesting a hydrocarbon has the potential for developing chemical pneumonitis.

○ **At what point can a patient who has ingested a hydrocarbon be safely discharged?**

After 6 hours, asymptomatic patients, with a normal chest X-ray and pulse oxygen, may be discharged to home.

○ **Chronic solvent abusers develop what metabolic complication?**

Renal tubular acidosis.

○ **Methylene chloride is metabolized to which toxin?**

Carbon monoxide.

○ **A 2-year-old child is asymptomatic after ingestion of a button battery. A KUB reveals the foreign body in his stomach. What is the disposition for this patient?**

Discharge to home. If the battery is lodged in the esophagus, an endoscopy must be performed immediately. Otherwise, reassure the patient's parents and instruct them to check their son's stools.

○ **What is the potent ingredient in Sarin?**

An organophosphate.

○ **What enzyme is inhibited by organophosphates?**

Acetylcholinesterase.

○ **How do organophosphates enter the body?**

They can be inhaled, ingested, or absorbed through the skin.

○ **What are the signs and symptoms of organophosphate poisoning?**

1 to 2 hours after poisoning patients may have GI upset, bronchospasm, miosis, bradycardia, excessive salivation and sweating, tremor, respiratory muscle paralysis, muscle fasciculations, agitation, seizures, coma and death. *Remember:* SLUDGE (**S**alivation, **L**acrimation, **U**rinary incontinence, **D**iarrhea, **G**astric upset, and **E**mesis).

○ **What antihypertensive agent may induce cyanide poisoning?**

Nitroprusside. One molecule of sodium nitroprusside contains five molecules of cyanide. To prevent toxicity with long duration infusions, sodium thiosulfate should be infused with sodium nitroprusside at a ratio of 10:1, thiosulfate to nitroprusside. Beware of thiocyanate toxicity!

○ **What is corn picker's pupil?**

Mydriasis from contact of the eye with Jimson weed. Jimson weed contains atropine, scopolamine, and hyoscyamine. It is a common plant and is available through health food stores.

○ **What is the most common cause of chronic heavy metal poisoning?**

Lead.

○ **Organophosphates are found in what kinds of compounds?**

Pesticides, flame retardants, and plasticizers.

○ **What is the rate-limiting step in the metabolism of ethanol?**

The conversion of ethanol to acetaldehyde by alcohol dehydrogenase.

○ **In a nondrinker, what blood ethanol level will cause confusion or stupor?**

180 to 300 mg/dL. The minimum blood alcohol level that can cause coma in a nondrinker is 300 mg/dL.

○ **In chronic alcohol users, alcohol withdrawal seizures occur approximately how many hours after cessation of heavy alcohol consumption?**

6 to 48 hours from the time of the last drink.

○ **Delirium tremens occurs how long after the cessation of alcohol consumption?**

On average, 3 to 5 days.

○ **Is there a role for phenytoin in the prevention or treatment of pure alcohol withdrawal seizures?**

No. Careful titration of benzodiazepines or phenobarbital should be used if necessary.

○ **True/False: Status epilepticus is commonly seen in alcohol withdrawal seizures.**

False. Status epilepticus is rare in alcohol withdrawal seizures and should suggest the need to find other causative pathology.

○ **What is the classic triad of Wernicke encephalopathy?**

Global confusion, oculomotor disturbances, and ataxia.

○ **What constellation of findings should prompt consideration of ethylene glycol toxicity?**

Ethanol-like intoxication (with no odor), large anion gap acidosis, increased osmolal gap, altered mental status leading to coma, and calcium oxalate crystals in the urine.

○ **In life-threatening theophylline overdose, what is definitive management?**

Charcoal hemoperfusion.

○ **True/False: Lithium has a narrow therapeutic toxic range.**

True. Therapeutic lithium levels are between 0.5 and 1.5 mEq/L and must be monitored closely.

○ **How is lithium eliminated after metabolism?**

By renal excretion.

○ **Name five herbal remedies associated with bleeding.**

Ginger, garlic, ginkgo, ginseng, and feverfew.

○ **If a patient has a sulfa or ASA allergy, can they be prescribed a COX II inhibitor?**
No.

○ **Which opiate combination is associated with arrhythmias, pulmonary edema, and hepatic failure?**
Propoxyphene N 100 plus APAP.

○ **Ethylene glycol is the alcohol that is present with hypocalcemia in one-third of the cases. Where does the calcium go?**

Oxalic acid is one of the metabolites of ethylene glycol. Calcium precipitates with oxalate and forms calcium oxalate crystals. The positive birefringent calcium oxalate dihydrate crystals are pathognomonic of this ingestion.

○ **Methanol intoxication causes early death as a result of:**

Respiratory arrest. The pathophysiology is unknown.

○ **Activated charcoal is not an effective treatment for which poisonous substances?**

Alcohols, ions, acids, and bases.

○ **Describe the clinical characteristics of carboxyhemoglobin concentrations, specifically for ranges of 10% to 70%.**

10%: Frontal headache
20%: Headache and dyspnea
30%: Nausea, dizziness, visual disturbance, fatigue, and impaired judgment
40%: Syncope and confusion
50%: Coma and seizures
60%: Respiratory failure and hypotension
70%: May be lethal

○ **What is the appropriate treatment for cyanide poisoning?**

Amyl nitrite and sodium nitrite IV, followed by sodium thiosulfate IV.

○ **What is the most common cause of chronic heavy metal poisoning?**

Lead. Arsenic is the most common cause of acute heavy metal poisoning.

○ **Cyanide binds to metals and disrupts the function of metal-containing enzymes. Which is the most important of these enzymes?**

Cytochrome A (also known as cytochrome oxidase) is necessary for aerobic metabolism.

○ **Why administer nitrites for cyanide poisoning?**

Nitrites form methemoglobin which strongly bind to cyanide.

○ **Why prescribe sodium thiosulfate for cyanide poisoning?**

Rhodanese, an intrinsic enzyme, transfers cyanide from its attachment to methemoglobin to sulfur, thereby forming thiocyanate. Thiocyanate is excreted. Sodium thiosulfate acts as a sulfur donor for this process.

○ **What is the antidote for ethylene glycol?**

Ethanol and dialysis.

○ **What is the antidote for gold?**

British anti-Lewisite (BAL).

○ **What are the potential complications of excess sodium bicarbonate?**

Cerebral acidosis, hypokalemia, hyperosmolality, and an increased binding of hemoglobin to oxygen.

○ **What are common entities in the differential diagnosis of pinpoint pupils?**

Narcotic overdose, clonidine overdose, and sedative hypnotic overdose, including alcohol, cerebellar pontine angle infarct, and subarachnoid hemorrhage.

○ **What mnemonic may assist in recalling the signs of life-threatening cholinergic poisoning?**
DUELS:

Diaphoresis
Urination
Eye changes (miosis)
Lacrimation
Salivation

○ **Name six common drugs that can cause hyperthermia:**
SANDS-PCP:

1. **S**alicylates
2. **A**nticholinergics
3. **N**euroleptics
4. **D**initrophenols
5. **S**ympathomimetics
6. **P**hencyclidine (**PCP**)

○ **What drugs cause an acetone odor on the breath?**

Ethanol, isopropanol, and salicylates. Ketosis is often accompanied by the same odor.

Substances or drugs that have an induced odor on breath:

Type of Odor on Breath	Drugs or Substances that Induce the Abnormality
Almonds	Cyanide, laetrile, and apricot pits (latter two contain amygdalin)
Garlic	DMSO, organophosphates, phosphorus, arsenic, arsine gas, and thallium
Peanut	Vacor (RH-787)
Pear	Chloral hydrate and paraldehyde
Rotten eggs	Hydrogen sulfide, mercaptans, and sewer gas

○ **What is the mnemonic for remembering drugs that are radiopaque?**

BAT CHIPS:

Barium
Antihistamines
Tricyclic antidepressants
Chloral hydrate, calcium, cocaine
Heavy metals
Iodine
Phenothiazine, potassium
Slow-release (enteric-coated)

○ **What three toxicologic emergencies require immediate dialysis?**

Ethylene glycol, methyl alcohol, and Amanita phalloides.

○ **What is the antidote for isoniazid?**

Pyridoxine.

○ **What drugs are commonly excreted by using alkaline diuresis?**

Long-acting barbiturates, INH, tricyclic antidepressants, salicylates, and less commonly, lithium.

○ **What are the signs and symptoms of a cyanide overdose?**

Dryness and burning in the throat, air hunger, and hyperventilation. If the individual is not removed from the toxic environment, loss of consciousness, seizures, bradycardia, and apnea will occur followed by asystole.

○ **What drugs can cause methemoglobinemia?**

Nitrites, local anesthetics, silver nitrate, amyl nitrite and nitrites, benzocaine, commercial marking crayons, aniline dyes, sulfonamides, and phenacetin.

○ **For which type of overdoses is atropine used?**

Organophosphate and carbamate.

○ **For which type of an overdose may the drug pralidoxime (2-PAM) be used?**

Organophosphate.

○ **Chronic bromism is treated with what drug?**

Sodium chloride.

○ **Isoniazid and *Gyromitra* mushroom poisoning is best treated with what drug?**

Pyridoxine.

○ **Name some side effects of alkalization of the urine.**

Hypernatremia and hyperosmolality.

○ **What is the antidote for phosphorus poisoning?**

Copper sulfate, 1% solution. Remove phosphorus within 30 minutes of exposure. Phosphorus may be identified by the formation of an insoluble black precipitate when swabbing with copper sulfate.

○ **What local anesthetics may cause anaphylaxis?**

The ester derivatives containing para-aminobenzoic acid (PABA) are known to stimulate IgE antibody formation and thereby cause anaphylaxis. Such anesthetics include procaine and tetracaine.

○ **What is the best diluent for treating the ingestion of solid lye?**

Milk.

○ **What is the most commonly abused volatile substance?**

Toluene.

○ **A patient presents with hypokalemia of 2.0, hyperchloremia, and acidosis. What is the most likely toxicologic cause?**

Chronic toluene abuse.

○ **A patient has been abusing nitrous oxide for a long time. What symptoms might be expected?**

Paresthesias and motor weakness may be present in chronic abusers. Such symptoms are often mistaken for symptoms of multiple sclerosis.

○ **A patient presents with belladonna alkaloid poisoning resulting in anticholinergic effects. Explain the dangers of treating this patient with physostigmine.**

Physostigmine acts to increase acetylcholine levels. In doing so, it can precipitate a cholinergic crisis resulting in heart block and asystole. As a result, it is recommended to reserve physostigmine for life-threatening anticholinergic complications.

○ **What is the ferric chloride test and what toxic ingestion does it detect?**

Add a few drops of 10% ferric chloride solution to a few drops of urine. A purple color indicates presence of salicylic acid. Ketones or phenothiazine can lead to falsely positive results.

○ **What is the treatment for chloral hydrate overdose?**

Hemodialysis and/or charcoal hemoperfusion will clear the active metabolite, trichloroethanol.

○ **What are the common effects of barbiturate overdose?**

Hypothermia, hyperventilation, vasodilation with hypotension, and negative inotropic effect on the myocardium. Clear vesicles and bullae may also be seen.

○ **What is the pediatric dose of naloxone?**

0.01 to 0.8 mg/kg; may need to repeat.

○ **What is the antidote for magnesium sulfate overdose?**

Calcium gluconate infusion.

○ **What are the effects of using ketamine in a pediatric patient?**

The child's eyes will be wide open with a glassy stare. He or she will have nystagmus, hyperemic flush, and hypersalivation. There will also be a slight rise in the heart rate. A very rare complication of ketamine use is laryngospasm. Hallucinations are a common side effect in children older than 10 years; as a consequence, ketamine should be restricted to use only in patients younger than 10 years.

Note: Ketamine may also cause sympathetic stimulation, which increases intracranial pressure and may cause random movements of the head and extremities. Thus, it is not a good sedative for children going to CT scan.

○ **You are having a hard time remembering which anesthetics are amides and which anesthetics are esters. What is a fairly easy way of telling these two classifications apart?**

With the exception of the suffix -caine, the anesthetics only in the amide classification include the letter I.

Amides esters

Lidocaine (Xylocaine)

Bupivacaine (Marcaine)

Mepivacaine (Carbocaine)

Procaine (Novocain)

Cocaine Tetracaine (Pontocaine)

Benzocaine

○ **Activated charcoal is not indicated for which types of overdose?**

Alcohol ingestion, electrolytes, heavy metals, lithium, hydrocarbons, and caustic ingestions.

○ **How should barbiturate poisoning be treated?**

Support, charcoal, alkalinization of the urine, charcoal hemoperfusion, or hemodialysis.

○ **A heroin addict presents with pulmonary edema. What is the best treatment?**

Naloxone, O_2, and ventilatory support (not diuretics).

○ **What alcohol poisoning is suggested by a plasma bicarbonate level of zero?**

Methanol. It also produces a large osmolar gap and a large anion gap. Methanol poisoning is treated with IV ethanol and hemodialysis.

○ **Positive birefringent calcium oxalate crystals in the urine are pathognomonic for poisoning with what substance?**

Ethylene glycol. The lethal dose of ethylene glycol is 100 mL.

○ **What are the signs and symptoms of ethylene glycol poisoning?**

Hallucinations, nystagmus, ataxia, papilledema, and a large anion gap.

○ **How should ethylene glycol poisoning be treated?**

This should be treated with gastric lavage, sodium bicarbonate, thiamine and pyridoxine, IV ethanol, and hemodialysis.

○ **A patient presents with ataxia, altered mental status, and sixth nerve palsy. What is your diagnosis?**

Wernicke encephalopathy.

○ **Alkalinization of urine will increase the excretion of which drugs?**

Cyclic antidepressants, salicylates, and long-acting barbiturates.

○ **What laboratory test can aid in the evaluation of a possible toxic iron ingestion?**

Total iron-binding capacity measured 3 to 5 hours after ingestion. If serum iron level is significantly less than the total iron-binding capacity, a toxic iron ingestion is less likely.

○ **What is the antidote for a toxic ingestion of iron?**

Deferoxamine chelates only free iron. It should be given if the iron level is greater than 350 µg/dL.

○ **Which type of hydrocarbons are most toxic?**

Substances with low viscosities (measured in Saybolt Seconds Universal [SSU]) are more toxic than compounds with high viscosities. Gasoline, kerosene, and paint thinner (all aliphatic hydrocarbons with SSUs < 60) are all more toxic than motor oil, tar, and petroleum jelly, which all have SSUs > 100.

Of the compounds with SSUs < 60, the most toxic are those that are not aliphatic, including benzene, toluene, xylene, and tetrachloroethylene.

○ **Where is the most reliable site for detecting central cyanosis?**

The tongue.

○ **What are two frequently observed organisms causing septic arthritis in drug addicts?**

Serratia and *Pseudomonas*. These are rare causes in nonaddicts.

○ **An alcoholic patient presents with complaints of abdominal pain and blurred vision. The patient is very photophobic, and blood gases reveal a metabolic acidosis. Diagnosis?**

Methanol poisoning. Patients may describe seeing something resembling a snowstorm.

○ **What is the lethal dose of methanol?**

30 mL. Formate levels in methanol poisoning are greatest in vitreous humor.

○ **What is clonidine mechanism of action?**

Clonidine is a centrally acting α-agonist. It leads to decreased sympathetic outflow and lowers catecholamine levels.

○ **What is a common complication of pancuronium?**

Tachycardia from its vagolytic action.

○ **Of the following anesthetics, which has the shortest duration of action—lidocaine, procaine, bupivacaine, or mepivacaine?**

Procaine.

○ **Hepatic failure is commonly associated with what anticonvulsant?**

Valproic acid.

○ **What are the end products of methanol, ethylene glycol, and isopropyl alcohol metabolism?**

Methanol: Formate
Ethylene glycol: Oxalate and formate
Isopropyl alcohol: Acetone

○ **Which type of alcohol ingestion is associated with hypocalcemia?**

Ethylene glycol.

○ **Which type of alcohol ingestion is associated with hemorrhagic pancreatitis?**

Methanol.

○ **Name some hydrocarbons that are considered to be the most toxic and have SSUs under 60.**

Aromatic hydrocarbons, halogenated hydrocarbons, mineral seal oil, kerosene, naphtha, turpentine, gasoline, and lighter fluid. Those considered less toxic (with SSUs over 100) include grease, diesel oil, mineral oil, petroleum jelly, paraffin wax, and tar.

○ **What drug is absolutely contraindicated when treating hydrocarbon poisoning?**

Epinephrine, as it sensitizes the myocardium and potentially leads to arrest.

○ **What drug is contraindicated in a glue-sniffing patient?**

Epinephrine. Like solvent abusers, these patients may be scared to death.

○ **What is a delayed complication of acid ingestion?**

Pyloric stricture.

○ **What is the difference between carbamates and organophosphates?**

Carbamates produce similar symptoms as organophosphates; however, the bonds in carbamate toxicity are reversible.

○ **A patient presents with miotic pupils, muscle fasciculations, diaphoresis, and diffuse oral and bronchial secretions. The patient has a garlic odor on his breath. What is your diagnosis?**

Organophosphate poisoning.

○ **What ECG changes may be associated with organophosphate poisoning?**

Prolongation of the QT interval, and ST-and-T wave abnormalities.

○ **What is the key laboratory finding in the diagnosis of organophosphate poisoning?**

Decreased RBC cholinesterase activity. The serum cholinesterase level (pseudocholinesterase) is more sensitive but less specific. RBC cholinesterase is regenerated slowly and can take months to approach normal levels.

○ **What is the treatment for organophosphate poisoning?**

Decontaminate, charcoal, atropine, and pralidoxime PRN.

○ **What signs and symptoms are expected after radiation exposures of 100 REM, 300 REM, 400 REM, and 2000 REM, less than 2 hours after exposure?**

100 REM: Nausea and vomiting

300 REM: Erythema

400 REM: Diarrhea

2000 REM: Seizures

○ **Psilocybin mushroom is associated with what?**

Hallucinations.

○ **How is pancuronium reversed?**

Atropine and neostigmine

○ **Of patients who die from CA overdose, what percent are awake and alert at the time of first prehospital contact?**

25%.

○ **What are the contraindications to TAC?**

Mucous membranes, burns, and large abrasions. TAC used on the tongue and mucous membranes has led to status epilepticus and patient death.

○ **What is the most reliable test for determining the severity of radiation poisoning 48 hours after exposure?**

Absolute lymphocyte counts. Presence or absence of GI symptoms following near lethal doses is a good indicator of mortality.

Lead poisoning (clinical features):

Learning disability

Encephalopathy

Anemia

Developmental

Poisoning (contraindications for charcoal use):

Cyanide

Hydrocarbon

Acid/alkali

Relative small compounds

Charged (iron, heavy metals)

Organophosphate

Alcohol

Lithium

○ **Match the poison with the antidote:**

1. **Acetaminophen**	a. Deferoxamine
2. Anticholinergics	b. Digoxin antibody
3. Arsenic	c. Dimercaptosuccinic acid or penicillamine
4. Carbon monoxide	d. Acetylcysteine (Mucomyst)
5. Digoxin	e. Oxygen
6. Iron	f. Atropine
7. Lead	g. Physostigmine
8. Mercury	h. Calcium EDTA or penicillamine
9. Methanol or ethylene glycol	i. Naloxone (Narcan)
10. Narcotics	j. Ethanol
11. Organophosphates	k. Penicillamine

Answers: (1) d, (2) g, (3) k, (4) e, (5) b, (6) a, (7) h, (8) c, (9) j, (10) i, and (11) f.

○ **What percentage of poisons have specific antidotes?**

5%.

○ **What agent usually causes anaphylactic reactions?**

Contrast media. Other causative agents include NSAIDs, thiamine, and codeine. Conversely, parenteral penicillin and hymenoptera stings are the most common causes of anaphylactic reactions. Anaphylactic reactions are IgE-mediated reactions in previously sensitized people, while anaphylactoid reactions are because of the direct release of mediators, including histamine and leukotriene.

○ **Describe the action and side effects of diazoxide:**

Action begins within 1 to 2 minutes and lasts up to 12 hours. Side effects may include nausea, vomiting, fluid retention, and hyperglycemia. Diazoxide is a direct arterial vasodilator. It is contraindicated in patients with aortic dissection or angina.

REFERENCES

Brunton L, Lazo J, Parker K. *Goodman and Gilman's the Pharmacological Basis of Therapeutics.* 11th ed. New York, NY: McGraw-Hill; 2006.

Fauci AS, Braunwald E, Kasper DL, et al., eds. *Harrison's Principles of Internal Medicine.* 17th ed. New York: McGraw-Hill; 2008.

McPhee SJ, Papadakis MA. *Current Medical Diagnosis and Treatment 2009.* New York, NY: McGraw-Hill; 2009.

Stringer J. *Basic Concepts in Pharmacology—A Students Survival Guide.* 3rd ed. New York, NY: McGraw-Hill; 2005.

INDEX

Note: Page numbers followed by *f*, indicates figure.

A

α-agonists, 438
A–a gradient, 80
ABCs approach, 7
Abdominal aortic aneurysm, 35, 403, 413
　indication for surgery for, 36
　X-ray study of, 35
Abdominal Compartment Syndrome, 435
Abdominal pain
　stimuli for, 158
Abdominal surgery, 408
ABI. *See* Ankle-brachial index
Abruption placentae, 226
Acalculous cholecystitis, 148
Acanthosis nigricans, 317
ACE inhibitors, 27, 29, 439–440
　and chronic cough, 444
　and heart failure, 441
Acetaminophen (APAP) poisoning, 467
Acetone odor, 475
Acetylcholine, 437
Achalasia, 141
Acid aspiration, 86
Acid/base disorders
　acid–base disturbance, 465–466
　metabolic acidoses, 185
　　increased anion gap, 186
　　treatment of, 187
　metabolic alkalosis, 187
　renal tubular acidosis
　　acid–base electrolyte abnormalities, 186–187
　　classification of, 186
　　mechanisms for, 186
　respiratory acidosis, 187–188
Acneiform lesions, 311–312
Acne rosacea, 312
Acoustic neuroma, 129, 130
Acromegaly, 109
ACS. *See* Abdominal Compartment Syndrome
Actinic keratosis, 313
Actinomycosis, 56
Activated charcoal, 474
Activities of daily living, 379
Acute abdominal pain, 160, 412
Acute adrenocortical insufficiency, 105
Acute anaphylactic shock, epinephrine for, 420
Acute aortic dissection, 35
Acute appendicitis, 393
Acute bowel obstruction, 412
Acute bronchitis
　causative agent of, 49
　and cigarette smokers, 49
　diagnosis of, 50
　diseases mimicking, 49
　symptoms of, 49
　treatment options for, 49
Acute cholecystitis, 147, 400, 413
Acute cor pulmonale, 80
Acute dyspnea, 80
Acute epiglottitis, treatment of choice for, 50
Acute gastritis, 145
Acute headaches, 270
Acute hemarthrosis, 250

Acute hematemesis, 157
Acute hypercapnia, 90
Acute hyperventilation, 91
Acute hypocapnia, 90
Acute iritis, 118
Acute ischemic stroke, 283, 283*f*
Acute liver failure, 152
Acute mesenteric ischemia, 159
　laboratory findings, 37
　source of, 37
Acute myocardial infarction (MI)
　angina pectoralis and prinzmetal angina,
　　difference between, 30
　arrhythmias with, 33
　aspirin reduced mortality from, 32
　cardiac rupture in, 31
　and cardiogenic shock, 32
　chest pain with, 32
　death related to, 32
　EKG interpretation, 22*f*, 23*f*
　myocardial deterioration following, 32
　papillary muscle dysfunction, 32
　with papillary muscle dysfunction, 42
　paroxysmal atrial fibrillation with, 33
　pericarditis following, 34
　PSVT treatment during, 31
　in pulmonary edema, 33
　with systolic ejection murmur, 31
　thrombolytic therapy for, 32
　treatment of, 34
　T waves invert in, 31
Acute narrow angle closure glaucoma, 123
Acute narrow angle glaucoma, 122
Acute necrotizing ulcerative gingivitis, 137
Acute optic neuritis, 125
Acute orchitis, 170
Acute otitis media, 129, 131, 376
Acute pancreatitis, 149–150, 159, 395–396, 413
Acute parotitis, 132
Acute prostatitis, 170–171
Acute renal failure, 176–177, 179
Acute respiratory distress syndrome, 85
Acute spinal cord injuries, 427
Acute stress disorder, 291, 302
Acute uncomplicated sinusitis, 139
Addison disease. *See* Chronic adrenocortical
　　insufficiency
Adenocarcinoma, 64, 65
Adenocarcinoma of colon, 405
Adenomatous polyps, 405
Adenomyosis, 195
Adenovirus pneumonia, 58
ADHD. *See* Attention-deficit hyperactivity disorder
Adjustment disorder, 293–294
Adjustment reactions, 306
ADLs. *See* Activities of daily living
Adrenal carcinoma, 397
Adrenal cortex, 105
Adrenal cortex hormones, 105
Adrenal crisis. *See* Acute adrenocortical insufficiency
Adrenal gland, diseases of, 105–108
Adrenal gland hormones, regulation of, 105
Adrenal insufficiency, 106

Adrenal medulla, 105
Adrenals glands, components of, 105
Adrenocortical insufficiency, 106
Adrenocortical insufficiency, acute and
　　chronic, 105
Adult acute sinusitis, 138
Adult airway, narrowest part of, 50
Adult Immunization Schedule, 380
Afferent pupillary defect, 126
AFP. *See* Alpha-fetoprotein
Age-related hearing loss, 381
Age-related macular degeneration, 118
Aging, 378–379
AIDS dementia, 267, 356
AIDS patients
　adverse effects of AZT in, 356
　CNS cryptococcal infection in, 354
　CNS lymphoma in, 355
　focal encephalitis in, 356
　gastrointestinal complaint in, 355
　immunizations for, 356
　malignancy associated with, 355
　opportunistic infection in, 354
　prophylactic regime for, 356
　retinitis in, 354
　visual acuity in, 355
AIDS-related oropharyngeal diseases, 137
Airway obstruction in trauma, 420
Albendazole, 459
Albuterol regimen for asthma, 68–69
Alcoholic liver disease, 152
Aldosterone, 105
Alkaline diuresis, 476
Alkalinization of urine, 479
Allergic bronchospasm, 49
Allergic rhinitis, 139
Alopecia areata, 314
Alpha-fetoprotein, 153, 174, 398
Alveolar and dead space ventilation, minute
　　ventilation related to, 89
Alveolar–arterial oxygen (A-ao$_2$) gradient, 88
Alveolar osteitis, 136
Alveolar ventilation, 90, 91
Alzheimer disease, 385
　manifestations of, 265
　medications for, 266
　pathologic features, 265
　risk factors for, 265
　treatment of, 447
　vs. vascular dementia, 266
Amaurosis fugax, 120, 281
Aminoglycosides, 457
Amiodarone, 442
Amniocentesis, 214
Amniotic fluid embolism, 227
Amphotericin B, 458
Ampicillin, 50, 55
Amputated extremity, transporting, 425
Amputation, 419
Anaerobic bacteria, antibiotics against, 55–56
Anaerobic lung abscess, 63
Anaerobic lung infection, 63
Anaerobic respiratory infection, 56

Anal fissure, 406
Anaphylactic reactions, 482
Anatomic dead space, 89
Anemia, 321–322
Angina pectoralis, 30
Angiodysplasia, 404
Angiotensin-converting enzyme inhibitor, 135
Animal bite infection, 336, 338
Ankle and foot, disorders of
   Achilles' tendon ruptures, 253
   ankle injuries, 252, 255*f*
   ankle sprains, 252
   anterior talofibular ligament injury, 252
   calcaneus fracture, 253
   cavus foot (pes cavus), 254
   Charcot joint, 254
   compartment syndrome, 253
   disrupted tarsal–metatarsal joint, 253
   distal tibial (medial malleolus) fractures, 254
   gout, 254
   hallucis valgus, 254
   injury to deltoid ligaments, 254
   Jones fracture, 253
   metatarsal fracture, 253
   Morton's foot, 254
   peroneal tendon subluxation, 252
   pes planus foot, 255
   plantar fasciitis, 254
   tarsal tunnel syndrome, 254
Ankle-brachial index, 37, 408
Ankylosing spondylitis, 247
Anorexia nervosa, 292–293
Antepartum corticosteroids in premature babies, 219
Anterior and posterior pituitary hormones, 108
Anterior cerebral artery stroke, 281
Anterior cord syndrome, 424
Anterior epistaxis, 138
Anterior hip dislocation, 247
Anterior hypopituitarism, 110
Anterior–posterior compression pelvic fracture, 248
Antiarrhythmic drugs, 15, 441–442
Antibiotic therapy, 456–460
   for anaerobic bacteria, 55–56
   uncomplicated pregnancy, 216
Anticancer drugs, 460
Anticholinergic poisoning, 439, 471
Anticholinergics therapy, 68, 438, 448
Anticoagulants, 216
Antiepileptic medications, 447
Antihypertensive therapy, 29
Antipsychotic drugs, 448
Antisocial personality disorder, 296–297
Antitussant, 62
Antiviral medications for viral pneumonia, 59
Anuria, 176
Anxiety disorders, 289–291
AOM. *See* Acute otitis media
Aortic aneurysms, 35–36
   abdominal. *See* Abdominal aortic aneurysm
   prognosis for, 37
   thoracic. *See* Thoracic aortic aneurysm
Aortic dissection
   acute proximal thoracic, 37
   prognosis of, 36
   site of occurrence, 36
   Stanford classification of, 36
   symptom of, 36
   treatment of, 36
   X-ray of patient with, 35
Aortic regurgitation, 39, 43–44

Aortic stenosis, 39–40, 42–43
Aortic valve, 418
APC. *See* Anterior–posterior compression
        pelvic fracture
Aperistalsis, 159
Aphthous ulcer, 137
Aphthous ulcers, 132
Appendicitis, 157, 412
ARDS. *See* Acute respiratory distress syndrome
ARF. *See* Acute renal failure
Arrhythmias, nonpharmacologic treatments for, 441
Arterial blood gas, 91
Arterial catheterization, complications from, 47
Arterial occlusive disease, artery affected by, 36
Arteriovenous malformations, 403
Asbestos exposure, malignancy associated with, 65
Asbestosis, 84
Ascites, 151
ASD. *See* Acute stress disorder; Atrial septal defect
Aseptic meningitis, 274
Aseptic necrosis, 248
Aspergillosis infection, 58, 329
Aspiration, 57
Aspiration pneumonitis, 57
Aspirin, 30, 32, 319, 464
Aspirin-induced bronchospasm, 465
Asthma, 49, 223
   bronchial, 68
   diagnosis of, 68
   pulmonary function test for, 68
   refractory, 70
   risk factors for, 67
   symptoms, 67
   treatment for, 68–70
Asymptomatic carotid bruit, 283
Asystole, differential diagnosis for, 15
Atelectasis, pleural effusions associated with, 76
Atopic dermatitis, 309
Atresia of bowel, 402
Atrial fibrillation
   cardiac arrhythmia, 16*f*
   causes of, 11, 12
   converted to sinus rhythm, 13
   EKG interpretation, 22*f*
   risk calculation score, 13
   risk of CVA in patients with, 13
   treatment of, 11, 13
Atrial flutter, 20*f*
   treatment of, 11
Atrial premature beats. *See* Premature atrial beats
Atrial septal defect
   murmur, 38
   symptoms of, 38
Atrial tachycardia
   with 2:1 conduction, 17*f*
   multifocal, 18*f*
Atrophy of palm, 243
Attention-deficit hyperactivity disorder, 291–292
Atypical mycobacterium, 341
Atypical pneumonia, 53
Auditory hallucination, 299
Augmentin, 55
Autistic disorders, 292
Autoimmune hepatitis, 151
Automatisms, 280
Autonomic nervous system, 437–439
AV blocks, 11–12, 14, 19*f*
   and inferior wall MIs, 15
   in perioperative period, 14
AVMs. *See* Arteriovenous malformations

Avoidant personality disorder, 297
Avulsion fractures, 250
AZT treatment of AIDS, 356

B
Babesia infection, 348
Back/spine, disorders of, 243–247
   ankylosing spondylitis, 247
   Cauda equina syndrome, 245
   cervical disk herniation, 244
   cervical flexion, 245
   chronic lower back pain, 243
   compression fractures, 243
   Down syndrome, 243
   hangman's fracture, 244
   Horner syndrome, 244
   Jefferson fracture, 244
   kyphosis, 246
   lumbar disk herniations, 244
   scoliosis, 246
   spinal stenosis, 246
   spinous process fractures, 245
   spondylolisthesis, 245, 245*f*
   spondylolysis, 244
   12th thoracic vertebrae, 247
Bacterial conjunctivitis, 118
Bacterial disease
   animal bite infection, 336, 338
   bacterial enterocolitis, 333
   botulism, 330
   brucellosis, 336
   cat-scratch disease, 336
   cellulitis, 336
   chancroid, 337
   Chlamydia trachomatis infections, 330–331
   coccidiomycosis, 341
   cutaneous abscesses, 336
   diphtheria, 331–332
   disseminated gonococcal infection, 332–333
   dog and cat bites, 336
   endocarditis in IV drug abusers, 337
   epizootic plague, 337
   gas gangrene, 336
   Giardia lamblia, 339
   gonococcal genital infections, 332
   gonorrhea, 332
   granuloma inguinale, 338, 341
   human plague, 337
   infectious diarrhea, 334
   leprosy, 342
   leptospirosis, 338
   lymphogranuloma venereum, 331
   pseudomonal infection, 336
   Pseudomonas aeruginosa infection, 338
   reactive arthritis, 338
   Reiter syndrome, 338
   rheumatic fever, 337
   salmonella enterocolitis, 333
   Salmonella infection, 333
   salmonellosis, 333
   shigella infection, 334
   strychnine, 335
   tetanus, 334–335
   tularemia, 335
   typhoid fever, 333
   vaginitis, 332
   Vibrio cholera outbreak, 331
   Vibrio parahaemolyticus, 339
   Weil syndrome, 338
   Yersinia sp., 337–338

Bacterial endocarditis, 46
Bacterial enterocolitis, 333
Bacterial infections, 316–317
Bacterial meningitis
    antibiotic treatment for, 273–274
    antibiotic treatment option for, 377–378
    causes of, 272–273
    complications associated with, 274
    and corticosteroids, 274
    CSF findings in, 273
    diagnosis of, 273
    incidence of, 377
    lumbar puncture for, 273
    in neonates, 377
    pathogens, 272
    prophylaxis indicated for, 274
    risk factors for, 273
    symptoms, 273
    vaccination for, 274
Bacterial parotitis, 135
Bacterial pneumonia, 52, 53
    and leukocytosis, 57
Bacterial sinusitis, 139
Bacterial vaginosis, 200–201
β-Adrenergic antagonists, 446
BAL. *See* British anti-Lewisite
Balloon valvuloplasty, indication for, 41
Ball-valve air trapping, 87
Barbiturates, 448–449, 455
Barlow maneuver, 249
Barrett esophagitis, 142
Bartholin gland abscess, 200
Basal body temperature (BBT) chart, biphasic
    curve on, 190
Basal cell carcinoma, 313–314
Basilar skull fracture, 417, 418, 423
BBB. *See* Blood brain barrier
β-blockers, 438–439
BCC. *See* Basal cell carcinoma
Beer potomania, 182
Bell palsy, 267
Benign esophageal neoplasm, 143
Benign gastric ulcers, 401
Benign gynecologic pelvic neoplasm, 194
Benign intraductal papilloma, 206
Benign positional vertigo, 128
Benign prostatic hyperplasia, 163
    first-line treatment of, 163
    surgical indications for, 163
    symptoms, 163
Benign salivary gland tumor, 392
Benign ulcerations, 146
Benzodiazepines, 448–449, 451, 452, 454,
    455, 464
Bereavement, 304
Berry aneurysms, 285
Beta-adrenergic agonists, 70
Beta-agonists, 69
Beta-blocker–induced bronchospasm, 70
Beta-blockers, 13, 29, 30
    and arrhythmias, 442
    and myocardial infarction, 31
Beta-blocking agents, 69
β-hCG levels and uncomplicated pregnancy,
    213–214
Bilateral mental fracture, 135
Bilateral nystagmus, 128
Bilateral sensory hearing loss, 130
Bile-stained emesis, 375
Biliary disease and dietary history, 148

Billroth I and II procedures, 390
Biophysical profile, 217
Bipolar disorder, 295–296
Bisphosphonates, 383
Black widow spider bite, 364
Bladder cancer, 172
Bladder rupture, 248, 436
Blast injury, 425
Bleeding peptic ulcer, 404
Bleeding ulcers, 146, 403
Bleomycin lung toxicity, 461
Blepharitis, 120
Blood brain barrier, 448
Blood donation, 326
Blood pressure, 28
Blood products and FFP, 422
"Blue bloater," 71
Blue dot sign, 168
Blunt chest trauma, 422
Blunt force thoracic trauma, 422
Blunt trauma, 420
Boerhaave syndrome, 144
    site of rupture in, 393
Bolus for dehydrated child, 390
Bone loss and osteoporosis, 209
Bone mineral density screening, 209
Bony articulations of elbow, 238
Borderline personality disorder, 297
Bornholm disease, 363
Botulism, 330
Boutonnière deformity, 240
Bowel obstruction
    and abdominal surgery, 412
    in children, 402
BPH. *See* Benign prostatic hyperplasia
BPP. *See* Biophysical profile
Bradycardia, 29
Brain abscesses, 394
Brain natriuretic peptide (BNP) levels, 82
Brain tumor in adults, 393
Breast abscess, 206
Breast cancer
    genetic markers, 207
    hematologic spread of, 410
    histologic type of, 207, 394
    prognosis in, 410
    prognostic indicator of, 208
    risk factors for, 207
    screening tool for, 207
    surgical treatment of, 207
Breast hyperplasia, 205
Breast infection, 206
Breast milk production, 208
Breathing, determinants of work of, 92
Breech presentation, 218
Brief psychotic disorder, 301
Bright red rectal bleeding. *See* Hematochezia
British anti-Lewisite, 475
Bronchial asthma, 68–69
Bronchiectasis, 70–71
Bronchiolitis, 374
    pathogen in, 50
    treatment for severe RSV documented, 50
Bronchodilators for COPD, 73
Bronchogenic carcinoma, 66, 429
Bronchopulmonary dysplasia, 374
Brown recluse spider, 312
Brown-Séquard syndrome, 429
Brucellosis, 336
Budd–Chiari syndrome, 36

Buerger disease, 393
Bulimia nervosa, 159, 293
Bullous myringitis, 130
Bullous pemphigoid, 311
BUN and creatinine, 216
Bupivacaine, 387
Burns of cornea, 121
Burn victim, fluid requirements for resuscitation
    of, 420
Bursitis, 237
BV. *See* Bacterial vaginosis
Bypass grafting
    revascularization with, 34
    vessel of preference in, 35

C

CABG. *See* Coronary artery bypass graft
Calcium channel blockers, 11, 13, 29, 30,
    440, 442
    poisoning, 445
Candida albicans, 310
Candidal disorders, 327–328
Carbon dioxide, 389
Carbon monoxide poisoning, 91, 428
Carboxyhemoglobin, 91, 474
Carbuncle, 316
Carcinoid syndrome, 155
Carcinoid tumors, 66, 155
Cardiac arrhythmia, 16–17, 16*f*, 17*f*
Cardiac catheterization with coronary
    angiography, 33
Cardiac cycle and nitrates, 440
Cardiac failure. *See* Congestive heart failure
Cardiac glycosides, 441
Cardiac output and PEEP, 92
Cardiac rupture, 31
Cardiac tamponade, pericardial effusion with, 37
Cardiogenic shock, 31
    and acute myocardial infarction, 32
Cardiomyopathies
    abnormality in 2D echocardiogram, 9, 9*f*
    dilated. *See* Dilated cardiomyopathies
    type of, 9
Cardiorespiratory collapse, 88
Cardiovascular disease, 47
Cardiovascular system, 216
    and norepinephrine, 438
Carotid massage, 12
Carpal tunnel syndrome, 239
Catatonia, 306
Cathepsin D level, 395
Cat-scratch disease, 336
Cauda equina syndrome, 245
Cavernous sinus thrombosis, 138
Cecal cancer, surgical treatment of, 405
Celiac disease, 154
Celiac sprue, 158
Cellulitis, 336, 405
Central cord syndrome, 424, 427, 429
Central facial palsy, 268
Central hypogonadism. *See* Gonadotropin
    deficiency
Central retinal artery occlusion, 122, 123
Central retinal vein occlusion, 117, 122
Central vertigo, 128
Cephalosporins, 50, 317, 456–457
Cerebral amebiasis, 342
Cerebral palsy, 267
Cervical cancer, 199
    and oral contraceptive use, 211

Cervical disk herniation, 244
Cervical flexion, 245
Cervical fractures, MCT of, 415
Cervical intraepithelial neoplasia, 199
Cervical vertebra, 98
Cervix
    disorders of, 198–199
    physical changes in, 216
Cesarean section, 228
CHADS₂ score, 13
Chagas disease, 141, 346, 347
Chalazion, 117, 120
Chancroid, 202, 337
Charcot triad, 148, 399
Chemotherapeutic agents, 460–461
CHF. See Congestive heart failure
Chicken pox, 315, 362
Chilblain. See Pernio
Childhood diarrhea, 159
Childhood nasal polyps, 73
Child maltreatment, 302–303
Child sexual abuse, 303
Chlamydial pneumonia, 56, 57
Chlamydial urethritis, 171
Chlamydia trachomatis, 203
Chlamydia trachomatis infections, 330–331
Chloral hydrate overdose, treatment of, 477
Chloramphenicol, 322
Chloroquine, 345, 460
Chocolate cysts, 193
Cholangitis, 149, 399
Cholecystectomy, 148
Cholecystitis, 148, 149, 398, 399
Choledocholithiasis, 149, 399
Cholelithiasis, 149, 399
Cholestatic injury, 151
Cholesteatoma, 132
Cholesterol stones, 399
Cholinergic poisoning, 475
Chondrosarcomas, 257
Chronic adrenocortical insufficiency, 105
Chronic aortic regurgitation, 43–44
Chronic bromism, 476
Chronic bronchitis, 71, 72
Chronic cough, 62
Chronic diabetic nephropathy, 180
Chronic gastritis, 145
Chronic heavy metal poisoning, 474
Chronic hiccups, 162
Chronic lower back pain, 243
Chronic pancreatitis, 149
Chronic pancreatitis and pleural effusions, 77
Chronic renal failure, 177, 180
Chronic sinusitis, 139
Cigarette smoking
    and acute bronchitis, 49
    and COPD, 72
    and lung cancer, 64–65, 66
Cimetidine, 464
CIN. See Cervical intraepithelial neoplasia
Cirrhosis, 153
    pleural effusions associated with, 76
Clavulanate, 55
Clay-shoveler fracture, 417
Clindamycin, 317
Clonidine, 479
Clonidine-induced hypotension, 445
Clonidine poisoning, 445–446
Clopidogrel, 443
Clostridium difficile colitis, 157

Clostridium tetani, 334
Clozapine, 451
Cluster headaches, 272
CNS cryptococcal infection, 354
Coagulation disorders, 322–324
Coarctation of aorta, 38
cocaine-induced MI, 445
Cocaine toxicity, 468
Coccidioidomycosis pneumonia, 58
Coccidiomycosis, 341
Cogwheel rigidity, 276
Cold agglutinins and pneumonia, 55
Colles fracture, 241, 241f
Colon cancer, 156
    right-sided vs. left-sided, 405
Colorado tick fever, 348
Colorectal cancer, 156, 161, 398, 405
Colostrum, 208
Colovesicular fistula, 403, 407
Combined oral contraceptives
    estrogen-mediated side effects of, 211
    progesterone-mediated side effects of, 211
Comedonal acne, 312
Commissurotomy, 41
Common cold, 62
Community-acquired pneumonia, 6, 321
    causes of, 52
    complications associated with, 53
    risk factors for, 52
    treatment of, 53
Compartment syndrome, 233–234, 250
Compensated shock, 418
Complete rectal prolapse, 406
Complex partial seizures, 280
Compression fractures, 243
Concussion, 285–286
Conduction disorders, 11–26
Conductive hearing loss, 127
Condyloma acuminatum, 199
Condylomata acuminata, 200, 315
Congenital abnormalities, 369
Congenital growth hormone (GH) deficiency, 111
Congenital heart disease, 38–44
Congenital hydrocele, 164
Congestive heart failure, 26–27, 34
    pleural effusions associated with, 76
Constipation, 156, 161
    treatment of, 464
Contact dermatitis, 309
Conversion disorder, 306
COPD, 71–73
    postoperative respiratory complications, 94
    treatment of, 463
CO poisoning, 87
Coral snake bite, 426
Corneal reflex, 417, 429
Corn picker's pupil, 472
Coronary artery, 35
Coronary artery bypass graft, 30
Coronary artery disease
    with myocardial ischemia, 12
    revascularization with bypass grafting, 34
Coronary artery disease, treatment of, 440
Coronary vasospasm, 440
Cor pulmonale, 82
Corpus luteum, 190
Cortical dementias, 266
Corticosteroids, 268
    and bacterial meningitis, 274
Cortisol, 105

Cotton wool spots, 119
Cough, 51, 444
Courvoisier law, 397
Courvoisier sign, 150
COX inhibitor, 464
"Crack belly." See Acute mesenteric ischemia
Cranial nerves, 127
CRAO. See Central retinal artery occlusion
CRF. See Chronic renal failure
Cribriform plate fractures, 138
Cricothyroidotomy, 433
Crohn disease, 154, 464
Croup, 134, 374–375
    cough of, 51
    diagnosis of, 50
    pathogens, 51
    symptoms of, 51
    treatment of, 51
Cryptococcal Antigen Lateral Flow Assay
    (CrAg LFA), 328
Cryptococcosis, 364
Cryptococcus infection, 328
Cryptorchidism, 164
Cryptosporidium parvum, 342
CSF leakage, 433
C-spine
    injuries, 416
    precautions, 421
    radiographic imaging of, 415–416
Cullen sign, 150, 395
Curettage, performance of, 196
Currant jelly sputum, 57
Cushing disease, 106
    and hypokalemia, 183
Cushing reflex, 422, 428
Cushing syndrome, 106–107
Cutaneous abscesses, 336
Cutis marmorata, 318
Cyanide
    poisoning, 472, 474
    toxicity, 28
Cyanoacrylate, 122
Cyanosis and pulmonary embolism, 92
Cyclic antidepressant overdose, 451, 452
Cysteine stones, 166
Cystic fibrosis
    diagnostic criteria for, 74
    immunological defects in, 74
    pathology in, 74
    pulmonary complications of, 75
    radiographic manifestations of, 74
    reproductive abnormalities in, 74
    respiratory pathogens in, 74
    triad of, 73
    vaccinations, 75
Cystitis, 169
Cytomegalovirus (CMV) infections, 351

D

Dacryocystitis, 118
DAE. See Dysbaric air embolism
Damage Control Surgery, 434
Danazol, 194
Dantrolene, 389
Dapsone, 458
Dawn phenomenon, 114
Decubitus ulcers, 317
Deep vein thrombosis, 80–81, 414
Deferoxamine therapy, 471
Dehydration, 411

Delayed primary closure, 388
Delirium, 286–287, 384
Delivery
    movements of, 218
    perineal tears associated with, 219
    stages of, 217
Delphian node, 391
Delusional disorder, 299
Dementia, 384–385
    AIDS, 267
    causes of, 265
    with Lewy bodies, 266
    vascular, 266
DepoProvera use, 212
Depot medroxyprogesterone acetate, 211–212
Depression, 294–295
Derailment, 307
Dermacentor andersoni, 349
Dermatologic disorders, 317–319
Developmental milestones
    gross and fine motor, 370
    language and social/cognition, 370
DHEA, 105
Diabetes insipidus, 109, 110
Diabetes mellitus
    American Diabetes Association
        recommendations for, 114
    clinical manifestations, 112
    complications, 113
    diagnosis criteria, 112
    and gangrene, 113
    and hypertensive medications, 27
    and hypoglycemia, 112
    management, 114–11
    medications for, 114
    treatment goals, 115
    type 1 DM, 112
    type 2 DM, 112
Diabetic gastroparesis, 147
Diabetic ketoacidosis
    laboratory findings, 115
    signs and symptoms of, 115
    treatment, 116
Diabetic nephropathy, 113
Diabetic neuropathy, 270
Diabetic retinopathy, 381
Diabetic sensory neuropathy, 270
Diabetic sensory polyneuropathy, 270
Diagnostic peritoneal lavage, 420–421, 431
Dialysis, 178
Diaper dermatitis, 378
"DIAPPERS," 165
Diarrhea and protozoa, 342
Diazoxide, 482
DIC. *See* Disseminated intravascular coagulation
Diffuse punctate keratopathy, 120
Digibind administration, 445
Digitalis toxicity, SVT caused by, 11
Digoxin, 13, 441
Dilated cardiomyopathies
    clinical presentations of, 10
    physiologic characteristics of, 10
Dilated cardiomyopathy, 9
Dilation and curettage, performance of, 196
Diltiazem, 29
2,3-Diphosphoglycerate, 89
Diphtheria, 133, 331–332
Diphyllobothrium latum, 344
Direct extension, 394
Direct ophthalmoscopic examination, 126

Dislocations
    and ligamentous injuries, 231
    mandibular condyles, 136
Disseminated gonococcal infection, 332–333
Disseminated intravascular coagulation, 323–324
Distal femoral fracture, 251
Distally lodged foreign body, 86
Distended neck veins, 418
Diuretics, 439
Diverticular disease, 406
Diverticulitis, 156–157, 406
DKA. *See* Diabetic ketoacidosis
DM. *See* Diabetes mellitus
DMPA. *See* Depot medroxyprogesterone acetate
Dobutamine, 33, 441
Dog and cat bites, 336
Domestic violence, 303
Dopamine, 438, 446
Down syndrome, 243
2,3-DPG. *See* 2,3-Diphosphoglycerate
DPL. *See* Diagnostic peritoneal lavage
Dressler (post–myocardial infarction) syndrome, 32
Drug excretion from kidneys, 437
Drug-induced liver disease, 151
Drug-induced lupus, 93
Drug-labeling categories, 215
drug metabolism and breakdown, mechanisms
        of, 437
Dual-energy X-ray (DXA) absorptiometry, 382
Duodenal bleeding, 403
Duodenal injury, 429
Duodenal ulcers, 146, 401, 404
Dupuytren contracture, 240
DVT. *See* Deep vein thrombosis
Dying, Kübler-Ross stages of, 307
Dynamic tension, 388
Dysbaric air embolism, 428
Dysdiadochokinesia, 277
Dysfunctional uterine bleeding, pharmaceutical
        treatment options for, 193
Dyshidrotic eczema, 310
Dysthymic disorder, 295
Dystonic reaction, 469

E

Ear disorders, 127–132
    acoustic neuroma, 129, 130
    acute otitis media, 129, 131
    benign positional vertigo, 128
    bilateral nystagmus, 128
    bilateral sensory hearing loss, 130
    bullous myringitis, 130
    central vertigo, 128
    cholesteatoma, 132
    conductive hearing loss, 127
    hematoma of ear, 130
    labyrinthitis, 127, 128, 129
    mastoiditis, 129, 132
    Ménière disease, 128, 129
    nystagmus, 128
    otitis externa, 129
    perichondritis, 130
    peripheral vertigo, 128
    presbycusis, 131
    recurrent unilateral serous otitis media, 131
    Rinne test, 127
    syphilis and sensorineural hearing loss, 131
    tinnitus, 131
    tympanic hypomobility, 131
    tympanic membrane perforation, 130

    unilateral sensory hearing loss, 130
    vertebrobasilar insufficiency, 132
    vestibular schwannoma, 129
    Weber test, 127
Eating disorders, 292–293
ECG. *See* Electrocardiograms
Eclampsia, 225
Ectopic atrial rhythm, EKG interpretation, 24*f*
Ectopic pregnancy, 220–221
Eczema herpeticum, 316
Eczematous eruptions, 309–310
"Effacement" of cervix, 218
Effusions and malignancy, 66
EGD. *See* Esophagogastroduodenoscopy
Eggshell hilar node calcification, 83
EKG interpretation, 21, 21*f*, 22, 22*f*, 23, 23*f*, 31
    of pericarditis, 46
    of posterior MI, 34
EKG rhythm abnormality, 17, 17*f*, 18, 18*f*
Elbow and forearm, disorders of, 237–238
Elbow flexion, 238–239
Elderly
    causes of death in, 379
    in nursing homes, 378
Electrical cardioversion, 11
Electrocardiograms
    question based on, 6–7
Electrolyte disorder, 425
Electrolyte disorders
    beer potomania, 182
    ECF volume contraction, 181
    geophagia/pica, 183
    in hospitalized patients, 181
    hyperkalemia
        causes of, 183
        EKG changes in, 184
        symptoms, 184
        treatment options, 184
    hypernatremia, 182
    hypocalcemia, 184–185
    hypokalemia
        causes of, 183
        physical examination in, 183
    hypomagnesemia, 185
    hyponatremia
        reasons of, 181
        symptoms, 181
        treatment goals, 182
    syndrome of inappropriate antidiuretic
        hormone, 181
Elephantiasis, 347
Elevated sweat chloride, conditions associated
        with, 74
Ellis class II and III fractures, 136, 137, 425, 428
Embolus, 80
Emergent resuscitative thoracotomy, 435
Emphysema, 71, 72
Empyema, 54
Encephalitis, 274
Endocarditis, 45–47
    bacterial. *See* Bacterial endocarditis
    infective. *See* Infective endocarditis
    in IV drug abusers, 337
    prophylaxis, 44
Endolymphatic hydrops. *See* Ménière disease
Endometrial cancer, 194
Endometrial hyperplasia, 194
Endometrial shedding, 190
Endometriosis, 193
Endotracheal intubation, 92

End-stage renal disease, 178
Enlarged kidneys, 178
Entamoeba histolytica, 342–343
Enterobius infection, 345
Enterocutaneous fistula, 412
Enterotoxin-producing organisms, 364
Entropion, 117
Enuresis, 307
Epicondyle, 238
Epidemic keratoconjunctivitis, 363
Epidemic pleurodynia, 363
Epididymitis, 167, 170
Epidural analgesia and labor, 218
Epidural hematoma, 419
Epiglottitis, 133, 134, 374–375
   cough of, 51
   pathogen in, 50
Epinephrine, 26
   for acute anaphylactic shock, 420
   and local anesthetics, 387
Episiotomy, 219
Epizootic plague, 337
Epstein–Barr virus (EBV) infections, 351–352
Erectile dysfunction, 164
Erythema infectiosum, 315
Erythema multiforme, 310
Erythema nodosum, 310
Erythromycin, 55, 457
Esophageal cancer, 392
   and distant metastasis, 143
   risk factors for, 143
Esophageal candidiasis, 327
Esophageal disease, 141
Esophageal impaction, 409
Esophagogastroduodenoscopy, 412
Esotropia, 124
ESRD. *See* End-stage renal disease
Essential tremor, 275
Estrogen, 189, 462
   changes associated with depletion of, 208
   effect on Alzheimer disease, 210
   effect on colorectal cancer, 210
   effect on endometrium, 190
Estrogen replacement therapy
   and bone mass, 209
   contraindications to, 210
ESWL. *See* Extracorporeal shockwave lithotripsy
Ethylene glycol, 474, 480
Ethylene glycol poisoning, 470, 478
Etomidate, 433
ET tube size calculation, 421
Euthyroid syndrome, 103
Ewing Sarcoma, 257
Examination day tips, 3–4
Examination preparation, suggestions for, 3
Exotropia, 124
Extracellular fluid (ECF) volume contraction, 181
Extracorporeal circulation, complication of, 34
Extracorporeal shockwave lithotripsy
Exudate *vs.* transudate, 75
Exudative pleural effusion, 94
Eye disorders, 117–127
   acute iritis, 118
   acute narrow angle closure glaucoma, 123
   acute narrow angle glaucoma, 122
   acute optic neuritis, 125
   afferent pupillary defect, 126
   age-related macular degeneration, 118
   amaurosis fugax, 120
   bacterial conjunctivitis, 118

blepharitis, 120
burns of cornea, 121
central retinal artery occlusion, 122, 123
central retinal vein occlusion, 117, 122
chalazion, 117, 120
cotton wool spots, 119
cyanoacrylate, 122
dacryocystitis, 118
diffuse punctate keratopathy, 120
direct ophthalmoscopic examination, 126
entropion, 117
esotropia, 124
exotropia, 124
flare, 121
glaucoma, 119, 124–125
herpes keratitis, 126
herpes simplex keratitis, 118, 124
herpes zoster ophthalmicus, 126
hordeolum, 117, 120
hyperopia, 125
hyphema, 121, 123
hypopyon, 120
indirect ophthalmoscopic examination, 126
lid lacerations, 121
myopia, 125
ophthalmoplegic migraine, 124
optic disk swelling, 126
optic neuritis, 122, 123
orbital blowout fracture, 119
orbital cellulitis, 117
orbital floor fractures, 119
perforated cornea with extruded iris, 123
periorbital and orbital infections, 118
pinguecula, 117
post-traumatic iritis, 126
preventable vision loss, 126
pseudomonas, 122
pterygium, 117
red eye, 123
retinoblastoma, 118
retrobulbar neuritis, 118
retrobulbar optic neuritis, 124
retro orbital hematoma, 120
Sjögren syndrome, 125, 127
strabismus, 124
subluxed or dislocated lens, 121
tonometry, 126

F
Face mask ventilation, oxygen flow rate for, 92
Facial paralysis, 267
Factitious disorder, 307–308
False-positive hematuria, 175
Familial polyposis, 405
FAST. *See* Focused Abdominal Sonography for Trauma
Fasting hypoglycemia, 112
Fatigue fracture, 232
Febrile seizure, 378
Fecaliths, 393
Fecal occult blood test, 158
Felon, 240
Felty syndrome, 262
Female puberty, normal course of, 189
Femoral hernia, 409
Femoral neck fracture, 247, 248
Fetal heart, 215, 219
Fetal lung maturity, 85, 219
Fetal movement, 215
Fever pattern in malarial infections, 345
FFP. *See* Fresh frozen plasma

Fibrates, 443
Fibroadenoma, 205–206, 395
Fibrocystic breast changes, 206
Fibromuscular dysplasia, 400
Fibromyalgia, 263
Finkelstein test, 239
Firearm injury, 304
Fish consumption and mercury poisoning, 213
Flare, 121
Flexion teardrop fracture, 429
Fluid overload, 391
Fluid requirements for resuscitation, 420
Fluid resuscitation, 432
Fluoroquinolone, 53
Focused Abdominal Sonography for Trauma,
   434, 435
Folate deficiency, 215
Follicle-stimulating hormone, 190
Foodborne illnesses, 363
Foodborne viral gastroenteritis, 363
Foreign-body aspiration, 86–87
Foreign-body removal procedure, 86
Fournier gangrene, 171, 413
Fresh frozen plasma, 422
Frostbite, 424–425
Frostnip, 424
FSH. *See* Follicle-stimulating hormone
Fungal disease, 327–329
   aspergillosis infection, 329
   candidal disorders, 327–328
   Cryptococcus infection, 328
   histoplasmosis, 328–329
   pneumocystis carinii pneumonia, 329
   pneumocystis infection, 329
   pneumocystis pneumonia, 329
   zygomycosis, 329
Fungal esophagitis, 143

G
GAD. *See* Generalized anxiety disorder
Galeazzi fracture/dislocation, 240
Gallbladder cancer, 399
Gallbladder emptying, drug impairing, 147
Gallbladder perforation, 148
Gallbladder polyps, 148
Gallstone ileus, 413
Gallstones, 147, 399, 400
Gamekeeper thumb, 240, 242
Ganglion cyst, 242
Gardner disease, 405
Gas gangrene, 336
Gastric acid aspiration, 86
Gastric cancer, 145–146
Gastric emptying, 453
Gastric ulcers, 404
Gastritis, 144–145
Gastroenteritis, 159
Gastroesophageal reflux disease
   complications from, 142
   diagnostic study of, 141
   extraesophageal manifestations of, 142
   and LES pressure, 142
   symptom of, 141–142
Gastroesophageal reflux, surgical methods for, 410
Gastrografin, 392
Gastroparesis, 147
General anesthesia for cholecystectomy, 389
Generalized anxiety disorder, 290
Generalized tonic–clonic seizure, 280
Genital warts. *See* Condylomata acuminata

Geophagia/pica, 183
GERD. *See* Gastroesophageal reflux disease
Geriatric disorders, 381–385
  Alzheimer disease, 385
  delirium, 384
  dementia, 384–385
  diabetic retinopathy, 381
  large bowel obstruction, 383
  presbycusis, 381
  pressure ulcers, 383–384
  sepsis, 384
  stage 1 hypertension, 381–382
  stress and urge incontinence, 383
  systemic skeletal disease, 382
  urinary incontinence, 383
  visual impairment, 381
Gestational choriocarcinoma, 222
Gestational diabetes, 223
Ghon lesion, 61
Giant cell arteritis, 36
Giardia, 339, 342
Gigantism, 109
Glasgow coma scale, 422–423
Glaucoma, 119, 124–125
Glioblastoma multiforme, 393
Glomerulonephritis, 179
Glomus jugulare tumors, 408
Glucagon, 445
Glucagonoma, 397
Glucocorticoid therapy, 323, 462
Glucose challenge test, 214
Gluten enteropathy. *See* Celiac sprue
GN. *See* Glomerulonephritis
Goiter, 98
Gonadotropin deficiency, 111
Gonadotropin levels after menopause, 208
Gonococcal genital infections, 332
Gonococcal infection, 171
Gonococcal urethritis, 171
Gonorrhea, 332
Goodpasture syndrome, 179
Gout, 261
Gram stain appearance of *Staphylococcus aureus*, 339
Granuloma inguinale, 338, 341
Graves disease, 99–100
Gray baby syndrome, 457
Grey–Turner sign, 395
Griseofulvin, 459
Group A beta-hemolytic streptococcus (GABHS)
  pharyngitis, 377
Group A hemolytic strep, 132
Group A Strep, 137
Growth hormone (GH) deficiency, 111
Guillain–Barré syndrome, 268, 349
GU tract, conditions of, 163–168
  benign prostatic hyperplasia, 163
  congenital hydrocele, 164
  cryptorchidism, 164
  erectile dysfunction, 164
  kidney stones, 165–167
  paraphimosis, 167
  phimosis, 167
  priapism, 168
  stress incontinence, 165
  testicular torsion, 167–168
  urinary incontinence, 165
  urinary retention, 164
  varicoceles, 164
Gynecoid pelvis, 190
Gynecologic disease of children, 200

Gynecologic malignancy, 194
Gynecomastia, 205

H
HAART. *See* Highly Active Antiretroviral Therapy
Haemophilus influenzae, 55
Haemophilus influenzae pneumonia, medical
  conditions associated with, 53
Haemophilus influenzae type B, 374
Hairy leukoplakia, 136
Hallucinations, 299
Haloperidol, 450
Hamman sign, 144, 393
Hamstrings, 252
Hangman fracture, 244, 416
Hantavirus, 58
HCG. *See* Human chorionic gonadotropin
Head lice. *See* Pediculosis capitis
Heart auscultation, 216
Heart failure
  and ACE inhibitors, 441
  and dobutamine, 441
  pharmacologic principles in treatment of, 440
Heart murmur of VSD, 373
Heat exhaustion, 426
Heat stroke, 426
Helicobacter pylori infection, 145
HELLP syndrome, 225
Hemangioma, 398
Hematochezia, 157
Hematogenous osteomyelitis, 256
Hematogenous spread, 394
Hematoma of ear, 130
Hemoccult, 158
Hemochromatosis, 152, 159
Hemodialysis, 178
Hemoglobin A1c and diabetes mellitus, 112
Hemoglobin concentration, 326
Hemolytic uremic syndrome, 175
Hemoptysis, 53
Hemorrhagic shock, 435
Hemorrhoids, 406
Hemostasis, 443
Hemostatic disorder, 323
Henoch-Schönlein purpura, 319
Heparin, 443
Hepatic cancer, 398
Hepatic metabolism of levothyroxine, 101
Hepatitis B surface antigen (HBsAg)-positive
  mother, 371
Hepatitis B vaccine, 365, 371
Hepatitis viruses, 151
Hepatocellular injury, 151
Hereditary hemorrhagic telangiectasia, 403
Hernia, 400–401, 408–409
Heroin, 468
Herpangina, 134
Herpes keratitis, 126
Herpes simplex I infection, 352–353
Herpes simplex keratitis, 118, 124
Herpes simplex virus, 202
  herpes simplex type 1, 133
  herpes simplex type 2, 133
Herpes zoster disease, 315
Herpes zoster ophthalmicus, 126
Hesselbach triangle, boundaries of, 401
Heterocyclics, 449
Heubner arteritis, 350
HHT. *See* Hereditary hemorrhagic telangiectasia
5-HIAA, 155

Hiatal hernia, 401
Hib. *See* Haemophilus influenzae type B
Hidradenitis suppurativa, 311
Highly Active Antiretroviral Therapy, 355
Hip and pelvis, disorders of
  anterior hip dislocation, 247
  aseptic necrosis, 248
  bladder rupture, 248
  femoral neck fracture, 247
  femoral neck fractures, 248
  instability of hip joints, 249
  intertrochanteric hip fracture, 247
  pelvic fractures, 247–248
  posterior hip dislocation, 247, 248
  pressure on first sacral root, 248
  slipped capital femoral epiphysis, 247, 248
  trochanteric bursitis, 249
Hirschsprung disease, 404
Hirsutism in menopausal women, 209
Histoplasma capsulatum, 57
Histoplasmosis, 57–58, 328–329
Histrionic personality disorder, 297–298
HIV-/AIDS-related pneumonia, 59–60
HIV-I encephalopathy, 356
HIV infection, 353–354, 459
HIV-related pulmonary infections, 59
HMD. *See* Hyaline membrane disease
Hoarseness, 62
"Home oxygen" therapy, 73
Homicide, 304
Hookworms, 343–344
Hordeolum, 117, 120
Hormonal-based contraceptive agents, 210
Horner syndrome, 244
Horseshoe kidneys, 181
HPO. *See* Hypertrophic osteoarthropathy
HPV associated with cervical cancer, 199
HPV vaccine for cervical cancer, 199
HSP. *See* Henoch-Schönlein purpura
Human chorionic gonadotropin, 174
Human leukocyte antigen (HLA) group, 99
Human papillomavirus (HPV) infections, 357
Human plague, 337
Huntington disease, 266, 276–277
HUS. *See* Hemolytic uremic syndrome
Hyaline membrane disease, 85, 369
Hydatidiform mole, 222
Hydrocarbons, 479, 480
Hydroxyindoleacetic acid. *See* 5-HIAA
Hymenolepis nana, 343
Hyperaldosteronism, 107
Hypercalcemia, 64
Hypercapnia, 90
Hypercholesterolemia, pharmacologic treatment
  of, 442
Hypercoagulability genetic disorders, 79–80
Hypercortisolism. *See* Cushing syndrome
Hyperemesis gravidarum, 213
Hyperkalemia
  causes of, 183
  EKG changes in, 184
  symptoms, 184
  treatment options, 184
Hypernatremia, 182
Hyperopia, 125
Hyperparathyroidism
  clinical manifestations of, 103
  diagnostic laboratory findings, 104
  etiologies of, 103
  indications for surgical treatment of, 104

Hyperphosphatemia, 178
Hypertension, 27–35
  and left ventricular hypertrophy, 28
  medication and diabetic patients, 27, 28
  in obese patients, first-line pharmacologic
    therapy for, 29
  secondary, 27–28
  stage 1, 381–382
Hypertensive emergency
  definition of, 28
  drug for treatment of, 28
  laboratory findings, 29
Hypertensive encephalopathy, 29
Hypertensive urgency, 28
Hyperthyroidism, 99, 222
Hypertrophic cardiomyopathy, 9
  clinical presentations of, 10
  management options for, 11
Hypertrophic osteoarthropathy, 64
Hyperventilation syndrome, 290
Hyphema, 121, 123
Hypocalcemia, 184–185
Hypocapnia, 90
Hypoglycemia
  management for, 112
  types of, 112
Hypokalemia
  causes of, 183
  physical examination in, 183
Hypomagnesemia, 185
Hyponatremia
  reasons of, 181
  symptoms, 181
  treatment goals, 182
Hypoparathyroidism
  clinical manifestations of, 104
  etiologies of, 104
  laboratory findings associated with, 104
  maintenance treatment for, 104
  treatment options for, 104
Hypopyon, 120
Hypotension, 28, 29
  orthostatic, 29
  treatment of, 453
Hypothyroidism, 100–101
Hypoventilation, 88, 91
Hypoxemia, 88–89, 90
Hysterectomy
  complications, 195
  types, 195

I

IADLs. *See* Instrumental activities of daily living
Iaundice in pregnancy, 153
ICP. *See* Intracranial pressure
Idiopathic achalasia, 141
Idiopathic enuresis, 307
Idiopathic obstructive hypertrophic
  cardiomyopathy, 34
Idiopathic pulmonary fibrosis, 83
Idiopathic thrombocytopenic purpura, 323
Idioventricular rhythm, 19*f*
  EKG interpretation, 25*f*
IHSS. *See* Idiopathic obstructive hypertrophic
  cardiomyopathy
Illusion, 299
Immunization
  before departing to Benin, 364
  healthy senior citizens, 365
  schedules for vaccines, 371–372

Immunocompromised patients, vaccines
  for, 357
Immunoprophylaxis, 374
Impetigo, 316
Indirect inguinal hernia, 400–401, 409
Indirect ophthalmoscopic examination, 126
Infectious arthritis, 255
Infectious diarrhea, 159, 334
Infectious digital flexor tenosynovitis, 241
Infectious disease, 255–256
Infectious disorders, 49–63
Infectious esophagitis, 143
Infectious gastroenteritis, 375
Infectious/inflammatory conditions, 168–171
  acute orchitis, 170
  acute prostatitis, 170–171
  cystitis, 169
  epididymitis, 170
  Fournier gangrene, 171
  gonococcal infection, 171
  inflammation of foreskin, 171
  prostatitis, 170
  pyelonephritis, 169–170
  urethritis, 171
  urinary tract infections
    pathogen of, 168
    by *Proteus mirabilis*, 169
    vesicoureteral reflux, 169
Infectious mononucleosis, 315, 352
Infective endocarditis, 45–46
Inferior wall myocardial infarction, 32
Infertility, 204–205
Infiltrating ductal carcinoma, 394
Inflammation of foreskin, 171
Inflammatory acne, 312
Influenza, 357–358, 459
  methods to detect, 52
  pneumonia in, 51
  treatment of, 52
Influenza A, 51
Influenza B virus, 51, 52
Influenza vaccine, 52, 365
Influenza virus, 51, 357–358
Inguinal (groin) hernia, 400
INH non resistant pulmonary TB, triple drug
  treatment for, 340
Instability of hip joints, 249
Instrumental activities of daily living, 379
Insulinoma, 397
Insulin preparations, 114
Intertrochanteric hip fracture, 247
Intestinal obstruction in newborn, 401–403
Intra-abdominal abscess, 63
Intra-abdominal malignancy, 159
Intracerebral hemorrhage, 284, 284*f*
Intracranial aneurysms, 285, 393
Intracranial pressure, 418
Intracranial toxoplasmosis, 346
Intracranial tumor, 271
Intrahepatic cholestasis of pregnancy, 153
Intrauterine gestational sac, 213
Intrauterine pregnancy, 213
Intravenous drug abuse, 46, 161
Intravenous immunoglobulin, 268, 319
Intravenous sodium nitroprusside, 33
Intubating patients, laboratory criteria for, 431
Intubation of neonate, 93
Intussusception, 376, 402, 410
Invasive or systemic candidiasis, 327
Involuntary movement disorder, 275

IPF. *See* Idiopathic pulmonary fibrosis
Iron deficiency anemia, 144
Iron poisoning, 471
Ischemic bowel disease, 411
Ischemic right leg, 35
Ischemic stroke, 281
Isoniazid, 458
Isopropanol poisoning, 446
IUD contraceptive devices, 212
IVIg. *See* Intravenous immunoglobulin

J

Jacksonian march, 279
Jarisch–Herxheimer reaction, 350, 364
Jefferson fracture, 244, 416
Jellyfish sting, treatment of, 364
JRA. *See* Juvenile rheumatoid arthritis
Junctional rhythm, 18*f*
Junctional rhythm with retrograde P waves, 16*f*
Juvenile rheumatoid arthritis, 263

K

Karnofsky scale, 322
Kawasaki disease, 319
Kegel exercises, 165
Kehr sign, 410
Kerley A and B lines, 93
Ketamine, 478
Kidney stones, 166–167, 399
  admission criteria for patients with, 166
  calcium oxalate, 166
  imaging option for, 166
  obstructing genitourinary tract, 167
  prevention of, 166
  radiolucent and radiopaque, 166
Kienböck disease, 240
Klebsiella granulomatis, 341
Klebsiella pneumoniae, 54
Kleinhauer–Betke test, 223
Knee and lower leg, disorders of, 249–252
  acute hemarthrosis, 250
  avulsion fractures, 250
  compartment syndrome, 250
  distal femoral fracture, 251
  knee dislocation, 251
  knee effusion, 251
  Lachman test, 251
  lower-extremity fractures, 250
  medial meniscus injury, 251
  Osgood–Schlatter disease, 250
  osteochondritis dissecans, 252
  patellar dislocations, 252
  patellofemoral pain syndrome, 249
  prepatellar bursitis, 251
  pseudogout, 251
  tibial plateau fracture, 251
  toddler fracture, 250
Koplik spots, 362
Krukenberg tumor, 146
Kübler-Ross stages of dying, 307
Kulchitsky cells, 407
Kyphosis, 246

L

Labor
  active phase of, 218
  and epidural analgesia, 218
  latent phase of, 217
  onset, 217
  stages of, 217–218

Labyrinthitis, 127, 128, 129
Lachman test, 251
Lactate dehydrogenase, 174
Lactated ringers IV solutions, 390
Lactic acidosis, 186
Lactose intolerance, diagnosis of, 158
Lacunar infarcts, 281
Laparoscopic cholecystectomy, complication associated with, 400
Large bowel obstruction, 383, 408, 409
Large cell carcinomas, 64
Laryngeal fracture, 420, 428
Laryngotracheitis. *See* Croup
LAs. *See* Local anesthetics
Laser bronchoscopy, 66
Lateral compression, 247
LC. *See* Lateral compression
LDH. *See* Lactate dehydrogenase
Left upper lobe consolidation, 54
Left ventricular aneurysms, complications of, 34
Left ventricular hypertrophy, 28
Left ventricular septum, rupture of, 33
Leg, compartments of, 250
Legionella pneumonia
    chest X-ray finding associated with, 55
    chest X-ray image of, 56
Legionella pneumophila, 55
Leiomyoma, 194–195
Leopold's maneuver, 219
Leprosy, 342
Leptospirosis, 338
Leriche syndrome, 407
Leukocytosis and bacterial pneumonia, 57
Levodopa, 448
Levodopa-carbidopa treatment, 276
Levothyroxine, 101, 462
Lewy bodies, dementia with, 266
LGV. *See* Lymphogranuloma venereum
LH. *See* Luteinizing hormone
Lhermitte sign, 278
Lichen simplex chronicus, 310
Lid lacerations, 121
Lidocaine, 45, 387
Lidocaine with epinephrine, 387
Life expectancy, 378
Ligament avulsion, 243
Lines of Langerhans, 387
Lipomas, 257
Lithium
    overdose, 452
    toxicity, 296, 453, 454
Liver abscess, 343
Liver injury, 151
LMWH. *See* Low-molecular-weight heparin
Local anesthetics, 387, 450
    and epinephrine, 387
Localized infection process, 411
Lochia, 229
Locked-in syndrome, 282
Lower esophageal sphincter (LES) pressure and GERD, 142
Lower-extremity fractures, 250
Lower GI bleeding, 157
Low-molecular-weight heparin, 443
Low output heart failure, 26
Ludwig angina, 133, 135
Lumbar disk herniations, 244
Lunate fracture, 241, 242
Lung abscesses, 63

Lung cancer
    associated with hypercalcemia, 64
    asymptomatic, 65
    and cigarette smoking, 64–65, 66
    and COPD, 64
    diagnostic test, 65
    incidence of, 63–64, 65
    and myopathic syndrome, 65
    in nonsmoking women, 65
    with paraneoplastic syndromes, 66
    screening programs, 64
    symptoms of, 63
    5-year survival for, 66
Lung/chest wall, compliance of, 92
Lung volumes, 216
Lupus pleuritis, 94
Luteinizing hormone, 190
LV. *See* Lymphogranuloma venereum
LV hypertrophy, drugs to regress, 10
LV mass, drugs to reduce, 10
Lyme disease, 347–348
Lymphatic filariasis, 459
Lymphogranuloma venereum, 203, 331
Lymphoma, 346

M
Macrocytic anemia, 160
Macrolide antibiotic, 53
Macrolide antibiotics, 457
Magnesium ammonium phosphate, 167
Maintenance IV fluid rate, 390
Malabsorption disorder, 153–154
Malaria, 344–345
Malignancies
    AML, 324
    and effusions, 66
    leukemia cutis, 324
    lymphoid, 325
    lymphoma, 324
    multiple myeloma, 325, 325*f*
    polycythemia vera, 324
Malignant pleural effusions, 65
Malignant transudative effusions, conditions associated with, 65
Malingering, 308
Mallet finger, 242, 242*f*
Mallory–Weiss tears, 144, 404
Malnutrition and respiratory failure, 92
Mammography, 207
Mandibular condyles, dislocation of, 136
Mandibular fracture, 135
MAOI. *See* Monoamine oxidase inhibitors
MAO inhibitors, 451
Massive transfusion protocol, 435
Mastitis, 206
Mastoiditis, 129, 132
MAT. *See* Multifocal atrial tachycardia
Maternal serum alpha-fetoprotein, 215
MCA. *See* Middle cerebral artery
McBurney point, 393
MCT. *See* Multislice Computed Tomography
Measles, 361–362
Mebendazole, 459
Meckel diverticulum, 158, 376, 404
Medial epicondyle fracture, 237
Medial meniscus injury, 251
Median nerve injuries, 243
Medroxyprogesterone acetate, 210
Medulloblastoma, 393

Meigs Syndrome, 198
Melancholia, 304
Melanoma, 313
Melanosis coli, 156
Membranoproliferative glomerulonephritis, 180
Ménière disease, 128, 129
Meningeal irritation, 273
Meningococcal conjugate vaccines, 371
Menometrorrhagia, 191
Menopause, 208–210
Menorrhagia, 191
Menstrual blood flow and OCP use, 210
Menstrual cycle, 189
Menstrual disorders
    menometrorrhagia, 191
    menorrhagia, 191
    metrorrhagia, 191
    oligomenorrhea, 191
    persistent vaginal bleeding, 191
    polymenorrhea, 191
    precocious puberty, 192
    premenstrual dysphoric disorder, 192
    Premenstrual Syndrome, 192
    primary amenorrhea, 191
    primary dysmenorrhea, 192
    secondary amenorrhea, 191
    secondary dysmenorrhea, 192
Mesenteric ischemia, 408, 411
Metabolic acidoses, 185
    increased anion gap, 186
    treatment of, 187
Metabolic alkalosis, 187
Metastatic bone tumors, 257
Methadone, 450, 468
Methanol poisoning, 470, 474
Methemoglobinemia, 444, 476
Methicillin resistant *Staphylococcus aureus* (MRSA), 317
Methotrexate (MTX) pulmonary toxicity, 461
Methylene blue, 446
Metronidazole, 157, 460
Metrorrhagia, 191
MI. *See* Myocardial infarction
"Mickey Finn," 470
Microscopic colitis, 155
Midazolam, 433
Midcycle spotting, 190
Middle cerebral artery, 283
Middle cerebral artery stroke, 282
Migraine headaches, 270–272
Mineralocorticoid, 462
Minute ventilation, 89
    at submaximal work rates, 93
Missed abortion, 221
Mitral regurgitation, 34, 42
Mitral stenosis, 40–41
Mitral valve prolapsed (MVP) syndrome, 40, 42, 43
Mitral valve reconstruction, 42
Mitral valve surgery, indication for, 41
Mittelschmerz, 190
M-mode echocardiogram, 44
MMR vaccine, immunization schedules for, 372
Mobitz II second-degree AV block, 11–12, 13, 17*f*
Mobitz I (Wenckebach) second-degree AV block, 11, 13, 15
Modified Ritgen maneuver, 218
Monoamine oxidase inhibitors, 449, 453
Mononeuropathy, 269, 270
Monteggia fracture, 237

Mood disorders, 293–296
  adjustment disorder, 293–294
  bipolar disorder, 295–296
  depression, 294–295
  dysthymic disorder, 295
  lithium toxicity, 296
  suicide, 296
  unipolar disorder, 296
Moraxella catarrhalis, 55
Morning sickness, 213
Morphine, 450
Motor innervation to diaphragm, 410
Motor neurons, 239
Mouth/throat disorders
  acute necrotizing ulcerative gingivitis, 137
  acute parotitis, 132
  AIDS-related oropharyngeal diseases, 137
  alveolar osteitis, 136
  angiotensin-converting enzyme inhibitor, 135
  aphthous ulcer, 137
  aphthous ulcers, 132
  bacterial parotitis, 135
  bilateral mental fracture, 135
  diphtheria, 133
  dislocation of mandibular condyles, 136
  Ellis class II and III fractures, 136, 137
  Ellis class II fracture, 137
  epiglottitis, 133, 134
  group A hemolytic strep, 132
  Group A Strep, 137
  hairy leukoplakia, 136
  herpangina, 134
  laryngotracheitis, 134
  Ludwig angina, 133, 135
  mandibular fracture, 135
  oral flora and anaerobes, 133
  oral thrush, 137
  parapharyngeal abscess, 134, 135
  peritonsillar abscess, 132, 133, 134
  post-extraction alveolitis, 133
  retropharyngeal abscess, 133, 134
  retropharyngeal abscesses, 135
  sialadenitis, 134
  sialolithiasis, 132
  strep throat, 137
  streptococcal infections, 136
  streptococcal pharyngitis, 134
  Streptococcus pyogenes, 132
  stridor, 133
  TMJ syndrome, 136
  ulcerative stomatitis, 137
  zygomatic arch fracture, 136
  zygomaticomaxillary complex fracture, 136
MPA. *See* Medroxyprogesterone acetate
Mucoepidermoid carcinoma, 392
Mucosal rectal prolapse, 406
Multiaxial diagnostic system, 306
Multifocal atrial tachycardia, 11, 12, 18*f*
Multiple myeloma, 258
Multiple sclerosis, 277, 278–279, 278*f*
Multislice Computed Tomography, 415
Mumps, 358–359
Munchausen syndrome, 307
Mural endocarditis, 47
Muscarinic antagonists, 438
Muscle viability, 234
Myasthenia gravis, 269
Myasthenic crisis, 269

Mycoplasma
  extrapulmonary manifestations of, 54
  treatment for, 55
Mycoplasma pneumonia, 56
Mycoplasma pneumoniae, 53, 55
Mycoplasma pneumoniae pneumonia, chest X-ray for, 53
Mycotic aneurysms, 408
Myocardial abscesses, 47
Myocardial contusions, 418
Myocardial deterioration, 32
Myocardial infarction. *See also* Acute myocardial infarction (MI)
  associated with thrombosis, 30
  and AV block, 15
  and beta-blockers, 31
  cause of death during, 31
  conduction defects, 15
  therapy for patients with large anterior, 34
Myocardial ischemia, 23*f*
Myocarditis, 45
Myopathic syndrome and lung cancer, 65
Myopia, 125
Myxedema crisis, 101

N

Nabothian cyst, 198
Naloxone, 470
Narcissistic personality disorder, 298
Narcotics, 450
Nasal disorders
  acute uncomplicated sinusitis, 139
  adult acute sinusitis, 138
  allergic rhinitis, 139
  anterior epistaxis, 138
  bacterial sinusitis, 139
  cavernous sinus thrombosis, 138
  chronic sinusitis, 139
  cribriform plate fractures, 138
  nasal fracture, 138
  nasal polyps and asthma, 139
  nasopharyngeal cancer, 139
  posterior epistaxis, 138, 140
  posterior nosebleeds, 138
  Pott puffy tumor, 138
  septal hematoma, 138, 140
  toxic shock syndrome, 138
  unilateral purulent rhinorrhea, 138
  vasomotor rhinitis, 139
Nasal fracture, 138
Nasal polyps and asthma, 139
NASH. *See* Nonalcoholic steatohepatitis
Nasopharyngeal cancer, 139
National Commission on the Certification of Physician Assistants, 1
NCCPA. *See* National Commission on the Certification of Physician Assistants
Necator americanus infection, 343
Necrobiosis lipoidica, 317
Neisseria gonorrhoeae, 203
Nematodes, treatment of, 459
Neologism, 307
Neonatal intestinal obstruction, 401–402
Neoplastic diseases, 63–67, 256–258, 313–314
  bladder cancer, 172
  prostate cancer
    definitive surgical treatment for, 173
    grading system, 173
    post-prostatectomy incontinence, 173
    risk factors for, 172

  site for distant metastases of, 172
  standard method for diagnosing, 172
  types of, 172
  renal cell carcinoma (RCC), 173–174
  testicular cancer, 174
  testicular teratomas, 174
  Wilms tumor, 174–175
Nephritic syndrome, 180
  pleural effusion in, 76
Neuraminidase inhibitors, 459
Neurapraxia, 233
Neurofibromatosis 1, 319
Neurogenic pulmonary edema, 94
Neuroleptic malignant syndrome, 448
Neuroleptics, 447, 454–455
Neuromuscular blockers, 438
Neurosyphilis, 350
Nevi, 313
Newborn infant
  Apgar score, 367
  Barlow maneuver, 368
  benign birthmarks, 368
  benign skin eruptions, 368
  birth weight, 375
  clavicle fracture, 368
  congenital abnormalities, 369
  genetic disorders, 368
  gonococcal ophthalmia neonatorum, 368
  infection transmission, 369
  kernicterus, 368
  neonatal jaundice, 368–369
  neonatal period, 367
  New Ballard Score, 367
  normal heart and respiratory rate ranges for, 367
  Ortolani test, 368
  painless lower GI bleeding in, 376
  postprandial spitting and vomiting, 375
  projectile vomiting, 375
  TORCH infections, 369–370
  volvulus (malrotation), 375–376
Newborn respiratory distress syndrome, 85
New onset headaches, 270
NF1. *See* Neurofibromatosis 1
Niacin, 442–443
Night blindness, 161
Nikolsky sign, 311
Nimodipine, 285
Nitrates and cardiac cycle, 440
Nocturnal bone pain, 257
Nodular basal cell carcinoma, 314
Nonalcoholic steatohepatitis, 153
Noncystic breast tumor, 395
Nonmetastatic carcinoid tumor, 66
Non–Q-wave infarctions, 31
Nonseminomatous germ cell tumors, 174
Nonsequiturs, 307
Nonsteroidal anti-inflammatory drugs, 443, 464
Nontraumatic cardiac death, 30
Nontraumatic subarachnoid hemorrhage, 284
Nontropical sprue, 322
Norepinephrine and cardiovascular system, 438
Nosocomial pneumonia, 54, 56
NSAIDs. *See* Nonsteroidal anti-inflammatory drugs
NSGCT. *See* Nonseminomatous germ cell tumors
"Nursemaid's elbow," 237
Nutrition and exercise, 3
Nystagmus, drugs causing, 128
Nystatin, 458

O

Obsessive-compulsive disorders, 298
Obstructive pulmonary disease, 67–75
Obturator hernia, 408
Obturator sign, 393
Occult rectal prolapse, 406
OCD. *See* Obsessive-compulsive disorders
OCP use
  and menstrual blood flow, 210
  noncontraceptive benefits of, 211
  side effect of, 211
  venous thromboembolic disease risk, 211
Odontoid fracture, 415
Olecranon bursa, 238, 238*f*
Oligomenorrhea, 191
Oliguria, 176
Onchocerciasis, 347
Onychomycosis, 314
Open mitral valvotomy, 41
Ophthalmologic changes, 217
Ophthalmoplegic migraine, 124
Opiate overdose, 455
Opioid pain medications, 408
Opportunistic infection in AIDS patients, 354
Optic disk swelling, 126
Optic neuritis, 122, 123, 278
OPV. *See* Oral polio vaccine
Oral contraceptive use
  and cervical cancer, 211
  DMPA, 211–212
  and ovarian cancer, 211
Oral decongestant, 62
Oral dissolution therapy, 400
Oral flora and anaerobes, 133
Oral hairy leukoplakia, 316
Oral polio vaccine, 372
Oral thrush, 137
Orbital blowout fracture, 119
Orbital cellulitis, 117
Orbital floor fractures, 119
Organophosphates, 472
Oropharyngeal dysphagia, 143
Orotracheal endotracheal tube, malposition
  of, 428
Ortolani maneuver, 249
Osgood–Schlatter disease, 250
Osler–Weber–Rendu syndrome, 403
Ossification centers in elbow, 237
Osteoarthritis
  diagnosis of, 259
  DIP joints in patients with, 258
  medication for, 259
  and osteophytes, 258
  risk factors for, 258
  surgical treatment options, 259
  symptoms and signs, 258
Osteochondritis dissecans, 252
Osteoid osteoma, 257
Osteomyelitis, 255–256
Osteoporosis, 382
  bony abnormalities in, 260
  diagnostic tests, 260
  prevention of, 261
  types of, 260
Osteosarcomas, 257
Otitis externa, 129
Ovarian cancer, 197–198, 211
Ovarian cysts, 196–197
Ovulation, 189
Oxygen content of blood, 89

Oxygen flow rate, face mask ventilation, 92
Oxyhemoglobin dissociation curve, 89
Oxytocin, 217

P

Pacemakers
  battery lifespan, 12
  fixed-rate demand modes of, 12
Paget disease, 82, 206
Painful third-trimester bleeding, 225
Palivizumab, 374
Pallor, 322
PAN. *See* Polyarteritis nodosa
PANCE. *See* Physician Assistant National
    Certification Examination
Pancoast syndrome, 66
Pancreatic cancer, 397
  periampullary lesions, 150
  risk factors for, 150
  site of, 150
  survival rate for, 151
  symptoms, 150
  tumor marker, 150
Pancreaticoduodenectomy, 390
Pancreatic pseudocysts, 396
Pancreatitis, 149–150, 395
Panic attacks, treatment for, 289
Panic disorders, 290
PANRE. *See* Physician Assistant National
    Recertification Examination
Pantaloon hernia, 409
Papillary muscle dysfunction, 32
Pap smear screening, 198
Papulosquamous diseases, 310–311
Paralytic ileus, 408
Paraneoplastic syndromes, 66
Paranoid personality disorder, 298
Paraparesis, 363
Parapharyngeal abscess, 134, 135
Paraphimosis, 167
Parapneumonic effusion, chest tube
    placement in, 76
Parasitic diarrhea infection, 159
Parasitic disease, 342–351
  babesia infection, 348
  cerebral amebiasis, 342
  Chagas disease, 346, 347
  Colorado tick fever, 348
  diarrhea and protozoa, 342
  elephantiasis, 347
  Enterobius infection, 345
  Giardia, 342
  hookworms, 343–344
  intracranial toxoplasmosis, 346
  liver abscess, 343
  Lyme disease, 347–348
  lymphoma, 346
  malaria, 344–345
  Necator americanus infection, 343
  neurosyphilis, 350
  onchocerciasis, 347
  periorbital edema, 343
  pinworms, 345
  RMSF, 349–350
  secondary syphilis, 350
  swimmer itch, 346
  tapeworms, 343–344
  tick paralysis, 349
  toxoplasmosis, 346
  Trichinella spiralis, 343

  Trichomonas vaginalis, 343
  Trichuris trichiura, 343
  trypanosomiasis, 347
  tularemia, 348
  vasculitis, 350
  wood tick, 349
Parathyroid gland
  diseases of, 103–104
  regulation of, 103
Parathyroid hormone, 103
Parietal pain, 391
Parkinson disease, 275–276
Paronychia, 243, 314
Paroxysmal atrial fibrillation, 33
Partial bowel obstruction, 412
Pasteurella multocida, 339
Patellar dislocations, 252
Patellofemoral pain syndrome, 249
Patent ductus arteriosus, 38, 373
PBC. *See* Primary biliary cirrhosis
PCO. *See* Polycystic kidney disease
PCP. *See* Pneumocystis carinii pneumonia
PDA. *See* Patent ductus arteriosus
PE. *See* Pulmonary embolism
PEA. *See* Pulseless electrical activity
Pearson Vue Testing Centers, 4
Peau d'orange, 206
Pediculosis capitis, 312
PEEP
  and cardiac output, 92
  and mechanical ventilation, 92
Pellagra, 160
Pelvic floor muscle exercises, 165
Pelvic fractures, 247–248
Pelvic inflammatory disease
  diagnosis criteria, 203
  organisms causing, 203
  risk factors for, 203
Pelvic organ prolapse, 195–196
Penetrating head trauma, 394
Penetrating injuries, evaluation of, 421
Penicillamine-induced lung toxicity, 456
Penicillin, 456
PEP. *See* Post Exposure Prophylaxis
Peptic ulcer disease, 146
Percutaneous transluminal coronary
    angioplasty, 30
Perforated cornea with extruded iris, 123
Periampullary lesions, 150
Perianal staphylococcal/streptococcal infection,
    317
Peribronchial pneumonia, 53
Pericardial effusion with cardiac tamponade, 37
Pericarditis, 45
  following acute MI, 34
Perichondritis, 130
Perimenopausal woman, laboratory work-up
    for, 193
Perineal tears, 219
Perioral dermatitis, 319
Periorbital and orbital infections, 118
Periorbital edema, 343
Peripheral aneurysms, 36
Peripheral cyanosis, 93
Peripheral facial palsy, 268
Peripheral nerve compression, 239
Peripheral tissues, oxygen delivery to, 89
Peripheral vertigo, 128
Peritonsillar abscess, 132, 133, 134
Pernio, 424

Perseveration, 307
Persistent vaginal bleeding, 191
Personality disorders, 296–299
  antisocial, 296–297
  avoidant, 297
  borderline, 297
  histrionic, 297–298
  narcissistic, 298
  OCD, 298
  paranoid, 298
  schizoidia, 298–299
  schizotypal, 299
Pertussis, 52
Phalenl's tests, 239
Phenothiazine, 469
Phenytoin, 447, 455, 473
Pheochromocytoma, 28, 107–108, 158, 397–398
Phimosis, 167
Phosphorus poisoning, antidote for, 477
Physician Assistant National Certification
      Examination
  examination day tips, 3–4
  framework of content, 1
    organ system, 2
    task areas, 2
  multiple choice questions, 1
  preparing for, 3
  test-taking strategy. See Test-taking strategy
Physician Assistant National Recertification
      Examination, 1
  examination day tips, 3–4
  framework of content, 1
    organ system, 2
    task areas, 2
  multiple choice questions, 1
  preparing for, 3
  test-taking strategy. See Test-taking strategy
Physiologic dead space, 89
Pica, 213
PID. See Pelvic inflammatory disease
PIH. See Pregnancy-induced hypertension
Pilonidal cyst, 317
Pinguecula, 117
"Pink puffer," 71
Pinworms, 345
Pituitary gland, diseases of, 108–111
Pituitary tumors, 108–109
Pit viper, 427
Pityriasis, 311
Placenta previa, 226–227
Plantar wart, treatment of, 405
Plaque psoriasis, 309
Plasmapheresis, 268
Plasmodium falciparum
  diagnosed on blood smear, 345
  lifecycle of, 344
Platelet inhibitors, 443
Pleural diseases, 75–79
Pleural effusion
  and atelectasis, 76
  and chronic pancreatitis, 77
  and cirrhosis, 76
  clinical features, 76
  and congestive heart failure, 76
  drugs associated with, 77
  in nephritic syndrome, 76
  and pneumonia, 56
  and pulmonary embolism, 77
Pleural fluid, 77
Pleuritic chest pain, 94

Pleurodesis, 78
PML. See Progressive multifocal
      leukoencephalopathy
Pneumococcal pneumonia, 52–53, 55
  pathogens, 53
  risk factors for, 52
  treatment of, 53
Pneumococcal vaccine, 57, 365
Pneumoconiosis, 83
Pneumocystis carinii pneumonia, 59–60, 329, 354
  intoxication, 468–469
  overdose, 468
Pneumocystis infection, 329
Pneumocystis jirovecii pneumonia, 59
Pneumocystis pneumonia, 329
Pneumonia
  in children, 54
  and cold agglutinins, 55
  by hantavirus, 58
  induced by Klebsiella pneumoniae, 54
  in influenza, 51
  and pleural effusions, 56
  and pneumothorax, 77
  in sickle cell disease, 55
  with single rigor, 57
  during summer, 56
  ventilator associated, 57
  X-ray findings, 54
Pneumoperitoneum, 389
Pneumothoraces, 78
Pneumothorax
  chest tube in patient with, 78
  and pneumonia, 77
  risk factors of, 79
  secondary, 78
  spontaneous, 77
  tension, 78
  traumatic, 78
  treatment for, 78
Polio, 363
Polio vaccine, 372
Poliovirus, 363
Polyarteritis nodosa, 263
Polycystic kidney disease, 180–181, 197
Polycythemia, 82
Polymenorrhea, 191
Polymyalgia rheumatic, 262
Polymyositis, 263
Polyneuropathy, 270
Porcelain gallbladder, 148
Portal hypertension, 398
Port wine stain, 318
Post concussion syndrome, 286
Posterior cerebral artery stroke, 282
Posterior column function, testing of, 418
Posterior epistaxis, 138, 140
Posterior hip dislocation, 247, 248
Posterior nosebleeds, 138
Post Exposure Prophylaxis, 355
Post-extraction alveolitis, 133
Postinfectious glomerulonephritis, 179
Postmenopausal bleeding, 208
Postpartum hemorrhage, 228
Postpartum psychosis, 302
Postpartum tubal ligation, 213
Postprandial hypoglycemia, 112
Postsplenectomy sepsis, 391
Postsplenectomy (postsplenic) sepsis, 411
Poststreptococcal glomerulonephritis, 179
Post-traumatic iritis, 126

Post-traumatic stress disorder, 290–291
Postvoid residual volume, 164
Pott puffy tumor, 138
PPROM. See Preterm premature rupture of
      membranes
Precocious puberty, 192
Pre-diabetes, criteria for, 112
Preeclampsia, 225
Pregnancy, complicated, 220–229
  abruption placentae, 226
  amniotic fluid embolism, 227
  asthma, 223
  cesarean section, 228
  eclampsia, 225
  ectopic pregnancy, 220–221
  gestational choriocarcinoma, 222
  gestational diabetes, 223
  HELLP syndrome, 225
  hydatidiform mole, 222
  hyperthyroidism, 222
  Kleinhauer–Betke test, 223
  lochia, 229
  missed abortion, 221
  painful third-trimester bleeding, 225
  placenta previa, 226–227
  postpartum hemorrhage, 228
  preeclampsia, 225
  pregnancy-induced hypertension, 224
  premature rupture of membranes, 224
  preterm delivery, 224
  preterm labor, 223
  preterm premature rupture of membranes, 224
  Rh isoimmunization, 223
  Rho-Gam administration, 223
  shoulder dystocia, 227–228
  spontaneous abortion, 221–222
  termination of, 222
  twins, 222
  uterine atony, 228
  uterine rupture, 227
  viral or protozoal infections, 223
Pregnancy-induced hypertension, 224
Pregnancy, uncomplicated, 213–220
  amniocentesis, 214
  antibiotics to use in, 216
  anticoagulant for, 216
  β-hCG levels, 213–214
  biophysical profile, 217
  BUN and creatinine, 216
  change in lung volumes in, 216
  changes in volume of cardiovascular system
      during, 216
  drug-labeling categories for use during, 215
  episiotomy, 219
  fetal heart, 215
  fetal heart rate, 219
  fetal lung maturity, 219
  fetal movement, 215
  fish consumption and mercury poisoning, 213
  folate deficiency, 215
  glucose challenge test, 214
  heart ausculation during, 216
  hyperemesis gravidarum, 213
  intrauterine gestational sac, 213
  intrauterine pregnancy, 213
  Leopold's maneuver, 219
  and maternal serum alpha-fetoprotein, 215
  modified Ritgen maneuver, 218
  morning sickness, 213
  normal P_{CO_2} in, 216

onset of labor, 217
ophthalmologic change during, 217
oxytocin, 217
perineal tears, 219
physical changes in cervix during, 216
pica, 213
progesterone levels, 214
routine screenings, 214
stages of labor and delivery, 217–218
vaginal–rectal culture, 214
weight gain in, 216
white blood cell count during, 216
Premature atrial beats, 12
Premature babies, antepartum corticosteroids in, 219
Premature menopause, 208
Premature rupture of membranes, 224
Premenstrual dysphoric disorder, 192
Premenstrual Syndrome, 192
Prepatellar bursitis, 251
Presbycusis, 131, 381
Pressure on first sacral root, 248
Pressure ulcers, 383–384
Pressure urticaria, 310
Preterm birth, 369
Preterm delivery, 224
Preterm infant, 85
respiratory distress in, 369
Preterm labor, 223
Preterm premature rupture of membranes, 224
Preventable vision loss, 126
Priapism, 168
Primary adrenal insufficiency
etiologies of, 105
management for, 106
Primary amenorrhea, 191
Primary biliary cirrhosis, 152
Primary carcinomas, 256
Primary dysmenorrhea, 192
Primary gastrointestinal cancer, 155
Primary hyperparathyroidism, 103
Primary hypothyroidism, 100–101
Primary sclerosing cholangitis, 152
Prinzmetal angina, 30
Procainamide loading infusion, 15
Proctalgia fugax, 406
Progesterone, 189, 214
Progestins, 462
Progressive multifocal leukoencephalopathy, 362–363
Prolactin, 190
Prolactinoma, 109
PROM. See Premature rupture of membranes
Prosopagnosia, 282
Prostate cancer
definitive surgical treatment for, 173
grading system, 173
post-prostatectomy incontinence, 173
risk factors for, 172
site for distant metastases of, 172
standard method for diagnosing, 172
types of, 172
Prostatitis, 170
Prosthetic vascular graft infection, 47
Proteinuria, 179
Proximal esophagus, cancer of, 143
PSC. See Primary sclerosing cholangitis
Pseudogout, 251, 262
Pseudohypoparathyroidism, 103
Pseudomonal infection, 336

Pseudomonas, 122
Pseudomonas aeruginosa, 54, 312
Pseudomonas aeruginosa infection, 338
PSGN. See Poststreptococcal glomerulonephritis
Psoas sign, 393
Psychiatric illness, 301
Psychoses, 299–302
brief psychotic disorder, 301
delusional disorder, 299
hallucinations, 299
illusion, 299
postpartum psychosis, 302
psychiatric illness, 301
psychosis, 301
schizophrenia, 299–301
schizophreniform disorder, 299
Psychosis, 301
Psychotropic agents, 382
PTCA. See Percutaneous transluminal coronary angioplasty
Pterygium, 117
PTH. See Parathyroid hormone
PTSD. See Post-traumatic stress disorder
PUD. See Peptic ulcer disease
Pulmonary abscess, 63
Pulmonary circulation, 79–83
Pulmonary embolism, 79–80
CXR findings in, 80
and cyanosis, 92
diagnostic test for, 81
and hypercoagulability genetic disorders, 79–80
and pleural effusions, 77
treatment of, 81
Pulmonary embolus, standard test for confirmation of, 6
Pulmonary hypertension
etiology of, 81
heart sounds, 82
mechanisms causing, 81
primary, 81
symptoms, 81
treatment plan for, 82
2-year survival rate, 82
Pulmonary infarction, 80
Pulmonary nodules, 66–67
Pulseless electrical activity, 15
Pulseless electrical activity, treatment of, 26
Pulseless ventricular tachycardia, treatment of, 26
Pulse oximetry, 87
PVCs in post-MI patients, 31
PVR. See Postvoid residual volume
PWS. See Port wine stain
Pyelonephritis, 169–170
Pyloric stenosis, 375
Pyogenic granuloma, 318
Pyogenic hepatic abscesses, 398
Pyridoxine, 476

Q
Q fever, 349
QRS complex tachycardia, 14
QRS widening, 452
Quadriceps, 252
Quervain tenosynovitis, 239
Quinolones, 458
Q wave, diagnostic criteria for, 30

R
Rabies, 359–360
Rabies virus, 360

Radial head fracture, 238
Radiation poisoning, 481
Radiation therapy, 199
Radical hysterectomy, 199
Ramsay Hunt syndrome, 268
Ranson criteria, 396
Rattlesnake bite, 427
RCC. See Renal cell carcinoma
Reactive arthritis, 338
Recreational drugs, hepatotoxicity of, 151
Rectal bleeding, 404
Recurrent unilateral serous otitis media, 131
Red eye, 123
Refractory asthma, 70
Reiter syndrome, 338
Renal calculi. See Kidney stones
Renal cell carcinoma, 173–174
Renal diseases
acute renal failure, 176–177, 179
anuria, 176
chronic diabetic nephropathy, 180
chronic renal failure, 177, 180
dialysis, 178
end-stage renal disease, 178
enlarged kidneys, 178
false-positive hematuria, 175
glomerulonephritis, 179
Goodpasture syndrome, 179
hemodialysis, 178
hemolytic uremic syndrome, 175
high levels of PTH, 178
horseshoe kidneys, 181
hyperphosphatemia, 178
membranoproliferative glomerulonephritis, 180
nephrotic syndrome, 180
oliguria, 176
polycystic kidney disease, 180–181
postinfectious glomerulonephritis, 179
poststreptococcal glomerulonephritis, 179
proteinuria, 179
rhabdomyolysis, 175
systemic lupus erythematosus, 180
uremic patient, 178
urinary obstruction, 176
Wegener granulomatosis, 179
Renal pedicle injury, 430
Renal tubular acidosis
acid–base electrolyte abnormalities, 186–187
classification of, 186
mechanisms for, 186
Reperfusion therapy, 34
Reproductive physiology, 189–190
Respiratory acidosis, 187–188
Respiratory failure and malnutrition, 92
Respiratory syncytial virus, 460
infection, 60
Respiratory tract aspirates, 86
Restrictive cardiomyopathy, 9
clinical presentations of, 10
common causes of, 10
physiological aspects of, 10
Restrictive pulmonary disease, 83–84
Retinoblastoma, 118
Retrobulbar neuritis, 118
Retrobulbar optic neuritis, 124
Retrocecal appendicitis, 393
Retrograde urethrogram, 430
Retro orbital hematoma, 120
Retropharyngeal abscesses, 63, 133, 134, 135
Revascularization with bypass grafting, 34

Reverse transcriptase, 355
Reverse transcriptase inhibitors, 459
Reyes syndrome, 51
Reynolds pentad, 399
Rhabdomyolysis, 175, 430
Rheumatic fever, 337
Rheumatic heart disease, 40
Rheumatic mitral stenosis, 41
Rheumatoid arthritis, 261, 321
Rheumatologic conditions, 261–263
    Felty syndrome, 262
    fibromyalgia, 263
    gout, 261
    juvenile rheumatoid arthritis, 263
    polyarteritis nodosa, 263
    polymyalgia rheumatic, 262
    polymyositis, 263
    pseudogout, 262
    rheumatoid arthritis, 261
    scleroderma, 262
    Sjögren syndrome, 262
    systemic lupus erythematous, 262
    ulnar deviation and subluxation, 261
Rhinocerebral zygomycosis, 329
Rh isoimmunization, 223
Rho-Gam administration, 223
Rhythm strip, abnormality in, 18, 18*f*, 19, 19*f*,
    20, 20*f*
Rib fracture, 430
Richter hernia, 409
Rickets, 160
Rifampin, 340, 458
Right middle lobe pneumonia, 54
Ring lesion, treatment of, 364
Rinne test, 127
RMSF. *See* Rocky Mountain spotted fever
Rocky Mountain spotted fever, 349–350
Roseola infantum, 316, 360–361
Rotator cuff, muscles of, 234
Routine screenings, 214
Roux-en-Y operative procedure, 390
Rovsing sign, 393
RSV. *See* Respiratory syncytial virus
Rubella, 361

S

Salicylate poisoning, 465–467
Salmonella enterocolitis, 333
Salmonella infection, 333
Salmonella osteomyelitis, 256
Salmonellosis, 333
Salter–Harris fracture, 232–234
Sarcoidosis, 84
Scabies, 312
Scaphoid (navicular) fracture, 240
Scar, 388
SCFE. *See* Slipped capital femoral epiphysis
Schilling test, 160
Schistosome dermatitis, 346
Schizoidia, 298–299
Schizophrenia, 298, 299–301
Schizophreniform disorder, 299
Schizotypal personality disorder, 299
Scleroderma, 262
Scoliosis, 246
Scurvy, 161
Seborrheic dermatitis, 309
Seborrheic keratoses, 313
Secondary amenorrhea, 191
Secondary bacterial infection, 59

Secondary dysmenorrhea, 192
Secondary hyperparathyroidism, 103
Secondary hypertension, 27–28
Secondary hypothyroidism, 101
Secondary intention, 388
Secondary pneumothorax, 78
Secondary syphilis, 350
Sedative hypnotics, 454
Seizures, 279–280, 447
Semen analysis, 205
Sensory innervation, 391
Sentinel loop, 391
Separation anxiety, average age at onset of, 289
Sepsis, 384
Septal hematoma, 138, 140, 419
Serotonin-selective reuptake inhibitors, 449
Serotonin syndrome, 454–455
Serum amylase, 395
Serum digoxin levels, 15
Serum osmolality, 390
Serum theophylline levels, 69
Severe diabetic gastroparesis, 115
Sexual desire, drugs decreasing, 451
Sexually transmitted infections
    chancroid, 202
    chlamydia trachomatis, 203
    herpes simplex virus, 202
    lymphogranuloma venereum, 203
    Neisseria gonorrhoeae, 203
    syphilis, 202
    trichomonas vaginitis, 202
Shaken baby syndrome, 425
Shigella infection, 334
Shingles, 315
Shoulder and upper arm, disorders of
    anterior dislocation, 234–236
    clavicle, 234
    glenohumeral dislocation, 235
    glenoid labrum, 235
    humeral shaft fracture, 235
    posterior shoulder dislocation, 235
    rotator-cuff tear, 234
    supraspinatus tendonitis, 235
Shoulder dystocia, 227–228
SIADH. *See* Syndrome of inappropriate
    antidiuretic hormone
Sialadenitis, 134
Sialolithiasis, 132
Sickle cell anemia, 321
Sickle cell disease, 55
Sigmoid volvulus, 410
Silicosis, 83–84
Simple partial seizures, 279
Sinus rhythm, conversion to, 13
Sister Mary Joseph node, 158
Sjögren syndrome, 125, 127, 262
SJS. *See* Stevens–Johnson syndrome
SLE. *See* Systemic lupus erythematosus
Sleep apnea, 94
Sliding hernia, 409
Slipped capital femoral epiphysis, 247, 248, 377
Small bowel obstruction in adults, 402
Small-cell lung cancer, 395
Smoking
    and Crohn disease, 154
    and ulcerative colitis, 154
Social phobia, 291
Sodium bicarbonate, 470
Sodium deficit, 182
Sodium nitroprusside, 28

Soft tissue sarcoma, 405
Solitary thyroid nodule, 392
Somatic hallucination, 299
Somatoform disorder, 302
Somogyi effect, 114
Spigelian hernia, 409
Spinal innervation, 432
Spinal (neurogenic) shock, 417
Spinal stenosis, 246
Spine, disorders of. *See* Back/spine, disorders of
Spinous process fractures, 245
Spondylolisthesis, 245, 245*f*
Spondylolysis, 244
Spontaneous abortion, 221–222
Spontaneous pneumothorax, 77
Spouse abuse, 303
Sprains, 231
Sputum sample, 57
Squamocolumnar junction, 198
Squamous cell carcinoma, 64
SSIs. *See* Surgical site infections
SSRI. *See* Serotonin-selective reuptake inhibitors
SSSS. *See* Staphylococcal scalded skin syndrome
Staphylococcal pneumonia, 54, 56, 57
Staphylococcal scalded skin syndrome, 317
Staphylococcus aureus, 314
Staples, 388
Static tension, 388
Statins, 442
Status epilepticus, 280, 473
ST depression, 23
STD pathogens, 353
"Steeple sign," 51
Steroid regimens for asthma, 68, 70
Stevens–Johnson syndrome, 311
Stomach cancer, 146
Stool cultures, 159
Strabismus, 124
Strain, 231
Strep throat, 137
Streptococcal infections, 136
Streptococcal pharyngitis, 134
Streptococcus pneumoniae, 55
Streptococcus pyogenes, 132
Streptokinase, 444
Stress
    laboratory abnormalities in, 430
    and urge incontinence, 165, 383
Stress fracture, 232
Stressful events of life, 308
Stridor, 87, 133
    treatment of, 51
Stroke, 281–283
Strychnine and tetanus poisoning, 335
Sturge—Weber syndrome, 318
Subacute headaches, 270
Subarachnoid hemorrhage, 285
Subclinical hypothyroidism, 101
Subcortical dementias
    causes of, 266
    manifestations of, 265
Subdural hematoma, 419, 431
Subglottic edema, 51
Subluxed or dislocated lens, 121
Subphrenic abscess, 391
Substance abuse disorders, 304–306
    alcoholism, 304–305
    antidepressants, 306
    CNS depressants, 305
    opiate, 305

Subungual melanoma, 313
Succinylcholine, 433, 438
Suicide, 296, 304
Sulbactam, 50
Supracondylar distal humerus fracture, 237
Supraventricular tachycardia
    common causes of, 10
    EKG interpretation, 25f
    mechanism responsible for, 10
    treatment for unstable, 15
    treatment of, 11, 26
Surgical infection, 388
Surgical procedures, tetanus after, 389
Surgical site infections, 413
Surgical wound infection, host for, 388
Suture, 387, 388
SVT. See Supraventricular tachycardia
Swimmer itch, 346
SWS. See Sturge—Weber syndrome
Sydenham chorea, 275
Sympathetic nervous system and cardiovascular
    system, 437
Sympathetic regional pain syndrome, 270
Sympathomimetic and cycloplegic medication,
    122
Symptomatic gallstones, 148
Syncope, 287
Syndrome of inappropriate antidiuretic
    hormone, 181
Syphilis, 202, 350
    and sensorineural hearing loss, 131
System emboli, 40
Systemic lupus erythematosus, 93, 94, 180,
    262
Systemic skeletal disease, 382

T
Tachycardia, 479
Tactile hallucination, 299
Tangential speech, 307
Tanner classification, 189
Tapeworms, 343–344
Tarsal–metatarsal joint, 253
TB. See Tuberculosis
TBI. See Traumatic brain injury
TCA-induced hypotension, 452
TCA-induced seizures, 452
Telogen effluvium, 314
TEN. See Toxic epidermal necrolysis
Tension headaches, 272
Tension pneumothorax, 78, 418, 421
Terbutaline, 69–70
Testicular cancer, 174
Testicular teratomas, 174
Testicular torsion, 167–168, 407
Testosterone, 209
Test-taking strategy
    ABCs approach, 7
    answer types, 5
    image to evaluate, 6–7
    types of questions, 4–5
Tetanus, 334–335
    after surgical procedures, 389
    prophylaxis, 389
Tetracycline, 452, 457
Tetralogy of Fallot, 38–39, 373–374
Theophylline, 68, 469
Thiazide diuretics, 28, 439
Thiocyanate toxicity, 28
Thioridazine, 450

Thoracic aortic aneurysm
    CXR findings, 35
    dissecting, CXR findings of, 37
    indication for surgery for, 36
Thoracic vertebrae, 247
Thought disorders, 307
Throat disorders. See Mouth/throat disorders
Thromboangiitis obliterans, 393
Thrombocytopenia, 322, 323
Thromboembolic events, prevention of, 13
Thrombolytic agents, 444
Thrombolytic therapy, 32, 283
Thrombosis, 30, 80
"Thumb print sign," 50
Thyroglossal duct cyst, 392
Thyroid carcinoma, 102–103, 392
Thyroidectomy, 392
Thyroid gland, diseases of, 98–103
Thyroiditis, 102
Thyroid nodules, 102
Thyroid replacement therapy, 101
Thyroid scintigraphy findings, 102
Thyroid stimulating hormone receptor
    antibodies, 100
Thyroid stimulating immunoglobulin, 100
Thyroid storm, 100
Thyrotoxicosis, 98–99
TIA. See Transient ischemic attack
Tibia, 249
Tibial plateau fracture, 251
Tick paralysis, 349
Ticlopidine, 443
Time management, 3
Tinea capitis, 315
Tinea versicolor, 310
Tinel's tests, 239
Tinnitus, 131
TMJ syndrome, 136
Toddler fracture, 250
Todd paralysis, 279
Tonometry, 126
Topical corticosteroids, 319
TORCH infections, newborn infant, 369–370
Torsades de pointes, 15
Tourette syndrome, 275
Toxic epidermal necrolysis, 311
Toxic iron ingestion, 479
Toxicologic emergencies, 476
Toxic shock syndrome, 138, 201
Toxoplasmosis, 346, 369
Tracheostomy, 88
Tranquilizer, 452
Transesophageal echocardiogram, 11
Transient ischemic attack, 281
Transudate vs. exudate, 75
Trauma
    airway obstruction in, 420
    assessment of, 433
    laparotomy, 434
    massive transfusion protocol, 435
    primary survey of, 434
Traumatic aortic injury, 419
Traumatic brain injury, 435
Traumatic pneumothorax, 78
Traumatic rupture of aorta, 429
Traumatic ventricular septal defect, 429
Tremor, 275
Trendelenburg test for varicose veins, 37
Treponema pallidum, 350
Trichinella spiralis, 343

Trichomonas, 200
Trichomonas vaginalis, 343
Trichomonas vaginitis, 202
Trichuris trichiura, 343
Tricuspid valve endocarditis, 44
Tricyclic antidepressant (TCA) poisoning, 452
Tricyclic toxicity, 456
Trigeminal neuralgia, 271
Trochanteric bursitis, 249
Tropical spastic paraparesis, 363
Trypanosomiasis, 347
T-score, 382
TSHrAb. See Thyroid stimulating hormone
    receptor antibodies
TSI. See Thyroid stimulating immunoglobulin
TSP. See Tropical spastic paraparesis
TSS. See Toxic shock syndrome
Tuberculosis, 60–61
    chest X-ray, 340
    lesions in, 340
    PPD response, 340
    relapse rate for, 62
    symptoms of, 340
    tests or, 61–62
    therapy for, 339
    treatment of, 61–62
    treatment regiments, 340
Tuberculous pleural effusion, 62, 76
Tularemia, 335, 348
Tumor markers, 174
Tumor of ampulla of Vater, 407
Tumor of appendix, 157
Tumors of jejunum and ileum, 404
Twins, 222
Tympanic hypomobility, 131
Tympanic membrane perforation, 130
Type 2 diabetes mellitus, medications for
    treatment of, 114
Typhoid fever, 333

U
Ulcerative colitis, 407
    extraintestinal manifestations of, 155
    risk factor for, 155
    signs and symptoms of, 155
    and smoking, 154
Ulcerative stomatitis, 137
Ulnar deviation and subluxation, 261
Unicameral bone cysts, 258
Unilateral bloody nipple discharge, 206
Unilateral purulent rhinorrhea, 138
Unilateral sensory hearing loss, 130
Unipolar disorder, 296
Upper gastrointestinal bleeding, 157
Upper GI bleeding, 403, 412
Upper lobe nodules, 83
Upper respiratory infectious agents, 62
Uremic acidosis, 186
Uremic patient, 178
Urethritis, 171
Urinary calculi. See Kidney stones
Urinary incontinence, 165, 383
Urinary obstruction, 176
Urinary retention, 164
Urinary tract infections
    pathogen of, 168
    by Proteus mirabilis, 169
    vesicoureteral reflux, 169
Urolithiasis. See Kidney stones
Urticaria, 318

Uterine atony, 228
Uterine bleeding, 193
Uterine rupture, 227
Uterus, 193–196
UTIs. *See* Urinary tract infections

V

Vaccine-associated paralytic poliomyelitis, 372
Vaccines
    administered to adults, 365
    for HPV prevention, 357
    immunization schedules for, 371–372
    for immunocompromised patients, 357, 365
    influenza, 358
    postsplenectomy patients, 365
Vagal maneuvers, 12
Vagina, normal pH of, 200
Vaginal atrophy, 209
Vaginal candidiasis infections, 200
Vaginal carcinoma, 201
Vaginal–rectal culture, 214
Vaginitis, 200, 209, 332
Valgus deformity, 231
Valsalva maneuver, 12
Vancomycin, 457
Varicella pneumonia, 59
Varicella rash, 362
Varicella vaccine, 362
Varicoceles, 164
Varus deformity, 231
Vascular dementia, 266
Vascular disease, 35–38
Vascular tumors of liver, 153
Vasculitis, 350
Vasodilator therapy, 42
Vasomotor rhinitis, 139
Vecuronium, 433
Venous air embolism, 83
Venous thromboembolic disease risk, 211
Ventilation–perfusion inequality, 88
Ventilation to compression ratio, 45
Ventilator associated pneumonias, 57
Ventilatory insufficiency, 94
Ventricular beats, 12
Ventricular fibrillation, 20f, 30, 33, 427
    treatment of, 12, 26
Ventricular pacemaker rhythm, 16, 16f
Ventricular rate control, 13
Ventricular remodeling, 32
Ventricular septal defect, 39, 373
Ventricular septal rupture, 31
Ventricular tachycardia
    causes of, 14
    degrading into ventricular fibrillation, 17f
    EKG interpretation, 21f, 24f
    with hyperkalemia, 21f
    procainamide loading infusion for, 15

Verapamil, 29
Verbigeration, 307
Verruca vulgaris, 315
Vertebrobasilar insufficiency, 132, 282
Vertical sheer pelvic fracture (VS), 248
Vestibular neuronitis. *See* Labyrinthitis
Vestibular schwannoma, 129
Vibrio cholera outbreak, 331
Vibrio parahaemolyticus, 159, 339
Violent behavior, prodromes of, 303
Viral disease
    chicken pox, 362
    CMV infections, 351
    cryptococcosis, 364
    EBV infections, 351–352
    epidemic keratoconjunctivitis, 363
    epidemic pleurodynia, 363
    foodborne illnesses, 363
    foodborne viral gastroenteritis, 363
    HIV infection, 353–354
    HPV infections, 357
    HSV infections, 352–353
    influenza, 357–358
    Jarisch–Herxheimer reaction, 364
    Koplik spots, 362
    measles, 361–362
    mumps, 358–359
    paraparesis, 363
    polio, 363
    poliovirus, 363
    progressive multifocal leukoencephalopathy, 362–363
    rabies, 359–360
    roseola infantum, 360–361
    rubella, 361
    STD pathogens, 353
    tropical spastic paraparesis, 363
    zoster, 362
Viral disorders, 315–316
Viral or protozoal infections, 223
Viral pneumonia, 52
Virchow node, 159
Virchow triad, 79
Visceral pain, 391
Visual impairment, 381
Vitamin K, 444
Volvulus, 375–376, 402, 409
von Willebrand disease, 323
VSD. *See* Ventricular septal defect
VT. *See* Ventricular tachycardia
Vulvar carcinoma, 201

W

Walking pneumonia, 55
Warfarin, 81, 181, 444
Weber test, 127
Wegener granulomatosis, 93, 179

Weight gain, 216
Weight loss, basic mechanisms of, 161
Weil syndrome, 338
Wernicke encephalopathy, 473
Westermark sign, 395
Wheezing and asthma, 68
Whipple disease, 154
Whipple procedure, 390
White blood cell count, 216
Wilms tumor, 174–175, 395
Wilson disease, 152
Wolff–Parkinson–White (WPW) syndrome, 14
Wood tick, 349
Wound closure, 388, 393
Wound infections, 389
Wound repair, hair removal before, 388
Wrist and hand, disorders of, 239–243
    atrophy of palm, 243
    boutonnière deformity, 240
    carpal tunnel syndrome, 239
    Colles fracture, 241, 241f
    Dupuytren contracture, 240
    felon, 240
    Finkelstein test, 239
    Galeazzi fracture/dislocation, 240
    gamekeeper thumb, 240, 242
    ganglion cyst, 242
    infectious digital flexor tenosynovitis, 241
    Kienböck disease, 240
    ligament avulsion, 243
    lunate fracture, 241, 242
    Mallet finger, 242, 242f
    median nerve injuries, 243
    paronychia, 243
    peripheral nerve compression, 239
    Quervain tenosynovitis, 239
    scaphoid (navicular) fracture, 240

X

Xanthomas, 318
X-rays, questions based on, 7

Y

Yellowish discoloration of skin, differential diagnosis of, 159
Yersinia sp., 337–338, 339

Z

Zenker diverticulum, 144
Zoster vaccine, 362
Zygomatic arch, 423
Zygomatic arch fracture, 136, 428
Zygomaticomaxillary complex fracture, 136
Zygomycosis, 329